Current Clinical Neurology

Series Editor

Daniel Tarsy
Beth Israel Deaconness Medical Center
Department of Neurology
Boston, MA, USA

Current Clinical Neurology offers a wide range of practical resources for clinical neurologists. Providing evidence-based titles covering the full range of neurologic disorders commonly presented in the clinical setting, the Current Clinical Neurology series covers such topics as multiple sclerosis, Parkinson's Disease and nonmotor dysfunction, seizures, Alzheimer's Disease, vascular dementia, sleep disorders, and many others. Series editor Daniel Tarsy, MD, is professor of neurology, Vice Chairman of the Department of Neurology, and Chief of the Movement Disorders division at Beth Israel Deaconness Hospital, Boston, Massachusetts.

More information about this series at http://www.springer.com/series/7630

Kathrin LaFaver • Carine W. Maurer
Timothy R. Nicholson • David L. Perez
Editors

Functional Movement Disorder

An Interdisciplinary Case-Based Approach

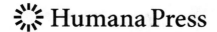 Humana Press

Editors
Kathrin LaFaver
Movement Disorder Specialist
Saratoga Hospital Medical Group
Saratoga Springs, NY, USA

Timothy R. Nicholson
Neuropsychiatry Research and
Education Group
Institute of Psychiatry Psychology &
Neuroscience
King's College London
London, UK

Carine W. Maurer
Department of Neurology
Renaissance School of Medicine at
Stony Brook University
Stony Brook, NY, USA

David L. Perez
Departments of Neurology and Psychiatry
Massachusetts General Hospital
Harvard Medical School
Boston, MA, USA

ISSN 1559-0585   ISSN 2524-4043   (electronic)
Current Clinical Neurology
ISBN 978-3-030-86497-2   ISBN 978-3-030-86495-8   (eBook)
https://doi.org/10.1007/978-3-030-86495-8

This Humana imprint is published by the registered company Springer Nature Switzerland AG
The registered company address is: Gewerbestrasse 11, 6330 Cham, Switzerland

Preface

Functional movement disorder (FMD), a subtype of functional neurological disorder (FND), is a prevalent, potentially disabling, and costly condition at the intersection of neurology and psychiatry. After being of significant interest to a number of early leaders across neurology, psychiatry, and psychology (e.g., Charcot, Freud, Janet, Briquet, Babinski), the late twentieth century was unfortunately marked by limited interest in the field of FND. Part of the difficulties arise from the notion that FND inherently challenges the conceptualization of modern-day medical specialties and societal views of physical health and mental health more broadly. Thankfully, interest in FMD and related conditions has renewed in the last 20 years. Improvements in diagnostic specificity, an expanding "toolbox" of evidence-based treatments, and an international, multidisciplinary professional society (www.FNDsociety.org) are all driving interest in this field among clinicians and researchers alike. Furthermore, FMD is scientifically compelling, teaching us about a range of cognitive-affective neuroscience principles, and when patients respond well to treatment, effect sizes rival those seen throughout the brain sciences.

In this case-based textbook on FMD, we offer readers a practical, evidence-based approach to the assessment and management of FMD presentations over 32 chapters. Chapter 1 provides a historical perspective on FMD and FND more broadly, with Chaps. 2 and 3 outlining emerging neural mechanisms and the importance of the biopsychosocial model, respectively. Chapter 4 offers an integrated clinical neuroscience approach to FMD. Thereafter, Chaps. 5, 6, 7, 8, 9, 10, 11, 12, and 13 detail case-based examples (including videos) and practical discussion on the assessment and management of the full range of functional movement symptoms – including but not limited to functional limb weakness, tremor, dystonia, parkinsonism, tics, jerks, gait difficulties, and speech/voice abnormalities. Non-motor symptoms found in patients with FMD are outlined in Chap. 14, while Chaps. 15 and 16 offer assessment recommendations for pediatric and elderly populations. Informed by the latest research and expert opinions, Chaps. 17, 18, 19, 20, 21, 22, 23, 24, 25, and 26 provide practical suggestions in regard to therapeutic approaches, including education, physical/occupational/speech and language therapies, and psychotherapy. The role of placebo treatment and transcranial magnetic stimulation are visited in Chaps. 27 and 28, respectively, potentially promising interventions requiring considerably more research. Chapters 29, 30, and 31 are also on noteworthy topics, including measuring symptoms, managing obstacles in longitudinal care, and the treatment of pediatric

FMD. Chap. 32 succinctly details the career narratives of the four co-editors, as a way of hopefully inspiring the next generation of clinicians and researchers toward the field of FMD and related conditions. Throughout the text, we advocate for a patient-centered, biopsychosocially informed clinical neuroscience perspective. Given that the clinical landscape of FMD and related conditions have undergone transformative changes in the last several decades, it can be expected that portions of the content put forth here will be updated in the coming decades.

Overall, we believe that this case-based textbook will be a valuable resource for trainees and seasoned clinicians alike across the fields of neurology, psychiatry, medicine, psychology, social work, allied mental health disciplines, and physical rehabilitation (including physical, occupational, and speech-language therapists). Given the overlap between FMD, other FND subtypes, chronic pain, and the range of functional disorders seen across medicine, clinicians working in these spaces will likely also find this text useful.

We would like to express our sincere and utmost gratitude to our chapter authors, who generously provided their expertise and time to help disseminate their knowledge and skills. We are also indebted to our patients, mentors, and current and former colleagues from whom we have learned so much. Lastly, we thank our families for their unwavering support and encouragement.

Saratoga Springs, NY, USA   Kathrin LaFaver
Stony Brook, NY, USA   Carine W. Maurer
London, UK   Timothy R. Nicholson
Boston, MA, USA   David L. Perez

Series Editor's Introduction

This volume, *Functional Movement Disorder: An Interdisciplinary Case Based Approach* provides a very useful and much needed comprehensive review of *functional movement disorder* as a subtype of *functional neurological disorder* which recently have become recognized as common and worthy of the serious attention of both neurologists and psychiatrists. The editors of this book, Drs. LaFaver, Maurer, Nicholson, and Perez, have collected many careful and thoughtful contributions from their colleagues, all of whom have taken a very serious interest in functional neurological disorder. In Part I of this book, the historical perspective provided by Richard Kanaan in Chap. 1 sets the stage for this discussion by reminding the reader of currently outmoded historical terms such as "conversion disorder", "psychogenic disorder", and "hysterical disorder" which have been of very limited value in characterizing, understanding, and treating patients with functional neurological disorder. In Chap. 2, the pathophysiologic underpinnings of functional movement disorder is imaginatively laid out by Dr. Mark Hallett, who has emphasized the concept of loss of "self-agency" by the patient as a way of understanding the occurrence of abnormal movements which closely resemble abnormal movements that arise from physical lesions of the brain. In Part II of the book, specific case descriptions will assist the clinician who may believe they are encountering a patient with functional tremors, jerky movements, tics, gait disorders, or some other functional movement disorder. Finally, Part III of the book provides a variety of useful approaches to the management of functional movement disorder by a variety of therapeutic techniques.

Daniel Tarsy
Department of Neurology
Harvard Medical School
Beth Israel Deaconess Medical Center
Boston, MA, USA

Contents

Contributors

Caitlin Adams Department of Psychiatry, North Shore Medical Center, Salem, MA, USA

Marine Ambar Akkaoui Centre Psychiatrique d'Orientation et d'Accueil (CPOA), GHU Paris - Psychiatry & Neurosciences, Paris, France

Psychiatric Emergency, CH Delafontaine, Etablissement Publique de Santé Mentale deVille Evrard, Paris, France

Jordan R. Anderson Psychiatry and Neurology, Oregon Health and Science University, Unity Center for Behavioral Health, Portland, OR, USA

Daruj Aniwattanapong Neuropsychiatry Research and Education Group, Institute of Psychiatry, Psychology & Neuroscience, King's College London, London, UK

Department of Psychiatry, Faculty of Medicine, Chulalongkorn University, Bangkok, Thailand

Selma Aybek Neurology, Inselspital, Bern, Switzerland

Gaston Baslet Division of Neuropsychiatry, Brigham and Women's Hospital, Boston, MA, USA

Harvard Medical School, Boston, MA, USA

Kim Bullock Department of Psychiatry and Behavioral Sciences, Stanford University School of Medicine, Stanford, CA, USA

Matthew J. Burke Neuropsychiatry Program, Department of Psychiatry, Sunnybrook Health Sciences Centre, University of Toronto, Toronto, ON, Canada

Division of Neurology, Department of Medicine, Sunnybrook Health Sciences Centre, University of Toronto, Toronto, ON, Canada

Hurvitz Brain Sciences Research Program, Sunnybrook Research Institute, Toronto, ON, Canada

Program in Placebo Studies, Beth Israel Deaconess Medical Center, Harvard Medical School, Boston, MA, USA

Alan Carson Centre for Clinical Brain Sciences, University of Edinburgh, Edinburgh, UK

W. Curt LaFrance Jr. Brown University, Providence, RI, USA

Providence Veterans Affairs Medical Center, Providence, RI, USA

Departments of Psychiatry and Neurology, Rhode Island Hospital, Providence, RI, USA

Bertrand Degos Neurology Unit, Avicenne University Hospital, Sorbonne Paris Nord University, Bobigny, France

Dynamics and Pathophysiology of Neuronal Networks Team, Center for Interdisciplinary Research in Biology, Collège de France, CNRS UMR7241/INSERM U1050, Université PSL, Paris, France

Benedetta Demartini Department of Health Sciences, "Aldo Ravelli" Research Center for Neurotechnology and Experimental Brain Therapeutics, Università degli Studi di Milano, ASST Santi Paolo e Carlo, Milan, Italy

Yasmine E. M. Dreissen Department of Neurology, Amsterdam University Medical Center, Amsterdam, the Netherlands

Joseph R. Duffy Department of Neurology, Mayo Clinic, Rochester, MN, USA

Barbara A. Dworetzky Division of Epilepsy, Brigham and Women's Hospital, Boston, MA, USA

Harvard Medical School, Boston, MA, USA

Mark J. Edwards St George's University of London, London, UK

Atkinson Morley Regional Neuroscience Centre, St George's University Hospital, London, UK

Alfonso Fasano Edmond J. Safra Program in Parkinson's Disease, Morton and Gloria Shulman Movement Disorders Clinic, Toronto Western Hospital, UHN, Toronto, ON, Canada

Division of Neurology, University of Toronto, Toronto, ON, Canada

Krembil Brain Institute, Toronto, ON, Canada

Jennifer Freeburn Department of Speech, Language, & Swallowing Disorders, Massachusetts General Hospital, Boston, MA, USA

Christos Ganos Department of Neurology, Charité University Medicine Berlin, Berlin, Germany

Béatrice Garcin Neurology Unit, Avicenne University Hospital, Sorbonne Paris Nord University, Bobigny, France

Faculty of Medicine of Sorbonne University, Brain and Spine Institute, INSERM U1127, CNRS UMR 7225, Paris, France

Paula Gardiner Royal Infirmary Edinburgh, Edinburgh, Scotland, UK

Jeannette M. Gelauff Department of Neurology, Amsterdam University Medical Center, Amsterdam, the Netherlands

Mark Hallett Human Motor Control Section, National Institute of Neurological Disorders and Stroke, National Institutes of Health, Bethesda, MD, USA

Kate Hayward Therapy Services Department, The National Hospital for Neurology and Neurosurgery, London, UK

Ingrid Hoeritzauer Centre for Clinical Brain Sciences, University of Edinburgh, Edinburgh, UK

Megan E. Jablonski Department of Psychology & Neuropsychology, Frazier Rehabilitation Institute, Louisville, KY, USA

Richard A. A. Kanaan Department of Psychiatry, University of Melbourne, Austin Health, Heidelberg, VIC, Australia

Kasia Kozlowska The Children's Hospital at Westmead, Westmead, NSW, Australia

Discipline of Psychiatry and Discipline of Child & Adolescent Health, University of Sydney, Medical School, Sydney, NSW, Australia

Westmead Institute for Medical Research, Westmead, NSW, Australia

Kathrin LaFaver Movement Disorder Specialist, Saratoga Hospital Medical Group, Saratoga Springs, NY, USA

Adrianne E. Lange Private Practice, Louisville, KY, USA

Sarah C. Lidstone Integrated Movement Disorders Program, Toronto Rehabilitation Institute, Toronto, ON, Canada

Edmond J. Safra Program in Parkinson's Disease and the Morton and Gloria Shulman Movement Disorders Clinic, Toronto Western Hospital, University Health Network, Toronto, ON, Canada

Division of Neurology, Department of Medicine, University of Toronto, Toronto, ON, Canada

Juliana Lockman Department of Psychiatry and Behavioral Sciences, Stanford University School of Medicine, Stanford, CA, USA

Lindsey MacGillivray Department of Psychiatry, University of Toronto, Toronto Western Hospital, University Health Network, Toronto, ON, Canada

Joel D. Mack Department of Psychiatry, Veterans Affairs Portland Health Care System, Portland, OR, USA

Northwest Parkinson's Disease Research, Education, and Clinical Center, Department of Neurology, Veterans Affairs Portland Health Care System, Portland, OR, USA

Departments of Psychiatry & Neurology, Oregon Health and Science University, Portland, OR, USA

Walter Maetzler Department of Neurology, University Hospital Schleswig-Holstein, Campus Kiel, Kiel, Germany

Julie Maggio Department of Physical Therapy, Massachusetts General Hospital, Boston, MA, USA

Tina Mainka Department of Neurology, Charité University Medicine Berlin, Berlin, Germany
Berlin Institute of Health, Berlin, Germany

Steve Martino Department of Psychiatry, Yale University School of Medicine, New Haven, CT, USA
Psychology Service, VA Connecticut Healthcare System, West Haven, CT, USA

Carine W. Maurer Department of Neurology, Renaissance School of Medicine at Stony Brook University, Stony Brook, NY, USA

Francesca Morgante Neurosciences Research Centre, Molecular and Clinical Sciences Research Institute, St. George's University of London, London, UK
Department of Clinical and Experimental Medicine, University of Messina, Messina, Italy

Mariana Moscovich Department of Neurology, University Hospital Schleswig-Holstein, Campus Kiel, Kiel, Germany

Clare Nicholson Therapy Services Department, The National Hospital for Neurology and Neurosurgery, London, UK

Timothy R. Nicholson Neuropsychiatry Research and Education Group, Institute of Psychiatry, Psychology & Neuroscience, King's College London, London, UK

Glenn Nielsen Neuroscience Research Centre, Institute of Molecular and Clinical Sciences, St Georges University of London, London, UK

David L. Perez Departments of Neurology and Psychiatry, Massachusetts General Hospital, Harvard Medical School, Boston, MA, USA

Susannah Pick Institute of Psychiatry, Psychology and Neuroscience, King's College London, London, UK

Bruce H. Price Neurology, McLean Hospital and Massachusetts General Hospital, Harvard Medical School, Belmont, MA, USA

Lucia Ricciardi Neurosciences Research Centre, Molecular and Clinical Sciences Research Institute, St George's University of London, London, UK

Mohammad Rohani Division of Neurology, Rasool Akram Hospital, School of Medicine, Iran University of Medical Sciences, Tehran, Iran

Petra Schwingenschuh Department of Neurology, Medical University of Graz, Graz, Austria

Jon Stone Centre for Clinical Brain Sciences, University of Edinburgh, Edinburgh, UK

Marina A. J. Tijssen Expertise Center Movement Disorders, Department of Neurology, University Medical Center Groningen, Groningen, the Netherlands

Benjamin Tolchin Comprehensive Epilepsy Center, Department of Neurology, Yale University School of Medicine, New Haven, CT, USA

Epilepsy Center of Excellence, Neurology Service, VA Connecticut Healthcare System, West Haven, CT, USA

Jeff L. Waugh Department of Pediatrics, University of Texas Southwestern, Dallas, TX, USA

Alison Wilkinson-Smith Department of Psychiatry, Children's Medical Center Dallas, Dallas, TX, USA

Part I
Framework

A Historical Perspective on Functional Neurological Disorder

Richard A. A. Kanaan

A history of one of mankind's oldest maladies would be a monumental work, but that is not this chapter. This chapter explores the history of functional neurological disorder (FND), a malady of much more recent birth. How recent? A search on PubMed for "functional neurological disorder" suggests its first English-language appearance was perhaps in 2015 [1]. That year there were 2 publications using the term; the following year there were 6, and a further 9 using the Americanized "neurologic". In 2016, mere months after this first appearance, the authoritative 700-page handbook of clinical neurology on the subject chose "Functional Neurologic Disorders" as its title [2]. Strikingly, for a term that was not the official choice of DSM-5, ICD-10, or the proposed ICD-11, it ("FND") was incorporated into the name of every patient group in the field. FND had very clearly arrived, seemingly out of the blue.

But this magical manifestation is of course an illusion, and in the following I will explore the history of its arrival and its conquest. In discussing 'FND' as opposed to 'hysteria', or 'conversion disorder', I am not indulging in mere pedantry: as any historian will tell you, one cannot simply transplant the concepts of the present into the past – and, make no mistake, the concept of FND involves profound changes from the past.

So, in addition to celebrating its birth, I will discuss what the differences in FND are, and what difference they may make.

The Way It Was

It would be hard to exaggerate how dire the situation of conversion disorder was at the turn of the millennium. After a burst of popularity 100 years earlier, when some of the greatest minds in medicine (including leading neurologists and psychiatrists) shared a fascination for the disorder at the Salpêtrière Hospital in Paris (Fig. 1.1), it had sunk into a prolonged and profound decline. Psychiatry seemed to have found a way to ignore it entirely, announcing its disappearance [3]; Neurologists could only wish it had disappeared, left grappling with a problem they did not understand, and did not think was really theirs [4]. Clinicians of all specialties would describe the disorder with dislike, or worse, and question whether it was really all just deliberate feigning [5, 6]. For a disorder of such prevalence and such morbidity, clinical research was astonishingly sparse, with not one single properly-powered clinical trial ever conducted during the twentieth century, and a medley of treatment approaches proliferated, based on the lowest grades of evidence [7]. The public, meanwhile, was barely aware of its existence: though 'hysteria' remained a popular cultural motif, it was viewed almost

R. A. A. Kanaan (✉)
Department of Psychiatry, University of Melbourne, Austin Health, Heidelberg, VIC, Australia
e-mail: richard.kanaan@unimelb.edu.au

© Springer Nature Switzerland AG 2022
K. LaFaver et al. (eds.), *Functional Movement Disorder*, Current Clinical Neurology,
https://doi.org/10.1007/978-3-030-86495-8_1

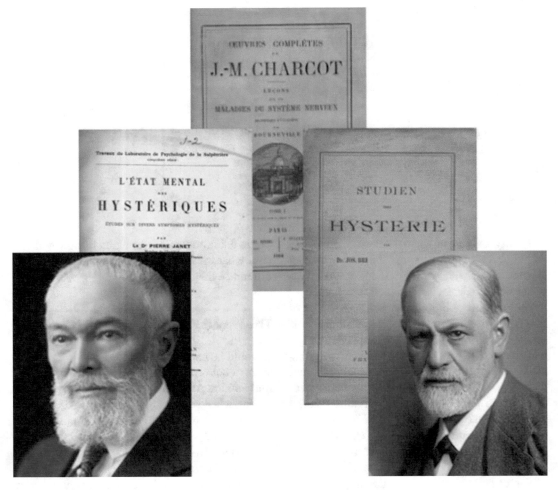

Fig. 1.1 Jean-Martin Charcot's *Lectures on the Diseases of the Nervous System* (1872), and two of the critical works of his students, Pierre Janet's *The Mental State of* *Hysterics* (1892) and Sigmund Freud's *Studies on Hysteria* (1895). (Images are available in the public domain)

exclusively as an historical artefact of medical misogyny [8] or Victorian absurdity [9]. The public shared in clinical suspicions of feigning [10], and patients newly diagnosed with conversion disorder would be so outraged they would go to any lengths to have the diagnosis overturned [11]. Unsurprisingly, there were no conversion disorder patient advocacy groups, and public demand for services in many places was non-existent [12].

Out With the Old…

The diagnostic criteria reflected these problems, and appeared to play a critical role. ICD-10 [13] and DSM-IV [14] shared the view that conversion disorder required the exclusion of both neurological and factitious alternatives, and the inclusion of a psychiatric explanation (see Box 1.1). There were real problems with each of these [15, 16].

Box 1.1 Comparison of the diagnostic criteria for Conversion Disorder in the Diagnostic and Statistical Manual (DSM), 4th and 5th editions

DSM-5 Conversion Disorder (Functional Neurological Symptom Disorder) - 2013

A. One or more symptoms of altered voluntary motor or sensory function.
B. Clinical findings provide evidence of incompatibility between the symptom and recognised neurological or medical conditions.
C. The symptom or deficit is not better explained by another medical or mental disorder.
D. The symptom or deficit causes clinically significant distress or impairment in social, occupational, or other important areas of functioning or warrants medical evaluation.

DSM-IV Conversion Disorder - 1994

A. One or more symptoms or deficits affecting voluntary motor or sensory function suggesting neurological or other general medical condition.
B. Psychological factors are judged to be associated to the symptom or deficit because conflicts or other stressors precede initiation or exacerbation of the symptom or deficit.
C. The patient is not feigning or intentionally producing his or her symptoms or deficits.
D. The symptom or deficit cannot, after appropriate investigation, be fully explained by a general medical condition, by the direct effects of a substance, or as a culturally sanctioned behaviour or experience.
E. The symptom is not limited to pain or to a disturbance in sexual functioning and is not better explained by another mental disorder.

The exclusion of neurological alternatives was not a problem in practice - despite the alarming reports of large-scale neurological misdiagnosis from the 1960s [17], overall, and particularly more recently, conversion disorder was not misdiagnosed more often than other disorders [18] - but it remained a serious problem in principle. For it meant that the neurologist would be required to exclude every alternative - known or unknown - something that appears impossible in principle, and a concerned patient could never be sure that something had not been overlooked, or had not yet been discovered. A patient's confidence in the diagnosis would depend on their confidence in their neurologist and second- or third- neurological opinions might seem only prudent.

The exclusion of feigning, or factitious disorder, was problematic both in principle and practice. In practice, it is usually impossible for a psychiatrist, or anyone else, to exclude feigning, particularly with neurological symptoms [19]. In principle, that this was an exclusion criterion for conversion disorder alone served to confirm all those suspicions that conversion disorder was uniquely close to feigning [20]. As far as a neurologist need be concerned [21], or anyone could prove, they might *all* be feigning [22].

The requirement for a psychiatric formulation was primarily a problem in practice. There were always patients in whom no plausible psychiatric explanation could be constructed, which meant the requirement was effectively ignored. Perhaps this was due to these patients' reluctance to disclose psychopathology [23], or clinician reluctance to explore it [24] – or perhaps because it was not present. But in almost every study, however it was studied, a relevant trauma history could not be identified in a significant minority of patients [25]. Though trauma was obviously still important, this also challenged the principle: it was difficult to support a monolithic, PTSD-type trauma model for conversion disorder when most studies appeared to provide evidence against it.

So, the diagnostic criteria brought the disorder into disrepute while being of little practical value. They drew heavily on psychodynamic ideas that, if not exactly disproven, were certainly old-fashioned, and perhaps no longer readily interpretable by most psychiatrists [9]. There was a once-in-a-generation opportunity for change, with both DSM-5 and ICD-11 in preparation.

... in With the New

For such 'old-fashioned' ideas to be so enduring suggests that replacing them would not be straightforward, however. They certainly had high-level endorsement, after all, and perhaps there were simply no better alternatives. That the neurological symptoms would not fit with identifiable pathology was established by Jean-Martin Charcot (Fig. 1.1), arguably the greatest neurologist of all time, in the nineteenth century [26]. The suspicions around feigning were part of the same discussion. Neurologists at the time were inclined to explain these apparently voluntary movements as malingering [27], since no better explanation was on offer [3]. The idea that these symptoms would be instead 'psychogenic' dates from the same era, most famously in Sigmund Freud's seminal "Studies on Hysteria", where he essentially argues for a post-traumatic aetiology – the novelty being that the traumas were 'emotional' ones (psychological conflicts), which became 'converted' into physical symptoms [28]. This construction survived largely intact for a century in conversion disorder, while all around it every other psychodynamic construction was being torn down [9]. Why it showed such unique longevity is unclear, given the ethos of the times was so strongly against aetiological criteria. Perhaps the loss of psychiatric interest allowed it to 'slip under the radar'. Or perhaps it just could not be understood psychiatrically without it. The symptoms, after all, were not psychiatric: what else was there about the disorder that would justify it being a psychiatric condition, if not its aetiology [29]? Suggestions for improving the criteria by simply removing the requirement for a psychiatric formulation [15] would have left it looking distinctly neurological, but a neurological syndrome for which no neurological explanation could be found.

There was a real reputational danger there, as outlined above: a criterion which depended on a neurologist's ability or zeal in finding an alternative explanation risked becoming the wastebasket for every patient the neurologist did not take seriously or whose symptoms they could not quite put together. The psychiatric aetiology requirement had protected against that, in theory, since the patient has to pass that test as well, and without it the risk would be clearly exposed. There was a solution, however: make the neurologist *prove* that the case was functional – make a 'positive diagnosis'. If they could identify features specific to the diagnosis that would mean they could demonstrate what it was, not just what it was not, and that risk would be removed.

Or nearly so. Unfortunately, distinguishing it from feigning would be as difficult as ever for most features of conversion disorder [30], but if excluding feigning was removed from the criteria, and feigning no longer considered as a likely alternative, the new criterion could still be considered 'positive' in regards to neurological alternatives. And this 'positive diagnosis' was to become the new principal diagnostic criterion in DSM-5 (Box 1.1).

But there were more changes in store. The name 'conversion disorder' still clearly harked back to Freud, and suggested a "one size fits all" psychodynamic process, even if the criteria did not. Neurologists had been using the term 'functional' to refer to these symptoms since at least the time of Charcot, who argued that any lesion invisible to his microscopes must be a 'functional' lesion of the underlying brain region [31]. Though the meaning of the term was opaque [32], it appeared to be a popular alternative with both patients and neurologists [33]. We, and others, suggested 'functional neurological symptoms' [15], or 'functional neurological symptom disorder' [16], which latter DSM-5 finally adopted. But in an early draft, perhaps following an earlier suggestion [34], it proposed 'functional neurological disorder' – a small difference, but one which shifted the emphasis from the *symptoms* being neurological to the *disorder* being neurological, a shift too far for most neurologists [20, 32]. Yet, this is the name that emerged triumphant, despite DSM-5's choice, and has become the standard bearer for the disorder: as of March 2020, a search on PubMed for "Functional Neurological Disorder" yields 55 references since 2019, while "Functional Neurological Symptom Disorder" yields only seven.

With regard to movement disorders more specifically, the subject of this book, similar changes were underway. Long known as 'psychogenic movement disorder', arguments were made on the same grounds [35] that they should instead be known as 'functional movement disorder' (FMD) [36]. Turning again to PubMed, 'functional movement disorder' first appears in 2012 [37], though a publication a year earlier uses the term with 'functional' in scare quotes [38]. But it has already come to dominate the field: since 2019, as of May 2020, "functional movement disorder" yields 25 references, and "psychogenic movement disorder" only six.

What Difference Does It Make?

Much has changed since the turn of the millennium. Clinical interest in the disorder has grown considerably – the first international conference (2017) open to all was hugely over-subscribed. A vibrant research community has developed and properly-powered clinical trials are finally underway. Public interest is increasing. Writing from Australia, FND has featured on 3 prime-time current affairs TV programs in the last few years, having never featured before. And patient attitudes are changing – most patients in my clinic have now actively sought an appointment in the clinic, instead of grudgingly accepting their neurologist's referral, or failing to attend once they understand what it's about – a position colleagues tell me is true more globally. The world of FND is a clearly different world to the world of Conversion Disorder. It's different in its appeal, to neurologists and patients in particular. We cannot be sure what caused these changes, and it seems unlikely that it was any one thing, but it is easy to see the new criteria and the new name as either causes or embodiments of this difference.

The embrace of the disorder by patient groups represents a tremendous advance for the field. As noted in the introduction, they have universally adopted FND into the names of their groups, which seems unlikely to be a coincidence. Patients have consistently expressed a preference for the term 'functional' over the more psychiatric sounding alternatives [33], but clearly the groups also preferred 'FND' over 'FNSD' - the advantage, other than perhaps euphony, presumably being that it more strongly implies the disorder is neurological. The stigma of a psychiatric diagnosis is unfortunately commonplace, and has very real consequences [39], but in the case of FND it appears bound up with the idea that the disorder is not real – is imaginary, or hallucinatory, or simply made up [10]. Though these attributions are not fixed [40], they are virtually absent from neurological disorders: a shift to a neurological disorder definitively makes the disorder seem more 'real'. Dropping the 'exclusion of feigning' criterion should also have helped in that regard. Patient groups also expressed concern with the psychogenic diagnostic criterion, and its implication that they had suffered a trauma, when not all reported such experiences [29] - so dropping that criterion should also be welcome. Finally, a 'positive' demonstration of FND could only help patient acceptance, alleviating doubts about the diagnosis being an excuse for medical incompetence or a way of dismissing unwelcome patients.

There were clear potential advantages for neurologists too. Conversion disorder was a source of great anxiety to neurologists, who found their patient encounters uniquely uncomfortable [4]. Their diagnostic approach of discovering inconsistency encouraged them to consider their patients as deceptive, while also involving the neurologist in a deception - of tricking their patients into revealing the truth [22]. But when it came to explaining their diagnosis, it involved them in discussions of such concepts as the subconscious, on which they felt unqualified; these could be interpreted as implying feigning, or dismissal, or incompetence, and greeted with anger [24]. The new criteria were in these areas a major advance. All mention of feigning was dropped, so that the 'positive' demonstration could be interpreted as of FND alone. Moreover, this meant the inconsistencies could be shown to the patient, removing any deception on the neurologists' part, and, in an inspired maneuver, turning these 'tricks' into ways of creating patient insight and support for the diagnosis [41]. Without the need to discuss some psychogenic aetiology, neurologists could stay within a zone more comfortable for them and the patient, so that their encounters need no longer be hostile [42].

So, Are the Problems All Over Now?

The above-discussed developments represent critical, and very welcome, changes. They have already transformed the disorder and have the potential to solve most of the problems that conversion disorder faced. But it would be naïve to think this most intractable of medical conundrums 'finally sorted', and these changes may yet lead to new problems.

Firstly, the thrust of the changes can be seen as rendering the disorder more neurological. The 'psychogenic' criterion is no longer essential; the diagnosis can now be made by neurologists alone; the diagnosis appears in the neurological section of ICD-11 as well [43]. The name FND, as we noted before, now appears to state that it is so. That initial alarm about the name has quietened. A steady stream of neuroimaging studies, while not, as a class, telling us anything we did not already know [44], make a neurological view of the disorder seem more comfortable, and more natural. This is no bad thing, inherently. The division of disorders into psychiatric and neurological has always been somewhat arbitrary, and many have suggested the two should be considered one. But it does encourage the view that the psychiatric aspects are secondary, and can perhaps be ignored in management. We are currently riding a wave of optimism that a neurological model will prevail [45], and that physical treatments may be enough, at least for most patients [46]. They may not, and the effect of that failure on 'FND' as a concept is hard to predict.

Secondly, not everyone will be happy. Among those who will be looking to the results of trials of transcranial magnetic stimulation (TMS) or physiotherapy most keenly may be the psychiatrists and psychologists who thought that 'conversion disorder' was fundamentally more valid, for all its flaws. Interviews with psychiatrists who specialize in the disorder suggests considerable discomfort with the new approach – that they certainly do not all think it is valid [47]. A survey of psychiatrists in the UK and Australia confirmed this, with respondents overwhelmingly reporting they think conversion disorder is psychogenic, and that a psychiatric formulation is not merely helpful for management, but essential to the diagnosis [48].

Thirdly, the new criteria will not diagnose the same patients as before. Any change in the sense of the criteria will inevitably affect their reference – the patients whom they do or do not fit. One obvious change from an aetiological criterion to a symptomatic criterion is that a larger number of seemingly straightforwardly neurological patients will now be included if they have any symptoms that are functional. Previously, the patient with a stroke who also developed a functional weakness need not have been diagnosed with conversion disorder if the psychiatrist did not formulate them as such: now, a 'positive sign' should be enough to make the diagnosis, as long as it is enough to cause distress. This view, of the symptom as sufficient, is not new [17], and not wrong, but it clearly broadens the number of potential FND patients enormously. Conversely, the diagnosis was 'positive' before, in theory, in terms of a 'positive psychiatric formulation', and removing this will exclude others. There will be patients who do have a positive psychiatric formulation but in whom no 'positive signs' are found, so would no longer be diagnosed with FND. Just how many of these there may be is not clear, as large-scale studies have not been conducted outside of specialist centres, but it could be a lot. One recent study, for example, suggested that most paediatric patients diagnosed with FND did not meet that criterion [49]. Some of the 'positive signs' are of doubtful discriminatory value [50], and certainty is typically rationed in neurological diagnoses: insisting on certainty, or on only the most valid signs, would doubtless lead to a more tightly defined, but inevitably smaller group, particularly in FMD [51]. Inevitably, some patients with Conversion Disorder diagnoses are going to miss out by the new criteria. Again, this is not necessarily wrong, and we cannot conclude from this that the new criteria are more or less valid than the old, but one of the problems with the old psychogenic criterion was that it could not be fulfilled in practice, and was therefore routinely ignored. The danger for the new criterion is precisely the same. And for FND, like Conversion disorder before it, the danger is that it may therefore become dependent on an idea that nobody really believes any longer.

This chapter has focused heavily on DSM-5 in the preceding. It is of course only one iteration of that classification system, and only one of the systems in use. ICD-11 has trodden a different path, in nomenclature and criteria, based on the principle of dissociation espoused by the great rival theorist from the Salpêtrière, Pierre Janet (Fig. 1.1). If anyone needed reminding, Freud's is not the only way to formulate a patient with 'Dissociative Neurological Symptom Disorder', as ICD-11 would have it [43], and this history is not simply of the struggle between the psychodynamic and biological views that is the particularly American history of psychiatry [9]. That struggle may obscure the extent of agreement. As the later chapters in this book will show, life events and the biopsychosocial model remain at the forefront of modern FMD conceptualizations. And even DSM-5 is perhaps less definitive than its criteria may suggest: the title of the disorder retains both Conversion Disorder and FNSD (indeed, with FNSD in parentheses), and the accompanying text make very clear the importance of psychiatric formulation. Perhaps the pendulum, restrained for so long, swung further than anyone quite intended with this version. Perhaps the next iteration will more faithfully capture the diversity of the disorder, and of opinion. Perhaps it will restore psychiatric formulation to an equal footing with neurological signs, as factors which contribute to, but do not define, FND - and confirm FND as a core, interdisciplinary neuropsychiatric disorder [52].

Summary

- Conversion Disorder was profoundly neglected and stigmatized by clinicians, patients and the public 20 years ago.
- The diagnostic criteria were a major contributor to this, based on principles established in the nineteenth century.
- The criteria of DSM-IV made a trauma history essential, which not all patients had, and required the exclusion of neuropathology and of feigning, which was not usually possible.
- The revised criteria for DSM-5 dropped these requirements, instead requiring the diagnostician to make a rule-in diagnosis, by demonstrating incompatibility or finding 'positive signs'.
- The name 'functional neurological disorder' is not the official name in DSM-5, but was proposed in an early draft, and has been adopted by the field despite concern that it suggests the disorder is solely a neurological disorder.
- The name and the new criteria have proven very popular, and the diagnosis is experiencing a transformation in public awareness and patient acceptability.
- As we consider the present and future of FND, an appreciation of neurological signs and psychiatric formulation are likely both to be important in the assessment and management of this condition at the interface of neurology and psychiatry.

References

1. Perez DL, Dworetzky BA, Dickerson BC, Leung L, Cohn R, Baslet G, et al. An integrative neurocircuit perspective on psychogenic nonepileptic seizures and functional movement disorders: neural functional unawareness. Clin EEG Neurosci. 2015;46(1):4–15.
2. Hallett M, Stone J, Carson A. Functional neurologic disorders. Amsterdam/New York: Elsevier; 2016. xviii, 662 pages p
3. Kanaan RA, Wessely SC. The origins of factitious disorder. Hist Hum Sci. 2010;23(2):68–85.

4. Kanaan R, Armstrong D, Barnes P, Wessely S. In the psychiatrist's chair: how neurologists understand conversion disorder. Brain. 2009;132(Pt 10):2889–96.

5. Ahern L, Stone J, Sharpe MC. Attitudes of neuroscience nurses toward patients with conversion symptoms. Psychosomatics. 2009;50(4):336–9.

6. Edwards MJ, Stone J, Nielsen G. Physiotherapists and patients with functional (psychogenic) motor symptoms: a survey of attitudes and interest. J Neurol Neurosurg Psychiatry. 2012;83(6):655–8.

7. Ruddy R, House A. Psychosocial interventions for conversion disorder. Cochrane Database Syst Rev. 2005;(4):CD005331.

8. Micale MS. Approaching hysteria : disease and its interpretations. Princeton/Chichester: Princeton University Press; 1995. xii, 327p

9. Kanaan RA. Freud's hysteria and its legacy. Handb Clin Neurol. 2016;139:37–44.

10. Stone J, Wojcik W, Durrance D, Carson A, Lewis S, MacKenzie L, et al. What should we say to patients with symptoms unexplained by disease? The "number needed to offend". Br Med J. 2002;325(7378):1449–50.

11. Crimlisk HL, Bhatia KP, Cope H, David AS, Marsden D, Ron MA. Patterns of referral in patients with medically unexplained motor symptoms. J Psychosom Res. 2000;49(3):217–9.

12. Kanaan RA. Conversion disorder: who cares? Australas Psychiatry. 2018;26(4):344–6.

13. WHO. The ICD-10 classification of mental and behavioural disorders : clinical descriptions and diagnostic guidelines. WHO; 1992.

14. APA. Diagnostic and statistical manual of mental disorders : DSM-IV. 4th ed. Washington, DC: American Psychiatric Association; 1994. xxvii, 886 p

15. Kanaan RA, Carson A, Wessely SC, Nicholson TR, Aybek S, David AS. What's so special about conversion disorder? A problem and a proposal for diagnostic classification. Br J Psychiatry. 2010;196(6):427–8.

16. Stone J, LaFrance WC Jr, Brown R, Spiegel D, Levenson JL, Sharpe M. Conversion disorder: current problems and potential solutions for DSM-5. J Psychosom Res. 2011;71(6):369–76.

17. Slater E. Diagnosis of "Hysteria". Br Med J. 1965;5447:1395–9.

18. Stone J, Smyth R, Carson A, Lewis S, Prescott R, Warlow C, et al. Systematic review of misdiagnosis of conversion symptoms and "hysteria". BMJ. 2005;331(7523):989.

19. Kanaan RA, Wessely SC. Factitious disorders in neurology: an analysis of reported cases. Psychosomatics. 2010;51(1):47–54.

20. Kanaan RA, Armstrong D, Wessely SC. Neurologists' understanding and management of conversion disorder. J Neurol Neurosurg Psychiatry. 2011;82(9):961–6.

21. Hallett M. Psychogenic movement disorders: a crisis for neurology. Curr Neurol Neurosci Rep. 2006;6(4):269–71.

22. Kanaan RAA. Conversion disorder and illness deception. In: Rogers R, Bender SD, editors. Clinical assessment of malingering and deception. 4th ed. New York: The Guilford Press; 2018. p. 236–42.

23. Stone J, Warlow C, Sharpe M. The symptom of functional weakness: a controlled study of 107 patients. Brain. 2010;133(Pt 5):1537–51.

24. Kanaan R, Armstrong D, Wessely S. Limits to truth-telling: neurologists' communication in conversion disorder. Patient Educ Couns. 2009;77(2):296–301.

25. Ludwig L, Pasman JA, Nicholson T, Aybek S, David AS, Tuck S, et al. Stressful life events and maltreatment in conversion (functional neurological) disorder: systematic review and meta-analysis of case-control studies. Lancet Psychiatry. 2018;5(4):307–20.

26. Charcot JM. Clinical lectures on diseases of the nervous system. London: New Sydenham Society; 1889.

27. Freud S. Charcot. In: Freud S, Freud A, Strachey A, Strachey J, Tyson AW, editors. The standard edition of the complete psychological works of Sigmund Freud. III. London: Hogarth Press; 1953.

28. Breuer J, Freud S. Studies on Hysteria. In: Freud S, Freud A, Strachey A, Strachey J, Tyson AW, editors. The standard edition of the complete psychological works of Sigmund Freud. II. London: Hogarth Press; 1953.

29. Kanaan RAA, Craig TKJ. Conversion disorder and the trouble with trauma. Psychol Med. 2019;49(10):1585–8.

30. Stone J, Mutch J, Giannokous D, Hoeritzauer I, Carson A. Hurst revisited: are symptoms and signs of functional motor and sensory disorders "dependent on idea"? J Neurol Sci. 2017;381:188–91.

31. Trimble MR. Functional diseases. Br Med J. 1982;285:1768–70.

32. Kanaan RA, Armstrong D, Wessely SC. The function of 'functional': a mixed methods investigation. J Neurol Neurosurg Psychiatry. 2012;83(3):248–50.

33. Ding JM, Kanaan RA. Conversion disorder: a systematic review of current terminology. Gen Hosp Psychiatry. 2017;45:51–5.

34. Stone J, LaFrance WC Jr, Levenson JL, Sharpe M. Issues for DSM-5: conversion disorder. Am J Psychiatry. 2010;167(6):626–7.

35. Stone J, Edwards MJ. How "psychogenic" are psychogenic movement disorders? Mov Disord. 2011;26(10):1787–8.

36. Edwards MJ, Stone J, Lang AE. From psychogenic movement disorder to functional movement disorder: it's time to change the name. Mov Disord. 2014;29(7):849–52.

37. Czarnecki K, Thompson JM, Seime R, Geda YE, Duffy JR, Ahlskog JE. Functional movement disorders: successful treatment with a physical therapy rehabilitation protocol. Parkinsonism Relat Disord. 2012;18(3):247–51.

38. Das P, Shinozaki G, McAlpine D. Post-pump chorea-choreiform movements developing after pulmonary thromboendarterectomy for chronic pulmonary hypertension presenting as "functional" movement disorder. Psychosomatics. 2011;52(5):459–62.

39. Sykes R. Medically unexplained symptoms and the Siren "Psychogenic Inference". Phil Psychiatr Psychol. 2010;17(4):289–99.

40. Kanaan RAA, Ding JM. Who thinks functional neurological symptoms are feigned, and what can we do about it? J Neurol Neurosurg Psychiatry. 2017;88(6):533–4.

41. Stone J, Edwards M. Trick or treat? Showing patients with functional (psychogenic) motor symptoms their physical signs. Neurology. 2012;79(3):282–4.

42. Carson A, Lehn A, Ludwig L, Stone J. Explaining functional disorders in the neurology clinic: a photo story. Pract Neurol. 2016;16(1):56–61.

43. WHO. ICD-11: international statistical classification of disease and related health problems: eleventh revision. World Health Organisation; 2018.

44. Kanaan RAA, McGuire PK. Conceptual challenges in the neuroimaging of psychiatric disorders. Philos Psychiatry Psychol. 2011;18(4):323–32.

45. Edwards MJ, Adams RA, Brown H, Parees I, Friston KJ. A Bayesian account of 'hysteria'. Brain. 2012;135(Pt 11):3495–512.

46. Nielsen G, Stone J, Buszewicz M, Carson A, Goldstein LH, Holt K, et al. Physio4FMD: protocol for a multi-centre randomised controlled trial of specialist physiotherapy for functional motor disorder. BMC Neurol. 2019;19(1):242.

47. Kanaan RA, Armstrong D, Wessely S. The role of psychiatrists in diagnosing conversion disorder: a mixed-methods analysis. Neuropsychiatr Dis Treat. 2016;12:1181–4.

48. Dent B, Stanton B, Kanaan RA. Psychiatrists' understanding and management of conversion disorder: a bi-national survey and comparison with neurologists. Neuropsychiatr Dis Treat. in press

49. Watson C, Sivaswamy L, Agarwal R, Du W, Agarwal R. Functional neurologic symptom disorder in children: clinical features, diagnostic investigations, and outcomes at a Tertiary Care Children's Hospital. J Child Neurol. 2019;34(6):325–31.

50. Daum C, Hubschmid M, Aybek S. The value of 'positive' clinical signs for weakness, sensory and gait disorders in conversion disorder: a systematic and narrative review. J Neurol Neurosurg Psychiatry. 2014;85(2):180–90.

51. Morgante F, Edwards MJ, Espay AJ, Fasano A, Mir P, Martino D, et al. Diagnostic agreement in patients with psychogenic movement disorders. Mov Disord. 2012;27(4):548–52.

52. Perez DL, Aybek S, Nicholson TR, Kozlowska K, Arciniegas DB, LaFrance WC Jr. Functional neurological (conversion) disorder: a core neuropsychiatric disorder. J Neuropsychiatry Clin Neurosci. 2020;32(1):1–3.

Free Will, Emotions and Agency: Pathophysiology of Functional Movement Disorder

Mark Hallett

Introduction

In many movement disorders, the brain is hijacked by a neurodegenerative process or a structural lesion and does not function normally. In some neuropsychiatric conditions, the brain is so altered that it is not capable of normal function in certain domains. In a severe stroke, for example, so many neurons are lost that full recovery is impossible. In functional movement disorder (FMD) the brain also is not functioning normally, but, at least in some circumstances normal function is possible. Patients may present with weakness or involuntary movements, but these symptoms may only occur some of the time, and other instances the patient can be normal. Even during the physical examination, certain maneuvers can reverse the weakness or dampen the involuntary movements. Thus, the manifestations are a product of the disordered central nervous system function; hence the name of *functional movement disorder*. In group analyses comparing patients with FMD to those without, some subtle structural differences have been found which might represent one end of the normal distribution and, in any event, do not prevent normal function [1]. It is important to note

that patients with FMD can have another disorder as well, and the FMD would refer to only those symptoms due to reversibly altered brain function.

Abnormal movements in FMD are perceived as involuntary; generally, patients will say that they have no control over the symptoms. There are two other entities that may look somewhat similar, with the patients saying that the symptoms are involuntary, but the individuals are feigning, and the movements are actually voluntary. These are factitious disorder, that has an underlying psychiatric disorder, and malingering, that does not [2]. In most medical practice settings, such patients are not commonly encountered. Better clinical tools and physiological tests are needed to help differentiate between these entities. This chapter will not discuss these other diagnoses further, and the pathophysiology of FMD is certainly distinct from factitious disorder and malingering.

The underpinning of any disorder rests on the two pillars of etiology and pathophysiology [3]. The etiology is the fundamental causes, and the pathophysiology (neural mechanisms), which is a direct result of the etiology, is what produces the symptoms. This chapter will focus on the pathophysiology, and the next chapter will focus on etiological factors. Suffice to say for here that the etiology is best understood to be multifactorial within the context of the biopsychosocial formulation. These factors can predispose,

M. Hallett (✉)
Human Motor Control Section, National Institute of Neurological Disorders and Stroke, National Institutes of Health, Bethesda, MD, USA
e-mail: hallettm@ninds.nih.gov

© Springer Nature Switzerland AG 2022
K. LaFaver et al. (eds.), *Functional Movement Disorder*, Current Clinical Neurology,
https://doi.org/10.1007/978-3-030-86495-8_2

precipitate or perpetuate the FMD. Predisposing factors, such as early life stress, can influence the developing central nervous system and render a person less resilient to stress later-on in life [4].

Normal Function

In order to understand the pathophysiology, it is necessary to understand the normal processes for making movement [5] (Fig. 2.1). Movement is generated by muscles, and the muscles are under control of the spinal cord (or for the cranial muscles, the brainstem). The spinal cord receives controlling signals in the corticospinal tract and

the reticulospinal tract. The rubrospinal tract, present in monkeys, has disappeared in humans. The reticulospinal tract is primitive and generally just deals with automatic and reflex movements. It also receives input from the cortex. The cortex is the main controller of voluntary movement. A small stroke involving just the corticospinal tract will produce a severe hemiplegia.

The motor part of the corticospinal tract originates in the primary motor cortex (M1, area 4) with contributions from the premotor cortex (PMC, lateral area 6) and the supplementary motor area (SMA, medial area 6). Contributions to the corticospinal tract from the post-central cortex go mostly to the dorsal horn of the spinal

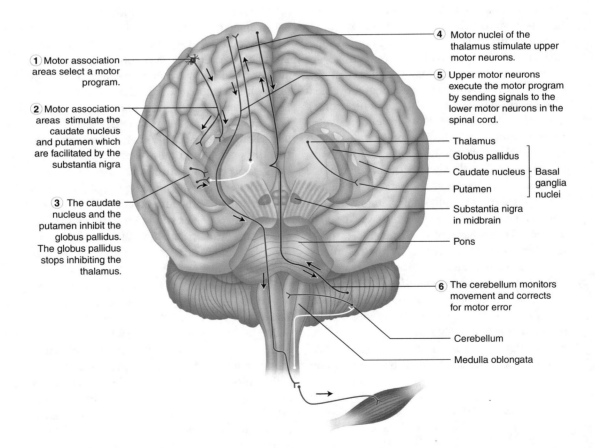

Fig. 2.1 Illustration of the parts and pathways of the brain that generate the movement command (see text for details). (Redrawn with modifications from Tortora and Derrickson [6])

cord and gate sensory information rather than adding to the motor command. What controls the motor cortex, controls movement. Such influences come from subcortical and cortical connections.

The two major subcortical networks involve the basal ganglia and the cerebellum. Both get important input from the cortex and then have their principal output back to the cortex via the thalamus. The loop involving the basal ganglia appears to help the cortex in controlling when and what will be moved, including both whole motor programs and the individual muscles that contribute to the motor programs. Abnormal function of the basal ganglia can lead to symptoms such as bradykinesia and dyskinesias. The loop involving the cerebellum appears to help the cortex in the precise control of the spatial-temporal features of movement, and the principal result of abnormality is ataxia. There are important connections between these loops and the functions may not be as distinct as was once thought. Also, relevant for aspects covered below, both the basal ganglia and cerebellum are involved in non-motor cognitive and affective processes.

The entire cortex provides direct or indirect input to the motor areas. Thus, the motor output at any one time reflects a complex calculation of an enormous number of competing influences. M1 receives strong input from PMC and SMA, and the latter two structures appear to synthesize much of this information for M1 as well as contribute to the corticospinal tract. As a generality, the posterior part of the brain provides information about the external world while the anterior part of the brain provides information about the internal world, the body and its regulation. The posterior part of the brain does receive all the sensory input, visual, somatosensory and auditory. Information is then routed from there to prefrontal and premotor areas where it can influence motor actions. The anterior part of the brain receives information about body function, homeostasis, emotions, and drives such as hunger, thirst, sex, reward, and therefore is likely to develop long and short-term goals. Information from the anterior part of the brain funnels to the anterior midline structures, the anterior/middle cingulate, pre-SMA, SMA and then to PMC and M1.

If you are hungry and felt rewarded recently in this situation when eating a chocolate bar, you might go toward the kitchen to find some chocolate. This is top down control [7]. Seeing the chocolate bar then triggers picking it up and eating it. If the chocolate bar is moldy, then this would discourage eating it. This is bottom up control. The details of skilled movements like picking up the chocolate bar are stored in parietal-motor pathways, perhaps because they are learned with trial and error feedback from the periphery [8].

The brain events associated with an internally triggered, top down movement, activation of the SMA and PMC, can be identified in the EEG as the Bereitschaftspotential (BP), also known, in the English translation, as the readiness potential (RP) [9]. This is a slowly rising negative potential over the anterior midline of the brain. It can be identified in the 1 to 2 seconds prior to the onset of movement.

Some brain events have correlates in consciousness. We do not understand how the contents of consciousness arise, but we are all aware of them. Each content element is a quale. Goals of behavior are appreciated as intentions, and the final command signal for making a movement is appreciated as willing. The quale of willing often has the sense that the action has been freely chosen by the person. This is the sense of free will [10]. When the brain generates goals and motor commands, there are feedforward signals to the inferior parietal lobule and temporoparietal junction (TPJ) in the posterior part of the brain. If these same regions get sensory input in accord with what was willed, this can be an indication that the brain caused that movement. This will be appreciated as the quale of agency, the person is the agent of the movement, and this is another aspect of the sense of free will. In one study of agency, the amount of control of a representation of a hand on a computer screen by the subject's hand was systematically varied. The right TPJ is an important node in the multimodal integration network that identifies the match of command

and result [11]. When there is a match, all is well, and the TPJ is relatively quiet; it becomes more active with mismatch. Other relevant areas in the network concerned with bodily awareness are the right anterior insula, right precuneus, and several regions in the frontal lobe [12].

The brain can focus on only one (or perhaps a few) thing at a time. This includes the qualia. The focusing mechanism is called attention, and this is a distributed system in the brain with at least two networks that have been defined, dorsal and ventral [13]. The dorsal attention network is bilateral including the intraparietal sulcus and the junction of the precentral and superior frontal sulcus (in the region of the frontal eye fields) and is said to be involved with voluntary or "top-

down" goal-oriented attention. The ventral attention network is right lateralized and includes the TPJ and the ventral frontal cortex and is thought to be involved, bottom-up, with orienting to salient stimuli. In relation to salience, there is a separate, but related [14], salience network including the anterior insula and dorsal anterior cingulate as well as some subcortical structures including the amygdala, substantia nigra and periaqueductal gray. For an illustration of these and other brain circuits implicated in the pathophysiology of FMD, see Fig. 2.2.

There is another important aspect to brain function that appears relevant. The brain creates reality for each person on an individual basis, framed as its predictive capabilities. Perception

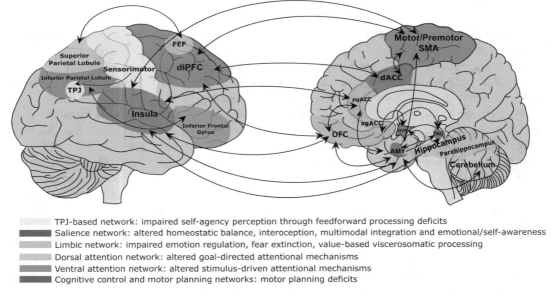

TPJ-based network: impaired self-agency perception through feedforward processing deficits
Salience network: altered homeostatic balance, interoception, multimodal integration and emotional/self-awareness
Limbic network: impaired emotion regulation, fear extinction, value-based viscerosomatic processing
Dorsal attention network: altered goal-directed attentional mechanisms
Ventral attention network: altered stimulus-driven attentional mechanisms
Cognitive control and motor planning networks: motor planning deficits

Fig. 2.2 Display of brain circuits (and related constructs) that are emerging as important in the pathophysiology of functional neurological disorder (FND). As depicted, FND is a multi-network disorder involving abnormalities within and across brain circuits implicated in self-agency, emotion processing, attention, homeostatic balance, interoception, multimodal integration, and cognitive/motor control among other functions. Circuits are described by their related dysfunction in the pathophysiology of FND. It should also be noted that several areas cut across multiple networks; for example, the dorsal anterior insula is most strongly interconnected with the dorsal anterior cingulate cortex (dACC), while the posterior insula receives afferent projections from the lamina I spinothalamocortical pathway and somatosensory cortices.

Similarly, the amygdala is part of both the salience and limbic networks. Prefrontal brain regions are interconnected with striatal-thalamic areas (not shown), and these pathways should also be factored into the neural circuitry of FND. TPJ indicates temporoparietal junction, FEF frontal eye fields, dlPFC dorsolateral prefrontal cortex, pgACC perigenual anterior cingulate cortex, sgACC subgenual anterior cingulate cortex, OFC orbitofrontal cortex, SMA supplementary motor area, AMY amygdala, HYP hypothalamus, PAG periaqueductal gray. (From: Drane DL, Fani N, Hallett M, Khalsa SS, Perez DL, Roberts NA, A framework for understanding the pathophysiology of functional neurological disorder [15], published with permission) of external and internal stimuli depend not only on the stimulus but on a person's current belief (expectations). Beliefs can be, but are not necessarily, updated by the stimuli. Someone nervous about catching a cold, when feeling hot may believe they have a fever, but might change their belief when they find out that the room they are in has a high temperature. This can be called predictive coding [16]; there is an *a priori* probability of how to interpret a stimulus, but after the stimulus, the probabilities might be modified. A hypothetical extension of this is called active inference where a movement can be generated by the brain in order to modify the environment to generate sensory data that would be in accord with an *a priori* belief [17]. How predictive coding is instantiated in the brain is not well established but appears to include broadly distributed brain areas, including frontal areas and multimodal integration brain areas (TPJ, dorsal anterior cingulate cortex, anterior insula) [18, 19]. Shifting of a belief utilizes dopaminergic mechanisms [19] and may involve the anterior insula [20].

A summary of normal motor function as described in this section is illustrated in a block diagram in Fig. 2.3.

Pathophysiology of FMD

The involuntary movements in patients with FMD look like voluntary movements but lack the sense of willing and self-agency [21]. For example, they never have the quick, simple appearance of cortical myoclonus or a tremor faster than 10 Hz. A tremor in one arm will either entrain or stop with rhythmic tapping of the other arm as would happen with voluntary production of alternating movements [21]. The EMG of the muscle activity looks like that of voluntary movement. Stimulus sensitive functional myoclonus is at the latency, and has the variability, of a voluntary reaction time movement. With functional weakness, improved strength can be demonstrated by changing the task and shifting the focus of attention. A patient who does not have any plantar flexion force might be able to walk on his toes. Additionally, exam findings such as a positive

Hoover sign will show normal strength when the muscle is acting as an automatic synergist. All these clinical features indicate that the motor command (M1) and its most proximal control (SMA and PMC) are largely working normally.

Cortical Motor Areas

In patients with functional weakness, transcranial magnetic stimulation (TMS) of M1 will produce a normal response in the somatotopic muscle, a motor evoked potential (MEP) with normal latency and amplitude [22]. This further confirms the integrity of the pathway from M1 to the muscle as anticipated from the clinical observations. However, modulation of the MEP is abnormal. Normally, if a person thinks about moving a muscle (without moving it), the MEP gets larger. In patients with functional weakness, the MEP gets smaller [23, 24]. Thinking about a movement should increase M1 activity, but in patients the activity decreases. A similar phenomenon can be seen with fMRI; trying to make a movement produced a deactivation of the motor cortex [25]. Thus, there is some top down process that is inhibiting M1. There have been other functional imaging studies in patients attempting to make movements that have not occurred. In these studies, dysfunctional activation is seen in the frontal lobes [26], and the frontal areas are particularly strongly connected to the "paretic" motor cortex [27].

The physiology of motor preparation in patients with functional weakness has been studied with the contingent negative variation (CNV), a widespread cortical negativity measured with EEG in between a warning stimulus (S1) and the go stimulus (S2). Patients with unilateral functional weakness were compared to normal subjects performing normally and normal subjects feigning weakness [28]. A low amplitude CNV was found only for the symptomatic hand of the FMD patients. The CNV was analyzed in patients with hyperkinetic FMD and the CNV was also low in that situation, even if the movement did not affect the limb being studied [29]. Interestingly, the CNV normalized in those

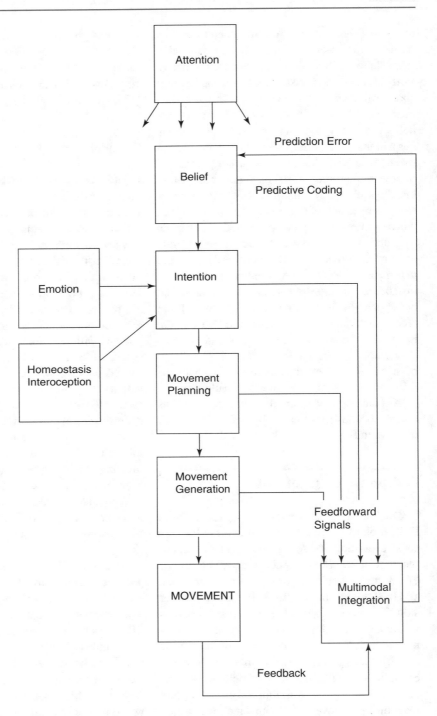

Fig. 2.3 Block diagram
of normal brain function
for making movements.
Attention is distributed
to all parts of the
system. See text for
additional details

patients who improved with treatment. Although
the interpretation of this finding is not completely
clear, it could be indicative of suppressed motor
preparation in frontal midline structures such as
the cingulate area, pre-SMA, and SMA.

In patients with functional myoclonus, a
hyperkinetic movement, analysis of the EEG just
prior to the movement shows a potential that
looks like a normal BP, in timing, morphology,
and amplitude [30]. This indicates that the final

common pathway to the motor command is similar to that of voluntary movement. Thus, not only M1, but SMA and PMC are functioning normally, pushing the origin of the disorder even further up in the hierarchy of motor control. Paradoxically, the BP was absent in 59% of the FMD patients for their normal voluntary movements. A possible explanation for this is discussed below.

Loss of Self-Agency

In FMDs, the patient feels that the abnormal excessive movement (or limb weakness) is involuntary – that is, there is no perceived self-agency. For other types of involuntary movements seen in movement disorder patients, the motor command is not produced in a normal fashion. In hemiballismus or Huntington chorea, the movements are thought to arise in the basal ganglia (although definitive proof is lacking). In cortical myoclonus, an epileptic-like event occurs in the motor cortex causing a quick movement but apparently not generating a normal feedforward signal despite the origin in M1. It is also the case that in most FMD patients, sensation is normal, so there is no abnormality of the pathway from the periphery to the primary sensory cortices. Therefore, there are two main possibilities; there is either an abnormal feedforward signal considering that it does not arise solely in M1 or there is an abnormality in the agency network.

As noted earlier, a particularly important node in the agency network is the right TPJ. The first indication that this was an area of abnormal activity in FMD was in a study of functional tremor. A group of patients were identified that could trigger their involuntary movement by moving their arm into a certain position, and they were also able to voluntarily mimic their involuntary tremor [31]. The movements looked the same to external observers, but they had a clear sense of when it was voluntary and when involuntary. These patients were studied in the two conditions with fMRI, and the biggest difference in the two conditions was in the right TPJ. The TPJ was less active with the involuntary tremor, clearly an

important finding, but paradoxical since it might be expected that involuntary tremor might be more of a mismatch. Additionally, there were some areas in the frontal lobe that were more active with the involuntary tremor. Another group of patients were studied with resting state fMRI (Fig. 2.4) [32]. Using the right TPJ as a region of interest, it was found to have decreased functional connectivity to the right sensorimotor cortex, cerebellar vermis, bilateral SMA, and right insula. The connection to the sensorimotor cortex and SMA might be part of the feedforward pathway. The connection to the insula might be part of the ventral attention/salience networks. In a study of normal movements in patients with FMD in the same paradigm described above where the amount of control of a representation of a hand on a computer screen by the subject's hand was systematically varied, all the appropriate areas were activated but the modulation by the percent control was poor [33]. Like the resting state fMRI study, this result shows abnormal network function even in the absence of abnormal movements.

Loss of Willing

An involuntary movement is characterized by a loss of intention or willing as well as a loss of agency. Indeed, if there is no willing, there cannot be any agency. No willing means no feedforward signaling. However, we already know in FMD, that the processes of motor cortex activation in the involuntary movements are normal. Hence, there appears to be aberrant willing whereby movement occurs normally, but the feedforward signal is abnormal. This is compatible with evidence about the TPJ just discussed, input from the sensorimotor area and SMA are deficient.

Further evidence for a failure of feedforward signaling comes from studies of sensory gating. Sensory gating is the reduction of sensation and somatosensory evoked potentials (SEPs) from a limb at the onset of, and during, self-generated movement. Studied in a mix of FMD patients, sensory gating was decreased in the patients [34,

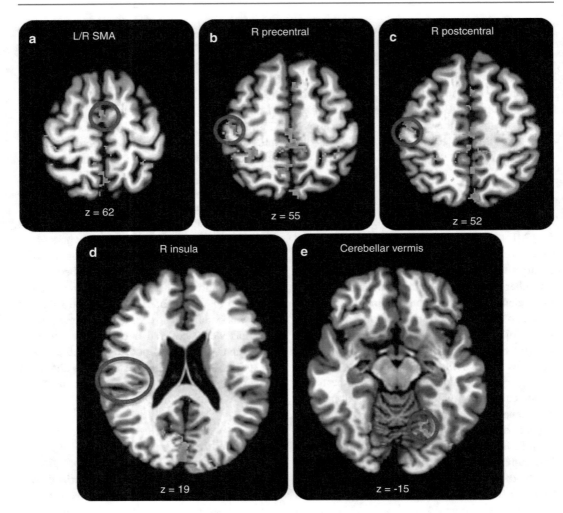

Fig. 2.4 Decreased functional connectivity (FC) between the right temporoparietal junction (rTPJ) and bilateral sensorimotor regions in patients with functional movement disorders (FMD). Maps demonstrate group differences in rTPJ resting-state FC between patients with FMD and healthy controls. Images show decreased FC in patients with FMD between the rTPJ (seed) and the (**a**) bilateral supplementary motor area (SMA) (circled), (**b**) right precentral gyrus (circled), (**c**) right postcentral gyrus (circled), (**d**) right insula (circled), and (**e**) cerebellar vermis (circled). The threshold for display was set at p < 0.02; cluster size .28 voxels. (Republished with permission from Maurer et al. [32])

35]. In one study of force matching, patients did not overestimate the force required as the normal controls did, indicating that they did not have normal gating [35]. In the other study of SEPs, the N20 and N30 potentials were not suppressed as they should have been [34]. Gating must be due to feedforward signaling from the motor command to the sensory system, thus dampening the sensory feedback from the movement. A possible function of gating is to reduce sensory input from expected sensory events. There are two important implications. First, this is evidence for abnormal feedforward signaling. Second, a loss of the gating function would mean that the movement related to the sensation would be more likely to be interpreted as externally generated rather than internally generated; this would foster a loss of the sense of agency.

Thus, one of the main problems in FMD may be in the premotor structures where intentions develop. As noted earlier, there are many excitatory and inhibitory inputs to these structures, and in the next sections some of these will be explored. Abnormalities of one or more of these inputs could be fundamental to FMD.

Emotion Processing

The limbic network of the brain centers on the amygdala and its connections, particularly to the orbitofrontal cortex, ventromedial prefrontal cortex and hypothalamus (see Fig. 2.2). Additionally, the salience network described above is also implicated in emotion processing. As noted earlier, emotion processing is one of the major factors influencing movement choice and often thought to be important in FMD [36]. Limbic structures, such as the amygdala, can be influenced by genetic factors and/or early life stress, important factors in the biopsychosocial model of FMD. In an fMRI study of faces showing different affects, patients with FMD showed increased activation of the right amygdala [37]. There was a pattern consistent with impaired amygdala habituation even when controlling for depressive and anxiety symptoms. Using psychophysiological interaction analysis, patients with FMD had greater functional connectivity between the right amygdala and the right SMA, and Granger Causality Modeling showed a directional influence from the right amygdala to the right SMA. Overactivity of the amygdala was confirmed in other studies [38, 39], and increased activity in the SMA was also seen in one of these studies [38]. In another study of emotional face processing in a group of patients with functional tremor, overactivity was seen in the cingulate/paracingulate region, and not in the amygdala [40], but this region is also part of the limbic sys-

tem. Incidentally, it can be noted that increased emotional activity can affect other movement disorders also; for example, increasing tremor in patients with Parkinson disease.

In another study, patients with FMD performed either an internally or externally generated 2-button action selection task in a functional MRI study [41]. During both types of movement, patients relative to normal volunteers had higher right amygdala, left anterior insula, and bilateral posterior cingulate activity and lower left SMA activity. During internally versus externally generated action in patients, the left SMA had lower functional connectivity with bilateral dorsolateral prefrontal cortices.

A quantitative structural MRI study using voxel-based morphometry in patients with FMD compared with healthy controls exhibited increased volume of the left amygdala, left striatum, left cerebellum, left fusiform gyrus, and bilateral thalamus, and decreased volume of the left sensorimotor cortex – abnormalities of the limbic and motor systems [42]. More work is needed to understand the role of laterality in limbic-related brain areas across the structural and functional neuroimaging literature.

One influence of the amygdala is on the startle reflex. Patients with FMD show an increased startle response to positive affective pictures as well as negative ones, indicating abnormal regulation of the startle response [43]. Even the simple startle reflex is increased [44].

The data are clear that there is limbic system hyperactivity and increased influence on the motor system. In resting state fMRI study using graph theory-based analyses [45], increased functional connectivity in FMD patients was found involving motor regions to the bilateral posterior insula, TPJ, middle cingulate cortex and putamen. From the right laterobasal amygdala, the patients showed enhanced connectivity to the left anterior insula, periaqueductal grey and hypothalamus among other areas. Symptom severity correlated with increased information flow from the left anterior insula to the right anterior insula and TPJ.

While there is strong evidence for hyperactivity of the limbic and salience networks, it is curious that many patients with FMD have alexithymia, a psychopathological trait characterized by the inability to identify and describe emotions experienced by one's self or others. Thus, this hyperactivity, which might be translated as representing the increased influence of emotion on action, is not recognized in consciousness. This might be due to a lack of attention to this function of the brain. There are problems with attention, which will be considered next. Other patients conversely do recognize that heightened arousal and negative affective states amplify symptoms such as functional tremor, which suggests an alternative framing for how to contextualize amygdala, cingulo-insular, and periaqueductal gray hyperactivations.

Attention

From clinical assessment alone it is clear that there is an important problem with attention [46]. Maintenance of functional movements or paresis might well depend on attending to the malfunctioning body part. If the patient's attention is distracted away from the abnormal movement by, for example, by asking a patient to do a task with a different body part, the abnormality might disappear. A tremor in the left arm might stop when a patient is asked to do a task with the right arm or solve a mathematical problem. Abnormalities in sustained and selection attention have characterized patients with functional neurological disorders, best identified in functional seizures [47].

Interoception

Interoception is the ability to appreciate the internal state of body functioning. This would include aspects such as hunger, thirst, or beating of the heart. Interoception and emotional awareness may also be partially inter-related constructs.

Interoceptive deficits based on use of a heartbeat detection task have been described in individuals with FMD [48]. The likely locus of abnormality is the insula, which is well known to process such information, particularly in its posterior segments. Deficits in interoception could also be considered as a problem with bodily-related attention.

Belief and Predictive Coding

One of the hypotheses about the genesis of FMD is abnormal belief and predictive coding deficits [49]. In simple terms, let's say that a man has the belief that he is sick and that despite feedback that all is well, the belief does not change. The prior does not update. From a clinical point of view, this often seems the case. A patient may feel that there is some structural brain disorder, such as a brain tumor, and refuses to drop that belief even after normal studies and a doctor's reassurance. The patient goes on to find another doctor. While normal movement should update the prior, abnormal movement verifies the prior and helps maintain it. It becomes circular. The patient believes he/she has a tremor disorder and the fact that he/she has tremor confirms that belief. To go one step further, if active inference is an actual function, then the belief itself might generate the tremor in order to maintain the belief. If this is occurring, the process cannot be conscious since the movement is felt to be involuntary. If this process creates involuntary movements, while the person is also able to generate voluntary movements, the involuntary process would seem dissociated from the brain mechanisms that are functioning normally. Indeed, for many patients there is a sense that the FMD is dissociated from their normal selves. There are two modes of operation, normal and abnormal. Perhaps this is most apparent with paroxysmal involuntary movements, such as functional seizures, which are often called dissociative seizures for this reason. Additionally, the brain must focus attention on this belief. If attention is diverted to normal function, the abnormal function disappears. The excessive attention to the abnormal belief deprives other brain function of attention, possibly including emotion and interoception.

How does an abnormal belief develop? If there is a temporary abnormal condition of the body, for example, a heightened emotion, the predictions about what the body should be like are incorrect. A prediction error is then fed back and the underlying probability for a new prediction is altered. A new model of the body might then develop after several iterations.

The last paragraphs contain many hypotheticals, but as a model has some explanatory power for some paradoxical phenomena discussed here previously. In patients with functional myoclonus, there is a BP before the involuntary movements, but often not before normal voluntary movements [30]. The involuntary movement generates movements via the usual pathway including the SMA, while the voluntary movement does not have such access. That might explain also why patients with FMD do not improve reaction time in response to a cue that has high validity for predicting the required movement [50], and why there is not the normal beta desynchronization prior to movement [51]. Additionally, it could explain why TPJ activation is less for involuntary tremor than for voluntary tremor [31]; the involuntary tremor creates less mismatch rather than more.

Synthesis of the Pathophysiology

Certainly, there is more to learn, but a picture is emerging (Fig. 2.5). The fundamental building blocks of normal movement are established, and that provides a basis for understanding the pathophysiology of FMD. An overactive limbic system disrupts brain function including a heightened influence on the motor system. Prediction errors arise and gradually develop a belief that the person is sick due to abnormal movements. Excessive

attention to the belief helps maintain it. The new predictive coding from the abnormal belief hijacks the normal motor apparatus. Movements (or paresis) may be generated either from the limbic system or an active inference process stemming from the belief. This abnormal generation does not create a quale of willing or a proper feedforward signal to the multimodal network of the TPJ, and no quale of agency develops either. The original normal motor system either exists in parallel with the new abnormal network or toggles back and forth with it. The two systems can give rise to the sense of dissociation. Attention is reduced to other brain functions such as interoception and emotion awareness. Additionally, it is possible that across FMD patient populations, distinct aspects of the neurobiology may play more prominent roles in one patient sub-group over another. In the end, it is no longer only a belief, the patient is truly sick.

Implications for Treatment

If these hypotheses are correct, or even partially correct, the only way of curing the patient at a fundamental level is to dampen down the limbic system and adjust its functioning to be more homeostatic. This may not be easy since its development may have been disrupted by factors such as early life stress that has left it less resilient [52, 53]. A fundamental change is not likely to happen quickly and may require a multipronged approach. Better understanding about the cellular and molecular neurobiology, and their detailed connections, will be helpful in the development of individually targeted approaches to treatment of FMD.

A second approach which might help reverse the disorder, but will likely still leave the patient vulnerable, would be to correct the illness belief and its top down influence on the motor system. Develop methods to encourage the brain to function more in its normal mode. Deprive the "sick mode" of attention and possibly even shift

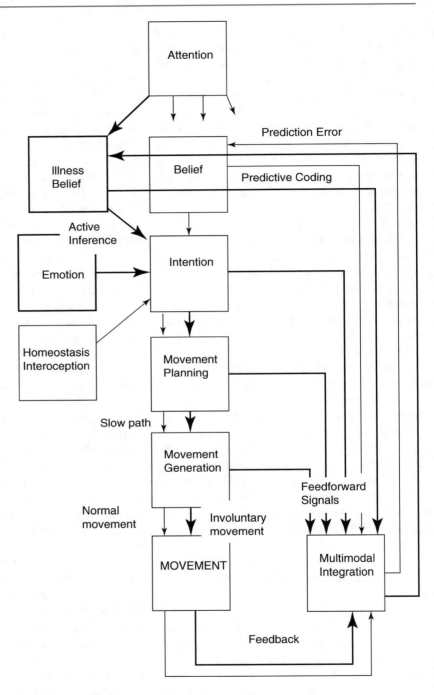

Fig. 2.5 Pathophysiology model of functional movement disorders. The normal mechanism for making movements is pushed aside in favor of an abnormal mechanism (indicated with bolder text and lines). Attention is co-opted for the abnormal mechanism. See text for additional details

it back to the normal mode by utilizing prediction error. There is some evidence, quoted above, that shifting of predictive coding is supported by dopaminergic mechanisms. Thus, using reward or even dopamine itself in an appropriate fashion could support shifting. To a certain extent, that is what psychologically supported physical therapy can provide by encouraging patients to understand that they can function normally.

Summary

- In functional movement disorder, instances of normal movement can be appreciated.
- Core constructs implicated in the pathophysiology of FMD include loss of self-agency, altered emotion processing, biased attentional mechanisms, altered beliefs/predictive coding, and impaired interoception.
- Emerging evidence suggests that FMD is a multi-network brain disorder with the right temporal parietal junction-based network implicated in disturbances in self-agency.
- An overactive limbic system disrupts brain function in FMD, including a heightened influence on the motor system.
- More research is needed to bridge neural mechanisms and disease etiologies within the context of the biopsychosocial model, as well as further investigating the neural mechanisms of treatment response.

Acknowledgement Dr. Hallett is supported by the NINDS Intramural Program.

References

1. Begue I, Adams C, Stone J, Perez DL. Structural alterations in functional neurological disorder and related conditions: a software and hardware problem? Neuroimage Clin. 2019;22:101798.
2. Galli S, Tatu L, Bogousslavsky J, Aybek S. Conversion, factitious disorder and malingering: a distinct pattern or a continuum? Front Neurol Neurosci. 2018;42:72–80.
3. Hallett M, Stone J, Carson A. Functional neurologic disorders. In: Aminoff MJ, Boller F, Swaab DF, editors. Handb Clin Neurol. Amsterdam: Elsevier; 2016. p. 662.
4. Lecei A, van Winkel R. Hippocampal pattern separation of emotional information determining risk or resilience in individuals exposed to childhood trauma: linking exposure to neurodevelopmental alterations and threat anticipation. Neurosci Biobehav Rev. 2020;108:160–70.
5. Hallett M. Motor control: physiology of voluntary and involuntary movements. In: Fahn S, Jankovic J, Hallett M, editors. Principles and practice of movement disorders. Second ed. Philadelphia: Elsevier Saunders; 2011.
6. Tortora GJ, Derrickson BH. Principles of Anatomy and Physiology. 15th ed. Hoboken: Wiley; 2017.
7. Corradi-Dell'Acqua C, Fink GR, Weidner R. Selecting category specific visual information: top-down and bottom-up control of object based attention. Conscious Cogn. 2015;35:330.
8. Wheaton LA, Hallett M. Ideomotor apraxia: a review. J Neurol Sci. 2007;260:1–10.
9. Shibasaki H, Hallett M. What is the Bereitschaftspotential? Clin Neurophysiol. 2006;117:2341–56.
10. Hallett M. Physiology of free will. Ann Neurol. 2016;80:5–12.
11. Nahab FB, Kundu P, Gallea C, Kakareka J, Pursley R, Pohida T, et al. The neural processes underlying self-agency. Cereb Cortex. 2011;21:48–55.
12. Sperduti M, Delaveau P, Fossati P, Nadel J. Different brain structures related to self- and external-agency attribution: a brief review and meta-analysis. Brain Struct Funct. 2011;216:151–7.
13. Vossel S, Geng JJ, Fink GR. Dorsal and ventral attention systems: distinct neural circuits but collaborative roles. Neuroscientist. 2014;20:150–9.
14. Parr T, Friston KJ. Attention or salience? Curr Opin Psychol. 2019;29:1–5.
15. Drane DL, Fani N, Hallett M, Khalsa SS, Perez DL, Roberts NA. A framework for understanding the pathophysiology of functional neurological disorder. CNS Spectr. 2021;26:555–61.
16. Siman-Tov T, Granot RY, Shany O, Singer N, Hendler T, Gordon CR. Is there a prediction network? Meta-analytic evidence for a cortical-subcortical network likely subserving prediction. Neurosci Biobehav Rev. 2019;105:262–75.
17. Brown H, Adams RA, Parees I, Edwards M, Friston K. Active inference, sensory attenuation and illusions. Cogn Process. 2013;14:411–27.
18. Kleckner IR, Zhang J, Touroutoglou A, Chanes L, Xia C, Simmons WK, et al. Evidence for a large-scale brain system supporting Allostasis and Interoception in humans. Nat Hum Behav. 2017;1:0069.
19. Schwartenbeck P, FitzGerald THB, Dolan R. Neural signals encoding shifts in beliefs. NeuroImage. 2016;125:578–86.
20. Wang BA, Schlaffke L, Pleger B. Modulations of insular projections by prior belief mediate the precision of prediction error during tactile learning. J Neurosci. 2020;40(19):JN-RM-2904-19.
21. Hallett M. Physiology of psychogenic movement disorders. J Clin Neurosci. 2010;17:959–65.
22. Liepert J, Hassa T, Tuscher O, Schmidt R. Electrophysiological correlates of motor conversion disorder. Mov Disord. 2008;23:2171–6.
23. Liepert J, Hassa T, Tuscher O, Schmidt R. Abnormal motor excitability in patients with psychogenic paresis. TMS study. J Neurol. 2009;256:121–6.

24. Liepert J, Hassa T, Tuscher O, Schmidt R. Motor excitability during movement imagination and movement observation in psychogenic lower limb paresis. J Psychosom Res. 2011;70:59–65.

25. Matt E, Amini A, Aslan T, Schmidhammer R, Beisteiner R. Primary motor cortex deactivation as a new mechanism of motor inhibition in conversion paralysis. Mov Disord. 2019;34:148–9.

26. Nowak DA, Fink GR. Psychogenic movement disorders: Aetiology, phenomenology, neuroanatomical correlates and therapeutic approaches. NeuroImage. 2009;47:1015–25.

27. Cojan Y, Waber L, Carruzzo A, Vuilleumier P. Motor inhibition in hysterical conversion paralysis. NeuroImage. 2009;47:1026–37.

28. Blakemore RL, Hyland BI, Hammond-Tooke GD, Anson JG. Deficit in late-stage contingent negative variation provides evidence for disrupted movement preparation in patients with conversion paresis. Biol Psychol. 2015;109:73–85.

29. Teodoro T, Koreki A, Meppelink AM, Little S, Nielsen G, Macerollo A, et al. Contingent negative variation: a biomarker of abnormal attention in functional movement disorders. Eur J Neurol. 2020;27:985.

30. van der Salm SM, Tijssen MA, Koelman JH, van Rootselaar AF. The bereitschaftspotential in jerky movement disorders. J Neurol Neurosurg Psychiatry. 2012;83:1162–7.

31. Voon V, Gallea C, Hattori N, Bruno M, Ekanayake V, Hallett M. The involuntary nature of conversion disorder. Neurology. 2010b;74:223–8.

32. Maurer CW, LaFaver K, Ameli R, Epstein SA, Hallett M, Horovitz SG. Impaired self-agency in functional movement disorders: a resting-state fMRI study. Neurology. 2016;87:564–70.

33. Nahab FB, Kundu P, Maurer C, Shen Q, Hallett M. Impaired sense of agency in functional movement disorders: An fMRI study. PLoS One. 2017;12(4):e0172502. https://doi.org/10.1371/journal.pone.0172502.

34. Macerollo A, Chen JC, Parees I, Kassavetis P, Kilner JM, Edwards MJ. Sensory attenuation assessed by sensory evoked potentials in functional movement disorders. PLoS One. 2015;10:e0129507.

35. Parees I, Brown H, Nuruki A, Adams RA, Davare M, Bhatia KP, et al. Loss of sensory attenuation in patients with functional (psychogenic) movement disorders. Brain. 2014;137:2916–21.

36. Pick S, Goldstein LH, Perez DL, Nicholson TR. Emotional processing in functional neurological disorder: a review, biopsychosocial model and research agenda. J Neurol Neurosurg Psychiatry. 2019;90:704–11.

37. Voon V, Brezing C, Gallea C, Ameli R, Roelofs K, LaFrance WC Jr, et al. Emotional stimuli and motor conversion disorder. Brain. 2010a;133:1526–36.

38. Aybek S, Nicholson TR, O'Daly O, Zelaya F, Kanaan RA, David AS. Emotion-motion interactions in conversion disorder: an FMRI study. PLoS One. 2015;10:e0123273.

39. Hassa T, Sebastian A, Liepert J, Weiller C, Schmidt R, Tuscher O. Symptom-specific amygdala hyperactivity modulates motor control network in conversion disorder. Neuroimage Clin. 2017;15:143–50.

40. Espay AJ, Ries S, Maloney T, Vannest J, Neefus E, Dwivedi AK, et al. Clinical and neural responses to cognitive behavioral therapy for functional tremor. Neurology. 2019;93:e1787–e98.

41. Voon V, Brezing C, Gallea C, Hallett M. Aberrant supplementary motor complex and limbic activity during motor preparation in motor conversion disorder. Mov Disord. 2011;26:2396–403.

42. Maurer CW, LaFaver K, Limachia GS, Capitan G, Ameli R, Sinclair S, et al. Gray matter differences in patients with functional movement disorders. Neurology. 2018;91:e1870–e9.

43. Seignourel PJ, Miller K, Kellison I, Rodriguez R, Fernandez HH, Bauer RM, et al. Abnormal affective startle modulation in individuals with psychogenic [corrected] movement disorder. Mov Disord. 2007;22:1265–71.

44. Dreissen YEM, Boeree T, Koelman J, Tijssen MAJ. Startle responses in functional jerky movement disorders are increased but have a normal pattern. Parkinsonism Relat Disord. 2017;40:27–32.

45. Diez I, Ortiz-Teran L, Williams B, Jalilianhasanpour R, Ospina JP, Dickerson BC, et al. Corticolimbic fast-tracking: enhanced multimodal integration in functional neurological disorder. J Neurol Neurosurg Psychiatry. 2019;90:929–38.

46. Baizabal-Carvallo JF, Hallett M, Jankovic J. Pathogenesis and pathophysiology of functional (psychogenic) movement disorders. Neurobiol Dis. 2019;127:32–44.

47. Simani L, Roozbeh M, Rostami M, Pakdaman H, Ramezani M, Asadollahi M. Attention and inhibitory control deficits in patients with genetic generalized epilepsy and psychogenic nonepileptic seizure. Epilepsy Behav. 2020;102:106672.

48. Ricciardi L, Demartini B, Crucianelli L, Krahe C, Edwards MJ, Fotopoulou A. Interoceptive awareness in patients with functional neurological symptoms. Biol Psychol. 2016;113:68–74.

49. Edwards MJ, Adams RA, Brown H, Parees I, Friston KJ. A Bayesian account of 'hysteria'. Brain. 2012;135:3495–512.

50. Parees I, Kassavetis P, Saifee TA, Sadnicka A, Davare M, Bhatia KP, et al. Failure of explicit movement control in patients with functional motor symptoms. Mov Disord. 2013;28:517–23.

51. Teodoro T, Meppelink AM, Little S, Grant R, Nielsen G, Macerollo A, et al. Abnormal beta power is a hallmark of explicit movement control in functional movement disorders. Neurology. 2018;90:e247–e53.

52. Diez I, Larson AG, Nakhate V, Dunn EC, Fricchione GL, Nicholson TR, et al. Early-life trauma endophenotypes and brain circuit-gene expression relationships in functional neurological (conversion) disorder. Mol Psychiatry. 2021;26:3817–28.

53. Spagnolo PA, Norato G, Maurer CW, Goldman D, Hodgkinson C, Horovitz S, et al. Effects of TPH2 gene variation and childhood trauma on the clinical and circuit-level phenotype of functional movement disorders. J Neurol Neurosurg Psychiatry. 2020;91:814.

The Biopsychosocial Formulation for Functional Movement Disorder

Lindsey MacGillivray and Sarah C. Lidstone

Case Vignette 1

Mr. S is a pleasant 54-year-old gentleman. He lives with his wife and 2 teenaged children and is financially supported by his work as a project manager for a large national firm. His medical history is significant for irritable bowel syndrome but is otherwise unremarkable. He has no formal psychiatric history, but family and friends describe him as stoic and at times "aloof." He tells you that his childhood was "normal and happy enough" and denies any history of trauma, though on probing you discover that when he was a child his father often physically struck him for minor discretions. "That's just the way it was back then," he says. Mr. S was unfortunately involved in a motor vehicle accident in his early 50s. He was struck from behind and though he sustained only minor musculoskeletal injuries, he never seemed to fully recover. Years later, he continues to complain of persistent low back and neck pain. Routine blood work, brain and spinal MRIs and nerve conduction studies are all normal.

Two months ago, Mr. S developed sudden onset jerks in his truncal region. He is referred to a movement disorders neurologist who, after a thorough neurological examination, diagnoses him with functional myoclonus on the basis of positive examination signs including prominent variability and distractibility. He is unable to self-identify any precipitating factors but indicates that his jerks are more frequent and debilitating on days in which he is more fatigued or experiencing increased pain. He admits that his abnormal movements make him feel self-conscious and that he has started to limit his social interactions and is working from home whenever possible. He brought disability application paperwork to his appointment today.

L. MacGillivray (✉)
Department of Psychiatry, University of Toronto, Toronto Western Hospital, University Health Network, Toronto, ON, Canada
e-mail: lindsey.macgillivray@uhn.ca

S. C. Lidstone
Integrated Movement Disorders Program, Toronto Rehabilitation Institute, Toronto, ON, Canada

Edmond J. Safra Program in Parkinson's Disease and the Morton and Gloria Shulman Movement Disorders Clinic, Toronto Western Hospital, University Health Network, Toronto, ON, Canada

Division of Neurology, Department of Medicine, University of Toronto, Toronto, ON, Canada

Case Vignette 2

Mrs. V is a 42-year-old married female and mother to three children. She works as a human resources manager and much of her time is spent navigating disputes among employees. She is skilled at this work and reports that she finds her position rewarding, but stressful. She

© Springer Nature Switzerland AG 2022
K. LaFaver et al. (eds.), *Functional Movement Disorder*, Current Clinical Neurology,
https://doi.org/10.1007/978-3-030-86495-8_3

balances her paid work with volunteering roles that she has accumulated over the years— for instance, the local parent teacher association and community food bank. At home, she is the primary caregiver for the children and takes most of the responsibility for managing the household, as her husband is CEO of a sales agency and has to travel frequently. She wishes her husband was able to be home more often but is proud of his success at work and reports that they have a mutually loving and supportive relationship. Her medical history is significant for dysmenorrhea and migraine headaches throughout her 20s, but she has been generally healthy since. She has no formal psychiatric history and denies any past or current symptoms of anxiety, depression or trauma-related disorders. Despite this, a possible generalized anxiety disorder is suspected given her descriptions of being "always on the go," "being a worrier" and having difficulties "turning my brain off." On interview, she presents as animated and anxious. She talks quickly and you have a sense of her being on 'overdrive.' Her body appears tense, with mild psychomotor agitation. She describes a one-year history of shaking in her right arm, starting after a bout of flu-like symptoms. The shaking comes and goes but seems to be worsening in intensity and frequency and she also notices that she is increasingly forgetful. "It feels like my brain is in a fog." Her grandfather suffered from Parkinson's disease and related dementia and she is worried that she, too, is developing a neurodegenerative condition. She now pays much more attentive to her body so that she can be on the lookout for new symptoms or other worrisome signs. She continues to push through at work, emphasizing that her employees rely on her.

Mrs. V is referred to a neurologist who diagnoses her with a functional movement disorder (FMD), after observing that her arm tremor was both readily distractible and entrainable (positive signs for functional tremor). The interviewer remembers from medical school that these disorders are likely connected to psychological trauma, and as such is surprised when she denies *any history of emotional, sexual or physical abuse. Of note, she has been chronically high achieving. She was an academic gold medalist in high school and is a former national-level dancer. Her friends describe her as being "the nice one who is always willing to help" and "a bit of a perfectionist." They wonder how she manages to do it all.*

Introduction to the Biopsychosocial Model and Formulation

In 1977, George Engel postulated a model that aimed to transform the way clinicians conceptualize disease [1]. By contrast to the dominant biomedical model that suggested disease could be fully accounted for by measurable biological variables, Engel offered us a more holistic way of understanding our patients, suggesting that we instead simultaneously consider the biological, psychological and social dimensions of illness (including cultural and spiritual aspects where relevant) [1]. While in some respects this **biopsychosocial model** could inadvertently reinforce a false mind-body dualism by encouraging clinicians to consider biological factors as discrete from psychological and social factors, it is important to remember that psychological experience has biological underpinnings and, in turn, that biological phenomena often have psychological correlates. Nonetheless, so long as we are mindful that brain, body and mind are parts of an integrated whole, the biopsychosocial framework can help guide us to a holistic understanding of our patients and to better identify a range of treatment targets.

To understand and treat patients with FMD, you must endeavor to learn their *story*, i.e. not simply the phenomenology of their symptoms, but the context in which those symptoms evolved, and how those symptoms affect the person before you. You should also seek to identify factors that potentially render your patient at risk for developing FMD and to explore their strengths; awareness of these will help clinicians to engage with patients and to assist in treating their symptoms. This information is often best obtained through open-ended qualitative interviews rather than exclusive reliance on clinical scales or symptom-checklists [2, 3].

The standard way to apply the biopsychosocial model is to generate a list of **predisposing**, **precipitating** and **perpetuating** factors that align with biological, psychological and psychosocial categories. Many use a three-by-three square grid to organize this list (see Fig. 3.1). Importantly, any given factor can apply to one of more categories (e.g. alexithymia may be both a predisposing vulnerability and a precipitating factor).

FMD is a complex neuropsychiatric disorder that is best understood as arising in the context of predisposing vulnerabilities (risk factors), acute precipitants and perpetuating factors. Rarely is there one identified *cause* for FMD and, by contrast to early psychodynamic theories of conversion, we now recognize that FMD is not exclusively a psychiatric disorder. For some patients, prominent psychological stressors are not readily apparent or are not the most relevant factors in understanding their illness [4–6]. Accordingly, the most recent version of the Diagnostic and Statistical Manual for Mental Disorders (DSM-5) has removed the diagnostic requirement for a psychological stressor to precede symptom onset [7]. In general, we suggest that clinicians de-emphasize an upfront search for a specific cause and instead focus on the rationale for the FMD diagnosis and the evidence-based treatments that may help the patient in their recovery journey. However, while an initial focus on "why" someone has developed FMD may be better left for exploration in the context of engagement in rehabilitation and psychological treatments, assessing the basic components of the biopsychosocial model to formulate clinical cases aids the development of a patient-centered treatment plan.

Formulation is an active process that requires more than collecting discrete biopsychosocial data points. To formulate, one uses information gleaned from a holistic interview to generate a tentative hypothesis about *how* and *why* a patient developed symptoms at this juncture in their lives. A formulation should be individualized to your patient and is not meant to identify a singular etiology for FMD (there are typically numerous or many relevant factors)— one size does not fit all. And remember, a formulation is merely a hypothesis, not conclusive fact. It should not be delivered in a top-down fashion as a certainty, but rather is best developed over time in active collaboration with the patient [8].

Predisposing Vulnerabilities (Risk Factors) for FMD

Predisposing factors confer vulnerability to later development of FMD. They include demographic and characterological factors, comorbid medical/neurological/psychiatric illnesses and influential events occurring throughout development. Typically, these vulnerabilities are remote from the onset of the FMD and while they do not necessarily have any direct (proximal) etiological relevance, they do foster risk.

Biological

Women are more frequently affected by FMD than men, representing an estimated 60-75% of the patient population [9]. This difference may vary by FMD phenomenology; functional myoclonus, for instance, appears to be equally or more common in men [10].

Comorbid neurological and psychiatric disorders may play a predisposing role; a broad range of pre-existing conditions have been reported in the FMD population, including but not limited to multiple sclerosis, Parkinson's disease, history of head injury, epilepsy, intellectual disability, anxiety and depression [4, 11–15]. Sensory processing difficulties have been reported in some patients with FMD [16]. Commonly, patients with FMD also have a history of somatic symptoms of unclear etiology. These, too, are broad ranging, but often include conditions such as chronic fatigue, fibromyalgia, pelvic pain and irritable bowel syndrome [17–19]. Whether these conditions are part of a larger "functional syn-

	Biological	Psychological	Social
Predisposing Vulnerabilities (Risk Factors)	Female gender Comorbid neurological and psychiatric conditions Sensory processing difficulties Chronic fatigue, pain gastrointestinal conditions	Comorbid psychiatric disorders Health anxiety and somatic vigilance Alexithymia Insecure attachment style Maladaptive personality traits	Physical, sexual or emotional trauma; neglect Low socioeconomic status; financial strain Major lossess such as bereavement or divorce Chronic interpersonal challenges
Acute Precipitants	Physical injury or surgery Preceding illness Accidents (e.g., motor vechicle accident) Autonomic hyperarousal event (e.g., panic attack) Sleep deprivation	Dissociation; panic attacks Events (e.g., losses, failures) that activate insecure attachment patterns, distorted cognitions Unprocessed guilt and anger Emotional impact of injury	Relationship stressors Significant losses– death, separation or divorce Interpersonal conflict Job loss or employment-related stressors
Prepetuating Factors	Chronic pain and/or fatigue Chronic medical conditions Physical deconditioning Entrenched abnormal motor programs	Invalidation by the healthcare system; stigma Maladaptive illness beliefs; Lack of diagnostic agreement Anxiety and hypervigilance around symptoms Avoidance patterns	Family dysfunction Interpersonal or work-related stressors Pending litigation Unconscious secondary gains Poor communication amongst health care providers

Fig. 3.1 Depiction of the biopsychosocial model for clinical formulation of patients with functional movement disorder. Note — other themes not addressed in this model may be relevant at the individual patient level. Also, a given factor may cut across multiple levels, such as alexithymia in a given patient being both a predisposing vulnerability and a perpetuating factor

drome" that exists on a continuum is the subject of debate, but they are nonetheless important to screen for in your intake assessment because they may also be relevant perpetuating factors that should be addressed in a comprehensive treatment plan. Notably, associated pain, fatigue and psychological symptoms are reported to account for more disability and impaired quality of life than do the motor symptoms themselves [20, 21].

Psychological

Categorical psychiatric disorders (e.g. generalized anxiety, panic, major depression, post-traumatic stress and personality pathology) have both biological and psychological substrates and are present in some individuals that develop FMD [2, 5, 13]. Health anxiety and a pattern of somatic vigilance are sometimes prominent [22]. More frequently, individuals with FMD have relational frameworks, personality traits and patterns of behavior that, while not necessarily pathological, may render them vulnerable to FMD. These dimensional considerations include factors such as alexithymia (difficulty identifying and labeling emotions), insecure attachment patterns and chronic challenges with affect regulation, neuroticism and/or obsessionality [23–25]. There is no singular personality style associated with FMD, but traits we see in some patients include excessive responsibility taking, chronic high achievement and perfectionism, tendencies to put the needs of others before oneself, and conflict avoidance [26–28]. Some individuals have a propensity to distance from emotion, to dissociate in the context of stress or to adopt a highly active "always on the go" lifestyle that might serve to distract from underlying feelings—a manic defense, of sorts [23].

Social

The most frequently reported predisposing factors are psychosocial in nature. Among these are a history of adverse life experiences, including trauma, significant interpersonal difficulties in one's family or social environment, or a major loss [6, 29–32]. Chronic pre-existing stressors in the form of financial strain, low socioeconomic status in general and limited psychosocial supports may also predispose individuals to later development of FMD [30, 32].

Historically, functional neurological disorder (FND) was ascribed in entirety to a psychological stressor or emotional conflict. Psychodynamic theory held that emotionally-laden stress was subconsciously repressed and "converted" to physical form [33] and previous versions of the DSM included a preceding psychological stressor as necessary for the diagnosis of conversion disorder [34]. This requirement has been removed from DSM-5 given that a substantial proportion of patients with FND do not report having experienced traumatic events in their history [5]. We caution clinicians against making any direct supposition to patients that their symptoms are "caused" by trauma or stress, especially if they themselves deny any such history. When present, however, trauma and other psychological factors often play important predisposing and perpetuating roles in FMD and correlate with symptom severity [5]. This is also a good example of the inter-relatedness of various components of the biopsychsocial model; childhood maltreatment has been linked to plastic changes in the brain that may help explain links between life events and the later development of FMD [35, 36].

Acute Precipitants for FMD

Acute precipitants are proximal factors that temporally associate with onset of FMD. They may or may not be identifiable. Like predisposing factors, precipitants are not "causes" of FMD. They should instead be considered as triggers or "tipping-point" variables. It is likely that precipitants set in motion FMD symptom onset only in the setting of predisposing vulnerabilities.

Biological

Inciting events are often physical in nature [4, 37–39]. Patients commonly tell us about flu-like illnesses or exacerbations of other underlying medical conditions preceding their FMD. Events that trigger acute autonomic hyperarousal— a panic attack, motor vehicle accident, mild head trauma or unexpected pain, for instance— or a period of prolonged sleep deprivation might contribute to FMD symptom onset [40–42].

Physical injury and surgery are common precipitants for FMD and include such presentations as ipsilateral hand dystonia following carpel tunnel surgery and functional leg weakness following lumbar radiculopathy [37, 39, 40, 43]. The pathophysiological correlates of these associations are not especially clear but might relate to abnormally directed somatic attention or a context of fear and uncertainty [42].

Psychological

Psychological precipitants might include panic attacks or acute dissociative events; these are likely to be experienced as frightening and often lead to a pattern of somatic vigilance and avoidance [22, 41, 44]. A major loss, perceived failure or interpersonal rejection might trigger insecure attachment patterns and activate early life maladaptive schemas and automatic negative cognitions [6, 32]. Unprocessed guilt and anger might also play a precipitating role. The psychological ramifications of mild head injuries, e.g. heightened anxiety, adjusting to the impact of cognitive dysfunction and uncertainty regarding recovery, may lay groundwork for an evolving FMD syndrome [45].

Social

Many individuals with FMD have faced and struggled to cope with recent upheavals in their relationships, health or employment [6, 14, 30]. These could include events such as bereavement or other losses, divorce, infidelity or losing one's job. Again, the connection between life events and FMD is not straightforward: anxiety, altered arousal patterns and a diminished sense of agency may be intermediaries, but conclusive evidence is lacking. We explain to our patients that the nervous system is extraordinarily complex and that the environment, cognitive processes and emotions can affect how the body functions (or dysfunctions) and that conversely, feedback from the body and nervous system can influence how we feel and behave. We explain that as best we can understand, FMDs represent "glitches" or breakdowns in this multifaceted and complex system.

Perpetuating Factors for FMD

Perpetuating factors impede recovery and foster maintenance of functional neurological symptoms. These factors are an especially important area of focus for the clinician because they often represent accessible treatment targets.

Biological

As mentioned previously, chronic pain and chronic fatigue often precede evolution of FMD. Persistence of pain and fatigue, especially that of a debilitating nature often limits participation in motor retraining or psychotherapy treatment programs [15, 20, 46]. Comorbid medical conditions or deconditioning stemming from prolonged motor disuse/reliance on gait aids might pose similar barriers [47].

High baseline sympathetic arousal, whether stemming from untreated anxiety, sequalae of post-traumatic stress disorder, persistent pain or genetic predisposition often contributes to motor hyperactivity, bodily tension and direct perpetuation of functional neurological symptoms [22, 48, 49]. The role of motor learning is also important: our motor systems can learn and maintain complex and dysfunctional ways of operating (e.g. maintenance of functional tremor), just as they can learn to execute "normal" motor programs (e.g. riding a bike). For patients with FMD who have developed these abnormal motor habits, motor-retraining physiotherapy is often a helpful treatment option, provided pain and fatigue do not impede participation [50].

Psychological

Patients with FMD often endure a convoluted and difficult journey through the healthcare system. The average time to an accurate diagnosis is typically prolonged and the patient experience with clinicians is often one of invalidation and incomplete explanation of their symptoms [51]. This trying experience, coupled with the stigma associated with the generally unhelpful explanation of physical symptoms as entirely attributable to psychological factors, serves to further entrench maladaptive illness beliefs and creates barriers for diagnostic agreement and subsequent treatment.

Expectations of symptom progression and irreversibility, or lack of agreement with the diagnosis altogether are also likely to perpetuate functional movement symptoms [52]. Ongoing anxiety, self-consciousness about symptoms and fears of secondary injuries or falls tend to foster a pattern of behavioral avoidance and disengagement, which are themselves likely to activate more anticipatory anxiety, symptom exacerbations and subsequent avoidance, in a vicious-cycle fashion [53]. Because symptoms are often unusual and debilitating, they typically have a high threat value. Many patients are anxious about the meaning of symptoms and start to hyper-attend to their bodily sensations so that they can gauge whether action is needed. If clinicians are themselves uncertain of the symptom etiology, the patient's state of hypervigilance and functional neurological symptoms often exacerbate, again in a vicious-cycle pattern.

Locus of control is another important psychological factor to consider. Individuals with an internal locus of control have a greater sense of self-efficacy and ability to change their circumstances; those with an external locus of control are more inclined to formulate that external factors beyond their control play important roles in determining outcome [54, 55]. This is relevant given that while patients with FMD are not in any way "doing this to themselves", they play an active role in their own recovery in the context of rehabilitative and psychological guidance from the treatment team. This is in contrast to medications where the "agent of change" is a clear external factor.

Social

Perpetuating psychosocial factors are wide ranging and can include family dysfunction, interpersonal or work-related stressors, or pending litigation [46]. If, for example, much of the clinical encounter is spent discussing and completing disability related paperwork, less attention is being given to catalyzing treatment engagement and clinical improvement. Unconscious secondary gains in the form of newly met emotional needs may also be relevant [32]. Poor communication amongst health care providers can be problematic— even if an individual initially has diagnostic agreement, if other clinicians postulate alternative diagnoses or order unnecessary investigations at the patient's behest, this may compromise recovery. This is not to say that additional diagnoses cannot arise, or that new investigations are never merited, but it is important that clinicians are operating from an open and collaborative model that promotes cohesive care.

Integration: Creating a Cohesive Biopsychosocial Formulation

As noted earlier in this chapter, a formulation is more than a list of potentially relevant factors. It is a hypothesis that postulates how and why your patient developed a given illness. The formulation can help guide the development of a patient-centered treatment plan, but remember that it is a "work in process" effort. It is important for the patient to become aware of their own formulation during their participation in treatment rather than having a detailed formulation presented to them after only an initial visit. Such attempts to share an overly detailed formulation with a patient can "fall flat" in large part because the clinician has not had the sufficient time to understand the many nuances regarding the factors that are at play for a given patient.

For patients who suffer from FMD, we aim to generate an individualized and holistic understanding of the context in which the movement disorder developed, *potential* etiological contributions and identifiable treatment targets. As examples, let us return to our opening case vignettes for consideration.

Case Vignette 1: Mr. S

Though our history is still limited, we can postulate that Mr. S was predisposed to FMD by his early-life exposure to physical trauma and pattern of emotional-distancing that may have defensively developed in the context of an insecure attachment with his father. His irritable bowel syndrome is an additional risk factor.

Mr. S's unfortunate involvement in a motor vehicle accident is the most likely precipitant for his FMD and as his treatment evolves, we should explore this event further; it could be that the suddenness of the event set in motion a pattern of hyperarousal or hypervigilance or compromised his sense of control. Reflecting back on his history, we wonder whether his experience of childhood physical abuse dysregulated his autonomic arousal system, fostering a nervous system that is chronically on "high alert" for threat. His trust and ability to be emotionally vulnerable with others might be compromised— it may take some time to build rapport with him.

His chronic pain and fatigue are perpetuating factors, as are the patterns of self-consciousness and avoidance that are developing in response to his symptoms. Assess for muscle tension in his body; tension commonly arises from pain "guarding" and you are unlikely to make much headway

treating his functional myoclonus until it is reduced. Education regarding pain and FMD will be important and a graded exercise plan might be a good initial step. Exposure therapy might help to target his self-consciousness and avoidance. Over time, psychotherapy work to facilitate an increased capacity to tolerate and express difficult emotions would likely serve him well. See Fig. 3.2 for graphic depiction of the biopsychosocial formulation for this vignette.

Case Vignette 2: Mrs. V

Mrs. V, by virtue of being female, is more at risk for developing an FMD. Notably, she has no history of trauma that predisposes her to FMD, but does demonstrate longstanding patterns of perfectionism, over-achievement and excessive responsibility taking— personality traits more common in the FMD population. Exploring whether she tends to prioritize the needs of others over herself will likely be helpful; she may benefit from encouragement to introduce more self-care activities into her lifestyle.

Mrs. V's history of dysmenorrhea and migraine headaches may have been harbingers for her later FMD. Her anxious predisposition also renders her vulnerable. Of note, it is com-

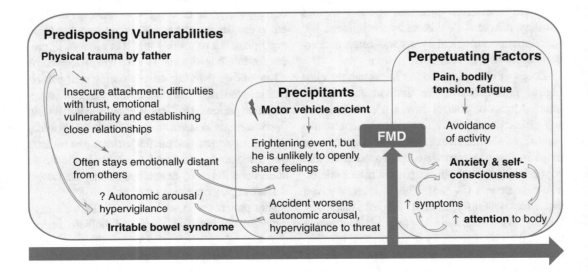

Fig. 3.2 Example of biopsychosocial formulation for Mr. S. FMD indicates functional movement disorder

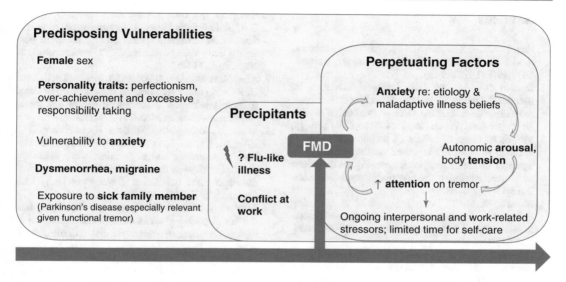

Fig. 3.3 Example of biopsychosocial formulation for Mrs. V. FMD indicates functional movement disorder

mon for patients with FMD to have difficulty identifying and labeling the psychological aspects of anxiety; look for bodily signs and work with those first.

Precipitants for Mrs. V's FMD are less obvious than with Mr. S. Her flu-like illness many have played a contributing role. We speculate that the onset of her tremor, perhaps a normal physiological event in the beginning, triggered a cascade of anxiety, somatic hypervigilance and worsening abnormal movements as she remembered her grandfather's Parkinson's disease and feared she was developing the same. This pattern of anxiety and hypervigilance manifests as autonomic hyperarousal and bodily tension, which likely serve to perpetuate her functional tremor. The stress of managing discord at work and the limited support she has when her husband is away may also be relevant perpetuating factors. We would potentially start with education regarding FMD and highlight the importance of brain, body and mind connections. We could provide her with some introductory breathing and muscle relaxation exercises to target autonomic hyperarousal. Motor-retraining strategies for her tremor might be helpful, as could CBT and/or pharmacotherapy for her anxiety, if she was open to this. Over time, exploring her behavioral patterns, emotional needs and defenses might provide etiological clues and

additional treatment targets for her FMD. See Fig. 3.3 for graphic depiction of the biopsychosocial formulation for this vignette.

Summary
1. Formulation is more than a collection of data points— it is the process of generating an individualized *hypothesis* about how and why your patient developed FMD.
2. A rich formulation requires a nuanced intake assessment, best accomplished by an open-ended qualitative interview.
3. The biopsychosocial model is a useful framework for ascertaining a holistic understanding of your patient and their FMD symptoms.
4. One size does not fit all in clinical formulations for patients with FMD. FMD is best understood in the context of predisposing, precipitating and perpetuating factors that are specific to a given patient.
5. A well-constructed biopsychosocial formulation is an important step in identifying potential patient-centered treatment targets.

References

1. Engel GL. The need for a new medical model: a challenge for biomedicine. Science. 1977;196(4286):129–36.
2. Epstein SA, Maurer CW, LaFaver K, Ameli R, Sinclair S, Hallett M. Insights into chronic functional movement disorders: the value of qualitative psychiatric interviews. Psychosomatics. 2016;57(6):566–75.
3. McKee K, Glass S, Adams C, Stephen CD, King F, Parlman K, et al. The inpatient assessment and management of motor functional neurological disorders: an interdisciplinary perspective. Psychosomatics. 2018;59(4):358–68.
4. Stone J, Warlow C, Deary I, Sharpe M. Predisposing risk factors for functional limb weakness: a case-control study. J Neuropsychiatry Clin Neurosci. 2020;32(1):50–7.
5. Roelofs K, Pasman J. Stress, childhood trauma, and cognitive functions in functional neurologic disorders. In: Handbook of clinical neurology. Elsevier; 2016. p. 139–55.
6. Ludwig L, Pasman JA, Nicholson T, Aybek S, David AS, Tuck S, et al. Stressful life events and maltreatment in conversion (functional neurological) disorder: systematic review and meta-analysis of case-control studies. Lancet Psychiatry. 2018;5(4):307–20.
7. American Psychiatric Association Diagnostic and statistical manual of mental disorders (DSM-5®). American Psychiatric Pub; 2013. 1520 p
8. Cabaniss DL, Moga DE, Oquendo MA. Rethinking the biopsychosocial formulation. Lancet Psychiatry. 2015;2(7):579–81.
9. Carson A, Lehn A. Epidemiology. In: Handbook of clinical neurology. Elsevier; 2016. p. 47–60.
10. Cubo E, Hinson VK, Goetz CG, Garcia Ruiz P, Garcia de Yebenes J, Marti MJ, et al. Transcultural comparison of psychogenic movement disorders. Mov Disord. 2005;20(10):1343–5.
11. Stone J, Carson A, Duncan R, Roberts R, Coleman R, Warlow C, et al. Which neurological diseases are most likely to be associated with "symptoms unexplained by organic disease". J Neurol. 2012;259(1):33–8.
12. Hallett M. Patients with Parkinson disease are prone to functional neurological disorders. J Neurol Neurosurg Psychiatry. 2018;89(6):557.
13. Elliott JO, Charyton C. Biopsychosocial predictors of psychogenic non-epileptic seizures. Epilepsy Res. 2014;108(9):1543–53.
14. Reuber M, Howlett S, Khan A, Grünewald RA. Non-epileptic seizures and other functional neurological symptoms: predisposing, precipitating, and perpetuating factors. Psychosomatics. 2007;48(3):230–8.
15. Carson A, Stone J, Hibberd C, Murray G, Duncan R, Coleman R, et al. Disability, distress and unemployment in neurology outpatients with symptoms "unexplained by organic disease". J Neurol Neurosurg Psychiatry. 2011;82(7):810–3.
16. Ranford J, MacLean J, Alluri PR, Comeau O, Godena E, Curt LaFrance W, et al. Sensory processing difficulties in functional neurological disorder: a possible predisposing vulnerability? Psychosomatics. 2020;61(4):343–52.
17. Afari N, Ahumada SM, Wright LJ, Mostoufi S, Golnari G, Reis V, et al. Psychological trauma and functional somatic syndromes: a systematic review and meta-analysis. Psychosom Med. 2014;76(1):2–11.
18. Matin N, Young SS, Williams B, LaFrance WC, King JN, Caplan D, et al. Neuropsychiatric associations with gender, illness duration, work disability, and motor subtype in a U.S. functional neurological disorders clinic population. J Neuropsychiatry Clin Neurosci. 2017;29(4):375–82.
19. Teodoro T, Edwards MJ, Isaacs JD. A unifying theory for cognitive abnormalities in functional neurological disorders, fibromyalgia and chronic fatigue syndrome: systematic review. J Neurol Neurosurg Psychiatry. 2018;89(12):1308–19.
20. Gelauff JM, Kingma EM, Kalkman JS, Bezemer R, van Engelen BGM, Stone J, et al. Fatigue, not self-rated motor symptom severity, affects quality of life in functional motor disorders. J Neurol. 2018;265(8):1803–9.
21. Věchetová G, Slovák M, Kemlink D, Hanzlíková Z, Dušek P, Nikolai T, et al. The impact of non-motor symptoms on the health-related quality of life in patients with functional movement disorders. J Psychosom Res. 2018;115:32–7.
22. Bakvis P, Roelofs K, Kuyk J, Edelbroek PM, Swinkels WAM, Spinhoven P. Trauma, stress, and preconscious threat processing in patients with psychogenic nonepileptic seizures. Epilepsia. 2009;50(5):1001–11.
23. Brown RJ, Bouska JF, Frow A, Kirkby A, Baker GA, Kemp S, et al. Emotional dysregulation, alexithymia, and attachment in psychogenic nonepileptic seizures. Epilepsy Behav. 2013;29(1):178–83.
24. Jalilianhasanpour R, Ospina JP, Williams B, Mello J, MacLean J, Ranford J, et al. Secure attachment and depression predict 6-month outcome in motor functional neurological disorders: a prospective pilot study. Psychosomatics. 2019;60(4):365–75.
25. Williams B, Ospina JP, Jalilianhasanpour R, Fricchione GL, Perez DL. Fearful attachment linked to childhood abuse, alexithymia, and depression in motor functional neurological disorders. J Neuropsychiatry Clin Neurosci. 2019;31(1):65–9.
26. Ekanayake V, Kranick S, LaFaver K, Naz A, Frank Webb A, LaFrance WC, et al. Personality traits in psychogenic nonepileptic seizures (PNES) and psychogenic movement disorder (PMD): neuroticism and perfectionism. J Psychosom Res. 2017;97:23–9.
27. Jalilianhasanpour R, Williams B, Gilman I, Burke MJ, Glass S, Fricchione GL, et al. Resilience linked to personality dimensions, alexithymia and affective symptoms in motor functional neurological disorders. J Psychosom Res. 2018;107:55–61.

28. Reuber M. Multidimensional assessment of personality in patients with psychogenic non-epileptic seizures. J Neurol Neurosurg Psychiatry. 2004;75(5):743–8.
29. Nicholson TR, Aybek S, Craig T, Harris T, Wojcik W, David AS, et al. Life events and escape in conversion disorder. Psychol Med. 2016;46(12):2617–26.
30. Levita L, Mayberry E, Mehmood A, Reuber M. Evaluation of LiNES: a new measure of trauma, negative affect, and relationship insecurity over the life span in persons with FND. J Neuropsychiatry Clin Neurosci. 2020;32(1):43–9.
31. Reuber M. Trauma, traumatisation, and functional neurological symptom disorder—what are the links? Lancet Psychiatry. 2018;5(4):288–9.
32. Carson A, Ludwig L, Welch K. Psychologic theories in functional neurologic disorders. In: Handbook of clinical neurology. Elsevier; 2016. p. 105–20.
33. Breuer J, Freud S. Studies on Hysteria. In: Basic books; 2009. 378 p.
34. Association AP. Diagnostic and statistical manual of mental disorders, 4th edition, text revision (DSM-IV-TR). American Psychiatric Association; 2000. 915 p.
35. Diez I, Larson AG, Nakhate V, Dunn EC, Fricchione GL, Nicholson TR, et al. Early-life trauma endophenotypes and brain circuit–gene expression relationships in functional neurological (conversion) disorder. Mol Psychiatry. 2021;26(8):817–28.
36. Teicher MH, Samson JA, Anderson CM, Ohashi K. The effects of childhood maltreatment on brain structure, function and connectivity. Nat Rev Neurosci. 2016;17(10):652–66.
37. Pareés I, Kojovic M, Pires C, Rubio-Agusti I, Saifee TA, Sadnicka A, et al. Physical precipitating factors in functional movement disorders. J Neurol Sci. 2014;338(1–2):174–7.
38. Stone J, Carson A, Aditya H, Prescott R, Zaubi M, Warlow C, et al. The role of physical injury in motor and sensory conversion symptoms: a systematic and narrative review. J Psychosom Res. 2009;66(5):383–90.
39. Schrag A, Trimble M, Quinn N, Bhatia K. The syndrome of fixed dystonia: an evaluation of 103 patients. Brain. 2004;127(10):2360–72.
40. Stone J, Warlow C, Sharpe M. Functional weakness: clues to mechanism from the nature of onset. J Neurol Neurosurg Psychiatry. 2012;83(1):67–9.
41. Goldstein LH. Ictal symptoms of anxiety, avoidance behaviour, and dissociation in patients with dissociative seizures. J Neurol Neurosurg Psychiatry. 2006;77(5):616–21.
42. Edwards MJ, Adams RA, Brown H, Parees I, Friston KJ. A Bayesian account of "hysteria". Brain. 2012;135(11):3495–512.
43. Stone J, Warlow C, Sharpe M. The symptom of functional weakness: a controlled study of 107 patients. Brain. 2010;133(5):1537–51.
44. Dimaro LV, Dawson DL, Roberts NA, Brown I, Moghaddam NG, Reuber M. Anxiety and avoidance in psychogenic nonepileptic seizures: the role of implicit and explicit anxiety. Epilepsy Behav. 2014;33:77–86.
45. Popkirov S, Carson AJ, Stone J. Scared or scarred: could 'dissociogenic' lesions predispose to non-epileptic seizures after head trauma? Seizure. 2018;58:127–32.
46. Gelauff J, Stone J, Edwards M, Carson A. The prognosis of functional (psychogenic) motor symptoms: a systematic review. J Neurol Neurosurg Psychiatry. 2014;85(2):220–6.
47. Nielsen G, Stone J, Edwards MJ. Physiotherapy for functional (psychogenic) motor symptoms: a systematic review. J Psychosom Res. 2013;75(2):93–102.
48. Roelofs K, Spinhoven P. Trauma and medically unexplained symptoms. Clin Psychol Rev. 2007;27(7):798–820.
49. Perez DL, Matin N, Barsky A, Costumero-Ramos V, Makaretz SJ, Young SS, et al. Cingulo-insular structural alterations associated with psychogenic symptoms, childhood abuse and PTSD in functional neurological disorders. J Neurol Neurosurg Psychiatry. 2017;88(6):491–7.
50. Nielsen G, Ricciardi L, Demartini B, Hunter R, Joyce E, Edwards MJ. Outcomes of a 5-day physiotherapy programme for functional (psychogenic) motor disorders. J Neurol. 2015;262(3):674–81.
51. Lidstone SC, MacGillivray L, Lang AE. Integrated therapy for functional movement disorders: time for a change. Mov Disord Clin Pract. 2020;7(2):169–74.
52. Sharpe M, Stone J, Hibberd C, Warlow C, Duncan R, Coleman R, et al. Neurology out-patients with symptoms unexplained by disease: illness beliefs and financial benefits predict 1-year outcome. Psychol Med. 2010;40(4):689–98.
53. Bakvis P, Spinhoven P, Zitman FG, Roelofs K. Automatic avoidance tendencies in patients with psychogenic non epileptic seizures. Seizure. 2011;20(8):628–34.
54. Stone J, Binzer M, Sharpe M. Illness beliefs and locus of control. J Psychosom Res. 2004;57(6):541–7.
55. Vizcarra JA, Hacker S, Lopez-Castellanos R, Ryes L, Laub HN, Marsili L, et al. Internal versus external frame of reference in functional movement disorders. J Neuropsychiatry Clin Neurosci. 2020;32(1):67–72.

Integrating Neurologic and Psychiatric Perspectives in Functional Movement Disorder

Jordan R. Anderson, David L. Perez, and Bruce H. Price

Clinical Vignette

A 17-year-old high school senior was involved in an accident during a soccer game when another player stepped on her right foot. She was medically cleared in Urgent Care with only a superficial laceration and no fractures, but over the next several weeks her foot pain continued despite wound healing. She also experienced inward turning of her foot, especially in the evenings. In the subsequent months, she underwent an extensive evaluation by her primary care physician and a general neurologist. Her examination showed, in addition to intermittent posturing of her right foot and pain to light touch, collapsing/ give-way weakness on right foot dorsiflexion. Diagnostic studies were normal including magnetic resonance imaging (MRI) of her brain, lumbar spine, and distal leg where the initial injury had occurred. Electromyogram, nerve conduction studies and skin biopsy for possible small

fiber neuropathy were also normal. She was diagnosed with dystonia and complex regional pain syndrome. Over several months, her abnormal right leg posture spread to involve a similar dystonia of her left leg with increasing ambulation difficulties. She was evaluated by a movement disorders specialist who noted variability and distractibility in her foot postures, including normal gait when concurrently performing serial 7 subtractions. She was diagnosed with a functional movement disorder (FMD) and referred to psychiatry with the explanation that the problem was "stress-related" and needed to be addressed by mental health professionals. No neurologic follow-up was offered.

The patient and her parents were confused by the diagnosis and the psychiatric referral, as she had no prior mental health history. While awaiting the psychiatric evaluation, her parents took her to a chiropractor and a naturopathic specialist as suggested by a neighbor. She received only mild benefit from musculoskeletal manipulations and naturopathic supplements prescribed. At her psychiatric consultation (which the patient and family almost cancelled), she was diagnosed with a generalized anxiety disorder and obsessive-compulsive personality disorder. Her interview revealed that the patient had previously excelled scholastically and at sports, with several years of increased home stress related to in her parents' marital difficulties. She was prescribed an antidepressant, which she took inconsistently for 2

J. R. Anderson (✉)
Psychiatry and Neurology, Oregon Health and Science University, Unity Center for Behavioral Health, Portland, OR, USA
e-mail: andejord@ohsu.edu

D. L. Perez
Departments of Neurology and Psychiatry, Massachusetts General Hospital, Harvard Medical School, Boston, MA, USA

B. H. Price
Neurology, McLean Hospital and Massachusetts General Hospital, Harvard Medical School, Belmont, MA, USA

© Springer Nature Switzerland AG 2022
K. LaFaver et al. (eds.), *Functional Movement Disorder*, Current Clinical Neurology,
https://doi.org/10.1007/978-3-030-86495-8_4

months but stopped due to lack of benefit. Psychotherapy was also recommended, but the patient had difficulty getting a new patient appointment given the complexity of her physical symptoms. The psychiatrist, who had not encountered a similar case before, was also perplexed by the severity of the patient's physical symptoms. Given the absence of a trauma history, he wondered whether the diagnosis she had received was incorrect.

As symptoms did not improve, the patient and her parents became increasingly frustrated. Her pediatrician suggested referral for a second opinion to a center with a FMD clinic. As part of the assessment, a detailed neuropsychiatric evaluation was performed and her FMD diagnosis based on examination features was confirmed. Time was spent discussing the diagnosis with the patient and her parents, including noting that the condition was common, real, brain-based, and potentially treatable. The analogy that the patient had more of a "software" rather than a hardware problem was emphasized. When discussing treatment options, it was mentioned that physical treatments (physical and occupational therapy), as well as talk therapy (psychotherapy), are generally helpful ways of "updating the software" and allowing normal movements to re-emerge. It was also discussed that it is possible that at times the "software crashes" because of worries and stressful life factors, and that these possibilities could be explored more in psychotherapy. She and her parents were engaged, and accepted referrals to physical therapy, occupational therapy and a psychotherapist affiliated with the center.

In physical and occupational therapy, the patient learned that distraction techniques were helpful in normalizing her foot posture, and she was empowered to identify ways to focus on normal movements. When experiencing setbacks, she learned to tolerate distress and use breathing techniques to help control muscle tension. In cognitive behavioral therapy, she explored connections between her physical symptoms, thoughts, behaviors, emotions and other life factors. In particular, she discussed that she was struggling to stay in all honors classes prior to getting sick and that she was working towards obtaining a college scholarship for soccer given her parents' financial difficulties. Patterns of "all-or-none" behaviors and emotional avoidance were observed, whereby she would push herself for several days followed by periods of crashing with increased physical symptoms. She increasingly recognized her triggers and received guidance in relaxation and grounding techniques. Over the next 6 months, she regained normal walking and started to practice with her soccer team again. She did have brief relapses that she was able to manage on her own using rsraction techniques. She continued to follow-up with her neuropsychiatrist regularly.

The Origins of the Divide: Shifting Foundations, Dualism and Stigma

In modern medicine, specialty care is commonly delivered by professionals trained in the medical or surgical treatment of a single organ system. The culture and standard of care within each medical subspecialty have been crafted and honed over decades of focused study and the accumulation of knowledge about its organ system. These cultures and standards, of course, develop uniquely in this way. Subspecialty medicine has advantages, but can create narrowness that clinicians should be mindful of. In the care of complex conditions that affect multiple different organs, subspecialties are generally able to work separately, in parallel, toward recovery and health for the patient. The subspecialties of neurology and psychiatry are a clear exception, as there are two disciplines for the same organ system: the brain (See Fig. 4.1). Notably, neurology and psychiatry each have their own culture and standard of care, and a unique perspective on the brain and its maladies. For diagnoses that challenge this artificial separation, including FMD, the fragmentation of care causes practical challenges that can impede patient engagement and negatively impact recovery.

Historically, neurology and psychiatry had a greater level of integration, and we recommend as detailed later in this chapter that going "back to the future" with updates to revive an integrated neuropsychiatric viewpoint is an approach that can help move the FMD field forward. To provide some historical context, neurology and psychiatry share common foundations in the works of important figures such as Jean-Martin Charcot, Sigmund Freud (a neurologist that studied under Charcot) and Emil Kraepelin, a psychiatrist and neuropathologist regarded as the founder of modern psychiatry [1]. Arnold Pick (a psychiatrist) and Alois Alzheimer (a psychiatrist and neuropathologist) were also early visionaries whose work defined certain neurologic conditions [2, 3]. However, these subspecialties diverged from one another with limited cross training by the mid twentieth century. The reasons for this divergence are complex, but exemplified by conditions in which the assumed etiology was greatly influenced by the presence or absence of objective findings. As discussed by Joseph Martin in his 2002 seminal article, fundamental observations of Alzheimer's were made in a psychiatric setting, though "once seen under a microscope… Alzheimer's disease was

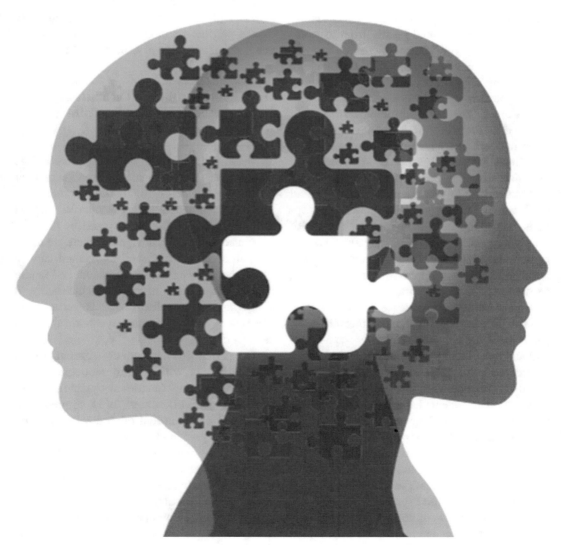

Fig. 4.1 Neurology and psychiatry depicted as two distinct subspecialties that both care for the same organ system: the brain. (From Perez et al. Neurology: Clinical Practice 2018 with permission)

assigned to the neurological category of disease" [2]. By contrast, in Tourette syndrome, "the absence of evidence of brain pathology resulted in vacillation between neurological and psychiatric explanations and persistent controversy about the nature of the illness" [2]. This focus on objective data grew stronger with the development of magnetic resonance imaging (MRI), the electroencephalogram and cerebrospinal fluid analyses, serving to "reinforce an unfortunate and artificial mind/brain dichotomy" [1]. If there existed objective data to demonstrate anatomic (etiologic) pathology, it was more likely to be under the purview of neurology. This "lesion-based" approach differed greatly from psychiatry that dealt in "gray" areas centered on some of the more complex aspects of brain (dys)function. In psychiatric conditions, disturbances in emotion regulation, behavioral control, perception, higher-order cognitive abilities and insight emerged as the result of distributed (dynamic) brain network alterations, which is more complex than traditional lesional neurology [4]. Psychiatrists do not generally have robust objective biomarkers to rely upon, but rather careful observations and subjective symptom descriptions. Thus, the false dichotomy of "organic" (implying neurological origins) versus "psychogenic" (implying psychiatric origins) was born — akin to the implausible and confusing separation of brain and mind.

An unfortunate consequence of this Cartesian dualism is the stigmatization of mental illness [5]. If there was not a clear link between a symptom and focal brain pathology, it may have been considered colloquially "all in your head" [6]. The divergence between neurology and psychiatry was further cemented after World War II when the *Archives of Neurology and Psychiatry*, originally founded in 1918, separated into two journals. In 1948, the American Academy of Neurology was founded, and with it came its own clinical practice, research, and culture that has remained separate from Psychiatry [2].

This separation is confusing (and deleterious) for the approach needed in many neuropsychiatric disorders. Such disorders impact sensorimotor functioning, behavior, emotion regulation, perception, higher-order cognition, awareness, and other faculties that require an integration of neurologic and psychiatric perspectives for patient-centered diagnostic assessments and treatments. Conditions in the borderlands between neurology and psychiatry include neurodegenerative disorders, traumatic brain injury, neurodevelopmental disorders, movement disorders, epilepsy, and many others [7–19]. FMD and other functional neurological disorder subtypes are core neuropsychiatric conditions directly at the intersection of neurology and psychiatry [20]. FMD presents with physical symptoms, yet etiological and treatment approaches appropriately rely in part on the biopsychosocial formulation that is foundational to psychiatry [21, 22].

Operationalizing the Difficulties Across Neurology and Psychiatry

FMD is a quintessential example of the need for an integrated, interdisciplinary approach. The approach to FMD, which has taken shape over the last few decades, highlights several shortcomings of neurologists and psychiatrists relying solely on traditional clinical practices [23]. As illustrated in the clinical vignette, there are many difficulties that ensue with fragmented care in FMD, mostly notably that the patient and family receive inconsistent messages. Additionally, it highlights the complexity that is common to these cases, and how a neuropsychiatric approach can be effective.

The patient in our vignette suffered from a physical injury with painful sequelae shortly before developing functional dystonia, weakness and gait difficulties. It is common for functional dystonia and other FMD presentations to be preceded by physical injury [24]. However, the presence of such a physical event near the onset of symptoms can potentially undermine the inherent complexity of FMD, as it can be misattributed as a primary etiology by patients, families, and providers alike. This has the potential to create confusion around the diagnosis or delay the diagnosis while an extensive medical workup is being pursued.

Additionally, FMD can coexist with other neurologic conditions [25–27], and making proper distinctions amongst comorbid conditions can also be time consuming, adding to the neurological challenges. Furthermore, neurologists have historically expressed other difficulties when assessing and managing patients with FMD, and may feel that in the absence of an obvious neurological lesion and with a treatment approach emphasizing psychotherapy, this condition is not their problem to solve [23, 28]. Part of the issue here is that neurologists are not generally trained in the use of the biopsychosocial model (the social and psychological determinants of health), which is foundational to clinical formulation and longitudinal care in FMD. This dilemma can leave the neurologist feeling frustrated and ill equipped, particularly given how common FMD is in clinical practice [29]. Furthermore, neurologists' lack of training in psychotherapy can make it difficult for them to answer the question "how is talk therapy going to help me move my leg and walk better?" [30].

While met with distinct challenges, psychiatrists and allied mental health professionals have their own difficulties in guiding the assessment and management of FMD. The neurological examination with "rule in" physical signs are the basis for diagnosing FMD, which places psychiatrists with less neurological training at a disadvantage. Additionally, patients with a FMD can report new neurological symptoms over the course of treatment, and the ability to assess those symptoms efficiently is critical to ensuring that treatment moves forward. Conceptual models for FMD have also moved beyond a singular focus on Freudian conversion disorder, and reliance on this framework alone can be detrimental to the therapeutic alliance. Notably, many well-trained psychotherapists (including psychologists and social workers) do not have prior experience working with FMD populations. This is a notable training gap, yet, many of the modalities of skills-based psychotherapy treatment (e.g., cognitive behavioral therapy) showing promise in treating FMD rely on principles that are well known to psychotherapists. The important adjustment is that while physical symptoms are front and center in clinical discussions, guiding the patient in understanding how physical symptoms interact with potentially unhelpful cognitive, behavioral, and affective responses is essential [31]. Lastly, illness beliefs are another consideration that offer challenges to psychotherapy. It is quite common for patients with FMD early in their treatment engagement to believe that their symptoms are a mystery never to be solved, or to reject psychological mechanisms when initially proposed to them [32, 33]. This may lead to patients getting lost to follow-up, not attending their psychotherapy appointments, or seeking multiple re-evaluations.

The nuanced perspective needed to contextualize etiological factors also offers unique challenges. The etiological role of adverse life experiences, including childhood maltreatment, is at the origins of early conceptual frameworks for FMD as detailed by Freud, Briquet and Janet among others [34]. High rates of childhood abuse are a well-documented risk factor for FMD, with several studies detailing associations between increased functional neurological symptom severity and the magnitude of previously experienced adverse life events [15, 35]. Recent neuroimaging studies are also working towards bridging etiological factors and the neural mechanisms underlying FMD [36, 37]. Despite the above evidence, not all patients with a FMD report childhood maltreatment and/or other traumatic experiences [38]. This suggests that there is a "balancing act" that is needed, recognizing the importance of psychiatric and psychosocial factors for some patients as predisposing vulnerabilities, acute precipitants and perpetuating factors [39]. For others, physical factors such as injury and pain (generally in combination with more subtle psychological factors) play important roles in precipitating and perpetuating a FMD [40]. Additionally, those without prominent trauma histories may have other psychiatric/psychological factors that are relevant to their development of an FMD, such as limited stress coping, alexithymia and personality traits [41, 42].

Beyond the clinical assessment, there are challenges in guiding the longitudinal management of patients with a FMD. Some neurologists may be reluctant to longitudinally follow FMD patients, and the neurological complexity of the patients' presentations can at times have psychiatrists and psychotherapists question the diagnosis [43]. There is also the issue of which provider is overall managing the direction of care [23]. For the vast majority of neurological conditions, neurologists take the lead in both diagnosing and guiding treatments. An approach whereby the neurologist makes the diagnosis and the psychiatrist and/or psychotherapist guides treatment generally does not prove as effective as one would like due to heightened fragmentation of care [44]. In the following section, we discuss a way forward, one that encourages the cultivation of shared (partially overlapping) expertise and close interdisciplinary collaborations across the clinical neurosciences.

The Path Forward: "Back to the Future" Using an Integrated Neuropsychiatric Perspective

The notion that psychiatric disorders are disorders of the mind while neurological disorders are disorders of the brain is outdated and problematic for patient care. Rather, a more helpful perspective is that psychiatric and neurologic conditions are both disorders of mind *and* brain. An early proponent of this perspective was Stanley Cobb. He was trained in Neurology, Psychiatry and Neuropathology, became Chief of Neurology at Boston City Hospital in 1925, and founded the Psychiatry department at the Massachusetts General Hospital in 1934. Troubled by the separation of mind and body, he stated,

> "I solve the mind-body problem by stating that there is no such problem. There are, of course, plenty of problems concerning the "mind", and the "body", and all intermediate levels of integration of the nervous system. What I wish to emphasize is that there is no problem of 'mind' versus 'body,' because biologically no such dichotomy can be made. The dichotomy is an artifact; there is no

truth in it, and the discussion has no place in science in 1943" [45].

Cobb went on to author a textbook in which he discussed the "mind-body" problem further, pointing to the separation of two entities as arbitrary when they can be better understood on a continuum. He used the examples of agnosia, apraxia and aphasia along with their associated lesions and anatomical connections to "form the transition, as it were, between the well understood lower mechanism for sensation and locomotion, and the higher intellectual function. Their zone is the no-man's-land where psychology and neurology meet" [46].

More recently, the "mind-body" or "brain-mind-body" connection has been demonstrated in studies on neuroplasticity characterizing the effects of environmental and social influences on the brain [47, 48]. Brain – behavior relationships are no longer thought of as unidirectional, but rather bidirectional, with life experiences interacting actively with a plastic brain [49]. Using this integrated and interdisciplinary perspective can broaden the understanding and treatment of FMD and many other conditions at the intersection of neurology and psychiatry. Of relevance, anxiety, depression and obsessive-compulsive disorder are common in "classic" movement disorders such as Parkinson's disease, Huntington's disease and Tourette syndrome [3]. Figure 4.2 illustrates the range of specialties across the clinical neurosciences and rehabilitation fields that can and should come together to holistically assess and manage patients with FMD and related functional neurological disorder subtypes [20].

To promote fundamental shifts toward a more integrated approach across the clinical neurosciences, important educational and cultural changes are needed at the medical school, residency, fellowship training, and departmental levels. A JAMA 2020 publication summarized the need to move "from a lesion-based model (s) towards a network based one (s), from a uni-directional toward a bi-directional framework of interactions, from exclusive reliance on categorical diagnoses towards trans-diagnostic dimensional perspectives, from silo-based toward interdisci-

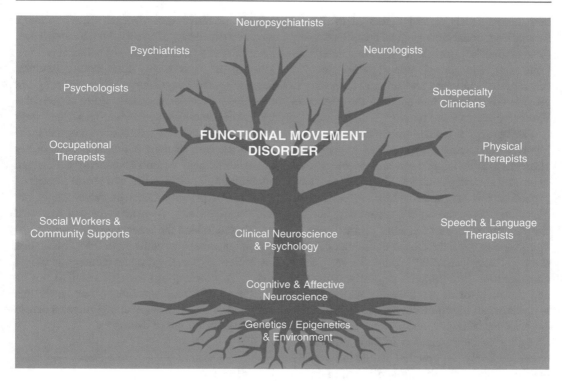

Fig. 4.2 The interdisciplinary and multidisciplinary tree of clinical neuroscience and allied rehabilitation specialties highlights the need for patient-centered assessments and management in functional movement disorder

plinary approaches, and from biologically-isolated methodologies towards integration of neuroscience with psychosocial and cultural factors" [50]. Additionally, traditional "lesion localization" that is the hallmark of neurological training is being complemented by "network lesion mapping" that incorporates principles of network science [51]. Practically, this includes neurologists-in-training receiving more teaching in performing psychiatric and social history screenings, and for psychiatrists-in-training to receive more instruction in neurological examination and the use of adjunctive diagnostic tests. At the fellowship training level, education and research pursuits within a neuropsychiatric framework should be encouraged throughout neurology and psychiatry subspecialities, including movement disorders, epilepsy, behavioral neurology – neuropsychiatry and consultation-liaison (medical) psychiatry. As one example, it is now well-recognized that non-motor features of Parkinson's disease, including cognitive,

affective and perceptual symptoms, are important to assess and manage within subspecialty movement disorder clinics. Now, movement disorder fellowship training programs are increasingly incorporating neuropsychiatric elements into standard training experiences. It is precisely an expansion of this effort that is needed for patients with a FMD. An alternative training opportunity in the United States is the Behavioral Neurology – Neuropsychiatry fellowship [3]. Similar opportunities are available internationally, for example, educational opportunities through the British Neuropsychiatry Association. This allows a pathway for both neurologists and psychiatrists to train together and develop shared expertise across the clinical neurosciences, while also working towards strengthening areas of relative weakness for each discipline. Dual training in both neurology and psychiatry is also an option, however, such training programs are rare and generally best suited for trainees that have a clear, well-established desire to work at the intersection of both fields. Lastly, a major goal of the newly formed Functional Neurological Disorder Society (www.fndsociety.org) is to promote collaborations and educational opportunities for the full range of clinicians and scientists working to provide clinical care and advance the science of FMD and related conditions.

Facilitating a neuropsychiatric perspective involves enhancing education to improve the clinician's knowledge base and comfort level regarding certain principles. For instance, "neurophobia" has become a subject of concern in psychiatry given the brain's complexity and the challenging nature of learning clinical neurology [52–54]. As Schildkrout et al. stated, however, "neuroscientific knowledge adds consideration of a patient's cognitive substrate and the focal or network brain localization of symptoms, all of which contribute to subjective experience, behavior, and mental status" [52]. Learning to incorporate a bedside neurologic exam routinely in practice would also assist psychiatrists in identifying additional manifestations of what are otherwise considered psychiatric disorders. Conversely, incorporating a mental status examination during a patient encounter can provide an enriched perspective for a neurologist treating complex neurobehavioral conditions. There is also a need for neurologists to develop a renewed appreciation of the importance of the psychosocial history and consider the biopsychosocial formulation to optimize treatment planning and outcomes for patients [49]. These perspectives are summarized eloquently by Schildkrout and colleagues, as a clinician may ask "What person has this brain? How does this brain make this person unique? How does this brain make this disorder unique? What treatment will help this disorder in this person with this brain?" [52].

To bring the discussion back to the clinical vignette, it is important to recognize that the patient's overall improvement was not reliant upon being evaluated by a "neuropsychiatrist." In fact, the patient's care could have been advanced at earlier stages had the general neu-

rologist or movement disorder specialist taken greater ownership of the patient's care. Thus, the clinician's training path—whether it is a fellowship in movement disorders, behavioral neurology-neuropsychiatry, dual training in neurology-psychiatry, or neurology or psychiatry alone—matters somewhat less than their dedication to a shared interdisciplinary perspective in the care of their patients. It is precisely those clinicians, neurologists with a nuanced appreciation of psychiatric and social aspects of care and/or psychiatrists who have sought out additional training in neurology that are well positioned to lead the assessment and longitudinal management patients with FMD. Notably, we believe that cultivating an element of shared (partially overlapping) expertise should not be limited to FMD subspecialists, but rather this approach is likely to serve clinicians well across a range of brain-based disorders.

Conclusion

The divide between neurologic and psychiatric perspectives was, in some ways, a natural consequence of the era during which the specialties were born. What was technologically available at that time in medical research greatly impacted disease conceptualization. This was followed by the arbitrary separation and eventual stigmatization of psychiatric conditions that influenced the medical community as well as society at large. Such deep-rooted and widespread bias does not benefit the patients we care for, and this separation can be hard to overcome. We hope that readers will use information in this chapter and throughout this case-based textbook to feel empowered in working at this exciting clinical neuroscience intersection bridging brain, mind and body. Our hope is to engage forward-thinking neurologists, psychiatrists, psychologists, allied mental health professionals and rehabilitation specialists to work together with a unified message in the care of those diagnosed with FMD. We are confident that such a collaboration, bringing together overlapping expertise and mutual respect across disciplines, will greatly benefit our fields and the patients we care for.

Summary
- The origins of neurology and psychiatry are closely intertwined, with many early leaders in both fields identifying as neuropsychiatrists.
- In the mid twentieth century, the disciplines of neurology and psychiatry diverged, a separation that has not served well many patient populations at the intersection of both fields.
- An educational culture of shared (partially overlapping) expertise, empowering neurologists to develop greater expertise in psychiatric and social history interviews, while energizing psychiatrists to become more proficient in performing and interpreting neurological examinations and tests, will advance the care of many neuropsychiatric populations including FMD.
- To catalyze clinical integration, interdisciplinary team-based approaches involve respecting and learning from the diverse and nuanced perspectives that clinicians across the clinical neurosciences bring to patient care.
- One helpful way of framing FMD is that this condition lies at the intersection of neurology and psychiatry, a statement that is synonymous with describing FMD as a neuropsychiatric disorder.

References

1. Price BH, Adams RD, Coyle JT. Neurology and psychiatry: closing the great divide. Neurology. 2000;54(1):8–14.
2. Martin JB. The integration of neurology, psychiatry, and neuroscience in the 21st century. Am J Psychiatry. 2002;159(5):695–704.
3. Arciniegas DB, Kaufer DI, Joint Advisory Committee on Subspecialty Certification of the American Neuropsychiatric Association and The Society for Behavioral and Cognitive Neurology. Core curriculum for training in behavioral neurology and neuropsychiatry. J Neuropsychiatry Clin Neurosci. 2006;18(1):6–13.
4. Torous J, Stern AP, Padmanabhan JL, Keshavan MS, Perez DL. A proposed solution to integrating cognitive-affective neuroscience and neuropsychiatry in psychiatry residency training: the time is now. Asian J Psychiatr. 2015;17:116–21.
5. Yudofsky SC, Hales RE. Neuropsychiatry: back to the future. J Nerv Ment Dis. 2012;200(3):193–6.
6. Burke MJ. "It's all in your head"-medicine's silent epidemic. JAMA Neurol. 2019;76(12):1417–8.
7. Galts CPC, Bettio LEB, Jewett DC, Yang CC, Brocardo PS, Rodrigues ALS, et al. Depression in neurodegenerative diseases: common mechanisms and current treatment options. Neurosci Biobehav Rev. 2019;102:56–84.
8. Leroi I, O'Hearn E, Marsh L, Lyketsos CG, Rosenblatt A, Ross CA, et al. Psychopathology in patients with degenerative cerebellar diseases: a comparison to Huntington's disease. Am J Psychiatry. 2002;159(8):1306–14.
9. Rub U, Seidel K, Heinsen H, Vonsattel JP, den Dunnen WF, Korf HW. Huntington's disease (HD): the neuropathology of a multisystem neurodegenerative disorder of the human brain. Brain Pathol. 2016;26(6):726–40.
10. Jorge RE, Robinson RG, Moser D, Tateno A, Crespo-Facorro B, Arndt S. Major depression following traumatic brain injury. Arch Gen Psychiatry. 2004;61(1):42–50.
11. Koponen S, Taiminen T, Portin R, Himanen L, Isoniemi H, Heinonen H, et al. Axis I and II psychiatric disorders after traumatic brain injury: a 30-year follow-up study. Am J Psychiatry. 2002;159(8):1315–21.
12. Oquendo MA, Friedman JH, Grunebaum MF, Burke A, Silver JM, Mann JJ. Suicidal behavior and mild traumatic brain injury in major depression. J Nerv Ment Dis. 2004;192(6):430–4.
13. van Reekum R, Bolago I, Finlayson MA, Garner S, Links PS. Psychiatric disorders after traumatic brain injury. Brain Inj. 1996;10(5):319–27.
14. King BH. Psychiatric comorbidities in neurodevelopmental disorders. Curr Opin Neurol. 2016;29(2):113–7.
15. Perez DL, Matin N, Barsky A, Costumero-Ramos V, Makaretz SJ, Young SS, et al. Cingulo-insular structural alterations associated with psychogenic symptoms, childhood abuse and PTSD in functional neurological disorders. J Neurol Neurosurg Psychiatry. 2017;88(6):491–7.
16. Voon V, Cavanna AE, Coburn K, Sampson S, Reeve A, LaFrance WC Jr. Functional neuroanatomy and neurophysiology of functional neurological disorders (conversion disorder). J Neuropsychiatry Clin Neurosci. 2016;28(3):168–90.

17. Kanner AM, Rivas-Grajales AM. Psychosis of epilepsy: a multifaceted neuropsychiatric disorder. CNS Spectr. 2016;21(3):247–57.

18. Kanner AM. Psychiatric comorbidities in epilepsy: should they be considered in the classification of epileptic disorders? Epilepsy Behav. 2016;64(Pt B):306–8.

19. Gold JA, Sher Y, Maldonado JR. Frontal lobe epilepsy: a primer for psychiatrists and a systematic review of psychiatric manifestations. Psychosomatics. 2016;57(5):445–64.

20. Perez DL, Aybek S, Nicholson TR, Kozlowska K, Arciniegas DB, LaFrance WC Jr. Functional neurological (conversion) disorder: a core neuropsychiatric disorder. J Neuropsychiatry Clin Neurosci. 2020;32(1):1–3.

21. Engel GL. The need for a new medical model: a challenge for biomedicine. Science. 1977;196(4286):129–36.

22. Pick S, Goldstein LH, Perez DL, Nicholson TR. Emotional processing in functional neurological disorder: a review, biopsychosocial model and research agenda. J Neurol Neurosurg Psychiatry. 2019;90(6):704–11.

23. Perez DL, Haller AL, Espay AJ. Should neurologists diagnose and manage functional neurologic disorders? It is complicated. Neurol Clin Pract. 2019;9(2):165–7.

24. Stone J, Carson A, Aditya H, Prescott R, Zaubi M, Warlow C, et al. The role of physical injury in motor and sensory conversion symptoms: a systematic and narrative review. J Psychosom Res. 2009;66(5):383–90.

25. Wissel BD, Dwivedi AK, Merola A, Chin D, Jacob C, Duker AP, et al. Functional neurological disorders in Parkinson disease. J Neurol Neurosurg Psychiatry. 2018;89(6):566–71.

26. Onofrj M, Thomas A, Tiraboschi P, Wenning G, Gambi F, Sepede G, et al. Updates on somatoform disorders (SFMD) in Parkinson's disease and dementia with Lewy bodies and discussion of phenomenology. J Neurol Sci. 2011;310(1–2):166–71.

27. Ani C, Reading R, Lynn R, Forlee S, Garralda E. Incidence and 12-month outcome of non-transient childhood conversion disorder in the U.K. and Ireland. Br J Psychiatry. 2013;202:413–8.

28. Kanaan R, Armstrong D, Barnes P, Wessely S. In the psychiatrist's chair: how neurologists understand conversion disorder. Brain. 2009;132(Pt 10):2889–96.

29. Stone J, Carson A, Duncan R, Roberts R, Warlow C, Hibberd C, et al. Who is referred to neurology clinics?--the diagnoses made in 3781 new patients. Clin Neurol Neurosurg. 2010;112(9):747–51.

30. Adams C, Anderson J, Madva EN, LaFrance WC Jr, Perez DL. You've made the diagnosis of functional neurological disorder: now what? Pract Neurol. 2018;18(4):323–30.

31. Sharpe M, Walker J, Williams C, Stone J, Cavanagh J, Murray G, et al. Guided self-help for functional (psychogenic) symptoms: a randomized controlled efficacy trial. Neurology. 2011;77(6):564–72.

32. Stone J, Warlow C, Sharpe M. The symptom of functional weakness: a controlled study of 107 patients. Brain. 2010;133(Pt 5):1537–51.

33. Ludwig L, Whitehead K, Sharpe M, Reuber M, Stone J. Differences in illness perceptions between patients with non-epileptic seizures and functional limb weakness. J Psychosom Res. 2015;79(3):246–9.

34. Janet P. The major symptoms of hysteria; fifteen lectures given in the Medical School of Harvard University. New York: Macmillan; 1907.

35. Roelofs K, Keijsers GP, Hoogduin KA, Naring GW, Moene FC. Childhood abuse in patients with conversion disorder. Am J Psychiatry. 2002;159(11):1908–13.

36. Diez I, Larson AG, Nakhate V, Dunn EC, Fricchione GL, Nicholson TR, et al. Early-life trauma endophenotypes and brain circuit-gene expression relationships in functional neurological (conversion) disorder. Mol Psychiatry. 2021;26(8):3817–28.

37. Spagnolo PA, Norato G, Maurer CW, Goldman D, Hodgkinson C, Horovitz S, et al. Effects of TPH2 gene variation and childhood trauma on the clinical and circuit-level phenotype of functional movement disorders. J Neurol Neurosurg Psychiatry. 2020;91(8):814–21.

38. Ludwig L, Pasman JA, Nicholson T, Aybek S, David AS, Tuck S, et al. Stressful life events and maltreatment in conversion (functional neurological) disorder: systematic review and meta-analysis of case-control studies. Lancet Psychiatry. 2018;5(4):307–20.

39. Keynejad RC, Frodl T, Kanaan R, Pariante C, Reuber M, Nicholson TR. Stress and functional neurological disorders: mechanistic insights. J Neurol Neurosurg Psychiatry. 2019;90(7):813–21.

40. Parees I, Kojovic M, Pires C, Rubio-Agusti I, Saifee TA, Sadnicka A, et al. Physical precipitating factors in functional movement disorders. J Neurol Sci. 2014;338(1–2):174–7.

41. Jalilianhasanpour R, Williams B, Gilman I, Burke MJ, Glass S, Fricchione GL, et al. Resilience linked to personality dimensions, alexithymia and affective symptoms in motor functional neurological disorders. J Psychosom Res. 2018;107:55–61.

42. Ekanayake V, Kranick S, LaFaver K, Naz A, Frank Webb A, LaFrance WC Jr, et al. Personality traits in psychogenic nonepileptic seizures (PNES) and psychogenic movement disorder (PMD): neuroticism and perfectionism. J Psychosom Res. 2017;97:23–9.

43. Harden CL, Burgut FT, Kanner AM. The diagnostic significance of video-EEG monitoring findings on pseudoseizure patients differs between neurologists and psychiatrists. Epilepsia. 2003;44(3):453–6.

44. Baslet G, Prensky E. Initial treatment retention in psychogenic non-epileptic seizures. J Neuropsychiatry Clin Neurosci. 2013;25(1):63–7.

45. Cobb S. Borderlands of psychiatry. Cambridge: Harvard University Press; 1943.

46. Cobb S. Foundations of neuropsychiatry. 5th rev. and enl. ed. Baltimore: Williams & Wilkins; 1952.

47. Castro-Caldas A, Petersson KM, Reis A, Stone-Elander S, Ingvar M. The illiterate brain. Learning to read and write during childhood influences the functional organization of the adult brain. Brain. 1998;121(Pt 6):1053–63.

48. van Praag H, Kempermann G, Gage FH. Running increases cell proliferation and neurogenesis in the adult mouse dentate gyrus. Nat Neurosci. 1999;2(3):266–70.

49. Perez DL, Keshavan MS, Scharf JM, Boes AD, Price BH. Bridging the great divide: what can neurology learn from psychiatry? J Neuropsychiatry Clin Neurosci. 2018;30(4):271–8.

50. Keshavan MS, Price BH, Martin JB. The convergence of neurology and psychiatry: the importance of cross-disciplinary education. JAMA. 2020;324(6):554–5.

51. Fox MD. Mapping symptoms to brain networks with the human connectome. N Engl J Med. 2018;379(23):2237–45.

52. Schildkrout B, Benjamin S, Lauterbach MD. Integrating neuroscience knowledge and neuropsychiatric skills into psychiatry: the way forward. Acad Med. 2016;91(5):650–6.

53. Zinchuk AV, Flanagan EP, Tubridy NJ, Miller WA, McCullough LD. Attitudes of US medical trainees towards neurology education: "Neurophobia" – a global issue. BMC Med Educ. 2010;10:49.

54. Schon F, Hart P, Fernandez C. Is clinical neurology really so difficult? J Neurol Neurosurg Psychiatry. 2002;72(5):557–9.

Part II
Presentations

Functional Limb Weakness and Paralysis

Selma Aybek

1 Clinical Vignette: History

A 35-year old woman presented to the emergency room on a Saturday evening after noticing the abrupt onset of right-sided weakness in the middle of an argument with her partner. She noticed that her face was asymmetric, she had difficulties speaking clearly and she could not control movements of her right arm and leg. She described her right side as "heavy".

Upon arrival to the emergency room (ER) she was alert and oriented, and exhibited a discrete dysarthria and a clear deviation of the lower lip toward the right side without upper facial weakness. While she was initially able to lift her right arm, the arm dropped after 10 seconds; she was unable to lift her right leg at all. She also had complete loss of sensation of her right arm and leg. She did not exhibit ataxia, eye movement abnormalities, visual abnormalities or aphasia. She was evaluated by the Stroke Service, and found to have an NIHSS score of 7

and a normal CT head. The clinical team considered treating her for possible stroke with intravenous thrombolysis.

History

The case above illustrates the challenges of establishing a diagnosis of functional weakness, which can, and often does, mimic stroke given its abrupt onset. The patient's history is significant for the sudden onset of lateralized weakness and sensory loss in a young woman. The abrupt onset of symptoms is typical of functional weakness, occurring in nearly half of cases. In addition, patients with functional weakness most commonly present with a lateralized pattern of symptoms, and weakness may be accompanied by sensory loss. Moreover, functional weakness most commonly occurs in females between the ages of 30–50. Although the clinical presentation raises a high probability of stroke, functional limb weakness should remain in the differential diagnosis based upon the history alone. Functional weakness can present in a very similar manner to other causes of weakness, with patients reporting inability to control some parts of their body. The history and standard neurological exam alone are not sufficient to make the diagnosis of functional weakness and an additional search for positive signs is needed.

Supplementary Information The online version contains supplementary material available at [https://doi.org/10.1007/978-3-030-86495-8_5].

S. Aybek (✉)
Neurology, Inselspital, Bern, Switzerland
e-mail: Selma.aybek@unige.ch

This chapter will review, with the aid of the above clinical vignette, the demographic characteristics of patients with functional weakness, in addition to clinical features, specific diagnostic signs, and treatment options.

Symptom Presentation

Rather than describing a loss of strength, patients with functional limb weakness often describe that they cannot "control" their limb. When symptoms persist over weeks or months (not only as an acute setting as in our clinical vignette), patients often report significant fluctuations in symptoms; sometimes the limb will "obey" and perform the desired task but most of the time it does not seem to execute the desired motor action. In the case of arm weakness, patients may report being unable to properly use the arm to perform activities such as getting dressed and cooking, and may report dropping objects. Patients with leg weakness often complain that the leg suddenly "gives way" at the knee while walking or that they have to "drag" the leg. Some patients have to adopt a strategy to facilitate walking, such as stiffening their legs, which gives their gait a 'robotic' appearance. While isolated functional weakness exists, in the majority of cases a sensory loss is also noticed. This sensory loss often has a non-anatomical distribution (ie. the sensory loss does not follow a root or nerve territory) or involves half of the body with midline splitting (ie. there is an exact line of sensory loss in the middle of the body over the face and trunk).

Symptom Onset

About half of patients with functional limb weakness present with sudden onset of stroke-like symptoms occurring over seconds to minutes [1]. The remainder present with more gradual onset of symptoms over the course of hours or days, opening the differential diagnosis to multiple sclerosis or spinal lesions. Some have recurring episodic weakness, expanding the differential

diagnosis to include disorders such as myasthenia gravis or hypo/hyperkalemic periodic paralysis. In a study of 107 patients with acute onset of functional weakness, over 40% had identifiable triggers or associated symptoms [1] including physical injury to the same limb (20%), pain (8%), migraine (10%) and functional seizure (12%).

Prevalence and Incidence

Functional limb weakness is one of the most common presentations of functional neurological disorder (FND). Older studies found a lifetime prevalence of functional weakness to be 7% in psychiatric patients [2]. 9% of post-partum women and 12% of medically ill patients were noted to experience unexplained paralysis [3, 4]. A controlled study of 30 patients examined in a neurology setting with recent onset functional limb weakness found a minimum population incidence of 5/100,000 [5]. A larger study in the catchment area of Edinburgh, a city of one million inhabitants, found a minimal annual incidence of 3.7/100,000 [6]. Such numbers are similar to those cited for multiple sclerosis (3/100,000) and primary brain tumors (5/100,000). In another study from the same investigators, 15% of 3781 neurology outpatients were noted to have a functional or more largely a psychological diagnosis. This included 45 patients with functional limb weakness (1.2% of the total) [7]. Other studies of neurology inpatients have found frequencies of functional paralysis ranging between 1% and 18% [8–11], and frequencies after back surgery of up to 3% [12].

Gender and Age of Onset

An analysis of seven studies comprising a total of 167 patients with functional limb weakness found an overall proportion of 48% female [13]. In other studies, including consecutive cases, a preponderance of females was found, with females comprising between 60% and 80% of the total study populations [80% (n = 56) [14], 79% (n = 107) [6], 64% (n = 98) [15] and 60% (n = 30) [5]]. The reported average age of onset is in the mid to late thirties [5–7, 16], with age of onset ranging from early childhood to older age.

Distribution and Laterality

Unilateral symptoms, including either hemiparesis or monoparesis, are the most common, although any pattern of limb weakness can occur, including triparesis. Monoparesis was over-represented in some series [ie. 30% (n = 30) in [5] and 37% (n = 81) in [17]]. However, one controlled study found that monoparesis was not more common in patients with functional paresis than in a population of controls with other causes of paresis (16% vs 24%) [6]. Lateralized symptoms occur in most patients (e.g. 79% [6], 83% [15]. Historical account of symptoms more commonly involving the left side (implying a right hemispheric involvement in FND) led to a systematic review in 2002 including 584 patients and 82 studies, confirming that weakness tended to be more common on the left (58%) [18]. However there was a suggestion of recruitment bias, given that studies that set out to examine this question found a high frequency of left lateralized symptoms (69%) whereas those that did not found no difference (50%). Subsequent studies have tended to confirm that if there is a bias to left-sided symptoms it is small (54% (n = 107) [6]; 59% (n = 94) [15]).

Other Functional Disorders and Symptoms

Functional limb weakness is rarely found in isolation, and many comorbid complaints can be found upon history-taking. In a case-control study comparing 107 patients with functional weakness to 46 controls with other neurological diseases the following symptoms were more frequent in patients with functional weakness: fatigue (82% vs 65%), sleep disturbances (75% vs 41%), pain (64% vs 35%), memory symptoms

(6% vs 41%), gastrointestinal symptoms (49% vs 20%), headache (40% vs 9%) and back pain (36% vs 17%) [6]. Comorbidity with functional seizures has been reported in at least two series (14%) [6]; 23% [19] at rates that are much higher than the general population, suggesting a shared etiology or mechanism.

Other Neurological Disease

Like all FND presentations, the presence of functional limb weakness does not imply the absence of other neurological conditions; in a related example, epilepsy and functional seizures can co-exist. In a study of 73 patients with mixed functional motor disorders (half of whom had paralysis), 48% had another comorbid neurological disease [19]; half of these were peripheral neurological disorders.

Clinical Exam

2 Clinical Vignette: Neurological Exam
*Two days after initial presentation, a detailed clinical neurological examination was performed, revealing facial asymmetry with **lip pulling** and a right-sided sensorimotor hemisyndrome characterized by **drift without pronation** (see Video 5.1), **give-way weakness** for all tested limb segments, **Hoover's sign** (see Fig. 5.2), **midline splitting sensory loss** of the head, trunk, right arm and right leg, and a pattern of gait with a **dragging** right leg. Examination was also remarkable for normal tone, normal symmetric reflexes, and absence of a Babinski sign.*

A detailed clinical exam is crucial to make the diagnosis of FND. In fact, Criteria B of the DSM-5 requires that "*clinical findings provide evidence of incompatibility between the symptom and recognized neurological or medical conditions*". This evidence comes from the presence of 'positive signs' on neurological examination. While most of these signs were initially described in the nineteenth century, modern medicine has offered quantitative validation of the specificity, sensitivity and inter-rater reliabil-

Table 5.1 Sensitivity and specificity of positive signs for functional weakness

Test	Sensitivity	Specificity	Number Case	Number Control	Studies	Pitfalls/caution in interpretation
Motor inconsistency	98%	13%	15	40	Chabrol et al. [21]	
Give-way weakness	90%	100%	20	20	Daum et al. [22]	The sign cannot be evaluated if there is joint pain, which would explain the patient's voluntary give-way.
	69%	98%	107	46	Stone et al. [6]	
	20%	95%	15	40	Chabrol et al. [21]	
Co-contraction	40%	100%	20	19	Daum et al. [23]	
Hoover's sign	63%	100%	8	116	McWhirter et al. [24]	Can only be applied in cases of unilateral leg weakness
	75%	100%	16	17	Sonoo [25]	
	100%	100%	8	11	Tinazzi et al. [26]	
	95%	86%	63	7	Stone et al. [6]	
	76%	100%	17	18	Daum et al. [23]	
Hip abductor sign	100%	100%	16	17	Sonoo [25]	Can only be applied in cases of unilateral leg weakness
Elbow flex-ex sign	100%	100%	10	23	Lombardi et al. [27]	Requires significant expertise to correctly assess
SCM test	100%	30%	19	20	Daum et al. [23]	
	90%	63%	30	40	Horn et al. [28]	
Drift without pronation	93%	100%	26	28	Daum and Aybek [29]	The hands must be carefully positioned in supination before observing for at least 10 seconds
	11%	100%	19	19	Daum et al. [22]	
	47%	100%	19	20	Daum et al. [23]	
5th finger abduction	100%	100%	10	11	Tinazzi et al. [26]	Can only be applied in cases of severe hand plegia
Arm drop	83%	100%	2	7	Daum et al. [22]	Very rare sign, only in cases of severe arm plegia
Spinal injuries center test	90%	13%	15	20	Daum et al. [22]	
	98%	100%	14	48	Yugue et al. [30]	
Leg dragging gait	8%	100%	107	46	Stone et al. [6]	
	20%	100%	20	23	Baker and Silver [31]	
	100%	11%	19	19	Daum et al. [22]	
Knee buckling	95%	21%	19	19	Daum et al. [22]	

ity of many of these signs (see Table 5.1). Caution must be taken as individual signs are not enough to definitively establish the diagnosis; only a coherent history, absence of neurological signs that could explain the symptom, and the presence of one or more positive signs can ensure the correct diagnosis. Below are some frequent signs suggestive of the diagnosis of functional weakness:

- **Motor inconsistency.** A difference in motor performance is observed in different testing conditions. For example, there may a severe weakness of a limb during the clinical exam (ie. the leg cannot be lifted from the examina-

tion bed, or the hand cannot accomplish any fine motoric movement), contrasting with another time of the consultation when the patient is able to get dressed by standing on the weak limb or is able to manipulate objects such as shoes with the weak hand (see Fig. 5.1).

- **Give-way weakness.** A sudden loss of force is felt by the examiner after an initial good/normal strength response when a muscle is tested against resistance. This sign should be interpreted with caution when there is pain in the limb, especially in a joint. Myasthenia gravis can sometimes also present with give-way weakness.

Patient Observation

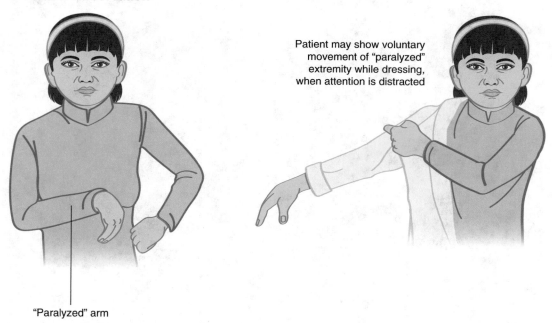

Patient may show voluntary movement of "paralyzed" extremity while dressing, when attention is distracted

"Paralyzed" arm

Fig. 5.1 Motor discordance. The patient shows inability to move the right arm (left panel) but is able, later in the same examination session, to use the arm almost normally (right panel): this illustrates the positive sogn of motor discordance or inconsistence. (Image with permission from Stone and Aybek [20])

- **Co-contraction**. When trying to move a limb, no movement at the joint is seen because both agonist and antagonist muscles are being recruited. For example, the examiner can feel a contraction in both the quadriceps and the harmstring, resulting in absence of movement at the knee.
- **Hoover's sign.** The examiner should first test the strength of hip extension, with the patient in either in a supine or seated position. The examiner will then ask the patient to flex their healthy hip against resistance, while continuing to assess hip extension of the weak leg by keeping their hand below the thigh if the patient is seated, or below the foot if the patient is supine. The examiner will feel an involuntary extension of the weak leg when the healthy contralateral leg is forced to flex against resistance. A discordance between voluntary hip extension and involuntary hip extension during contralateral hip flexion is considered a positive Hoover's sign (see Fig. 5.2). Other ways to interpret a positive

Hoover's sign are also described, including a failure to extend the healthy hip when attempting to flex the weak leg.
- **Hip Abductor Sign.** This is the equivalent of the Hoover's sign, but applies to abduction/adduction as opposed to flexion/extension of the hip. Involuntary abduction of the weak leg during contralateral abduction against resistance is noted.
- **The elbow flex-ex test.** This is the equivalent of the Hoover's sign for the upper limbs: involuntary elbow extension will occur during contralateral flexion against resistance. One caveat is that its testing requires significant experience and skill, and it has only been validated in a single study.
- **Sternocleidomastoid (SCM) test**. Even though this test does not directly address limb weakness, it is worth testing and as a positive test often accompanies functional arm or leg weakness. A weakness in head turning to the side is noted, often when turning towards the paralyzed arm or leg; this often presents with

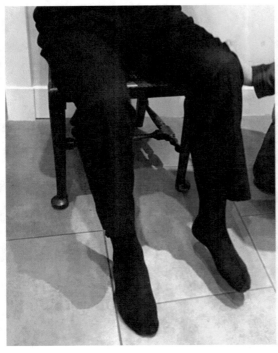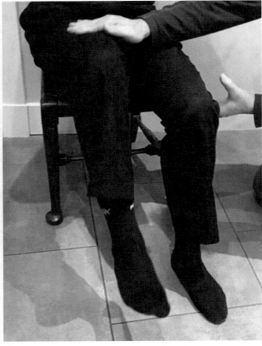

'Keep your left heel on the ground – don't let me lift it up'   *'Lift up your right leg. Don't let me push it down'*

LEFT hip extension is weak   **LEFT hip extension returns to NORMAL**

Fig. 5.2 Hoover's sign. Left panel: The patient shows weakness when performing hip extension (pushing the examiner's hand towards the chair) on the left side (left hip extension is weak). Right panel: This contrasts with better strength when the patient focuses on moving the right healthy leg upwards against resistance (left hip extension returns to normal). A positive Hoover's sign is present when such discordance is noted. (Image with permission from Stone and Aybek [20])

a give-way pattern. As the SCM has bilateral cortical innervation, such asymmetry would not be expected in hemispheric lesions such as stroke.

- **Drift without pronation.** When testing for pronator drift with the arms outstretched and the hands supinated, the hand will drop without pronating in cases of functional weakness. This is in contrast to the drift with pronation that is seen with pyramidal lesions.

- **Finger Abduction**. In rare cases of complete hand plegia, one can search for synkinetic movement of the weak hand, consisting of abduction of the fifth finger, during abduction of the healthy fingers of the contralateral hand against resistance.

- **Arm drop.** In cases of complete arm plegia, when the patient with functional weakness has their own arm dropped onto their face, the arm avoids the face. In other neurological weakness, the arm will drop on the face. Use caution with this test to avoid the patient actually hitting themselves regardless of etiology.

- **Spinal Injuries Center test**. In cases of complete unilateral leg weakness this sign can complement the Hoover sign. With the patient supine the weak legs are passively lifted in a flexed position on the bed. In functional hemiplegia they remain in that position instead of instantly falling to the side as they would in other neurological conditions.

- **Dragging monoplegic gait.** If functional leg weakness is marked, the patient will typically walk with a dragging gait in which the front part of the foot remains in contact with the floor through the step. The hip may be internally or externally rotated although sometimes will remain in the normal position. This pattern of dragging leg is different from circumduction of the leg seen in other cases of weakness with a spastic component.

- **Knee buckling.** In functional leg weakness, gait may be impaired by sudden give-way weakness at the knee (see Video 5.2).

2 Clinical Vignette: Neurological Exam Discussion

As illustrated by our vignette, in the case of stroke mimics, an abbreviated neurological examination such as the NIHSS, as typically performed during stroke triage, is not sufficient to rule out functional weakness from the differential diagnosis. Indeed, the symptoms of functional weakness can produce elevated NIHSS scores. The careful assessment for positive signs should complement the NIHSS scoring. One should also bear in mind that the diagnosis of stroke and FND are not mutually exclusive: both disorders can co-exist. The presence of positive signs confirms the diagnosis of FND but does not rule out an underlying stroke. This patient presented **6 positive signs** for FND. Based on clinical grounds a positive diagnosis of FND could be made; a comorbid stroke was excluded by the absence of pyramidal signs on clinical exam and the presence of a normal brain MRI.

Ancillary Testing

Rule-In Tests: Is There Ancillary Testing Available to Confirm the Diagnosis?

The diagnosis of functional limb weakness is a clinical diagnosis and no tests have been developed yet to assist with the diagnosis. A first step towards validation of a 5-minute resting-state brain MRI to differentiate FND patients from normal controls is promising – with 70% accuracy – [32] but further steps are needed before it can be applied in a clinical setting as a diagnostic tool.

Studies have quantified the motor discordance of the Hoover's sign [33, 34] and give-way weakness [35] in muscle strength but their use in clinical practice has not been validated. Abnormal EMG activation during voluntary ankle flexion has been suggested to help with the diagnosis but has only been tested in 2 cases of functional weakness [36].

Several studies looked at the utility of transcranial magnetic stimulation (TMS) studying motor excitability; normal central motor conduction time and motor evoked potentials (MEP) are expected in FND as opposed to other neurological conditions [12, 37–40]. A small controlled study [41] showed a greater intrasubject variance in MEP size in patients with functional weakness as compared those with amyotrophic lateral sclerosis or healthy controls in a study involving a cued ramp-and-hold contraction task; this tool has not been validated in routine clinical practice. A paradoxical decrease of cortical excitability during movement imagination has been found in functional weakness but not in healthy controls (for arm [42] and leg [43]), and is suggestive of the diagnosis.

Rule-Out Tests: Which Tests Are Necessary to Exclude Other Neurological Conditions?

Criteria C of the DSM-5 states the following: "*the symptom or deficit is not better explained by another medical or mental illness*". In clinical practice, this means that a comorbid underlying neurological condition can be masked by functional signs and should be investigated. In the example of our vignette, it means that even if the clinical picture is strongly suggestive of the diagnosis of FND a brain MRI should likely be done to rule out a co-existing stroke. Brain MRI is also potentially necessary in all cases presenting with midline splitting sensory loss to search for a thalamic lesion that could explain this pattern of sensory loss. In some cases the functional weakness can impair the examiner's ability to test for ataxia, and a brain MRI should also be performed to search for vascular or multiple sclerosis lesions.

Other tests, such as lumbar puncture or electromyography can be performed, depending on the differential diagnosis raised by the clinical findings.

As a general rule, it is advised to run tests that are necessary to reassure the clinician that FND is the sole diagnosis explaining the symptom. It is recommended that testing occur early in the diagnostic process. Patients may return from their initial consultation with many questions, and requests for additional testing. If a thorough initial investigation has been performed, the patient will have more trust and confidence in the diagnosis. This will avoid repeating unnecessary tests later on in the follow-up, avoid multiple medical consultations, and allow for the patient to engage early in the appropriate therapy.

Pitfalls in the Diagnosis of Functional Weakness

A fear of mislabeling weakness as functional and missing the diagnosis of another neurological disorder has always been strong among neurologists [44–46]. This has led to the false view that before making the diagnosis of functional weakness a thorough process of excluding other diagnoses must be performed. As discussed above, there are many specific signs that can and should be used to make a positive clinical diagnosis, which is now reflected since 2013 in the new DSM-5 criteria B. The rate of misdiagnosis of FND in general has been confirmed to be very low (below 1%), and is similar to that seen with other clinical neurological or psychiatric diagnoses [47].

Clinicians should always keep in mind the potential for a co-occurring neurological disorder. This is of utmost importance because such patients will need two different therapeutic paths (for example, a patient with both MS and FND will require immunomodulatory therapy for multiple sclerosis and an interdisciplinary approach for functional weakness).

Particular attention should be paid to patients with paroxysmal symptoms that are reported but not seen during the consultation (ie. when no positive signs can be elicited). In such cases, follow-up should be planned and the patient asked to film an episode and/or schedule a consult for a time when the symptoms are expected to re-occur so that the positive signs can be visualized by the examiner. When patients report particular triggers (fatigue, exercise, particular food intake, etc.) it may be useful to plan a second evaluation and ask the patient to self-trigger the episode before or during the neurological exam.

A misdiagnosis in the other direction (labelling a disorder as another neurological condition when it is actually functional) can also be an important pitfall [48], as it can lead to invasive, unnecessary and potentially dangerous treatments, as well as delay appropriate treatment for FND. In a study of 110 patients misdiagnosed with multiple sclerosis (due to various alternative conditions including functional weakness), 31% experienced unnecessary morbidities due often to side effects of unnecessary immunomodulatory therapy [49]. Inappropriately diagnosing patients with seronegative myasthenia gravis when FND should be considered may also lead to unnecessary immunomodulatory therapy and the adverse effects associated with this type of therapy [50]. In the case of our vignette, the patient received IV thrombolysis, which is not without risks. Fortunately, one series looking at hemorrhage risk among stroke mimics (including FND) who received thrombolysis [51] found low rates of complications, probably explained by demographics, as FND patients tend to be younger and have fewer cardiovascular risk factors.

Another diagnostic pitfall involves placing too much emphasis on comorbid psychiatric complaints, and inappropriately concluding that these complaints imply that a patient's symptoms must be secondary to a neuropsychiatric disorder such as FND. Of note, psychiatric complaints can be frequent in disorders such as myasthenia gravis [52]. It has been suggested that caution should be made in interpreting non-specific symptoms such as fatigue as psychiatric, and thus miss or delay a diagnosis of myasthenia. Along this vein, it is also important to note that the DSM-5 diagnostic criteria for FND no longer considers the presence of a psychological stressor as mandatory for the diagnosis.

Finally, disregarding a diagnosis of functional weakness and overdiagnosing other neurological conditions leads to a delay in proper therapy for FND [48].

3 Clinical Vignette: Therapy

The diagnosis was explained to the patient by telling her she had a "functional neurological disorder". It was explained that her brain suddenly lost control over the right side of her body, explaining why she could not move properly and why she exhibited altered sensation. This loss of control was due to a dysfunction in certain brain areas as opposed to permanent damage, as can happen in a stroke when a vessel does not bring enough blood and oxygen. The comparison was made to a software problem causing a computer to dysfunction; it was explained that no hardware damage was involved, such as cable or keyboard keys. It was explained that the brain needed to be retrained in order to regain appropriate motor and sensory function, and a program of physiotherapy was offered. The role of potential stressors, such as the argument with her partner, was discussed. The patient said she was under a lot of pressure at home and often disagreed with her partner regarding the education of their 4-year old and 2-year old children. She felt overwhelmed and feared losing her job as she had missed several days of work recently to take care of her kids without help from the partner. The role of stress in contributing to the impairment of normal brain function was discussed and psychotherapeutic help was offered. Multidisciplinary treatment, involving regular meetings between the patient, neurologist, psychotherapist and physiotherapist, was planned. After a three-day inpatient course the patient's symptoms improved dramatically and she was discharged. She continued outpatient multidisciplinary treatment for 3 months and recovered completely.

Treatment of Functional Weakness

The treatment of functional limb weakness has three main pillars: explanation of the diagnosis, physiotherapy and psychotherapy. Not all patients need all three steps but the explanation of the diagnosis is essential in every case. Studies have shown that a careful explanation by itself has therapeutic value [53]. In light of the fear of misdiagnosis dicussed above, many clinicians are reluctant to disclose the diagnosis of FND and prefer to remain cautious and provide a vague explanation, insisting on negative findings and reassuring the patients that no lesion has been found, that all tests were normal and that no serious condition was found. This is problematic, as patients still lack an explanation for their symptoms and they often distrust the physican and will seek a second outpatient opinion [54] or present to the emergency room. This approach also prevents patients from engaging in the appropriate therapy. The use of the term "functional "has been shown to be descriptive and neutral [55, 56]. It offers a rationale for why the symptoms occur and an explanation for how physiotherapy may be helpful in targeting the underlying mechanisms.

The second pillar, FND-specific physiotherapy programs, have shown good clinical outcomes in pilot controlled trials [57, 58]. Such specific FND-focused therapies use distractibility as their main strategy, retraining the motor program and diverting attention away from the weak limb(s). Practice recommendations are available [59], and larger controlled studies are underway [60]. Occupational therapy also plays an important role [61] in retraining activities of daily life and integrating the motor symptoms in normal day-to-day functioning.

The third pillar of treatment, psychotherapy, should always be kept in mind, but not necessarily offered to all patients [62]. Before psychotherapy is offered, a good understanding of the diagnosis is needed, and a link between motor function and emotion/stress factors should be explained (as described below). This may require several neurological follow-up consultations, and may enhance acceptance of psychotherapy. It is also important to keep in mind that some patients will recover with physiotherapy alone. When psychotherapy is considered, cognitive behavioural therapy (CBT) is usually the first line treatment for functional seizures [63, 64] but can also be of benefit in patients with functional weakness [65]. Other forms of individualized psychotherapies can be useful [66, 67].

For the sub-group of patients who will benefit from psychotherapy, it is important to offer this treatment at the appropriate time. Just like using terms such as "psychogenic" or "psychosomatic" may be offensive to some patients, offering psychotherapy too early in the diagnosis explanation phase may be counterproductive. Patients may feel stigmatized and feel that their symptoms are not taken seriously, because they may not understand how psychotherapy may help their symptoms. One way to introduce the potential benefits of psychotherapy is to address the link between emotions, thoughts and bodily symptoms while explaining the diagnosis. Highlighting the effectiveness of psychotherapy for FND as demonstrated by several controlled studies [68–71] can also facilitate acceptance to engage in psychotherapy. This approach presents psychotherapy as a proven treatment, and reduces the risk that a patient will feel stigmatized when psychotherapy is offered as part of the treatment course.

Most importantly, multidisciplinary approaches in an outpatient [72] or inpatient [73–75] setting offer optimal options to integrate care from different healthcare professionals. Neurologists should stay involved [76] in the long-term care of patients suffering from functional limb weakness, as symptoms may evolve, change or relapse and integrated care is essential.

Summary
1. Functional limb weakness is one of the most common presentations of FND.
2. The typical age of onset of functional limb weakness is between 30 and 40 years old; it is more common in women.
3. Many validated positive clinical signs can help with the diagnosis of functional limb weakness.
4. Functional limb weakness can co-exist with other neurological conditions.
5. Physiotherapy has proven to be effective in improving the symptoms of functional limb weakness.

References

1. Stone J, Warlow C, Sharpe M. Functional weakness: clues to mechanism from the nature of onset. J Neurol Neurosurg Psychiatry. 2012;83:67–9.
2. Farley J, Woodruff RAJ, Guze SB. The prevalence of hysteria and conversion symptoms. Br J Psychiatry. 1968;114(514):1121–5.
3. Woodruff RA Jr. Hysteria: an evaluation of objective diagnostic criteria by the study of women with chronic medical illnesses. Br J Psychiatry. 1968;114(514):1115–9.
4. Woodruff RA Jr, Clayton PJ, Guze SB. Hysteria: an evaluation of specific diagnostic criteria by the study of randomly selected psychiatric clinic patients. Br J Psychiatry. 1969;115(528):1243–8.
5. Binzer M, Andersen PM, Kullgren G. Clinical characteristics of patients with motor disability due to conversion disorder: a prospective control group study. J Neurol Neurosurg Psychiatry. 1997;63(1):83–8.
6. Stone J, Warlow C, Sharpe M. The symptom of functional weakness: a controlled study of 107 patients. Brain J Neurol. 2010;133(Pt 5):1537–51.
7. Stone J, Carson A, Duncan R, Roberts R, Warlow C, Hibberd C, Coleman R, Cull R, Murray G, Pelosi A, Cavanagh J, Matthews K, Goldbeck R, Smyth R, Walker J, Sharpe M. Who is referred to neurology clinics?--the diagnoses made in 3781 new patients. Clin Neurol Neurosurg. 2010;112(9):747–51.
8. Ewald H, Rogne T, Ewald K, Fink P. Somatisation in patients newly admitted to a neurological department. Acta Psychiatr Scand. 1994;89:174–9.
9. Marsden CD. Hysteria: a neurologist's view. Psychol Med. 1986;16(2):277–88.
10. Metcalfe R, Firth D, Pollock S, Creed F. Psychiatric morbidity and illness behaviour in female neurological in-patients. J Neurol Neurosurg Psychiatry. 1988;51(11):1387–90.
11. Schiffer RB. Psychiatric aspects of clinical neurology. Am J Psychiatry. 1983;140(2):205–7.
12. Janssen BA, Theiler R, Grob D, Dvorak J. The role of motor evoked potentials in psychogenic paralysis. Spine (Phila Pa 1976). 1995;20(5):608–11.
13. Stone J, Sharpe M, Binzer M. Motor conversion symptoms and pseudoseizures: a comparison of clinical characteristics. Psychosomatics. 2004;45(6):492–9.

14. Stone J, Carson A, Duncan R, Coleman R, Roberts R, Warlow C, Hibberd C, Murray G, Cull R, Pelosi A, Cavanagh J, Matthews K, Goldbeck R, Smyth R, Walker J, Macmahon AD, Sharpe M. Symptoms 'unexplained by organic disease' in 1144 new neurology out-patients: how often does the diagnosis change at follow-up? Brain J Neurol. 2009;132(Pt 10):2878–88.

15. Gargalas S, Weeks R, Khan-Bourne N, Shotbolt P, Simblett S, Ashraf L, Doyle C, Bancroft V, David AS. Incidence and outcome of functional stroke mimics admitted to a hyperacute stroke unit. J Neurol Neurosurg Psychiatry. 2017;88(1):2–6.

16. Ehrbar R, Waespe W. Functional gait disorders. Schweiz Med Wochenschr. 1992;122(22):833–41.

17. Lempert T, Dieterich M, Huppert D, Brandt T. Psychogenic disorders in neurology: frequency and clinical spectrum. Acta Neurol Scand. 1990;82(5):335–40.

18. Stone J, Sharpe M, Carson A, Lewis SC, Thomas B, Goldbeck R, Warlow CP. Are functional motor and sensory symptoms really more frequent on the left? A systematic review. J Neurol Neurosurg Psychiatry. 2002;73(5):578–81.

19. Crimlisk HL, Bhatia K, Cope H, David A, Marsden CD, Ron MA. Slater revisited: 6 year follow up study of patients with medically unexplained motor symptoms. BMJ. 1998;316(7131):582–6.

20. Stone J, Aybek S. Functional limb weakness and paralysis. Handb Clin Neurol. 2016;139:213–28.

21. Chabrol H, Peresson G, Clanet M. Lack of specificity of the traditional criteria for conversion disorders. Eur Psychiatry. 1995;10(6):317–9.

22. Daum C, Gheorghita F, Spatola M, Stojanova V, Medlin F, Vingerhoets F, Berney A, Gholam-Rezaee M, Maccaferri GE, Hubschmid M, Aybek S. Interobserver agreement and validity of bedside 'positive signs' for functional weakness, sensory and gait disorders in conversion disorder: a pilot study. J Neurol Neurosurg Psychiatry. 2015;86:425–30.

23. Daum C, Hubschmid M, Aybek S. The value of 'positive' clinical signs for weakness, sensory and gait disorders in conversion disorder: a systematic and narrative review. J Neurol Neurosurg Psychiatry. 2014;85(2):180–90.

24. McWhirter L, Stone J, Sandercock P, Whiteley W. Hoover's sign for the diagnosis of functional weakness: a prospective unblinded cohort study in patients with suspected stroke. J Psychosom Res. 2011;71(6):384–6.

25. Sonoo M. Abductor sign: a reliable new sign to detect unilateral non-organic paresis of the lower limb. J Neurol Neurosurg Psychiatry. 2004;75(1):121–5.

26. Tinazzi M, Simonetto S, Franco L, Bhatia KP, Moretto G, Fiaschi A, Deluca C. Abduction finger sign: a new sign to detect unilateral functional paralysis of the upper limb. Mov Disord. 2008;23(16):2415–9.

27. Lombardi TL, Barton E, Wang J, Eliashiv DS, Chung JM, Muthukumaran A, Tsimerinov EI. The elbow flex-ex: a new sign to detect unilateral upper extremity non-organic paresis. J Neurol Neurosurg Psychiatry. 2014;85(2):165–7.

28. Horn D, Galli S, Berney A, Vingerhoets F, Aybek S. Testing head rotation and flexion is useful in functional limb weakness. Mov Disord Clin Pract. 2017;4(4):597–602.

29. Daum C, Aybek S. Validity of the "drift without pronation" sign in conversion disorder. BMC Neurol. 2013;13:31.

30. Yugue I, Shiba K, Ueta T, Iwamoto Y. A new clinical evaluation for hysterical paralysis. Spine. 2004;29(17):1910–3; discussion 1913.

31. Baker JH, Silver JR. Hysterical paraplegia. J Neurol Neurosurg Psychiatry. 1987;50(4):375–82.

32. Wegrzyk J, Kebets V, Richiardi J, Galli S, de Ville DV, Aybek S. Identifying motor functional neurological disorder using resting-state functional connectivity. Neuroimage Clin. 2018;17:163–8.

33. Diukova GM, Ljachovetckaja NI, Begljarova MA, Gavrileyko GI. Simple quantitative analysis of Hoover's test in patients with psychogenic and organic limb pareses. J Psychosom Res. 2013;74(4):361–4.

34. Ziv I, Djaldetti R, Zoldan Y, Avraham M, Melamed E. Diagnosis of "non-organic" limb paresis by a novel objective motor assessment: the quantitative Hoover's test. J Neurol. 1998;245(12):797–802.

35. Knutsson E, Martensson A. Isokinetic measurements of muscle strength in hysterical paresis. Electroencephalogr Clin Neurophysiol. 1985;61(5):370–4.

36. McComas AJ, Kereshi S, Quinlan J. A method for detecting functional weakness. J Neurol Neurosurg Psychiatry. 1983;46(3):280–2.

37. Cantello R, Boccagni C, Comi C, Civardi C, Monaco F. Diagnosis of psychogenic paralysis: the role of motor evoked potentials. J Neurol. 2001;248(10):889–97.

38. Foong J, Ridding M, Cope H, Marsden CD, Ron MA. Corticospinal function in conversion disorder. J Neuropsychiatry Clin Neurosci. 1997;9(2):302–3.

39. Meyer BU, Britton TC, Benecke R, Bischoff C, Machetanz J, Conrad B. Motor responses evoked by magnetic brain stimulation in psychogenic limb weakness: diagnostic value and limitations. J Neurol. 1992;239(5):251–5.

40. Pillai JJ, Markind S, Streletz LJ, Field HL, Herbison G. Motor evoked potentials in psychogenic paralysis. Neurology. 1992;42(4):935–6.

41. Morita H, Shimojima Y, Nishikawa N, Hagiwara N, Amano N, Ikeda S. Size variance of motor evoked potential at initiation of voluntary contraction in palsy of conversion disorder. Psychiatry Clin Neurosci. 2008;62(3):286–92.

42. Liepert J, Hassa T, Tuscher O, Schmidt R. Abnormal motor excitability in patients with psychogenic paresis. A TMS study. J Neurol. 2009;256(1):121–6.

43. Liepert J, Hassa T, Tuscher O, Schmidt R. Motor excitability during movement imagination and movement observation in psychogenic lower limb paresis. J Psychosom Res. 2011;70(1):59–65.

44. LaFaver K, Lang AE, Stone J, Morgante F, Edwards M, Lidstone S, Maurer CW, Hallett M, Dwivedi AK, Espay AJ. Opinions and clinical practices related to diagnosing and managing functional (psychogenic) movement disorders: changes in the last decade. Eur J Neurol. 2020;27(6):975–84.

45. Slater E. Diagnosis of "hysteria". Br Med J. 1965;1(5447):1395–9.

46. Slater ET, Glithero E. A follow-up of patients diagnosed as suffering from "hysteria". J Psychosom Res. 1965;9(1):9–13.

47. Stone J, Smyth R, Carson A, Lewis S, Prescott R, Warlow C, Sharpe M. Systematic review of misdiagnosis of conversion symptoms and "hysteria". BMJ. 2005;331(7523):989.

48. Walzl D, Carson AJ, Stone J. The misdiagnosis of functional disorders as other neurological conditions. J Neurol. 2019;266(8):2018–26.

49. Solomon AJ, Bourdette DN, Cross AH, Applebee A, Skidd PM, Howard DB, Spain RI, Cameron MH, Kim E, Mass MK, Yadav V, Whitham RH, Longbrake EE, Naismith RT, Wu GF, Parks BJ, Wingerchuk DM, Rabin BL, Toledano M, Tobin WO, Kantarci OH, Carter JL, Keegan BM, Weinshenker BG. The contemporary spectrum of multiple sclerosis misdiagnosis: a multicenter study. Neurology. 2016;87(13):1393–9.

50. Al-Asmi A, Nandhagopal R, Jacob PC, Gujjar A. Misdiagnosis of myasthenia gravis and subsequent clinical implication: a case report and review of literature. Sultan Qaboos Univ Med J. 2012;12(1):103–8.

51. Kvistad CE, Novotny V, Naess H, Hagberg G, Ihle-Hansen H, Waje-Andreassen U, Thomassen L, Logallo N. Safety and predictors of stroke mimics in the Norwegian Tenecteplase Stroke Trial (NOR-TEST). Int J Stroke. 2019;14(5):508–16.

52. Nicholson GA, Wilby J, Tennant C. Myasthenia gravis: the problem of a "psychiatric" misdiagnosis. Med J Aust. 1986;144(12):632–8.

53. Stone J, Carson A, Hallett M. Explanation as treatment for functional neurologic disorders. Handb Clin Neurol. 2016;139:543–53.

54. Crimlisk HL, Bhatia KP, Cope H, David AS, Marsden D, Ron MA. Patterns of referral in patients with medically unexplained motor symptoms. J Psychosom Res. 2000;49(3):217–9.

55. Kanaan RA, Armstrong D, Wessely SC. The function of 'functional': a mixed methods investigation. J Neurol Neurosurg Psychiatry. 2012;83(3):248–50.

56. Stone J, Wojcik W, Durrance D, Carson A, Lewis S, MacKenzie L, Warlow CP, Sharpe M. What should we say to patients with symptoms unexplained by disease? The 'number needed to offend'. BMJ: Br Med J. 2002;325(7378):1449–50.

57. Nielsen G, Buszewicz M, Stevenson F, Hunter R, Holt K, Dudziec M, Ricciardi L, Marsden J, Joyce E, Edwards MJ. Randomised feasibility study of physiotherapy for patients with functional motor symptoms. J Neurol Neurosurg Psychiatry. 2017;88:484–90.

58. Nielsen G, Ricciardi L, Demartini B, Hunter R, Joyce E, Edwards MJ. Outcomes of a 5-day physiotherapy programme for functional (psychogenic) motor disorders. J Neurol. 2015;262(3):674–81.

59. Nielsen G, Stone J, Matthews A, Brown M, Sparkes C, Farmer R, Masterton L, Duncan L, Winters A, Daniell L, Lumsden C, Carson A, David AS, Edwards M. Physiotherapy for functional motor disorders: a consensus recommendation. J Neurol Neurosurg Psychiatry. 2015;86(10):1113–9.

60. Nielsen G, Stone J, Buszewicz M, Carson A, Goldstein LH, Holt K, Hunter R, Marsden J, Marston L, Noble H, Reuber M, Edwards MJ. Physio4FMD: protocol for a multicentre randomised controlled trial of specialist physiotherapy for functional motor disorder. BMC Neurol. 2019;19(1):242.

61. Ranford J, Perez DL, MacLean J. Additional occupational therapy considerations for functional neurological disorders: a potential role for sensory processing. CNS Spectr. 2018;23(3):194–5.

62. Vermeulen M, de Haan RJ. Favourable outcome without psychotherapy in patients with functional neurologic disorder. J Clin Neurosci. 2020;71:141–3.

63. Goldstein LH, Robinson EJ, Mellers JDC, Stone J, Carson A, Reuber M, Medford N, McCrone P, Murray J, Richardson MP, Pilecka I, Eastwood C, Moore M, Mosweu I, Perdue I, Landau S, Chalder T, CODES Study Group. Cognitive behavioural therapy for adults with dissociative seizures (CODES): a pragmatic, multicentre, randomised controlled trial. Lancet Psychiatry. 2020;7(6):491–505.

64. LaFrance WC, Baird GL, Barry JJ, Blum AS, Webb AF, Keitner GI, Machan JT, Miller I, Szaflarski JP NES Treatment Trial (NEST-T) Consortium. Multicenter pilot treatment trial for psychogenic non-epileptic seizures: a randomized clinical trial. JAMA Psychiatry. 2014;71(9):997–1005.

65. Dallocchio C, Tinazzi M, Bombieri F, Arno N, Erro R. Cognitive behavioural therapy and adjunctive physical activity for functional movement disorders (conversion disorder): a pilot, single-blinded, randomized study. Psychother Psychosom. 2016;85(6):381–3.

66. Hubschmid M, Aybek S, Maccaferri GE, Chocron O, Gholamrezaee MM, Rossetti AO, Vingerhoets F, Berney A. Efficacy of brief interdisciplinary psychotherapeutic intervention for motor conversion disorder and nonepileptic attacks. Gen Hosp Psychiatry. 2015;37(5):448–55.

67. Kompoliti K, Wilson B, Stebbins G, Bernard B, Hinson V. Immediate vs. delayed treatment of psychogenic movement disorders with short term psychodynamic psychotherapy: randomized clinical trial. Parkinsonism Relat Disord. 2014;20(1):60–3.

68. Gelauff JM, Dreissen YEM, Tijssen MAJ, Stone J. Treatment of functional motor disorders. Curr Treat Options Neurol. 2014;16(4):1–19.

69. Hinson VK, Weinstein S, Bernard B, Leurgans SE, Goetz CG. Single-blind clinical trial of psychotherapy for treatment of psychogenic movement disorders. Parkinsonism Relat Disord. 2006;12(3):177–80.

70. Lehn A, Gelauff J, Hoeritzauer I, Ludwig L, McWhirter L, Williams S, Gardiner P, Carson

A, Stone J. Functional neurological disorders: mechanisms and treatment. J Neurol. 2016;263(3):611–20.

71. Reuber M, Burness C, Howlett S, Brazier J, Grunewald R. Tailored psychotherapy for patients with functional neurological symptoms: a pilot study. J Psychosom Res. 2007;63(6):625–32.

72. Aybek S, Lidstone SC, Nielsen G, MacGillivray L, Bassetti CL, Lang AE, Edwards MJ. What is the role of a specialist assessment clinic for FND? Lessons from three national referral centers. J Neuropsychiatry Clin Neurosci. 2019:appineuropsych19040083.

73. Demartini B, Batla A, Petrochilos P, Fisher L, Edwards MJ, Joyce E. Multidisciplinary treatment for functional neurological symptoms: a prospective study. J Neurol. 2014;261:2370–7.

74. Jordbru AA, Smedstad LM, Klungsoyr O, Martinsen EW. Psychogenic gait disorder: a randomized controlled trial of physical rehabilitation with one-year follow-up. J Rehabil Med. 2014;46(2):181–7.

75. McKee K, Glass S, Adams C, Stephen CD, King F, Parlman K, Perez DL, Kontos N. The inpatient assessment and management of motor functional neurological disorders: an interdisciplinary perspective. Psychosomatics. 2018;59(4):358–68.

76. Perez DL, Haller AL, Espay AJ. Should neurologists diagnose and manage functional neurologic disorders? It is complicated. Neurol Clin Pract. 2019;9(2):165–7.

Functional Tremor

Petra Schwingenschuh

Clinical Vignette

The patient is a 27-year old woman who suffers from a tremor mainly affecting her right arm. About 6 months ago, the tremor began suddenly 5 days after the delivery of her first child.

She had mild anxiety upon learning that she was pregnant, but had remained fit and well during the course of the pregnancy. She continued her job as a waitress in a busy restaurant until the beginning of her maternity leave. At 39 weeks of gestation, the young woman presented to the delivery unit following the spontaneous onset of labor. Her husband, who was present throughout the delivery, noticed that the patient's whole body was shivering from exhaustion, but they were told this was normal. A caesarian section was performed without complications due to prolonged and obstructed labor. She was discharged home 4 days later, and remembers feeling happy to be bringing her healthy baby boy home.

The following day, she developed sudden onset of shaking of her right (dominant) arm after drinking her morning coffee. The tremor has fluctuated in intensity since this time, but it has never disappeared completely. The tremor is reported to be worse when she is tired; on "bad days" it is reported to affect both the right and left arms. She is unable to suppress the tremor voluntarily. She and her husband report that symptoms are present to some degree the whole day but subside during sleep. The tremor sometimes interferes with the patient's ability to care for her baby, thus she has needed the help of her husband and her mother. She has not noticed improvement with alcohol consumption, and has had unsuccessful trials with propranolol and clonazepam. She denies a family history of tremor. She has no past history of psychiatric, neurologic or functional somatic disorders. She reports mild stress incontinence since the delivery and 3-month history of intermittent dizziness. MRI of the brain performed 1 month before her initial presentation was reported as normal. She denied feeling anxious or depressed, although she endorsed feeling worried about her health and her future. She was also concerned about being unable to adequately care for her child on her own and about being unable to return to her job.

On examination, she exhibited tremor of the right arm at rest, with posture, and with voluntary movements; tremor amplitude was similar at rest, with posture and with action. The tremor interfered with writing and drawing spirals with her right hand. While drawing spirals with her left hand, her right hand tremor stopped. There

Supplementary Information The online version contains supplementary material available at [https://doi.org/10.1007/978-3-030-86495-8_6].

P. Schwingenschuh (✉)
Department of Neurology, Medical University of Graz, Graz, Austria
e-mail: petra.schwingenschuh@medunigraz.at

was no clear distractibility of her right hand tremor during mental distraction maneuvers such as counting backwards or performing simple arithmetic. Concentrating on the tremor resulted in increased tremor amplitude. Tremor fluctuated between flexion-extension and pronation-supination patterns. Tapping as fast as possible with the thumb and fingers III, V, II, and IV in subsequent order with the left hand induced breaks in the contralateral upper limb tremor. When instructed to tap to a slow rhythm with her left hand, the tremor of the right hand adopted this new rhythm and at times ceased altogether. The remainder of the neurological examination was normal.

Tremor recordings showed a 5 Hz tremor of the right arm, with pauses during ballistic movements performed with the left arm. While tapping with the left hand to a metronome at a frequency of 3 Hz, the tremor of the right arm adopted the same frequency (entrainment).

In summary, this woman suffered from a tremor mainly affecting her right arm that began abruptly 5 days after the uncomplicated birth of her first son. Based on positive signs on history and clinical examination we made the diagnosis of functional tremor. When communicating the diagnosis, we demonstrated distractibility and entrainment to the patient and focused on the potential reversibility of her symptoms. This was reinforced during a follow-up appointment 4 weeks later. After her second visit, she endorsed acceptance of the diagnosis, and agreed to an intensive outpatient treatment plan and to psychiatric evaluation. She was referred for outpatient cognitive-behavioral therapy, specialist physiotherapy, and occupational therapy. At her follow-up appointment 3 months later, she reported a near-remission of her tremor and felt confident about her future.

Introduction

Tremor is defined as an involuntary, rhythmic, oscillatory movement of a body part and is classified along two axes, namely clinical characteristics and etiology. Axis 1 describes the classical

features of functional tremor such as sudden tremor onset, fluctuating course, inconsistency of symptoms and variable features [3]. A differentiation between involuntary tremor, like functional tremor, and voluntary tremor, like malingering, is made. Their differentiation remains difficult, but malingering is considered uncommon in clinical practice [1].

Functional tremor is the most commonly reported functional movement disorder (FMD), accounting for more than 50% of patients in published cohorts [4]. There is a large variability in the reported incidence of functional tremor, ranging from a rare disorder to 11% of all tremor referrals to a movement disorder clinic [4, 7].

At the present time, there is no gold standard for diagnosis of functional tremor apart from clinical criteria [3, 16]; as a result, many patients undergo a large number of diagnostic and therapeutic procedures until the final diagnosis is established. The importance of making a positive diagnosis based upon findings on neurological examination has been repeatedly emphasized [7, 10, 20, 48].

When making a diagnosis of a functional tremor the overall clinical picture needs to be taken into consideration. There are several features of the history, positive signs on physical examination and electrophysiological testing that help make the diagnosis (see Table 6.1) [48].

Approach to Diagnosis: Clues from the History

Tremor Onset

The history of the patient's complaints frequently reveals important information. Patients often present with a history of sudden tremor onset, sometimes even within seconds to minutes. Similar to the patient described in this chapter, patients with functional tremor can often provide the exact day, time and circumstances of tremor onset. In many patients symptoms start with maximal intensity.

Many patients describe physical events that precede the onset of functional symptoms.

Table 6.1 Characteristics of functional tremor

Clues from the history:

Sudden onset of the condition

Precipitating factors (e.g. a physical trauma)

Remissions

Variability of symptoms over time

Psychological comorbidity

Other functional symptoms and unspecific symptoms such as pain and fatigue

Clinical examination and positive signs:

Unusual clinical combinations of rest, postural and kinetic tremors

Increased attention toward the affected limb

Change or even suppression of tremor during distraction (distractability)

Shift of tremor frequency to contralateral voluntary tapping frequency (entrainability)

Variability of tremor phenomenology

Suggestibility

Presence of the "whack-a-mole" sign (suppression of the tremulous body part leads to reemergence or worsening of tremor in another body part)

Co-contraction

Excessive exhaustion during examination or "La belle indifference"

Appearance of additional and unrelated functional neurologic signs

Physical trauma is regarded as a very common precipitating factor [53]. Other common precipitating physical events include surgery (as in the case described here), infections, drug reactions or other illnesses [44]. Physical triggers may play an important role in symptom development by providing initial sensory data, which along with psychological factors such as panic, might drive subsequent functional symptoms [44]. It is of course important to keep in mind that these triggers are not always readily identifiable in patients with functional tremor. Similarly, when present, these features do not exclude the presence of another neurological disorder. In addition, functional overlay in movement disorders is not rare and neurological disorders such as Parkinson's disease are regarded as risk factors for functional neurological symptoms [22].

The onset of functional tremor may be temporally related to a stressful life event, but very often an association to a psychological stressor is unable to be identified. It is thus important not to insist on heightened stress levels when caring for patients with FMD [33].

Variability Over Time

The patient in the above clinical vignette describes having good and bad days. Such variability in tremor severity is another characteristic of functional tremor, with some patients experiencing full remissions in between episodes of tremor. In other patients, the disease course can be rather static. Rarely, functional tremor presents as a paroxysmal movement disorder [17]. Variability of the affected body parts is commonly reported [7, 10, 25].

Discrepancy Between Subjective and Objective Symptoms

Taking the patient's history can sometimes reveal a mismatch between impairment and reported level of disability. Patients with functional tremor may overestimate their daily tremor duration, thus a history from a caregiver is useful. One study using actigraphy and patient self-report to compare duration and severity of tremor in a real-life ambulatory setting in patients with functional and neurogenic tremor found that patients with functional tremor dramatically overestimated their tremor duration [43].

The pathophysiology of this mismatch between the patient's actual versus perceived tremor duration and tremor severity is only partly understood. Important roles are attributed to altered attention, abnormal predictions and expectations related to the symptoms, and an abnormal sense of agency [11, 34]. These pathophysiological features might lead to altered symptom perception in patients with functional tremor, resulting in the observed discrepancy between self-reported symptoms and objective recordings. In contrast to the findings of the study described above [43], a recent validation study using wrist-worn accelerometry and patient self-report found that patients with functional tremor had a similar association between subjective and objective tremor symptoms as patients with other types of tremor [28].

Other Functional Symptoms

Careful history often reveals multiple other functional neurological symptoms (e.g. weakness, seizures or sensory symptoms) and less specific symptoms such as generalized fatigue, nonspecific pain, memory disturbance and impaired vision [4]. In some patients a history or the presence of other functional symptoms, such as bladder problems or changes in speech and gait can be diagnostic clues. Patients may have past or present psychological comorbidity, especially depression, anxiety, panic, or post-traumatic stress disorder. A history of unresponsiveness to medications, response to placebos, and remission with psychotherapy may also be present.

It is important to keep in mind that the neurological examination begins when a patient enters the room. History-taking provides a good opportunity to start the examination by observing the tremor and its variability and distractibility during spontaneous speech and behavior.

Approach to Diagnosis: Clinical Examination and Positive Signs

Symptom Patterns

Distinguishing between functional tremor and other types of tremor requires a careful clinical examination by a neurologist or neuropsychiatrist experienced in movement disorders. Functional tremor often presents with a complex clinical presentation and marked variability in tremor phenomenology can often be observed within one consultation [31].

Most patients suffer from a tremor of the hands and arms. Functional upper limb tremor may present as rest, postural, or kinetic tremor and commonly is present in all three conditions. While most other etiologies for tremor present with either predominant action or predominant resting tremor, functional tremors often have

similar tremor amplitude in all three conditions. In bilateral tremors synchronous movements are characteristic [48].

Other body parts frequently affected include the head, legs, and the trunk [7, 10, 25]. Some patients present with a tremor while standing [7]. The lower limbs can be involved in a variety of tremor disorders. However, if tremor of the lower limbs occurs in essential tremor, Parkinson's disease or dystonic tremor, it is usually associated with a longer disease duration. A whole body distribution involving the lower limbs at the initial onset of symptoms is another possible clue to the diagnosis of functional tremor [47].

Facial functional tremors are uncommon. However, it is now thought that many cases of essential palatal tremor represent a FMD. Essential palatal tremor presents with the symptom of an ear click, mostly attributed to rhythmic 0.5–3 Hz palatal movements produced by contractions of the tensor veli palatini. Other throat muscles may be involved, but there are no additional neurological abnormalities. Magnetic resonance imaging of the inferior olives is normal, and extremity or eye muscles are not involved [8]. A functional neurological origin has been supported by the fact that the movements in many of these cases are incongruous, variable, entrainable, and distractible on electromyographic recordings [52]. Recently, combined electroencephalography and electromyography with time-locked video recordings has been suggested as another useful tool supporting the FMD origin in a patient diagnosed with essential palatal tremor [58]. In contrast to this, symptomatic palatal tremor usually does not present with an ear click and involves the levator veli palatini and other muscles innervated by brainstem nuclei (eye movements, face) or spinal motoneurons (trunk and extremity tremor) and often is accompanied by ataxia. Symptomatic palatal tremor is usually caused by a lesion in the dentato-olivary pathway and MRI usually reveals olivary pseudohypertrophy [8].

Role of Attention

The patient described in the clinical vignette at the beginning of this chapter exhibited an increase in tremor severity with increased attention. Indeed, simple observation of patients with functional tremor has revealed excessive attention to their affected limbs and to movements of these limbs during examination compared to patients with other etiologies of tremor [57]. In concordance with this clinical observation, functional imaging studies FMD have reported increased activity in areas associated with "self-monitoring" [2, 6]. Visual attention to the limb may be a marker of explicit control of movement, usually seen during the performance of novel tasks [60]. Sometimes focused attention causes re-emergence of the functional tremor if previously absent.

Distractability

Distraction of attention away from the affected limb forms the basis for most of the clinical tests used to diagnose functional tremor [12]. Typically, tremor dramatically improves, subsides, or changes frequency and amplitude during distraction tasks. In some patients such distractibility of the tremor may already become obvious by simple inspection of the tremor during history-taking or during standard neurological examination.

Distraction tasks can be cognitive or motor. Cognitive distraction maneuvers may include mental arithmetic (counting backwards from 100, serial sevens, etc.), listing days of the week or months of the year in reverse order, or recognizing a number drawn on the dorsum of the contralateral hand by the examiner's finger.

Motor distraction tasks need to be adapted based upon the tremor distribution. In clinical practice, the most frequently used distraction task to assess for functional arm tremor is the sequential finger tapping method (see Video 6.1). The patient is asked to tap with the thumb and fingers II, III, IV, and V in subsequent order. The difficulty level is subsequently raised by instructing the patient to change the tempo of the task. Finally, the patient is instructed to perform complex tapping sequences. The tremor of the contralateral hand is simultaneously observed to assess for distractibility. Finger-to nose-test with a mov-

ing target performed with the contralateral hand may also help to reveal distractibility of the tremor. Additionally, patients may be asked to perform sudden ballistic movements with the contralateral upper limb; in the case of functional tremor this may trigger a brief pause in tremor.

Some patients describe other maneuvers that induce amelioration or exacerbation of their symptoms. The patient should be asked to demonstrate this. For example, a patient may have noticed that being touched at a certain trigger point may induce exacerbation of tremor. Other patients may mention that listening to a certain song can stop the tremor.

Importantly, distraction maneuvers can only be successful when they sufficiently reduce the attention directed towards the tremulous limb. Before establishing that a tremor is unable to be distracted, the level of difficulty and the type of distraction task may need to be adapted. The "difficulty level" required for distraction tasks may vary from patient to patient. Additionally, tremor in different body parts warrants different distracters. Appropriate maneuvers for the lower limbs include foot tapping tasks or drawing on the floor with the contralateral foot. For head tremor, a task using repetitive eye or tongue movements may be helpful [48].

An unexplained poor performance on tasks of distraction while the functional tremor is maintained may be suggestive of functional tremor [48].

While distractibility is a prominent feature of functional tremors, in some patients with functional tremor distractibility cannot be demonstrated on clinical grounds, even when an appropriate examination maneuver is used. Functional tremor should not necessarily be excluded when a tremor is unable to be distracted [7].

Entrainability

In addition to demonstrating motor distraction, finger tapping at a given frequency can also be used to demonstrate entrainment, which represents another clinical hallmark of functional tremor. The patient is asked to tap voluntarily at various frequencies set by the examiner with a body part unaffected or less affected by tremor; the patient may, for example, be instructed to tap with a finger on a table at a given frequency. Entrainment occurs if the tremor adapts the same frequency (or a harmonic of this frequency) as the contralateral movements (see Video 6.1).

Variability

Variability is another red flag suggestive of functional tremor. This variability can present as a change in frequency, amplitude, direction (e.g. changing from pronation/supination to flexion/extension pattern), or as fluctuation of anatomic tremor distribution. Such tremor variability may occur spontaneously or only become obvious with a change in the level of attention towards the tremor [4].

However, it is important to recognize that tremor variability does not necessarily indicate functional tremor. Tremor secondary to other etiologies may also exhibit variable amplitude influenced by the level of anxiety and exhaustion, may be position-dependent, or may appear irregular in rhythm and may change direction (e.g. in the case of a dystonic tremor) [56].

Coactivation Sign

Functional tremors may show a "coactivation sign", i.e. some underlying antagonistic muscle activation whenever their tremor is present. If the increased muscle tone disappears, the tremor disappears too. This is demonstrated during slow, arrhythmic, passive movements, for example during assessment of tone. In functional tremor, fluctuations of muscle tone may be observed [7, 48].

Suggestibility

Some functional tremors are suggestible and may vary in response to certain stimuli. Suggestibility may be assessed with application of a vibrating

tuning fork to the affected body part, or application of pressure to a certain "trigger point" with the examiner's finger. This is performed while suggesting that the stimulus may reduce the symptoms [20, 56]. Of note, care must be taken when using suggestion as an exam maneuver as this may affect the physician-patient relationship.

"Whack-a-Mole" Sign

Tremor suppression in one body part by the examiner may cause an immediate appearance of tremor in another body part. If present, this "whack-a-mole" sign is regarded as another positive physical sign and diagnostic maneuver in patients with FMD [45].

Excessive Exhaustion or "La belle Indifference"

In patients with functional tremor voluntary movements can appear to be slow throughout the performance of rapid repetitive and alternating movements, albeit without the fatiguing and decreasing amplitude or the typical arrests that are seen in Parkinson's disease [32]. Some patients with functional tremor seem to struggle and put more effort than needed to perform the tasks. During examination they may demonstrate exhaustion and excessive fatigue and may use their whole body in order to perform a minor movement [4, 56]. Other patients with functional tremor may disregard their symptoms despite showing severe tremor on examination ("la belle indifference").

Other Functional Neurological Signs

Sometimes functional tremor may present as part of a mixed FMD or a mixed functional neurologic disorder. Patients may show other functional symptoms and signs including give-away weakness, functional gait disorder, non-anatomical sensory loss, or convergence spasm and other dysconjugate oculomotor abnormalities [20, 56].

It is important to keep in mind that the presence of other functional neurological signs does not confirm that the tremor itself is functional. It is possible for a patient with tremor secondary to another etiology, such as a parkinsonian tremor, to exhibit other functional features as well [48].

One clinical study has systematically compared the effects of various provocative tests on patients with essential tremor and functional tremor using a standardized protocol [24]. Functional tremor was able to be differentiated from essential tremor on the basis of negative family history, sudden onset, spontaneous remission, shorter duration of tremor, suggestibility, and distractibility. Interestingly, entrainment was not frequently seen in either tremor type. However, the method used to evaluate entrainment in this study (10 s of wrist extension and flexion in the unaffected arm) is probably not an adequate assessment of this feature [20].

Electrophysiology: The Role for Tremor Recordings

Clinical assessment remains the most important aspect in evaluating patients with functional tremor and in many patients a confident diagnosis can be made on the basis of clinical criteria alone. In some patients, however, the diagnosis may be more challenging. In these cases, electrophysiological characterization can provide a useful method to complement the history and physical exam, providing additional objective, reproducible, and diagnostic information [59]. The development of laboratory-supported criteria for functional tremor support this important diagnostic role [19, 20, 49, 50].

Standard Equipment

Tremor recordings require two accelerometers, a four-channel electromyography, a metronome, and a 500-g weight. Metronomes are easily accessible, and available as online tools and apps. Hand tremor is recorded at rest, at posture (with and without weight loading), and during move-ment. Recorded signals are analyzed in the time and frequency domains [50, 59].

A variety of electrophysiologic techniques have been proposed as useful in distinguishing functional tremor from other types of tremor. These are mainly used to demonstrate the same clues that are assessed during clinical examination, namely entrainability, distractability, co-contraction, and synchronicity [5, 21, 48, 59].

Entrainability and Distractability

Functional tremor may entrain at the frequency at which the patient is tapping, with significant coherence between the EMG spectra of the tremulous extremity and the tapping extremity at the tapping frequency [35, 49, 50]. It is important for tapping to be performed at a low amplitude to reduce the likelihood of mechanical transmission between the limbs, which could erroneously be reported as coherence. For the same reason, the coherence is calculated between EMG channels and not between accelerometers [59]. More common than true entrainment is a significant absolute change in tremor frequency and marked intraindividual variability with tapping [49, 61].

Less accurate tapping performance at requested frequencies is also considered suggestive of a functional etiology. Thus, it is mandatory to record the patient's tapping performance, in addition to recording the tremor [49, 50, 61].

If the original tremor frequency peak persists and is accompanied by a new tremor peak at the frequency of the tapping, this finding can correspond to a mirror movement and should not be confused with entrainment. Mirror movements are involuntary movements of homologous muscles during voluntary movements of contralateral body regions. While subtle mirror movements can occur in otherwise healthy adults, overt mirror movements are common in many movement disorders such as Parkinson's disease [36].

In the ballistic movement test the patient is asked to perform a quick movement with one hand, for example, a fast wrist extension. In contrast to tremor seen in essential tremor and Parkinson's disease, functional tremor transiently stops during ballistic contralateral hand movement [29, 49].

Other signs that may be observed in functional tremor include irregularities in the tremor frequency and amplitude, and an increase in tremor amplitude when weights are added to the limb [42, 49, 61].

Co-contraction

The electrophysiological equivalent of the clinical "coactivation sign" is a short (i.e., 300 ms) tonic coactivation phase on EMG before the onset of tremor bursts [7, 49].

Synchronicity

With the exception of orthostatic tremor, most patients with bilateral neurogenic tremor have independent tremor rhythms in different extremities. In contrast, approximately half of patients with functional tremor exhibit significant tremor coherence between the two hands [46, 49]. Recently, the percentage of time with significant coherence and the number of periods without significant coherence, as detected by wavelet coherence analysis, were suggested as useful parameters in discriminating functional tremor from other types of tremor [27]. Two possible mechanisms that have been suggested to underlie noncoherent functional

tremor include a clonus mechanism and presence of an "overtrained" tremor that runs automatically and is not perturbed by another voluntary movement [21, 46].

Test Battery

A simple test battery consisting of tremor recordings at rest, posture (with and without weight loading), action, while performing tapping tasks (1, 3, and 5 Hz), and while performing ballistic movements with the less-affected hand was able to distinguish functional tremor from other types of tremor with excellent sensitivity and specificity. Tonic muscular co-activation, tremor coherence, pause in tremor with contralateral ballistic movement, increased tremor frequency with weight loading, and incorrect tapping performance to a given frequency were regarded as positive functional signs (see Table 6.2) [49]. A score of at least 3 out of 10 points indicates a functional tremor. The test battery was validated in a prospective study including 40 patients with functional upper limb tremor and 72 patients with tremors of other etiologies, and had good sensitivity (89.5%), specificity (95.9%), and inter-rater reliability. This test battery may allow an earlier "confident" diagnosis of functional tremor in the setting of clinical diagnostic uncertainty, impacting the overall prognosis [18, 50]. In patients in whom the clinical diagnosis of a functional tremor is more obvious, the test battery can still provide

Table 6.2 Test battery

Task	Positive feature	Score
Tapping task at 1 Hz	Incorrect tapping performance	1 point
Tapping task at 3 Hz	Incorrect tapping performance	1 point
Tapping task at 5 Hz	Incorrect tapping performance	1 point
Contralateral tapping at 1, 3, and 5 Hz	Tremor suppression, pathological frequency shift or entrainment of tremor	1–3 points
Contralateral ballistic movement task	Tremor interruption	1 point
Tremor onset	Tonic coactivation	1 point
Bilateral tremors	Coherence	1 point
Loading with a weight	Increased postural tremor amplitude	1 point
Sum score		Maximum of 10 points

Reprinted from Schwingenschuh and Deuschl [48], with permission from Elsevier
Note that tapping and ballistic movement tasks are performed with the less affected hand; recordings are made from both arms; a sum score of at least three points indicates a functional tremor [49, 50]

objective evidence and help when conveying the diagnosis to a patient [50].

Management

Explanation/Education

Treatment starts with an explanation of the diagnosis, often aided by demonstration of functional exam findings, exploration of physical and psychological trigger factors and discussion of the potential for reversibility of symptoms [30]. Sharing positive clinical signs such as tremor entrainment or distractability illustrates how the diagnosis is made, and provides a powerful means of establishing a patient's confidence in the diagnosis as illustrated in the chapter's clinical vignette [54]. Visualized electrophysiological data can also be used as an objective tool to demonstrate how the diagnosis was made [50]. If present, the "whack-a-mole" sign can be described to patients as evidence in support of a "software" problem involving broader networks, as opposed to a "hardware" problem affecting a particular anatomical location [45].

There is increasing evidence for benefits of physical, occupational, as well as psychotherapeutic interventions, with treatment being tailored to individual symptoms and comorbidities [30]. Most prior treatment studies have included patients with mixed FMD. Only few treatment studies have focused on patients with functional tremor and will therefore be mentioned here along with studies that detailed the number of functional tremor patients in their mixed cohorts.

Physiotherapy

There is growing evidence that physiotherapy is an effective treatment for patients with FMD. A prospective uncontrolled study in 47 patients with functional tremor ($n = 9$) and other functional motor symptoms first provided evidence to support the use of specialist physiotherapy treatment in these patients [39]. These findings were supported by a subsequent randomized feasibility

trial that compared 5-day specialist physiotherapy to treatment as usual in 57 patients with functional motor symptoms (9 patients had a functional tremor). At 6 months, 72% of the intervention group rated their symptoms as improved, compared to 18% in the control group [38]. A larger randomized controlled trial of physical-based rehabilitation aiming to recruit 264 patients with a clinically definite diagnosis of functional motor disorders (Physio4FMD) is underway [40].

The intervention used in the above-mentioned trials uses a "movement retraining" model based on the consensus recommendation paper on physiotherapy for FMD [41]. The approach includes reducing abnormal self-directed attention by distraction techniques and breaking down learned patterns of abnormal movement to then retrain normal patterns, but recognizes the importance of education and entwining psychological approaches. A starting point for physiotherapy may be helping the patient to develop strategies to control or stop the tremor. Therefore, patients are instructed to actively produce a tremor, then increase the amplitude and decrease the frequency, and finally slow the movement to stillness. The patient can learn how the tremor can be stopped during distraction by performing competing movements (e.g. clapping to a rhythm or performing a large flowing movement of the symptomatic arm as if conducting an orchestra) [41]. These strategies can help patients develop a sense of control over movement without using potentially unhelpful passive coping strategies. Visual feedback from a mirror can be helpful in establishing control [41].

Physiotherapy should discourage habitual postures and movement patterns which can make the tremors worse. Functional tremor of the lower limbs is often triggered by a clonus mechanism when the patient sits with forefoot contact with the floor. Changing lower limb posture so the heel and forefoot have floor contact can stop the movement. Sometimes patients try to control a functional tremor by increasing the tension in their muscles, which may actually worsen the tremor. Therefore, patients often benefit if they learn how to relax their muscles. EMG feedback targeting muscles proximal to the tremor may help to reduce unhelpful attention to the tremulous limb [41].

Retrainment

Ten patients with functional tremor were included in an uncontrolled clinical trial investigating the efficacy of tremor retrainment. Retrainment was facilitated by tactile and auditory external cueing and real-time visual feedback on a computer screen. The primary outcome measure was the Tremor subscale of the Rating Scale for Psychogenic Movement Disorders. Functional tremor significantly improved at the end of retrainment. The benefits were maintained for at least 1 week and up to 6 months in 6 patients, with relapses occurring in 4 patients between 2 weeks and 6 months. Three subjects achieved tremor freedom [14]. The therapeutic use of retrainment strategies as adjunctive to psychotherapy or specialized physical therapy should be tested in larger studies.

Botulinum Toxin

Botulinum neurotoxin (BoNT) has also been evaluated for possible therapeutic role. In 48 patients with chronic jerky and tremulous FMD the effect of botulinum neurotoxin (BoNT) was assessed in a double-blind, randomized placebo-controlled trial with an open-label extension phase. Patients were assigned to two subsequent treatments with BoNT or placebo every 3 months with stratification according to symptom localization. Subsequently all patients were treated with BoNT in a 10 month open-label phase. The authors found no evidence of improved outcomes in patients treated with BoNT compared with placebo. The response to placebo, however, was very large. Interestingly, despite symptom improvement, there was no change in quality of life and disability [9].

Psychological Therapies

Cognitive behavioral therapy (CBT): CBT has been suggested as a useful tool in management of patients with FMD. In one recent study, 15 patients with functional tremor underwent 12 weeks of cognitive behavioral therapy (CBT), with before and after functional MRI (fMRI). Tremor severity improved significantly in 73% of patients after CBT and was associated with changes in anterior cingulate/paracingulate activity, which may represent a marker of emotional dysregulation in functional tremor as well as a predictor of treatment response. The lack of a control group and long-term follow-up were limiting factors [15].

Psychodynamic psychotherapy: In a small prospective trial on ten patients with FMD (eight had functional tremor), 3 months of weekly psychodynamic psychotherapy with adjunctive psychiatric medication significantly improved the FMD [23]. However, a randomized, cross-over design trial including 15 patients with FMD (6 patients with functional tremor) did not show a significant difference between psychodynamic psychotherapy versus neurological observation [26]. Patients with good insight and receptive of diagnosis might have the greatest likelihood for response to psychodynamic psychotherapy [51].

Hypnosis: In a randomized controlled trial including 45 patients with functional motor disorder (7 had functional tremor) who received a comprehensive 8-week inpatient treatment, the authors found no additional effect of hypnosis [37].

Transcranial Magnetic Stimulation

Recently, the effect of five consecutive daily sessions of active versus sham repetitive transcranial magnetic stimulation (rTMS) delivered over the primary motor cortex at a rate of 1 Hz was compared in a randomized, double-blind, parallel-armed controlled study including 18 patients with functional tremor. The study used validated rTMS parameters that are known to induce long-lasting inhibitory changes in motor cortex excitability. In a second open-label phase all patients underwent hypnosis combined with single sessions of active rTMS. In the active group, the mean Psychogenic Movement Disorder Rating Scale scores were significantly decreased after 1 and 2 months, with benefit maintained at months 6 and 12. In the sham group, a non-significant improvement was observed after 1 month, but scores had returned almost to its baseline by month 2 and remained unchanged at months 6 and 12. The authors concluded that the stronger and longer benefit observed in the active rTMS group may represent preliminary evidence of rTMS-induced neuromodulation of the motor cortex involving long-term depression-like synaptic plasticity mechanisms [55]. Although the addition of hypnosis in an open-label phase of the study may have been a confounding factor, further research in this area is of interest to test pathways involved in symptom genesis and identify new treatment targets [30]. This fits in with broader testing, with promising, but preliminary data, in other motor functional neurological disorders (see Chap. 28 for more details on the role of TMS).

Multidisciplinary Treatment Approaches

Multidisciplinary treatment is a common treatment approach for patients with functional tremor. The development of a patient-centered treatment plan benefits from interdisciplinary neurologic, psychiatric, allied mental health and rehabilitation perspectives. Comorbid mood disorders may be treated pharmacologically. The use of anti-tremor medication is not appropriate. Patients who have been severely or chronically impaired may benefit from intense inpatient treatment programs. However, clinical studies are needed to guide development of evidence-based treatment recommendations and determine the best setting, frequency, intensity, and length of interventions [13, 30].

For additional details regarding the treatment of patients with functional tremor see Part III of this book.

Conclusion

Functional tremor is a common and disabling movement disorder. It is diagnosed based on characteristic clues from history and positive features on clinical examination. In difficult cases, tremor recordings can be useful to differentiate functional tremor from other tremor disorders. There is growing evidence for effective treatment strategies for these patients, however large randomized controlled studies comparing and combining different treatment modalities and measuring long-term effects are needed.

Summary
- Functional tremor is the most common functional movement disorder.
- Diagnosis of functional tremor relies on positive signs on history and physical examination.
- Clues from the clinical examination include the presence of distractibility, entrainability, and variability in tremor frequency, axis, and/or topographical distribution.
- Sharing these clinical signs with the patient can provide a powerful means of establishing a patient's confidence in the diagnosis.
- If features of distractibility, entrainability and/or tremor variability are not clinically overt, electrophysiology can support an early positive diagnosis.

References

1. Bartl M, Kewitsch R, Hallett M, Tegenthoff M, Paulus W. Diagnosis and therapy of functional tremor a systematic review illustrated by a case report. Neurol Res Pract. 2020;2:35.
2. Bell V, Oakley DA, Halligan PW, Deeley Q. Dissociation in hysteria and hypnosis: evidence

from cognitive neuroscience. J Neurol Neurosurg Psychiatry. 2011;82(3):332–9.

3. Bhatia KP, Bain P, Bajaj N, Elble RJ, Hallett M, Louis ED, Raethjen J, Stamelou M, Testa CM, Deuschl G, Tremor Task Force of the International Parkinson and Movement Disorder Society. Consensus Statement on the classification of tremors. from the task force on tremor of the International Parkinson and Movement Disorder Society. Mov Disord. 2018;33(1):75–87.

4. Bhatia KP, Schneider SA. Psychogenic tremor and related disorders. J Neurol. 2007;254(5):569–74.

5. Brown P, Thompson PD. Electrophysiological aids to the diagnosis of psychogenic jerks, spasms, and tremor. Mov Disord. 2001;16(4):595–9.

6. de Lange FP, Roelofs K, Toni I. Increased self-monitoring during imagined movements in conversion paralysis. Neuropsychologia. 2007;45(9):2051–8.

7. Deuschl G, Koster B, Lucking CH, Scheidt C. Diagnostic and pathophysiological aspects of psychogenic tremors. Mov Disord. 1998;13(2):294–302.

8. Deuschl G, Toro C, Valls-Sole J, Zeffiro T, Zee DS, Hallett M. Symptomatic and essential palatal tremor. 1. Clinical, physiological and MRI analysis. Brain. 1994;117(Pt 4):775–88.

9. Dreissen YEM, Dijk JM, Gelauff JM, Zoons E, van Poppelen D, Contarino MF, Zutt R, Post B, Munts AG, Speelman JD, Cath DC, de Haan RJ, Koelman JH, Tijssen MAJ. Botulinum neurotoxin treatment in jerky and tremulous functional movement disorders: a double-blind, randomised placebo-controlled trial with an open-label extension. J Neurol Neurosurg Psychiatry. 2019;90(11):1244–50.

10. Edwards MJ, Bhatia KP. Functional (psychogenic) movement disorders: merging mind and brain. Lancet Neurol. 2012;11(3):250–60.

11. Edwards MJ, Fotopoulou A, Parees I. Neurobiology of functional (psychogenic) movement disorders. Curr Opin Neurol. 2013;26(4):442–7.

12. Edwards MJ, Schrag A. Hyperkinetic psychogenic movement disorders. Handb Clin Neurol. 2011;100:719–29.

13. Espay AJ, Aybek S, Carson A, Edwards MJ, Goldstein LH, Hallett M, LaFaver K, LaFrance WC Jr, Lang AE, Nicholson T, Nielsen G, Reuber M, Voon V, Stone J, Morgante F. Current concepts in diagnosis and treatment of functional neurological disorders. JAMA Neurol. 2018;75(9):1132–41.

14. Espay AJ, Edwards MJ, Oggioni GD, Phielipp N, Cox B, Gonzalez-Usigli H, Pecina C, Heldman DA, Mishra J, Lang AE. Tremor retrainment as therapeutic strategy in psychogenic (functional) tremor. Parkinsonism Relat Disord. 2014;20(6):647–50.

15. Espay AJ, Ries S, Maloney T, Vannest J, Neefus E, Dwivedi AK, Allendorfer JB, Wulsin LR, LaFrance WC, Lang AE, Szaflarski JP. Clinical and neural responses to cognitive behavioral therapy for functional tremor. Neurology. 2019;93(19):e1787–98.

16. Fahn S, Williams DT. Psychogenic dystonia. Adv Neurol. 1988;50:431–55.

17. Ganos C, Aguirregomozcorta M, Batla A, Stamelou M, Schwingenschuh P, Munchau A, Edwards MJ, Bhatia KP. Psychogenic paroxysmal movement disorders--clinical features and diagnostic clues. Parkinsonism Relat Disord. 2014;20(1):41–6.

18. Gelauff J, Stone J, Edwards M, Carson A. The prognosis of functional (psychogenic) motor symptoms: a systematic review. J Neurol Neurosurg Psychiatry. 2014;85(2):220–6.

19. Gironell A. Routine neurophysiology testing and functional tremor: toward the establishment of diagnostic criteria. Mov Disord. 2016;31(11):1763–4.

20. Gupta A, Lang AE. Psychogenic movement disorders. Curr Opin Neurol. 2009;22(4):430–6.

21. Hallett M. Physiology of psychogenic movement disorders. J Clin Neurosci. 2010;17(8):959–65.

22. Hallett M. Patients with Parkinson disease are prone to functional neurological disorders. J Neurol Neurosurg Psychiatry. 2018;89(6):557.

23. Hinson VK, Weinstein S, Bernard B, Leurgans SE, Goetz CG. Single-blind clinical trial of psychotherapy for treatment of psychogenic movement disorders. Parkinsonism Relat Disord. 2006;12(3):177–80.

24. Kenney C, Diamond A, Mejia N, Davidson A, Hunter C, Jankovic J. Distinguishing psychogenic and essential tremor. J Neurol Sci. 2007;263(1-2):94–9.

25. Koller W, Lang A, Vetere-Overfield B, Findley L, Cleeves L, Factor S, Singer C, Weiner W. Psychogenic tremors. Neurology. 1989;39(8):1094–9.

26. Kompoliti K, Wilson B, Stebbins G, Bernard B, Hinson V. Immediate vs. delayed treatment of psychogenic movement disorders with short term psychodynamic psychotherapy: randomized clinical trial. Parkinsonism Relat Disord. 2014;20(1):60–3.

27. Kramer G, Van der Stouwe AMM, Maurits NM, Tijssen MAJ, Elting JWJ. Wavelet coherence analysis: A new approach to distinguish organic and functional tremor types. Clin Neurophysiol. 2018;129(1):13–20.

28. Kramer G, Dominguez-Vega ZT, Laarhoven HS, Brandsma R, Smit M, van der Stouwe AM, Elting JWJ, Maurits NM, Rosmalen JG, Tijssen MA. Similar association between objective and subjective symptoms in functional and organic tremor. Parkinsonism Relat Disord. 2019;64:2–7.

29. Kumru H, Valls-Sole J, Valldeoriola F, Marti MJ, Sanegre MT, Tolosa E. Transient arrest of psychogenic tremor induced by contralateral ballistic movements. Neurosci Lett. 2004;370(2–3):135–9.

30. LaFaver K. Treatment of functional movement disorders. Neurol Clin. 2020;38(2):469–80.

31. Lidstone SC, Lang AE. How do I examine patients with functional tremor? Mov Disord Clin Pract. 2020;7(5):587.

32. Lang AE, Koller WC, Fahn S. Psychogenic parkinsonism. Arch Neurol. 1995 Aug;52(8):802–10.

33. Maurer CW, LaFaver K, Ameli R, Toledo R, Hallett M. A biological measure of stress levels in patients with functional movement disorders. Parkinsonism Relat Disord. 2015;21(9):1072–5.

34. Maurer CW, LaFaver K, Ameli R, Epstein SA, Hallett M, Horovitz SG. Impaired self-agency in functional

movement disorders: a resting-state fMRI study. Neurology. 2016;87(6):564–70.

35. McAuley J, Rothwell J. Identification of psychogenic, dystonic, and other organic tremors by a coherence entrainment test. Mov Disord. 2004;19(3):253–67.

36. Merchant SH, Haubenberger D, Hallett M. Mirror movements or functional tremor masking organic tremor. Clin Neurophysiol Pract. 2018;15;3:107–113.

37. Moene FC, Spinhoven P, Hoogduin KA, van Dyck R. A randomised controlled clinical trial on the additional effect of hypnosis in a comprehensive treatment programme for in-patients with conversion disorder of the motor type. Psychother Psychosom. 2002;71(2):66–76.

38. Nielsen G, Buszewicz M, Stevenson F, Hunter R, Holt K, Dudziec M, Ricciardi L, Marsden J, Joyce E, Edwards MJ. Randomised feasibility study of physiotherapy for patients with functional motor symptoms. J Neurol Neurosurg Psychiatry. 2017;88(6):484–90.

39. Nielsen G, Ricciardi L, Demartini B, Hunter R, Joyce E, Edwards MJ. Outcomes of a 5-day physiotherapy programme for functional (psychogenic) motor disorders. J Neurol. 2015a;262(3):674–81.

40. Nielsen G, Stone J, Buszewicz M, Carson A, Goldstein LH, Holt K, Hunter R, Marsden J, Marston L, Noble H, Reuber M, Edwards MJ, Physio4FMD Collaborative Group. Physio4FMD: protocol for a multicentre randomised controlled trial of specialist physiotherapy for functional motor disorder. BMC Neurol. 2019;19(1):242.

41. Nielsen G, Stone J, Matthews A, Brown M, Sparkes C, Farmer R, Masterton L, Duncan L, Winters A, Daniell L, Lumsden C, Carson A, David AS, Edwards M. Physiotherapy for functional motor disorders: a consensus recommendation. J Neurol Neurosurg Psychiatry. 2015b;86(10):1113–9.

42. O'Suilleabhain PE, Matsumoto JY. Time-frequency analysis of tremors. Brain. 1998;121(Pt 11):2127–34.

43. Pareés I, Saifee TA, Kassavetis P, Kojovic M, Rubio-Agusti I, Rothwell JC, Bhatia KP, Edwards MJ. Believing is perceiving: mismatch between self-report and actigraphy in psychogenic tremor. Brain. 2012;135(Pt 1):117–23.

44. Parees I, Kojovic M, Pires C, Rubio-Agusti I, Saifee TA, Sadnicka A, Kassavetis P, Macerollo A, Bhatia KP, Carson A, Stone J, Edwards MJ. Physical precipitating factors in functional movement disorders. J Neurol Sci. 2014;338(1–2):174–7.

45. Park JE, Maurer CW, Hallett M. The "whack-a-mole" sign in functional movement disorders. Mov Disord Clin Pract. 2015;2(3):286–8.

46. Raethjen J, Kopper F, Govindan RB, Volkmann J, Deuschl G. Two different pathogenetic mechanisms in psychogenic tremor. Neurology. 2004;63(5):812–5.

47. Rajalingam R, Breen DP, Chen R, Fox S, Kalia LV, Munhoz RP, Slow E, Strafella AP, Lang AE, Fasano A. The clinical significance of lower limb tremors. Parkinsonism Relat Disord. 2019;65:165–71.

48. Schwingenschuh P, Deuschl G. Functional tremor. Handb Clin Neurol. 2016;139:229–33.

49. Schwingenschuh P, Katschnig P, Seiler S, Saifee TA, Aguirregomozcorta M, Cordivari C, Schmidt R, Rothwell JC, Bhatia KP, Edwards MJ. Moving toward "laboratory-supported" criteria for psychogenic tremor. Mov Disord. 2011;26(14):2509–15.

50. Schwingenschuh P, Saifee TA, Katschnig-Winter P, Macerollo A, Koegl-Wallner M, Culea V, Ghadery C, Hofer E, Pendl T, Seiler S, Werner U, Franthal S, Maurits NM, Tijssen MA, Schmidt R, Rothwell JC, Bhatia KP, Edwards MJ. Validation of "laboratory-supported" criteria for functional (psychogenic) tremor. Mov Disord. 2016;31(4):555–62.

51. Sharma VD, Jones R, Factor SA. Psychodynamic psychotherapy for functional (psychogenic) movement disorders. J Mov Disord. 2017;10(1):40–4.

52. Stamelou M, Saifee TA, Edwards MJ, Bhatia KP. Psychogenic palatal tremor may be underrecognized: reappraisal of a large series of cases. Mov Disord. 2012;27(9):1164–8.

53. Stone J, Carson A, Aditya H, Prescott R, Zaubi M, Warlow C, Sharpe M. The role of physical injury in motor and sensory conversion symptoms: a systematic and narrative review. J Psychosom Res. 2009;66(5):383–90.

54. Stone J, Edwards M. Trick or treat? Showing patients with functional (psychogenic) motor symptoms their physical signs. Neurology. 2012;79(3):282–4.

55. Taib S, Ory-Magne F, Brefel-Courbon C, Moreau Y, Thalamas C, Arbus C, Simonetta-Moreau M. Repetitive transcranial magnetic stimulation for functional tremor: a randomized, double-blind, controlled study. Mov Disord. 2019;34(8):1210–9.

56. Thenganatt MA, Jankovic J. Psychogenic tremor: a video guide to its distinguishing features. Tremor Other Hyperkinet Mov (N Y). 2014;4:253.

57. van Poppelen D, Saifee TA, Schwingenschuh P, Katschnig P, Bhatia KP, Tijssen MA, Edwards MJ. Attention to self in psychogenic tremor. Mov Disord. 2011;26(14):2575–6.

58. Vial F, Akano E, Attaripour S, McGurrin P, Hallett M. Electrophysiological evidence for functional (psychogenic) essential palatal tremor. Tremor Other Hyperkinet Mov (N Y). 2020;10:10.

59. Vial F, Kassavetis P, Merchant S, Haubenberger D, Hallett M. How to do an electrophysiological study of tremor. Clin Neurophysiol Pract. 2019;4:134–42.

60. Willingham DB. A neuropsychological theory of motor skill learning. Psychol Rev. 1998;105(3):558–84.

61. Zeuner KE, Shoge RO, Goldstein SR, Dambrosia JM, Hallett M. Accelerometry to distinguish psychogenic from essential or parkinsonian tremor. Neurology. 2003;61(4):548–50.

Functional Dystonia

7

Francesca Morgante

Case Vignette 1

A 19-year old girl was referred to the Movement Disorders Clinic because of involuntary turning of the head to the left beginning 2 years prior. She did not have a family history for movement disorders or any other neurological condition. Past medical history was negative, and she did not take medications or use any recreational drugs. She was a high-school student and sang in the church choir. She mentioned that when singing, her symptoms resolved.

*At initial examination (Video 7.1, **Segment A**), her head was turned and tilted to the left. She had difficulty in turning the head to the right and pain in the posterior cervical region. When singing or being engaged in arithmetic tasks, she had marked improvement of head posture. Speaking did not improve her symptoms. She was diagnosed with cervical dystonia and injected with botulinum toxin without any benefit, despite repeated ses-*

sions over the course of 1 year. We saw her again 4 years later for re-evaluation of a complex clinical picture. Indeed, over the years, she had developed marked disability with onset of severe gait and balance difficulties, involuntary jerky movements of all limbs (more prominent on the left side), and urinary retention. She had been assessed by several other movement disorders neurologists and undergone many hospital admissions and investigations, including brain magnetic resonance imaging, evoked potentials, nerve conduction studies, electromyography, laboratory investigations, and genetic testing for genetic dystonias. She had been previously evaluated by two psychiatrists who did not find any evidence of psychopathology or apparent life stressors. She received multiple diagnoses, including "generalized dystonia", "dystonia-ataxia syndrome", "young onset extrapyramidal disorder with spasticity", "spastic paraplegia plus", "stress disorder", and "medically unexplained disorder".

*At our neurological examination in 2013 (Video 7.1, **Segment B**), she was in a wheelchair and catheterized. She could walk for less than 5 meters only with support, had fixed posturing of the left foot, and weakness associated with stiffness in both lower limbs. Fixed posturing of the left foot improved when she was distracted by motor tasks other than walking. When lying down, she had a slow tremor affecting both legs that was more prominent on the left. She had fixed posturing of the head which was turned and*

Supplementary Information The online version contains supplementary material available at [https://doi.org/10.1007/978-3-030-86495-8_7].

F. Morgante (✉)
Neurosciences Research Centre, Molecular and Clinical Sciences Research Institute, St. George's University of London, London, UK

Department of Clinical and Experimental Medicine, University of Messina, Messina, Italy
e-mail: fmorgant@sgul.ac.uk

tilted to the left with associated left shoulder elevation. She could not turn her head to the right, but she could passively turn it using her hand pushing on her left cheek. When engaged in alternate repetitive movements with both arms, she did not have any overflow of dystonia, but rather her abnormal head posture improved and shortly resolved. On neuropsychiatric interview complemented with self-report measures, she only endorsed mild depression and denied anxiety.

We made the diagnosis of FMD with prominent functional dystonia based on the demonstration of positive signs, including variability and improvement with distraction. We discussed the diagnosis and showed her how neurological symptoms could be improved by shifting her attention. A multidisciplinary in-patient rehabilitation program for FMD[1] was suggested. She underwent 2-months of multidisciplinary rehabilitation involving neuro-physiotherapy focused on sensation and attention. The program also included occupational therapy and sessions with a psychologist aimed to regain confidence and autonomy. This program resulted in marked improvement (Video7.1, **Segment C**), with resolution of gait abnormality, urinary disturbances, and involuntary movements affecting the upper and lower limbs. At 2-month follow-up, she continued to have turning of the head to the left side and left shoulder elevation associated with pain in the left shoulder. At 1-year follow-up, she showed persistent improvement of gait, balance and head posture (Video 7.1, **Segment D**). Over the subsequent 2 years, she underwent three additional in-patient rehabilitation admissions for FMD, which resulted in further gains. After regaining functional independence, she started working as a tour guide and had a daughter. Periodically, she complained of increased pain and spasms in the left upper trapezius which were treated with a small dose of incobotulinumtoxinA (20 U). She also continued to practice at home the physiotherapy exercises prescribed by the multidisciplinary rehabilitation team.

Case Vignette 2

A 41-year woman presented with a 4-year history of abnormal posturing of the left lower limb compromising her ability to walk. Symptoms started with painful inversion of the left foot occurring soon after a lower back trauma due to a fall. Within 3 months from onset, she rapidly worsened and developed a severe gait disorder. At our consultation, she reported severe disability, reporting that she needed help to perform all activities of daily living. She had severe pain localized to the whole left lower limb and also reported concentration difficulties and "brain fog".

On examination, she was in a wheelchair, unable to stand up or walk. She had inversion of the left foot and flexion of all toes. There was resistance to passive extension of the left leg and hip. Passive manipulation of the left ankle and passive extension of the left leg evoked unbearable pain. Complete extension of the left lower limb was limited by intense pain. When the examination was performed with the patient's eyes closed, the left leg was able to be passively extended without pain (Video 7.2). On mental status examination, she performed normally on the Montreal Cognitive Assessment. She endorsed moderate depression. All laboratory tests and investigations were normal. Specifically, brain and spinal magnetic resonance imaging did not identify any structural abnormalities. Motor and somatosensory evoked potentials showed normal conduction times within the central nervous system. A diagnosis of functional dystonia was reached based on the presence of the following features: (1) acute onset; (2) rapid progression; (3) presence of fixed dystonic posturing affecting the foot; (4) release of fixed posture of the lower limb upon eye closure, which served as a distractive task; (5) absence of brain structural lesions justifying fixed dystonia; (6) absence of any other movement disorders (i.e. parkinsonism) or neurological signs (i.e. apraxia) which might have supported the diagnosis of fixed dystonia associated with a neurodegenerative disease.

Delivery of the diagnosis included a careful discussion of all the clinical features supporting the diagnosis of functional dystonia. We explained the role of minor trauma as a frequent precipitating (triggering) factor for this condition, yet we highlighted that the trauma was not causative of *her symptoms. A 1-month in-patient multidisciplinary rehabilitation program was started, and repeated four times over 2 years. This treatment strategy was not successful in improving her motor symptoms due to the interference of pain during the physiotherapy program. However, the multidisciplinary rehabilitation program aided improvement of her mood and greater diagnostic acceptance of her condition.*

Introduction

Functional movement disorder (FMD) may manifest with fixed postures and/or torsional repetitive movements that are consistent with the phenotype of functional dystonia [2]. This is one of the most common phenotypes of FMD, together with weakness and tremor [3, 4]. Functional dystonia is typically fixed [5] and affects the lower limb more often than the upper limb, commonly arising shortly after a minor peripheral injury. However, within the clinical spectrum of functional dystonia, multiple clinical manifestations are described including paroxysmal or continuous phasic movements as well as focal involvement of neck and facial muscles [6]. Misdiagnosis and delay in diagnosis is frequent due to lack of validated positive signs. Moreover, the complexity of motor manifestations of isolated genetic and idiopathic dystonias may complicate the differentiation of

functional dystonia from these other conditions, despite a few clinical features aiding the narrowing of the differential diagnosis [7]. Finally, overlap of functional dystonia symptoms may occur in the context of idiopathic dystonia syndromes [8], adding to the complexity of therapeutic management. The two case vignettes above provide a description of the heterogenous clinical picture of functional dystonia and their impact on diagnosis and treatment. The following sections discuss the diagnostic and therapeutic approach to functional dystonia.

How to Diagnose Functional Dystonia

Functional dystonia is the second most common FMD. Despite similarities with idiopathic and isolated genetic dystonia, functional dystonia can be diagnosed based on specific phenomenological features (Table 7.1).

Functional dystonia predominantly affects young women, who comprise approximately 80% of the cases. Symptoms often start after a physical injury of minor/moderate severity (similar to the presentation outlined in the Case Vignette 2) or an emotional triggering event [9]. Yet, in a proportion of subjects, there are no clear triggering factors. Pain is a frequent associated non-motor symptom, and significantly impacts prognosis and management.

Table 7.1 Clinical features helpful in differentiating idiopathic or genetic dystonia from the three phenotypes of functional dystonia

	Idiopathic or genetic dystonia	Functional fixed dystonia	Functional mobile dystonia	Functional paroxysmal dystonia
Effect of voluntary action or exercise	↑	−	↑ or ↓ or −	↑ or ↓ or −
Overflow	+++	−	−	−
Variability during the examination	−	−/+	+++	+++
Change with distraction	−	−/+	+++	+/−
Effect of increased attention	−	−/+	↑	↑
Geste antagoniste	+++	−	−/+	NK
Spreading to distant body parts	−/+	+++	+++	+++
Presence of other movement disorders	−/+	+	+++	+++
Tremor	+	+	+	+
Abnormal posturing	+++	+++	+++	+++
Pain	+/−	+++	+/−	+/−

↑ = increase; ↓ = decrease; + = present; − = not present; +++ = prominent feature; NK = not known

Incorrect and delayed diagnosis of functional dystonia may lead to unnecessary investigations, increased healthcare costs, and inappropriate treatments with potential iatrogenic harm and poor prognosis, including limb amputation [10, 11]. Diagnostic delays and lack of treatment guidelines specific for functional dystonia, particularly for the fixed dystonia phenotype, additionally negatively impact the prognosis of these patients, which is generally poor [12].

Diagnostic Criteria

Several sets of clinical criteria have been developed to formalize the diagnostic process in people with FMD, and can be applied to functional dystonia. Indeed, the first official diagnostic criteria for FMD were developed by Fahn and Williams in 1988 for functional dystonia, formerly referred to as "psychogenic dystonia" [13]. These set of criteria have defined the level of certainty for this diagnosis based on the clinical incongruence or inconsistency of the movement disorder, with response to suggestion, placebo and psychotherapy defining the highest level of diagnostic certainty. Inconsistency of movement refers to variability over time or during clinical examination which is a common feature of all FMD presentations. As the "probable" and "possible" categories of diagnostic certainty yield overall low agreement for this and other diagnostic criteria [14], the importance of a phenotype-specific diagnostic approach has been encouraged [15] based on identifying positive clinical signs to support the diagnosis [2, 16]. Furthermore, the Gupta-Lang criteria for FMD incorporated electrophysiological findings toward a "laboratory supported" diagnosis [17]. Yet, there are no validated electrophysiology-based criteria for functional dystonia [18]. A few studies employing blink reflex [19], transcranial magnetic stimulation [20, 21] and psychophysiological testing of pain thresholds [22] and somatosensory tactile discrimination [23] have discriminated at group level between functional dystonia and other dystonia presentations, but specificity and sensitivity of such tests have not been performed so far.

Additionally, historical clues and specific positive phenomenological signs as outlined below represent the pillars of diagnosis for functional dystonia.

Historical Clues and Comorbidities

Although not diagnostic, one core element to consider in the clinical history of functional dystonia is the temporal evolution of the symptoms [24], which typically has a subacute onset with a development over days or weeks and a rapid progression, resulting in many cases in a tonic posture. This can be initially corrected but then may become fixed over a short time. Another feature of functional dystonia is the spreading to other body sites eventually being associated to other motor phenotypes (i.e. tremor, ataxia) or other functional neurological symptoms, as shown in Case Vignette 1. Such mixed FMD presentations tend to have a higher burden of non-motor symptoms and are more likely to be diagnosed by a movement disorders neurologist after a long illness duration [3].

The rapid progression and the tendency to spread and develop other neurological manifestations is highly supportive of the diagnosis of functional dystonia. In contrast to adult-onset dystonia whose spreading trajectories follow a cranio-caudal pattern and tend to affect two contiguous body parts [25, 26], in functional dystonia the spreading does not necessarily follow adjacent anatomical segments or manifest with the same motor phenomenology.

There are a number of comorbidities that may be identified and may represent predisposing, precipitating, and perpetuating factors for the development and maintenance of functional dystonia. Non-motor symptoms such as pain, headache, insomnia, and fatigue are often reported in patients with FMD [3, 27, 28]. Pain is localized either in regions affected by functional dystonia or in other body parts. Whereas the presence of pain in the neck muscles makes functional dystonia difficult to differentiate from idiopathic cervical dystonia, it should be recognized that pain is unusual in upper limb adult-onset idiopathic dystonias, which are often task-specific. Dystonia associated with corticobasal syndrome or Parkinson's disease, which respectively involve the upper and lower limbs, are often painful, but the combination with parkinsonism and/or apraxia, myoclonus and cortical sensory dysfunction allows differentiation of these conditions from functional dystonia. Pain is a major concern in 41% of patients with fixed dystonia who might also present with clinical features of complex regional pain syndrome type 1 (CRPS-1) [5]. Movement disorders associated with CRPS-1 have been a subject of controversy over the last 10 years regarding their nature, with an intense debate about the framing of this disorder [29–31]. CRPS-1 dystonia has many similarities with functional dystonia both in terms of clinical features and natural history. Indeed, recent research has also showed pathophysiological similarities between individuals with functional dystonia and patients with CRPS-1 and fixed hand postures [21]. Finally, it has been suggested that joint hypermobility syndrome might be a risk factor for the development and maintenance of functional dystonia [32].

Psychological or physical trauma might predate the onset of motor symptoms in about one third of patients with functional dystonia [27, 33]. Psychiatric comorbidities are reported more frequently in patients with fixed dystonia [5], particularly anxiety, depression, and apathy [34, 35]. Nevertheless, psychiatric symptoms are also a prominent component of idiopathic dystonia [36, 37], especially anxiety and depression. However, in functional dystonia other psychopathologies have been described such as substance-related disorders, schizophrenia, adjustment disorder, borderline personality disorder, post-traumatic stress disorder, psychotic depression, and delusional disorder. Patients with functional dystonia are also more likely to have high levels of alexithymia [38] as well as impaired emotional processing [39].

Finally, it should be highlighted that functional dystonia may arise in the context of other neurological disorders, including idiopathic dystonias [8]. Such overlap of functional neurological manifestations associated with other hyperkinetic disorders represents a great challenge and might lead to inappropriate interventions for "complex intractable dystonia", such as deep brain stimulation [40].

Basic Clinical Features

The phenomenology of functional dystonia may vary over time and the severity of symptoms might fluctuate with relapses and remissions. Remission of symptoms is very rare in idiopathic dystonia. However, it has to be acknowledged that this can still occur, especially in cervical dystonia and blepharospasm [41]. Phenotypic manifestations may vary by temporal pattern of movement (persistent, paroxysmal), types of dystonic manifestations (fixed, mobile), and body localization (cranial, upper and lower limbs, trunk).

In the majority of cases the clinical presentation is a unilateral fixed dystonia, mostly affecting the distal limb and more frequently the lower than the upper limb. When affecting the lower limb, the classical presentation is that of foot plantar flexion and inversion and curling of toes. In the hand, individuals classically present with wrist and finger flexion either with sparing of the thumb and the index fingers or more rarely with development of clenched fist [5] (Fig. 7.1). A few other positive signs have been described in people with fixed dystonia, but they have not validated [42]; these additional signs requiring further inquiry include the "swivel chair sign" [43], variable resistance to passive manipulation and the "psychogenic toe sign" [44].

Functional dystonia may also manifest with phasic rather than tonic dystonic movements, either with a paroxysmal or continuous presentation. Such mobile functional dystonia poses major diagnostic challenges as the phenomenological features are difficult to dissect from other forms of mobile dystonia [45]. Functional dystonia lacks the patterned manifestations typical of other dystonia syndromes [45], despite the fact that some movements might look stereotyped (for example, stereotyped and repetitive oscillatory movements of the upper limbs).

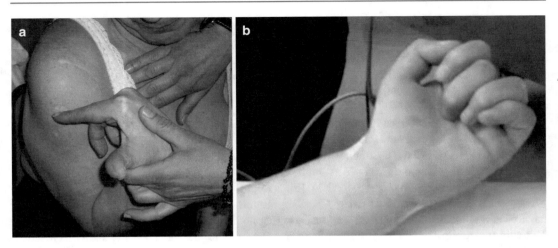

Fig. 7.1 (**a**) Fixed dystonia of the upper limb with sparing of the thumb and index; (**b**) Fixed dystonia of the upper limb with clenched fist

Gestes antagonistes might be also present in functional dystonia [46], or at least, an alternative motor pattern might act as a distractive maneuver, as in Case Vignette 1 in whom singing improved significantly torsional movements of the head. Indeed, modulation by distraction is an important phenomenological feature of functional dystonia that should be carefully probed for. Distractibility can be tested using specific clinical maneuvers such as finger tapping movements at different speeds, side-to-side tongue movements, serial-seven backward counting, and contralateral rhythmic ballistic movements. In addition, the effect of complex motor tasks such as running, jumping side to side, and walking backwards should be also evaluated, keeping in mind that the boundaries between these distractive maneuvers and *gestes antagonistes* may be difficult to define. One of the clinical features which may help to distinguish between the two conditions is lack of overflow of muscular activation [2]. Especially in idiopathic and genetic dystonia, the presence of overflow dystonia is very prominent and characterized by the appearance of involuntary movements at body sites distant from the primary dystonic movement when the patient is voluntarily moving.

Paroxysmal dystonia is another phenotype of functional dystonia and is typically characterized by a combination of abnormal postures and jerky movements. The differential diagnosis with genetic paroxysmal dyskinesia [47] remains a challenge. The following elements can help to differentiate functional dystonia from these conditions, which typically present in childhood: adult age of onset, presence of paroxysmal tremor, precipitation of attacks or/and variability during the examination (Fig. 7.2), atypical and variable duration of attacks, presence of multiple atypical triggers, altered level of responsiveness, presence of atypical precipitating factors, presence of unusual relieving maneuvers, and atypical response to medication [48, 49].

Finally, regardless of the phenotype of functional dystonia, a large number of patients may display positive clinical signs for other functional neurological disorder presentations [2].

Specific Phenotypes Based on Body Localization

Neck involvement is a less common presentation of functional dystonia. Most of the time it presents

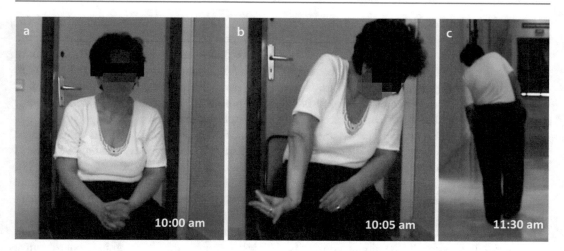

Fig. 7.2   In-clinic variability of phenotype in a patient with paroxysmal functional dystonia

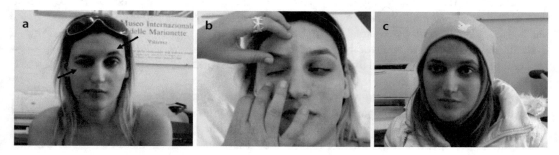

Fig. 7.3   Clinical features of functional facial spasm. (**a**) Contraction of the frontalis muscle contralateral to the side of contraction of the orbicularis oculi muscle. (**b**) Resistance to passive opening of the right eyelid. (**c**) Spontaneous remission 1 year after onset

with laterocollis, ipsilateral shoulder elevation and contralateral shoulder depression associated to pain [50]. Acute onset of retrocollis has been also described as a rare phenotype [49, 51].

Functional facial dystonia usually presents with unilateral lip and jaw deviation and ipsilateral platysma involvement [52]. Given that symptoms are often unilateral, the differential diagnosis includes hemifacial spasm, from which functional facial dystonia is distinguished by absence of the "other Babinski sign" [53] and presence of frontalis muscle contraction contralateral to spasm of the orbicularis oculi [54] (Fig. 7.3). Functional facial spasm may also present with alternating spasms from one side of the face to the other

and simultaneous involvement of multiple body regions at onset in 30% [52]. Further discussion of functional facial movements can be found in Chap. 10.

Two large studies have described the phenomenology of functional gait disorders either in isolation or in combination with another FMD presentation [55, 56]. In both studies, functional dystonic gait and the classic knee-buckling pattern were among the most common patterns. Another characteristic of functional dystonic gait is the lack of improvement of the abnormal posture when walking backwards or sideways, which is typically seen in other forms of dystonia [57]. Further discussion of functional gait can be found in Chap. 11.

Management of Functional Dystonia

As with other FMD phenomenologies, the treatment of functional dystonia starts with explaining the diagnosis. Acceptance of the diagnosis is required prior to initiation of therapeutic strategies, which mostly rely on non-pharmacological interventions such as physiotherapy [1, 58, 59]. Explaining the diagnosis successfully is based in part on accurate discussion of signs supporting the diagnosis of functional dystonia, which should be demonstrated to the patients during the consultation [60]. As shown in Case Vignette 1, diagnostic delay and/or diagnostic uncertainty is associated with disease progression.

In addition to the timing of diagnosis, phenotype also impacts prognosis in functional dystonia. Indeed, patients with paroxysmal functional dystonia seems to have a more favorable outcome [48] compared to those with fixed dystonia [12].

Data on efficacy of different treatments (physiotherapy, occupational therapy, cognitive behavioral therapy, pharmacological therapies) have not been robustly tested in functional dystonia cohorts and it is unknown whether different phenotypes may be more or less responsive to a specific intervention [61]. Case Vignette 1 shows the success of an in-patient rehabilitation multidisciplinary program which included physiotherapy, occupational therapy and psychological intervention [1, 2, 61]. In general, a multidisciplinary rehabilitation treatment (see Chap. 26) helps to address the complexity of the movement disorder and the multiple associated non-motor symptoms and comorbidities. More research is also needed to determine the optimal treatment setting for a given patient, across inpatient, intensive outpatient and conventional outpatient treatment settings. Management of pain is of paramount importance although this might be a limiting factor for physiotherapy [58], as shown by Case Vignette 2. Indeed, presence chronic pain, CRPS-1, depression and other functional somatic symptoms is associated with worse outcome in fixed dystonia [12].

In addition to non-pharmacological interventions, oral medications targeting psychiatric comorbidities might be used [62]. Indeed, a recent large cohort study of 410 patients with FMD revealed that oral medications, including antidepressants, benzodiazepines, antiepileptics and, rarely, antipsychotics are employed in clinical practice by neurologist experts in movement disorders. In the same study, botulinum toxin was employed as a treatment in 13% of cases. Yet, despite anecdotical reports [63], no large-scale studies have assessed the efficacy of botulinum toxin in patients with functional dystonia in whom it might have a potential benefit in treating tonic postures, thus preventing contractures. Accordingly, intractable contractures [5] represent a detrimental consequence of fixed dystonia, potentially requiring surgery.

Conclusions

Functional dystonia is characterized by a variety of phenotypes which can be mainly grouped into fixed, mobile, paroxysmal forms. More complex clinical pictures arise in those patients developing mixed FMD presentations in whom functional dystonia coexists with other motor symptoms or in those individuals that have both functional dystonia and other neurological conditions. Such complexities of clinical manifestations often lead to diagnostic delays and inappropriate treatments. Despite the great challenge in diagnosing functional dystonia, there are specific phenomenological features that support a diagnosis based on positive signs. Yet, many of these signs need further validation in larger cohorts. Another unmet need is the development of laboratory-based diagnostic criteria for functional dystonia. With growing knowledge of the pathophysiology of functional dystonia, it is conceivable that diagnostic biomarkers for functional dystonia might be incorporated in the future [64]. Such adjunctive biomarkers are also needed to test treatments specific for functional dystonia phenotypes, including fixed dystonia which has a guarded prognosis.

Summary
- Functional dystonia is a common functional movement disorder subtype.
- The three presentations of functional dystonia include fixed, mobile and paroxysmal forms.
- Historical clues can raise the index of suspicion for functional dystonia, while diagnosis is based on detection of rule-in phenotypic characteristics.
- While more research is needed on the treatment of functional dystonia, components of a multidisciplinary and interdisciplinary approach to care include physical rehabilitation, psychotherapy and treatment of comorbidities.

References

1. Nielsen G, Stone J, Matthews A, Brown M, Sparkes C, Farmer R, et al. Physiotherapy for functional motor disorders: a consensus recommendation. J Neurol Neurosurg Psychiatry. 2015;86(10):1113–9.
2. Espay AJ, Aybek S, Carson A, Edwards MJ, Goldstein LH, Hallett M, et al. Current concepts in diagnosis and treatment of functional neurological disorders. JAMA Neurol. 2018;75(9):1132–41.
3. Tinazzi M, Morgante F, Marcuzzo E, Erro R, Barone P, Ceravolo R, Mazzucchi S, Pilotto A, Padovani A, Romito LM, Eleopra R, Zappia M, Nicoletti A, Dallocchio C, Arbasino C, Bono F, Pascarella A, Demartini B, Gambini O, Modugno N, Olivola E, Di Stefano V, Albanese A, Ferrazzano G, Tessitore A, Zibetti M, Calandra-Buonaura G, Petracca M, Esposito M, Pisani A, Manganotti P, Stocchi F, Coletti Moja M, Antonini A, Defazio G, Geroin C. Clinical correlates of functional motor disorders: an Italian multicenter study. Mov Disord Clin Pract. 2020;7(8):920–9.
4. Stone J, Warlow C, Sharpe M. The symptom of functional weakness: a controlled study of 107 patients. Brain. 2010;133(Pt 5):1537–51.
5. Schrag A, Trimble M, Quinn N, Bhatia K. The syndrome of fixed dystonia: an evaluation of 103 patients. Brain. 2004;127(Pt 10):2360–72.
6. Frucht L, Perez DL, Callahan J, MacLean J, Song PC, Sharma N, et al. Functional dystonia: differentiation from primary dystonia and multidisciplinary treatments. Front Neurol. 2021;11:605262.
7. Fung VS, Jinnah HA, Bhatia K, Vidailhet M. Assessment of patients with isolated or combined dystonia: an update on dystonia syndromes. Mov Disord. 2013;28(7):889–98.
8. Tinazzi M, Geroin C, Erro R, Marcuzzo E, Cuoco S, Ceravolo R, et al. Functional motor disorders associated with other neurological diseases: beyond the boundaries of "organic" neurology. Eur J Neurol. 2021;28(5):1752–8.
9. Parees I, Kojovic M, Pires C, Rubio-Agusti I, Saifee TA, Sadnicka A, et al. Physical precipitating factors in functional movement disorders. J Neurol Sci. 2014;338(1–2):174–7.
10. Newby R, Alty J, Kempster P. Functional dystonia and the borderland between neurology and psychiatry: new concepts. Mov Disord. 2016;31(12):1777–84.
11. Edwards MJ, Alonso-Canovas A, Schrag A, Bloem BR, Thompson PD, Bhatia K. Limb amputations in fixed dystonia: a form of body integrity identity disorder? Mov Disord. 2011;26(8):1410–4.
12. Ibrahim NM, Martino D, van de Warrenburg BP, Quinn NP, Bhatia KP, Brown RJ, et al. The prognosis of fixed dystonia: a follow-up study. Parkinsonism Relat Disord. 2009;15(8):592–7.
13. Fahn S, Williams DT. Psychogenic dystonia. Adv Neurol. 1988;50:431–55.
14. Morgante F, Edwards MJ, Espay AJ, Fasano A, Mir P, Martino D. Diagnostic agreement in patients with psychogenic movement disorders. Mov Disord. 2012;27(4):548–52.
15. Espay AJ, Lang AE. Phenotype-specific diagnosis of functional (psychogenic) movement disorders. Curr Neurol Neurosci Rep. 2015;15(6):32.
16. Teodoro T, Edwards MJ. Functional movement disorders. Curr Opin Neurol. 2016;29(4):519–25.
17. Gupta A, Lang AE. Psychogenic movement disorders. Curr Opin Neurol. 2009;22(4):430–6.
18. Perez DL, Aybek S, Popkirov S, Kozlowska K, Stephen CD, Anderson J, et al. A review and expert opinion on the neuropsychiatric assessment of motor functional neurological disorders. J Neuropsychiatry Clin Neurosci. 2021;33(1):14–26.
19. Schwingenschuh P, Katschnig P, Edwards MJ, Teo JT, Korlipara LV, Rothwell JC, et al. The blink reflex recovery cycle differs between essential and presumed psychogenic blepharospasm. Neurology. 2011;76(7):610–4.
20. Quartarone A, Rizzo V, Terranova C, Morgante F, Schneider S, Ibrahim N, et al. Abnormal sensorimotor plasticity in organic but not in psychogenic dystonia. Brain. 2009;132(Pt 10):2871–7.
21. Morgante F, Naro A, Terranova C, Russo M, Rizzo V, Risitano G, et al. Normal sensorimotor plasticity in complex regional pain syndrome with fixed posture of the hand. Mov Disord. 2017;32(1):149–57.
22. Morgante F, Matinella A, Andrenelli E, Ricciardi L, Allegra C, Terranova C, et al. Pain processing in functional and idiopathic dystonia: an exploratory study. Mov Disord. 2018;33(8):1340–8.

23. Morgante F, Tinazzi M, Squintani G, Martino D, Defazio G, Romito L, et al. Abnormal tactile temporal discrimination in psychogenic dystonia. Neurology. 2011;77(12):1191–7.

24. Stephen CD, Perez DL, Chibnik LB, Sharma N. Functional dystonia: a case-control study and risk prediction algorithm. Ann Clin Transl Neurol. 2021;8(4):732–48.

25. Abbruzzese G, Berardelli A, Girlanda P, Marchese R, Martino D, Morgante F, et al. Long-term assessment of the risk of spread in primary late-onset focal dystonia. J Neurol Neurosurg Psychiatry. 2008;79(4):392–6.

26. Berman BD, Groth CL, Sillau SH, Pirio Richardson S, Norris SA, Junker J, et al. Risk of spread in adult-onset isolated focal dystonia: a prospective international cohort study. J Neurol Neurosurg Psychiatry. 2020;91(3):314–20.

27. Gelauff JM, Rosmalen JGM, Gardien J, Stone J, Tijssen MAJ. Shared demographics and comorbidities in different functional motor disorders. Parkinsonism Relat Disord. 2020;70:1–6.

28. Aybek S, Lidstone SC, Nielsen G, MacGillivray L, Bassetti CL, Lang AE, et al. What is the role of a specialist assessment clinic for FND? Lessons from three national referral centers. J Neuropsychiatry Clin Neurosci. 2020;32(1):79–84.

29. Verdugo RJ, Ochoa JL. Abnormal movements in complex regional pain syndrome: assessment of their nature. Muscle Nerve. 2000;23(2):198–205.

30. Lang AE, Chen R. Dystonia in complex regional pain syndrome type I. Ann Neurol. 2010;67(3):412–4.

31. Popkirov S, Hoeritzauer I, Colvin L, Carson AJ, Stone J. Complex regional pain syndrome and functional neurological disorders – time for reconciliation. J Neurol Neurosurg Psychiatry. 2019;90(5):608–14.

32. Kassavetis P, Batla A, Parees I, Saifee TA, Schrag A, Cordivari C, et al. Joint hypermobility syndrome: a risk factor for fixed dystonia? Mov Disord. 2012;27(8):1070.

33. Tinazzi M, Geroin C, Marcuzzo E, Cuoco S, Ceravolo R, et al. Functional motor phenotypes: to lump or to split? J Neurol. 2021; https://doi.org/10.1007/s00415-021-10583-w.

34. Tomic A, Petrovic I, Pesic D, Voncina MM, Svetel M, Miskovic ND, et al. Is there a specific psychiatric background or personality profile in functional dystonia? J Psychosom Res. 2017;97:58–62.

35. Pastore A, Pierri G, Fabio G, Ferramosca S, Gigante A, Superbo M, et al. Differences in psychopathology and behavioral characteristics of patients affected by conversion motor disorder and organic dystonia. Neuropsychiatr Dis Treat. 2018;14:1287–95.

36. Berman BD, Junker J, Shelton E, Sillau SH, Jinnah HA, Perlmutter JS, et al. Psychiatric associations of adult-onset focal dystonia phenotypes. J Neurol Neurosurg Psychiatry. 2017;88(7):595–602.

37. Lee S, Chung SJ, Shin HW. Neuropsychiatric symptoms and quality of life in patients with adult-onset idiopathic focal dystonia and essential tremor. Front Neurol. 2020;11:1030.

38. Demartini B, Petrochilos P, Ricciardi L, Price G, Edwards MJ, Joyce E. The role of alexithymia in the development of functional motor symptoms (conversion disorder). J Neurol Neurosurg Psychiatry. 2014;85(10):1132–7.

39. Espay AJ, Maloney T, Vannest J, Norris MM, Eliassen JC, Neefus E, et al. Dysfunction in emotion processing underlies functional (psychogenic) dystonia. Mov Disord. 2018;33(1):136–45.

40. Pauls KAM, Krauss JK, Kampfer CE, Kuhn AA, Schrader C, Sudmeyer M, et al. Causes of failure of pallidal deep brain stimulation in cases with pre-operative diagnosis of isolated dystonia. Parkinsonism Relat Disord. 2017;43:38–48.

41. Mainka T, Erro R, Rothwell J, Kuhn AA, Bhatia KP, Ganos C. Remission in dystonia – systematic review of the literature and meta-analysis. Parkinsonism Relat Disord. 2019;66:9–15.

42. Sokol LL, Espay AJ. Clinical signs in functional (psychogenic) gait disorders: a brief survey. J Clin Mov Disord. 2016;3:3.

43. Okun MS, Rodriguez RL, Foote KD, Fernandez HH. The "chair test" to aid in the diagnosis of psychogenic gait disorders. Neurologist. 2007;13(2):87–91.

44. Espay AJ, Lang AE. The psychogenic toe signs. Neurology. 2011;77(5):508–9.

45. Albanese A, Bhatia K, Bressman SB, DeLong MR, Fahn S, Fung VS, et al. Phenomenology and classification of dystonia: a consensus update. Mov Disord. 2013;28(7):863–73.

46. Munhoz RP, Lang AE. Gestes antagonistes in psychogenic dystonia. Mov Disord. 2004;19(3):331–2.

47. Erro R, Sheerin UM, Bhatia KP. Paroxysmal dyskinesias revisited: a review of 500 genetically proven cases and a new classification. Mov Disord. 2014;29(9):1108–16.

48. Ganos C, Aguirregomozcorta M, Batla A, Stamelou M, Schwingenschuh P, Munchau A, et al. Psychogenic paroxysmal movement disorders--clinical features and diagnostic clues. Parkinsonism Relat Disord. 2014;20(1):41–6.

49. Ganos C, Edwards MJ, Bhatia KP. The phenomenology of functional (psychogenic) dystonia. Mov Disord Clin Pract. 2014;1(1):36–44.

50. Sa DS, Mailis-Gagnon A, Nicholson K, Lang AE. Posttraumatic painful torticollis. Mov Disord. 2003;18(12):1482–91.

51. Cakmak MA, Sahin S, Cinar N, Tiyekli U, Karsidag S. Nine years with Munchausen syndrome: a case of psychogenic dystonia. Tremor Other Hyperkinet Mov (N Y). 2015;5:tre-5-297-6792-1.

52. Fasano A, Valadas A, Bhatia KP, Prashanth LK, Lang AE, Munhoz RP, et al. Psychogenic facial movement disorders: clinical features and associated conditions. Mov Disord. 2012;27(12):1544–51.

53. Varanda S, Rocha S, Rodrigues M, Machado A, Carneiro G. Role of the "other Babinski sign" in hyperkinetic facial disorders. J Neurol Sci. 2017;378:36–7.

54. Kaski D, Bronstein AM, Edwards MJ, Stone J. Cranial functional (psychogenic) movement disorders. Lancet Neurol. 2015;14(12):1196–205.

55. Baizabal-Carvallo JF, Alonso-Juarez M, Jankovic J. Functional gait disorders, clinical phenomenology, and classification. Neurol Sci. 2020;41(4):911–5.
56. Baik JS, Lang AE. Gait abnormalities in psychogenic movement disorders. Mov Disord. 2007;22(3):395–9.
57. Nonnekes J, Ruzicka E, Serranova T, Reich SG, Bloem BR, Hallett M. Functional gait disorders: a sign-based approach. Neurology. 2020;94(24):1093–9.
58. Nielsen G, Buszewicz M, Stevenson F, Hunter R, Holt K, Dudziec M, et al. Randomised feasibility study of physiotherapy for patients with functional motor symptoms. J Neurol Neurosurg Psychiatry. 2017;88(6):484–90.
59. Nielsen G, Stone J, Edwards MJ. Physiotherapy for functional (psychogenic) motor symptoms: a systematic review. J Psychosom Res. 2013;75(2):93–102.
60. Stone J, Edwards M. Trick or treat? Showing patients with functional (psychogenic) motor symptoms their physical signs. Neurology. 2012;79(3):282–4.
61. Nicholson C, Edwards MJ, Carson AJ, Gardiner P, Golder D, Hayward K, et al. Occupational therapy consensus recommendations for functional neurological disorder. J Neurol Neurosurg Psychiatry. 2020;91(10):1037–45.
62. Voon V, Lang AE. Antidepressants in the treatment of psychosis with comorbid depression in Parkinson disease. Clin Neuropharmacol. 2004;27(2):90–2.
63. Khachane Y, Kozlowska K, Savage B, McClure G, Butler G, Gray N, et al. Twisted in pain: the multidisciplinary treatment approach to functional dystonia. Harv Rev Psychiatry. 2019;27(6):359–81.
64. Thomsen BLC, Teodoro T, Edwards MJ. Biomarkers in functional movement disorders: a systematic review. J Neurol Neurosurg Psychiatry. 2020;91(12):1261–9.

Functional Parkinsonism

8

Marine Ambar Akkaoui, Bertrand Degos, and Béatrice Garcin

Clinical Vignette 1

A 50-year-old woman presented with a 15-year history of parkinsonian symptoms. She had no relevant family or personal medical history. Upon clinical examination, she exhibited resting tremor of the hands and slowness of her movements, affecting mostly the right side of the body. While her presentation was suggestive of a parkinsonian disorder, some features were atypical for idiopathic Parkinson's disease. Notably, she exhibited variable frequency resting and postural tremor of the right hand. Her right hand tremor was distractible as well as entrainable, with the frequency of tremor in the affected limb adapting to an

examiner-suggested frequency when the patient tapped in her less affected limb (see Video 8.1). Rigidity was noted to diminish with use of reinforcement maneuvers. Voluntary movements were very slow, and this slowness was distractible. Moreover, the patient complained about knee buckling when standing. Her gait was variable, ranging from very slow to normal, with a loss of arm swing even while running. There was no freezing and the patient did not report any falls. Although she endorsed subjective memory complaints, she did not exhibit objective cognitive impairment.

She had been diagnosed with Parkinson's disease (PD) 5 years earlier and had since been treated with levodopa, with rapid onset of dyskinesia appearing 2 years after treatment onset. Functional parkinsonism was strongly suspected due to the variability and distractibility of symptoms, and their atypical course. She underwent a dopamine transporter scan (DaTscan), which

---

All authors have contributed to and approved the submitted draft manuscript.

Supplementary Information The online version contains supplementary material available at [https://doi.org/10.1007/978-3-030-86495-8_8].

M. A. Akkaoui (✉)
Centre Psychiatrique d'Orientation et d'Accueil (CPOA), GHU Paris - Psychiatry & Neurosciences, Paris, France

Psychiatric Emergency, CH Delafontaine, Etablissement Publique de Santé Mentale deVille Evrard, Paris, France

B. Degos
Neurology Unit, Avicenne University Hospital, Sorbonne Paris Nord University, Bobigny, France

Dynamics and Pathophysiology of Neuronal Networks Team, Center for Interdisciplinary Research in Biology, Collège de France, CNRS UMR7241/INSERM U1050, Université PSL, Paris, France

B. Garcin
Neurology Unit, Avicenne University Hospital, Sorbonne Paris Nord University, Bobigny, France

Faculty of Medicine of Sorbonne University, Brain and Spine Institute, INSERM U1127, CNRS UMR 7225, Paris, France

© Springer Nature Switzerland AG 2022
K. LaFaver et al. (eds.), *Functional Movement Disorder*, Current Clinical Neurology,
https://doi.org/10.1007/978-3-030-86495-8_8

showed significant dopaminergic denervation of the left striatum.

We concluded that the patient had both neurodegenerative Parkinson's disease as well as functional parkinsonism. The diagnosis was explained to the patient. Her neurologist demonstrated the positive features leading to the diagnosis of functional parkinsonism, including entrainability and distractibility. She was referred for physiotherapy. She was educated on specific physiotherapy techniques using a motor learning approach as well as distraction techniques. She was continued on dopaminergic medication for treatment of her neurodegenerative Parkinson's disease.

Clinical Vignette 2

A 62-year-old man presented with a history of rapid onset slowness and rigidity of the left side of the body. The diagnosis of PD had been made 2 years prior, and he had been treated with levodopa, with a modest effect on his bradykinesia. He had no personal or family history of neurological or psychiatric disorders.

The patient went for a second opinion. The neurologist performing this evaluation questioned the diagnosis of PD given the presence of several atypical features (see Video 8.2). The history was notable for sudden onset of rapidly maximal symptoms. On examination, the patient exhibited bradykinesia without gradual decrement in amplitude, rigidity that diminished with reinforcement maneuvers, prominent distractibility, and variability in the severity and characteristics of these clinical signs. The patient reported frequent falls, but no fall was observed during the pull test. There was no freezing of gait, and there was a positive Hoover's sign of the left leg.

The patient underwent a DaTscan, which was interpreted as normal. A diagnosis of functional parkinsonism was suspected based on clinical signs and normal nuclear imaging. The functional origin of his symptoms was discussed with the patient and levodopa was discontinued. A single session of repeated single pulse transcranial magnetic stimulation (TMS) was performed at supramotor threshold (150% of resting motor threshold) and low frequency (0.5 Hz) with a circular coil over the motor cortex, leading to a partial recovery of symptoms (see section "Treatment" for additional details). Following TMS treatment, the patient was prescribed physiotherapy.

Introduction

Functional parkinsonism is defined by the presence of a combination of marked slowness of movement in the absence of progressive decrement and variable resistance against passive movement, that is not caused by neurodegeneration or dysfunction of the dopaminergic system. Other functional neurological phenotypes, including functional tremor and functional gait impairment, may also be present. Arriving at an accurate diagnosis of functional parkinsonism is essential for initiation of appropriate treatment.

Functional parkinsonism is often incorrectly diagnosed as idiopathic Parkinson's disease (PD). This is often the case in patients with scans without evidence of dopaminergic depletion (SWEDD). Most patients with SWEDD are incorrectly diagnosed as PD, and a proportion of these patients have undiagnosed functional parkinsonism. This misdiagnosis can lead to inappropriate treatment, including escalation of antiparkinsonian treatment and requests for alternative therapy such as deep brain stimulation [1]. These patients can also be inappropriately enrolled in PD clinical trials. It is also important to keep in mind that functional neurological symptoms (including functional parkinsonism) can occur comorbid with neurodegenerative parkinsonism including PD; the presence of neurodegenerative parkinsonism is in fact considered a risk factor for functional parkinsonism. This situation is sometimes called functional overlay, meaning that functional neurological symptoms co-occur with a concomitant neurological disease. The identification of both functional and neurodegenerative etiologies for a patient's symptoms is crucial, as the approach to treatment of these will differ.

At the present time, there are no specific diagnostic criteria for functional parkinsonism. Most studies use the diagnostic criteria for functional movement disorder (FMD) [2, 3] or the DSM-5 diagnostic criteria for functional neurological disorder (FND) [4]. These criteria include symptoms of altered voluntary motor or sensory function, with clinical findings providing evidence of incompatibility between the symptom and recognized neurological or medical conditions, known as "positive neurological signs". The symptoms should not be better explained by another medical or mental disorder, and should cause the patient clinically significant distress or impairment in social, occupational, or other important areas of functioning or warrant medical evaluation.

One of the first descriptions of functional parkinsonism was published in 1988 by Walter and colleagues [5], who reported the case of a 64-year-old man suffering from "hysterical parkinsonism" who exhibited dragging of both legs and atypical tremor that had been present for 3 years. In 1995, Lang and colleagues [6] published the first series of 13 cases of functional parkinsonism. Specific features of the tremor, rigidity, gait, weakness and evolution were described in this paper; these features are described in Table 8.1 and in the section below on "Clinical Presentation and Diagnosis".

Epidemiology

Functional parkinsonism is estimated to represent between 3% and 6% of patients with FMD [6, 7]. The overall prevalence of functional parkinsonism is unknown. One study [8] seeking to estimate the prevalence of functional parkinsonism in the Swiss population found the prevalence of functional parkinsonism to be 0.64 per 100,000. In previous studies, functional parkinsonism represented 0.24–1.5% of all patients with parkinsonism [8, 9], and 1.3% of cases of non-degenerative parkinsonism. Drug-induced parkinsonism (44%) and vascular parkinsonism (37%) were noted to be the most frequent causes of non-degenerative parkinsonism [8].

As previously mentioned, functional neurological symptoms, including functional parkinsonism, can co-occur comorbid with Parkinson's disease. Wissel and co-authors calculated a prevalence of 1.4% of PD patients also had comorbid functional neurological disorder [1]. One study performed on 1360 patients with neurodegenerative disorders ranging from PD to Alzheimer's found that patients with PD and dementia with Lewy bodies (DLB) exhibited a higher frequency of somatoform disorders than other neurodegenerative disorders, including Alzheimer's, multiple system atrophy (MSA), progressive supranuclear palsy (PSP) and frontotemporal dementia. Somatoform symptoms included functional motor symptoms such as paresis, abnormal postures, and functional parkinsonism, and sensory symptoms such as anesthesia, multilocalized pain and body deformation delusions. Of note, the frequency of somatoform disorders was also higher in PD and DLB than in a population of patients selected from a psychiatric clinic (1.5%) [10].

A recent review of the literature described 120 patients with functional parkinsonism [4]. In this review, the mean age at onset was 45.7 years old, with female predominance (62.1%). The mean duration of symptoms at diagnosis was 5.0 years, with an abrupt onset in half of the patients.

Pathophysiology

The pathophysiology of functional parkinsonism remains incompletely understood. As discussed in Chaps. 2 and 3, environmental factors (notably childhood psychological trauma and more recent physical and psychological stressors), cognitive factors (beliefs, self-agency impairment), and emotional factors may play a role as vulnerability or triggering factors. It is noteworthy that in one literature review, comorbid Parkinson's disease was diagnosed in 32.6% of patients with functional parkinsonism [4]. This rate is significantly

Table 8.1 Clinical differences between functional parkinsonism and Parkinson's disease

		Parkinson's disease	Functional parkinsonism
Tremor	*Type*	Rest	Rest/postural/action
	Finger tremor	+	Unusual
	Frequency	Slow, 4–6 Hz	**Variability** **Entrainability** (tremor adapts the same frequency and phase as voluntary tapping in another limb)
	Coherence of bilateral tremors	Lack of coherence between tremor in different limbs	Coherence between tremor in different limbs
	Effect of distraction	Increases with mental calculation or other distraction techniques	Decreases in amplitude or disappears (**distractibility**)
	Weight-loading	Tremor is not transmitted; tremor amplitude may decrease or stay the same	Tremor may be transmitted to other body segments Tremor amplitude may increase
Rigidity		Plastic rigidity	Variable resistance against passive movement
	Cogwheeling	+	Coactivation sign (oppositional rigidity "Gegenhalten" with no real cogwheeling)
	Effect of reinforcement maneuvers	Rigidity increases	Rigidity diminishes
Bradykinesia	*Sequence effect*	+	No
	Distractibility	No	Marked slowness of voluntary movements with **distractibility**
	Hypokinesia	+	No
			Difficulty performing everyday tasks/manual tasks; may be accompanied by grimacing, sighs. Exaggerated discrepancy between the difficulty in movement initiation and the actual speed of movement execution
Balance	*Pull test*	Variable retropulsion Patient may fall	May have bizarre response to the pull test with extreme response for very light pulls but usually no falls. Better balance observed compared to patient's complaints.
Gait	*Type*	Slow, stiff, with retropulsion or propulsion	Slow, stiff, may be painful
	Arm swing	Flexed posture with reduced arm swing	Diminished or absent on the most affected side; arm held stiffly extended and adducted to the side
		Reduced arm swing can improve with running	Reduced arm swing persists with running
	Freezing	Common	Uncommon
	Other		Buckling of the knees; astasia-abasia
Speech			Baby talk; gibberish
Writing		Micrographia with decrement	Slow but no micrographia with decrement
Other neurologic features			Give-way weakness, non-anatomic sensory loss, unusual diffuse muscle pain and tenderness, Hoover's sign

higher than what is usually reported in other FND subtypes [11]. Additionally, in cases of PD with comorbid functional parkinsonism, functional neurological symptoms have been shown to start before or at the time of onset of PD in 61 out of 99 patients (61.6%) [4]. This suggests the possibility of potential shared pathogenic mechanisms between both diseases.

Clinical Presentation and Diagnosis

Diagnosis

Clinical signs that guide the diagnosis of functional parkinsonism are commonly under-recognized. Indeed, in one study, only 25% of patients with functional parkinsonism received the correct diagnosis at the time of their initial visit [8]. This highlights the important need for training of neurologists in FND semiology. The search for positive signs of functional parkinsonism should be systematic when patients present with unusual features of PD, such as a sudden change in PD course, an unusual evolution of PD, or when atypical features are present during clinical examination. Better training and extended evaluations would help avoid the misdiagnosis of functional parkinsonism and likely improve patient prognosis. However, even for well-trained neurologists, the distinction between functional parkinsonism and PD may be challenging [12–17].

History

In contrast to PD, which progressively worsens over time, the onset of functional parkinsonism is commonly abrupt, with symptoms reaching a maximum intensity at their onset, and then remaining stable. However, it is important to note that although history may be suggestive, it is not specific. Patients with idiopathic PD can also describe sudden onset of symptoms on clinical history, and stable symptoms over an extended period of time. There is a lack of data about the evolution of functional parkinsonism over time.

Examination Features

Clinical signs of functional parkinsonism are summarized in Table 8.1 as well as below [4]. The diagnosis of functional parkinsonism is based on the presence of positive signs on clinical examination. Knowledge of these positive signs is critical for arriving at the correct diagnosis of functional parkinsonism.

Tremor

Tremor is the most frequently observed symptom in functional parkinsonism, detected in approximately 72% of patients (for additional details on functional tremor please see Chap. 6). It is often present at rest, but can also be present at posture and/or with action. In patients with functional parkinsonism, postural and action tremor may be present at the same amplitude as resting tremor [5, 9, 18] in contrast to the predominant resting tremor seen in PD. Re-emergent tremor, a postural tremor that appears after a variable delay in patients with PD, is not observed in functional parkinsonism. Tremor frequency in functional parkinsonism may be variable, in contrast to PD, which has a characteristic tremor frequency between 4 and 6 Hz. Entrainability of the tremor may be observed in functional parkinsonism; this refers to the phenomenon whereby the frequency of tremor in the affected limb adapts to an examiner-suggested frequency which the patient taps in an unaffected or less affected limb. Tremor may be distractible, and disappear or decrease in amplitude when the patient is asked to concentrate on another task [8, 19]. When present in different parts of the body, functional tremor is typically synchronous, meaning that it has the same frequency and is phase-synchronous in all affected body parts, as illustrated in vignette 1. When a tremulous limb is restricted by the examiner, the tremor can spread to other parts of the body, a phenomenon that has been termed the "whack-a-mole" sign [20]. Finally, the absence of finger tremor is an additional clue that can suggest a functional origin [21, 22].

Rigidity

In functional parkinsonism, rigidity is described as oppositional and noted to be variable. Rigidity may be distractible, with a decrease of rigidity when reinforcement maneuvers are used, as illustrated in vignette 2. This contrasts with the plastic rigidity of PD, which is usually constant, includes cogwheeling, and increases with reinforcement maneuvers such as the Froment maneuver. The Froment maneuver consists of applying passive movements to the patient's wrist while asking the patient to make a continuous gesture with the other hand, most commonly a large circle. In neurodegenerative parkinsonism, as soon as the contralateral voluntary movement is initiated, rigidity is noted to increase.

Bradykinesia

The slowness of movement in functional parkinsonism is effortful (sometimes called "pseudoslowness"), with difficulty in performing everyday tasks. There may be variability in bradykinesia across different tasks. Movements may also be accompanied by excessive demonstration of effort, consisting of grimacing, huffing, grunting, or sighing [22], which is known as the "huffing and puffing" sign. Slowness is distractible, without decrement in speed and amplitude and without arrests in movement during rapid successive movement tasks. This contrasts to the bradykinesia in PD, in which a "sequence effect" is observed, referring to the decrement in amplitude and speed of a repetitive movements over time. In functional parkinsonism, writing can be slow but is often without micrographia.

Gait and Balance

Most often, patients with functional parkinsonism do not fall during the pull test, although there can be an exaggerated response to very light pulls. The observed balance impairment may be less severe than what is reported by the patient. Gait in a patient with functional parkinsonism may be slow, stiff, and possibly painful. The arm swing may be diminished or absent on the most affected side (vignette 2), with the arm typically held stiffly extended and adducted to the side; this is in contrast to patients with PD who exhibit a flexed posture with reduced arm swing. There is usually no freezing of gait, a common feature in idiopathic PD. The swivel chair test may afford a means of assessing the inconsistency of gait by comparing two ways of ambulation. During this test, subjects are asked to walk forward and backwards; they are then asked to propel themselves forward and backwards in a swivel chair with wheels. Patients with functional gait were demonstrated to successfully propel themselves in the swivel chair despite difficulties when walking [23]; it is important to note that this sign has not

yet been validated to determine sensitivity and specificity. Additional positive signs may be present in the gait of patients with functional parkinsonism, including buckling of the knees, or astasia-abasia, which is defined as an inability to stand and walk in the presence of intact motor structures.

Psychiatric Comorbidities

Psychiatric history is frequently observed in patients with functional parkinsonism. In one study, 67.6% of patients with functional parkinsonism had a comorbid psychiatric disorder; while depression was noted to be the most frequent comorbid psychiatric disorder, anxiety, bipolar disorder, post-traumatic stress disorder, personality disorder and substance use disorders were also noted [4]. Triggering stressors can be identified in nearly half of the patients (46.8%), notably physical injury, stress at work, or loss of friend or family member [4]. It is however important to note that while psychiatric history or the presence of overt stressors may be identified, these are not requirements for the diagnosis of functional parkinsonism.

Functional Parkinsonism Overlapping with Parkinson's Disease

Some patients with functional parkinsonism may also have a comorbid neurodegenerative parkinsonism, [6, 8, 12, 18, 19, 24], as illustrated in clinical vignette 1.

FND is associated with comorbid neurological disorders in approximately 12% of cases [10]. Interestingly, prior studies of patients with functional parkinsonism report rates of comorbid PD that vary between 7.1% and 66.6%, with a mean rate of comorbid PD of 32.6% [4]. When the diagnosis is uncertain, DaTscan testing may be requested to assess for striatal dopaminergic loss as is characteristic of neurodegenerative parkinsonism. As discussed earlier, similar pathophysiology may explain the high comorbidity of both diseases. Alternatively, although the clinical presentation is similar, "pure" functional parkinsonism may be relying on distinct mechanisms than functional parkinsonism with comorbid PD, or may also rely on only partially shared mechanisms, along with a possible bidirectional relationship. Further prospective studies are necessary to verify the high rate of PD comorbidity in functional parkinsonism and to better characterize the differences and similarities between pure functional parkinsonism, functional parkinsonism with comorbid PD, and PD with comorbid FND.

Additional Testing

A positive diagnosis is based on clinical features. However, as seen in vignettes 1 and 2, ancillary testing can be helpful to confirm the positive diagnosis of functional parkinsonism and to search for underlying neurodegenerative parkinsonism.

DaTscan

Striatal dopamine transporter imaging (DaTscan) involves a ligand that binds to the presynaptic dopaminergic transporter in the brain and can be used to assess the degeneration of the dopaminergic pathway seen in PD and other neurodegenerative parkinsonisms. In functional parkinsonism, DaTscan shows normal nigrostriatal dopaminergic function [18, 24–26]. DaTscan, when normal, may be useful to rule out an underlying PD. However, it should always be interpreted with caution, given the possibility of false-negative results. Of note, one study found that about 2.1% of cases of neurodegenerative parkinsonism had a normal DaTscan [27]. Moreover, the absence of denervation does not prove a functional origin, given that some other parkinsonian syndromes may have a normal DaTscan, including neuroleptic-induced parkinsonism as well as some vascular and some genetic parkinsonisms. Parkinsonian syndromes caused by enzyme abnormalities in the BH4 (tetrahydrobiopterin)

pathway, which is a cofactor in the dopamine synthesis pathway, for example, may present with a normal DaTscan. It is also important to note that an abnormal DaTscan does not rule out functional parkinsonism, as some patients with functional parkinsonism may have comorbid PD, as described above.

Electrophysiology

The diagnosis of functional parkinsonism may be documented by EMG/accelerometry, which can help demonstrate and quantify variability in frequency, entrainability, and distractibility of the tremor [29]. Functional tremor also typically has a higher frequency (6–11 Hz) than the characteristic parkinsonian tremor (4–6 Hz) [28]. Electrophysiology can also be used to demonstrate the coactivation sign, which refers to a short tonic coactivation of agonist and antagonist muscles occurring before the onset of tremor bursts. Moreover, loading a tremulous limb with a weight often increases the amplitude of a functional tremor. It is important to note that electrophysiological testing is not available in most centers, and only a few experts have sufficient training to conduct this assessment. For further description of the role of electrophysiology in assessment of functional tremor, please see Chap. 6.

Role of Medication Response

Previous authors [7] have used carbidopa 25 mg, which does not cross the blood-brain barrier, as a placebo to treat patients with functional parkinsonism, suggesting that a dramatic improvement in symptoms after carbidopa would support the diagnosis of functional parkinsonism. However, this strategy should not be used as a diagnostic test, and more generally, diagnostic tests based on placebo treatments should be interpreted with caution because patients with PD can also demonstrate an important placebo response [30].

The absence of levodopa-responsiveness is similarly not a useful test of functional parkinsonism, given that there are many other causes of parkinsonism that may be levodopa non-responsive.

Treatment

The treatment of functional parkinsonism should proceed in a similar manner to that of other FMD. Treatment relies upon providing an effective explanation of the diagnosis [34], and offering follow-up with a neurologist and/or psychiatrist. Showing the patient with functional motor symptoms their physical signs is actually one of the most useful things a neurologist can do to persuade patients of the accuracy of their diagnosis and the potential reversibility of their symptoms [31]. The medical follow-up should be multidisciplinary, involving a combination of neurology, psychiatry and psychology, and rehabilitative medicine. The effectiveness of management by both psychiatrists and neurologists has been demonstrated [32, 33], and recommendations for the care of patients with FND have been proposed [31].

Physiotherapy and Psychotherapy

There are no specific data on the role of physiotherapy in treating functional parkinsonism, but several studies have shown the effectiveness of specialized physiotherapy in FMD in general [35]. The role of physiotherapy and occupational therapy in FMD are further described in Chaps. 23 and 24, respectively. As mentioned in Part III of this book, FMD symptoms can also improve with psychotherapy [36–40]; although there are no specific studies at the present time assessing the efficacy of psychotherapy in functional parkinsonism.

Dopaminergic Treatment

After effective explanation of the diagnosis, dopaminergic treatment should be progressively discontinued in cases of pure functional parkinsonism.

TMS

TMS applied at supraliminal intensities (120–150% of the motor threshold) and at low frequency (0.25–0.5 Hz) has been shown to significantly improve motor symptoms in patients with FMD [41]. There are currently three reported cases of patients with functional parkinsonism who significantly improved with TMS. One patient with a 25-year history of functional parkinsonism improved by more than 50%, as assessed using a modified version of the Abnormal Involuntary Movement Scale and the walking subscore of the disability score from the Burke–Fahn–Marsden Scale [41]. Another patient with a 6-year history of functional parkinsonism improved by approximately 70% after TMS [42]. The third patient, who had a 7-year history of functional parkinsonism, had a full recovery after TMS, which persisted at 6-month follow-up [14]. Although usually attributed to neuromodulation, the effect of TMS here may more likely rely on suggestion and placebo effect as well as relearning normal movement and changing of illness model induced by the brief interruption of tremor during the TMS session [42, 43]. This therapeutic effect remains to be validated in randomized controlled trials.

Treating Functional Parkinsonism Accompanied by Comorbid Neurodegenerative Parkinson's Disease

When functional parkinsonism is associated with comorbid PD, explanation of both diseases and their potential pathophysiological link is particularly important. Additional explanation is usually necessary regarding comorbid functional parkinsonism. This can be facilitated by showing and explaining clinical signs such as entrainability and distractibility to patients. Specific physiotherapy techniques for functional parkinsonism may be explained and physiotherapy may be prescribed. It is also important that treatments for PD are continued with the usual follow-up.

Summary

- Functional parkinsonism should be considered if a patient exhibits sudden onset of symptoms with maximal severity at onset, and if there is no improvement with dopaminergic therapy.
- Clinical signs suggesting a functional neurological origin include distractibility, tremor entrainment, oppositional stiffness without cogwheel rigidity, and bradykinesia without decreased amplitude.
- DaTscan can be used as an adjunctive tool in the evaluation of functional parkinsonism. It may be useful in providing evidence either for or against a comorbid neurodegenerative parkinsonism (in the case of a positive or negative scan, respectively).
- Treatment should involve a multidisciplinary team including neurologists and psychiatrists and may include TMS, physical therapy, and psychotherapy.

Conflict of Interest Statements: Marine Ambar Akkaoui and Béatrice Garcin declare no conflicts of interest. Bertrand Degos received honoraria from IPSEN and travel funding from Merz-Pharma, Elivie, Orkyn.

References

1. Wissel BD, et al. Functional neurological disorders in Parkinson disease. J Neurol Neurosurg Psychiatry. 2018;89(6):566–71. https://doi.org/10.1136/jnnp-2017-317378.
2. Fahn S, Williams DT. Psychogenic dystonia. Adv Neurol. 1988;50:431–55.
3. Gupta A, Lang AE. Psychogenic movement disorders. Curr Opin Neurol. 2009;22(4):430–6. https://doi.org/10.1097/WCO.0b013e32832dc169.
4. Ambar Akkaoui M, Geoffroy PA, Roze E, Degos B, Garcin B. Functional motor symptoms in Parkinson's disease and functional parkinsonism: a systematic review. J Neuropsychiatry Clin Neurosci. 2020;32:4–13. https://doi.org/10.1176/appi.neuropsych.19030058.
5. Walters AS, Wright D, Boudwin J, Jones K. Three hysterical movement disorders. Psychol Rep. 1988;62(3):979–85. https://doi.org/10.2466/pr0.1988.62.3.979.
6. Lang AE, Koller WC, Fahn S. Psychogenic parkinsonism. Arch Neurol. 1995;52(8):802–10. https://doi.org/10.1001/archneur.1995.00540320078015.
7. Jankovic J. Diagnosis and treatment of psychogenic parkinsonism. J Neurol Neurosurg Psychiatry. 2011;82(12):1300–3. https://doi.org/10.1136/jnnp-2011-300876.
8. Frasca Polara G, et al. Prevalence of functional (psychogenic) parkinsonism in two Swiss movement disorders clinics and review of the literature. J Neurol Sci. 2018;387:37–45. https://doi.org/10.1016/j.jns.2018.01.022.
9. Sage JI, Mark MH. Psychogenic parkinsonism: clinical spectrum and diagnosis. Ann Clin Psychiatry. 2015;27(1):33–8.
10. Onofrj M, et al. Updates on somatoform disorders (SFMD) in Parkinson's disease and dementia with Lewy bodies and discussion of phenomenology. J Neurol Sci. 2011;310(1–2):166–71. https://doi.org/10.1016/j.jns.2011.07.010.
11. Stone J, et al. Which neurological diseases are most likely to be associated with "symptoms unexplained by organic disease". J Neurol. 2012;259(1):33–8. https://doi.org/10.1007/s00415-011-6111-0.
12. Umeh CC, Szabo Z, Pontone GM, Mari Z. Dopamine transporter imaging in psychogenic parkinsonism and neurodegenerative parkinsonism with psychogenic overlay: a report of three cases. Tremor Other Hyperkinet Mov (N Y). 2013;3:4.
13. Factor SA, Podskalny GD, Molho ES. Psychogenic movement disorders: frequency, clinical profile, and characteristics. J Neurol Neurosurg Psychiatry. 1995;59(4):406–12. https://doi.org/10.1136/jnnp.59.4.406.
14. Bonnet C, Mesrati F, Roze E, Hubsch C, Degos B. Motor and non-motor symptoms in functional parkinsonism responsive to transcranial magnetic stimulation: a case report. J Neurol. 2016;263(4):816–7. https://doi.org/10.1007/s00415-016-8061-z.
15. Pourfar MH, Tang CC, Mogilner AY, Dhawan V, Eidelberg D. Using imaging to identify psychogenic parkinsonism before deep brain stimulation surgery: report of 2 cases. J Neurosurg. 2012;116(1):114–8. https://doi.org/10.3171/2011.10.JNS11554.
16. Kumar R, Kumar R. A case of psychogenic Parkinsonism: late age of onset should not be a barrier to make the diagnosis. Aust N Z J Psychiatry. 2018;52(11):1098. https://doi.org/10.1177/0004867418804068.
17. Langevin J-P, Skoch JM, Sherman SJ. Deep brain stimulation of a patient with psychogenic movement disorder. Surg Neurol Int. 2016;7(Suppl 35):S824–6. https://doi.org/10.4103/2152-7806.194063.
18. Gaig C, et al. 123I-Ioflupane SPECT in the diagnosis of suspected psychogenic Parkinsonism. Mov Disord. 2006;21(11):1994–8. https://doi.org/10.1002/mds.21062.
19. Benaderette S, et al. Psychogenic parkinsonism: a combination of clinical, electrophysiological, and [123I]-FP-CIT SPECT scan explorations improves

diagnostic accuracy. Mov Disord. 2006;21(3):310–7. https://doi.org/10.1002/mds.20720.

20. Park JE, Maurer CW, Hallett M. The "whack-a-mole" sign in functional movement disorders. Mov Disord Clin Pract. 2015;2(3):286–8. https://doi.org/10.1002/mdc3.12177.

21. Deuschl G, Köster B, Lücking CH, Scheidt C. Diagnostic and pathophysiological aspects of psychogenic tremors. Mov Disord. 1998;13(2):294–302. https://doi.org/10.1002/mds.870130216.

22. Thenganatt MA, Jankovic J. Psychogenic (functional) parkinsonism. In: *Handbook of clinical neurology*, vol. 139. Elsevier; 2016. p. 259–62.

23. Okun MS, Rodriguez RL, Foote KD, Fernandez HH. The "chair test" to aid in the diagnosis of psychogenic gait disorders. Neurologist. 2007;13(2):87–91. https://doi.org/10.1097/01.nrl.0000256358.52613.cc.

24. Felicio AC, et al. Degenerative parkinsonism in patients with psychogenic parkinsonism: a dopamine transporter imaging study. Clin Neurol Neurosurg. 2010;112(4):282–5. https://doi.org/10.1016/j.clineuro.2009.12.010.

25. Ba F, Martin WRW. Dopamine transporter imaging as a diagnostic tool for parkinsonism and related disorders in clinical practice. Parkinsonism Relat Disord. 2015;21(2):87–94. https://doi.org/10.1016/j.parkreldis.2014.11.007.

26. Rodriguez-Porcel F, Jamali S, Duker AP, Espay AJ. Dopamine transporter scanning in the evaluation of patients with suspected Parkinsonism: a case-based user's guide. Expert Rev Neurother. 2016;16(1):23–9. https://doi.org/10.1586/14737175.2015.1120160.

27. Nicastro N, Burkhard PR, Garibotto V. Scan without evidence of dopaminergic deficit (SWEDD) in degenerative parkinsonism and dementia with Lewy bodies: a prospective study. J Neurol Sci. 2018;385:17–21. https://doi.org/10.1016/j.jns.2017.11.039.

28. Vial F, Kassavetis P, Merchant S, Haubenberger D, Hallett M. How to do an electrophysiological study of tremor. Clin Neurophysiol Pract. 2019;4:134–42. https://doi.org/10.1016/j.cnp.2019.06.002.

29. Schwingenschuh P, et al. Validation of "laboratory-supported" criteria for functional (psychogenic) tremor. Mov Disord. 2016;31(4):555–62. https://doi.org/10.1002/mds.26525.

30. Lidstone SC, et al. Effects of expectation on placebo-induced dopamine release in Parkinson disease. Arch Gen Psychiatry. 2010;67(8):857–65. https://doi.org/10.1001/archgenpsychiatry.2010.88.

31. Stone J, Edwards M. Trick or treat?: Showing patients with functional (psychogenic) motor symptoms their physical signs. Neurology. 2012;79(3):282–4. https://doi.org/10.1212/WNL.0b013e31825fdff63.

32. Aybek S, Hubschmid M, Mossinger C, Berney A, Vingerhoets F. Early intervention for conversion disorder: neurologists and psychiatrists working together.

Acta Neuropsychiatr. 2013;25(1):52–6. https://doi.org/10.1111/j.1601-5215.2012.00668.x.

33. Hubschmid M, et al. Efficacy of brief interdisciplinary psychotherapeutic intervention for motor conversion disorder and nonepileptic attacks. Gen Hosp Psychiatry. 2015;37(5):448–55. https://doi.org/10.1016/j.genhosppsych.2015.05.007.

34. Stone J, Carson A, Hallett M. Explanation as treatment for functional neurologic disorders. Handb Clin Neurol. 2016;139:543–53. https://doi.org/10.1016/B978-0-12-801772-2.00044-8.

35. Nielsen G, Stone J, Edwards MJ. Physiotherapy for functional (psychogenic) motor symptoms: a systematic review. J Psychosom Res. 2013;75(2):93–102. https://doi.org/10.1016/j.jpsychores.2013.05.006.

36. Kompoliti K, Wilson B, Stebbins G, Bernard B, Hinson V. Immediate vs. delayed treatment of psychogenic movement disorders with short term psychodynamic psychotherapy: randomized clinical trial. Parkinsonism Relat Disord. 2014;20(1):60–3. https://doi.org/10.1016/j.parkreldis.2013.09.018.

37. Reuber M, Burness C, Howlett S, Brazier J, Grünewald R. Tailored psychotherapy for patients with functional neurological symptoms: a pilot study. J Psychosom Res. 2007;63(6):625–32. https://doi.org/10.1016/j.jpsychores.2007.06.013.

38. Hinson VK, Weinstein S, Bernard B, Leurgans SE, Goetz CG. Single-blind clinical trial of psychotherapy for treatment of psychogenic movement disorders. Parkinsonism Relat Disord. 2006;12(3):177–80. https://doi.org/10.1016/j.parkreldis.2005.10.006.

39. Sharpe M, et al. Guided self-help for functional (psychogenic) symptoms: a randomized controlled efficacy trial. Neurology. 2011;77(6):564–72. https://doi.org/10.1212/WNL.0b013e318228c0c7.

40. Dallocchio C, Tinazzi M, Bombieri F, Arnó N, Erro R. Cognitive behavioural therapy and adjunctive physical activity for functional movement disorders (conversion disorder): a pilot, single-blinded, randomized study. Psychother Psychosom. 2016;85(6):381–3. https://doi.org/10.1159/000446660.

41. Garcin B, et al. Transcranial magnetic stimulation as an efficient treatment for psychogenic movement disorders. J Neurol Neurosurg Psychiatry. 2013;84(9):1043–6. https://doi.org/10.1136/jnnp-2012-304062.

42. Garcin B, et al. Impact of transcranial magnetic stimulation on functional movement disorders: cortical modulation or a behavioral effect? Front Neurol. 2017;8:338. https://doi.org/10.3389/fneur.2017.00338.

43. McWhirter L, Carson A, Stone J. The body electric: a long view of electrical therapy for functional neurological disorders. Brain J Neurol. 2015;138(Pt 4):1113–20. https://doi.org/10.1093/brain/awv009.

Functional Jerky Movements

9

Yasmine E. M. Dreissen, Jeannette M. Gelauff, and Marina A. J. Tijssen

Clinical Vignette

Case 1

A 52-year old man with a history of ankylosing spondylitis presented after developing jerking movements of the abdomen and legs, which predominantly occurred in the supine position and started after a period of severe lower back pain (Video 9.1). Symptoms typically occurred in the evening before falling asleep, and could last for hours, with jerks occurring every few seconds. The symptoms waxed and waned over the years, but worsened again in the past year. Due to these symptoms, the patient was significantly impaired, and declared unable to work as a journalist. Symptoms also contributed to social isolation, which took its toll on his family as well. An MRI scan of the spine was normal. On polymyographic electromyography (pEMG) the jerks were preceded by a readiness potential (RP). The patient was treated with botulinum toxin (BoNT) injections with complete symptom resolution 1 week after treatment. The treating physicians and the patient made the joint decision to not pursue additional treatment. At 1 year follow-up visit, the patient's symptoms had returned to their prior severity.

Case 2

A 56-year old woman with hypertension presented complaining of jerky movements of the left leg accompanied by dystonic posturing with inward positioning of the ankle and foot; this movement was especially prominent when she was seated (Video 9.2). Her symptoms started after arthroscopic surgery of the left knee; the patient perceived that local anesthetic of the femoral nerve during this procedure "went wrong". Touching the left leg and assessing reflexes elicited the movements. The patient could resolve the dystonic posturing by tapping the upper leg at a certain spot. EMG/nerve conduction study (NCS) of the femoral nerve was normal. One year after these complaints started, the patient experienced an exaggerated startle reaction after a client at work made a loud noise by slapping his hand on a table. This evolved into a generalized attack with uncontrollable non-synchronous

Supplementary Information The online version contains supplementary material available at [https://doi.org/10.1007/978-3-030-86495-8_9].

Y. E. M. Dreissen · J. M. Gelauff
Department of Neurology, Amsterdam University Medical Center, Amsterdam, the Netherlands

M. A. J. Tijssen (✉)
Expertise Center Movement Disorders, Department of Neurology, University Medical Center Groningen, Groningen, the Netherlands
e-mail: m.a.j.de.koning-tijssen@umcg.nl

© Springer Nature Switzerland AG 2022
K. LaFaver et al. (eds.), *Functional Movement Disorder*, Current Clinical Neurology,
https://doi.org/10.1007/978-3-030-86495-8_9

movement of the arms and legs, vocalizations, preservation of consciousness and hyperventilation. The patient was admitted to a neurology ward for several days, where an electroencephalogram (EEG) performed during a similar episode was negative for epileptiform activity. She was discharged from the hospital, but remained extremely sensitive to startling noises. The auditory startle reflex was assessed, which revealed an exaggerated startle reaction with enlarged and prolonged (minutes) muscle activity mainly in stereotypical movements, vocal utterings and predominantly prolonged onset latencies (>100 ms). BoNT treatment of the left leg resulted in considerable improvement in symptoms and the startle reflex normalized 1 year after treatment.

Functional Jerky Movements

Functional jerky movements (also known as functional myoclonus) are a heterogenous group of involuntary abrupt movements that are mostly paroxysmal and can involve the limbs, trunk and/or neck. While the prevalence of functional jerky movements within general neurology is unknown, they represent one of the more common functional movement disorder (FMD) subtypes [1–4]. In a tertiary movement disorder clinic specialized in myoclonus, more than one third of patients seen suffered from a functional jerky movement disorder [5]. They can be challenging to diagnose, mainly due to their paroxysmal nature and their heterogeneous presentation, as highlighted by the above cases. Indeed, the diagnostic accuracy for functional jerky movements based on review of video recordings by movement disorder specialists showed moderate inter-rater agreement (kappa = 0.56 ± 0.1) [6]. The diagnosis can be made with the help of clinical criteria [7–9] and supported by neurophysiological tests. In this chapter we will discuss the clinical presentation, positive signs in history and physical examination for the diagnosis, additional testing and the most important differential diagnoses.

Clinical Presentation

Although the clinical presentation is heterogeneous in terms of localization of the jerks, age at onset, associated symptoms and disease course, there are a number of factors that characterize functional jerky movements and can support the diagnosis.

History

There are a number of relevant features on clinical history that are typical for functional jerky movements. There is often an abrupt onset, triggered by either a physical or psychological trigger, after which the symptoms deteriorate [1, 10, 11]. Furthermore, like in other FMD subtypes, attention plays an important role [12], and patients either spontaneously report or confirm noticing that symptoms improve with distraction and worsen during relaxation (for example before falling asleep). Usually there is a discrepancy between the severity of the symptoms as observed by the examiner and their influence on daily functioning. Previous episodes of somatization and/or functional symptoms are relevant, but do not have high specificity, since FMD is comorbid with other non-functional movement disorders more often than expected by chance [13–15].

Although functional jerky movements can occur in any body part, their localization is helpful in distinguishing them from the differential diagnosis of tics and non-functional ("organic") myoclonus. Generally, we find that axial jerks are likely to represent functional jerks. Facial and neck jerks point more often towards tics, especially when they start at a young age. Distal limb jerks are more likely to reflect non-functional myoclonus (see below). Functional jerks may be present continuously or episodically [10, 16, 17]. The episodic variant can be challenging to diagnose as it can be absent during the outpatient clinic visit.

In terms of non-motor symptoms in patients with functional jerky movements, similar to other FMD, high rates of pain and fatigue are found

[18, 19]. Interestingly, non-motor symptoms were equally common in patients with cortical myoclonus as in those with functional myoclonus, while pain was the only symptom that significantly occurred more commonly in the functional myoclonus group [5]. In general, hyperkinetic FMD are often accompanied by high proportions of psychiatric co-morbidity. Specifically, patients with functional dystonia, tremor and myoclonus exhibit high rates (50–80%) of DSM IV axis I disorders (mostly mood and anxiety disorders) and moderate rates (18–45%) of DSM IV personality disorders [1, 20–24].

Neurological Examination

Observation of the jerky movements may reveal variation in duration, localization, amplitude and/or direction of the movements within the same patient. High variability is suggestive of a functional etiology. The effect of attention and distraction can be tested during examination, but is not as reliable as in tremor as the jerks themselves are irregular and as previously mentioned can be paroxysmal. When distracted, the jerky movements can decrease or disappear [9]. Also, the examiner might induce adaptation of the patient's jerks to a certain frequency, a phenomenon called "entrainment", when asking the patient to perform a specific rhythmic task. Generally, if the character of the jerky movements can be influenced by the examiner, that argues in favor of a FMD.

Additional functional (motor) symptoms can be found, like functional weakness or dystonia, as patients commonly present with more than one functional neurological symptom [4, 19]. While this is supportive of the diagnosis of functional myoclonus, it does not rule out the possibility of a non-functional myoclonus being comorbid with a functional neurological disorder.

Abnormal stimulus-sensitivity can be observed in all FMD, and especially in functional jerky movements; this can present as exaggerated tendon reflexes or excessive startle reactions

[25]. Further supportive clues are a marked response to placebo or suggestion, although, again, this is also observed in other movement disorders [10, 26].

Additional Investigations

Neurophysiological testing is a useful diagnostic aid in jerky movement disorders.

The first step in this testing involves evaluating the jerky movements with *polymyographic surface EMG* (pEMG). This is helpful in establishing the burst duration and the muscle recruitment pattern. An EMG burst duration of <75 ms is very unlikely to represent a jerk of functional origin [27, 28]. In myoclonus-dystonia a longer burst duration can occur, so in these cases the duration is of less distinctive value. The pEMG muscle recruitment pattern can also help with the diagnosis, including findings of entrainment, distractibility, inconsistent recruitment pattern and stimulus-sensitivity supporting a functional origin [29], although this last feature can also be present in cortical myoclonus. In the case of axial jerks specifically, the recruitment pattern is of special interest. It is generally considered that patients with functional axial jerks reveal a more variable recruitment pattern. But even with a consistent pattern a functional origin cannot be ruled out and back-averaging of the electroencephalography (EEG) time-locked to the onset of the jerk (EEG-EMG co-registration) is essential [30, 31]. With this technique a Readiness Potential (RP) also known as the Bereitschaftspotential preceding the movements can be detected, which is a powerful diagnostic aid in functional jerky movements. The RP appears about 2 seconds prior to the movement as a slowly rising negative cortical potential (Fig. 9.1) and is especially useful in distinguishing functional jerks from other jerky movements. A drawback of this procedure is that it is a time-consuming procedure requiring at least 40 jerks in order to produce a reliable result. In a small study assessing the presence an RP preceding jerky

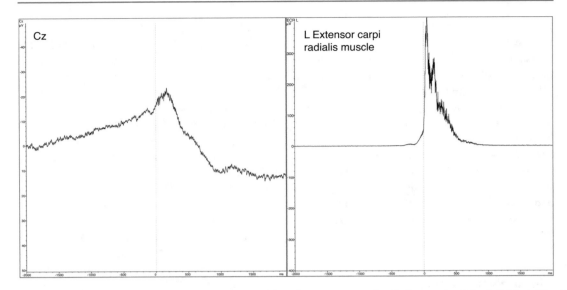

Fig. 9.1 Readiness potential, or "pre-motor" potential. Average traces from simultaneous electroencephalography (EEG) (left) and electromyography (EMG) (right) recordings, as derived from 75 extension movements of the extensor carpi radialis muscle of the left hand. The readiness potential is visible 1500–2000 ms prior to movement onset

movements, a RP was found in 25 of 29 patients with functional jerks, with a sensitivity and specificity of 0.86 [31]. When the RP is combined with event-related desynchronization (ERD) in the beta-range (13–45 Hz) prior to the jerks, even higher diagnostic certainty can be reached [32]. However the RP can also be found in a small proportion of patients with primary tics, albeit with shorter onset latencies [31].

Another important feature of functional jerks is their stimulus-sensitivity and the presence of exaggerated startle responses. Measuring the whole-body auditory startle reflex with surface EMG can be used to distinguish between functional and other types of jerks. The auditory startle reflex consists of two responses: a stereotyped first muscle response revealing a rostro-caudal recruitment pattern with short onset latencies (<100 ms) [33, 34] followed by a second response, which is more variable in pattern and associated with behavioral processing and autonomic changes [35]. Although normal first responses are seen in functional jerky movements, the rate of second responses (onset latency >100 ms) is higher and responses are enlarged compared to healthy controls [25].

Differential Diagnosis

The differential diagnosis of functional jerky movements includes tics, non-functional myoclonus, epilepsy, restless legs syndrome, and primary paroxysmal dyskinesias (see Table 9.1). Below we describe how these can be distinguished from functional jerky movements.

Tics

Tics are defined as sudden, repetitive, *non-rhythmic*, purposeless, irresistible muscle movements (motor tic) or vocalizations (vocal tic) which can be classified as simple or complex [36]. They are categorized into different tic disorders, including Tourette's syndrome. The diagnosis of these tic disorders is based on history and clinical examination, using DSM-V/ICD-10 criteria [37].

Although tics co-occur with functional tic-like jerks in a considerable number of patients [38] and pathophysiological mechanisms overlap [39], there are a number of features that can be used to support the diagnosis of primary tic.

Table 9.1 Differential diagnosis of functional jerky movements

	History	Localization	Examination	Neurophysiology
Functional jerky movements	Acute onset Precipitating (physical) event	Limbs/axial/face/neck	Stimulus-sensitive Entrainment Distractibility	pEMG EEG-EMG back-averaging RP Enlarged startle reflex with predominant second responses
Tics	Premonitory urge Childhood onset Vocalizations	Face/neck	Temporarily suppressible Rebound effect	Burst duration > 100 ms RP is rare, and shorter when present
Cortical myoclonus	Variable	Face/distal limbs	Stimulus-sensitive	Burst duration < 100 ms C-reflex Giant SSEP Corticomuscular coherence
Myoclonus-dystonia	Childhood onset Positive family history Alcohol-responsiveness	Limbs/axial	Dystonic features	Burst duration > 100 ms pEMG with brainstem recruitment pattern
Hyperekplexia	Stiffness at birth Exaggerated startle reactions with generalized stiffness	Generalized	Exaggerated startle with generalized stiffness Positive head-retraction reflex	Exaggerated startle reflex with rostro-caudal recruitment pattern
Propriospinal myoclonus	Acute onset	Axial/limbs	Features of myelopathy Stimulus-sensitive Present in supine position	pEMG EEG-EMG backaveraging RP MRI-spine, although most cases lack an underlying structural lesion
Restless legs	Presence when rested in evening/night	Lower limbs	Normal	Polysomnography
Paroxysmal dyskinesias	Childhood onset Positive family history Specific triggers	Usually unilateral	Mixed movement disorders	Not contributing

RP readiness potential (or Bereitschaftspotential), *SSEP* somatosensory evoked potential, *MRI* magnetic resonance imaging

Tics originate in most cases in childhood, with a mean age of onset of 5 years and male preponderance (male:female ratio 3:1) [36]. This is in contrast with functional jerks which usually start in adulthood [10, 16].

The most defining feature of tics is that the movements are intentional and, in line with this feature, suppressible, while functional jerky movements are perceived as involuntary [36, 40]. Most patients with tics experience an involuntary pre-motor urge, which is subsequently relieved by carrying out the tic. Patients are often able to suppress the tics for a certain period of time, in many cases resulting in a rebound of a temporary worsening of the tics. It is therefore not surprising that tics are more stereotyped and less variable compared to functional jerks. Recently it has been described that patients with functional paroxysmal motor symptoms, like jerky movements, may experience a pre-motor urge [16, 41], however they are considered to be much less common. Further, patients with tics may camouflage the movement by assimilating it into a purposeful movement whereas patients with functional jerks are not able to hide and/or suppress their movements [36, 42, 43]. Echophenomena like echolalia (repeating sounds) and echopraxia (repeating actions), and coprolalia (involuntary swearing) are present in up to 20% of patients with primary tics, while these are rare in patients with functional jerks [17].

The entity of "functional tics" has been described in small groups of patients [44, 45]. However, it remains unclear how to distinguish them from functional jerky movements, as they do not possess the typical characteristics of a tic. Notably, premonitory urge, childhood onset, suppressibility and positive family history are lacking. Therefore, it seems more appropriate to use the broader term of functional jerky movements instead of tic-like functional movements (for a more detailed description see Chap. 12).

For tics, clinical neurophysiological investigations do not add to the diagnosis. However, they are sporadically used to differentiate tics from other jerky movements, like functional jerky movements. The presence of a readiness potential before the movement is in favor of a functional neurological origin, while in tics the RP is seen less frequent and the configuration differs from FMD with shorter onset latencies (500–1000 ms) [31, 46, 47].

A correct diagnosis of either tics or functional jerky movements is important for choosing the right treatment strategy. The effect of treatment in tics is favorable, both for behavior therapy (either habit reversal or exposure to premonitory urges with response prevention) [48] with medium to large effect sizes [49] as well as for medication (dopamine D2-receptor-antagonists) with small to medium effect sizes [50].

Myoclonus

Non-functional myoclonus (denoted in this chapter as "myoclonus") has to be considered in the differential diagnosis of functional jerky movements. Myoclonus is defined as a brief, sudden, shock-like involuntary movement, resulting from a muscle contraction (positive myoclonus) or the short interruption of tonic muscle activity (negative myoclonus) [51]. There are several acquired and genetic causes for myoclonus [52, 53] but for this chapter we will focus on the different clinical phenotypes. Once the subtype/phenotype of myoclonus is established, determining the underlying etiology is the next step and beyond the scope of this chapter.

Clinically, myoclonus can be classified based on the anatomical localization: cortical, subcortical and spinal myoclonus. Neurophysiological testing plays an important tool in the classification of these subtypes [54].

Cortical Myoclonus
Cortical myoclonus is characterized by very short-lasting shock-like movements, manifesting in the limbs and the face which can be focal, mul-

tifocal or generalized. Although jerks can occur spontaneously, they can often be triggered by a stimulus such as tapping the fingers [55]. Its pathophysiology is based on pathologically enhanced excitability of motor neurons in the primary motor cortex. Causes of cortical myoclonus include inherited (genetic) as well as acquired (post-hypoxic, epileptic, toxic/metabolic) origins [55]. sEMG reveals short-lasting (<100 ms) jerks, which differentiates it from functional myoclonus [56]. More advanced neurophysiological testing in support of a cortical origin include giant somatosensory evoked potentials (SSEP's), coherence analysis and the C-reflex [54, 57, 58].

Subcortical Myoclonus
This form of myoclonus is generated between the cortex and the spinal cord, mainly in the basal ganglia or brainstem. We will discuss the most important forms here, starting with myoclonus-dystonia (DYT11). This is a form of subcortical myoclonus generated in the basal ganglia. It is characterized by jerks of the upper limbs and trunk accompanied by mild dystonia (usually cervical dystonia and writer's cramp) [59]. The key to the diagnosis is onset of symptoms in childhood, alcohol-responsiveness and a positive family history. High rates of psychiatric co-morbidity including anxiety, depression and obsessive-compulsive disorders are also found [60]. In 50% of cases a mutation in the SGCE gene is detected [61]. Neurophysiological testing typically shows a longer (>100 ms) burst duration and is further aimed to rule out any signs of a cortical origin as mentioned above.

Brainstem Myoclonus and Startle Syndromes
Brainstem, or reticular myoclonus is characterized by a generalized, synchronous axial jerks [62]. Post-hypoxia is usually the cause [63], but other causes such as anatomical anomalies have also been described [64]. The jerks are usually stimulus-sensitive and can be elicited by startling stimuli. A syndrome which is closely related is hyperekplexia (HPX). This is a pathological startle syndrome, which is caused by different gene mutations (GLRA1, GLRB, Glyt2) involving the glycine neu-

rotransmission pathway [65]. It is characterized by generalized stiffness at birth and non-habituating exaggerated startle reactions followed by short-lasting generalized stiffness in response to loud noises. Neurophysiological testing can be especially useful to distinguish the pathological startle reflex of hyperekplexia from a functional myoclonus. The startle reflex shows a consistent pEMG recruitment pattern, starting at the muscles innervated by the caudal brainstem (sternocleidomastoid), spreading in a rostro-caudal fashion with the intrinsic hand muscles showing a relatively long onset latency in the startle response [33, 65].

Spinal Myoclonus

This form of myoclonus can be differentiated into *spinal segmental myoclonus* and *propriospinal myoclonus*. Here, we will only discuss propriospinal myoclonus, since it is of particular interest in relation to functional jerky movements, and spinal segmental myoclonus is extremely rare. Propriospinal myoclonus is characterized by stereotyped rhythmic relatively slow axial jerks, which are often present in the supine position and elicited by tactile stimulation of the abdomen. Propriospinal myoclonus can be caused by pathology (e.g. tumor, infection) of the thoracic spine. However, most often an underlying structural lesion is lacking and it was shown that the typical movement pattern can easily be mimicked voluntarily [66]. The majority of cases of idiopathic propriospinal myoclonus have been shown to have a functional neurological origin [41, 67]. Neurophysiological testing including back-averaging in order to demonstrate the presence of a RP is especially useful.

Epilepsy

Repetitive jerky movements can also be seen in several forms of epilepsy. Functional jerky movement disorders show many overlapping features with functional seizures as well [68]. Functional seizures mimic epileptic seizures but lack an EEG-correlate. As in FMD, a substantial fraction (10–20%) of patients with functional seizures also have co-morbid epilepsy [69]. Despite well-

formulated diagnostic criteria based on the semiology of functional seizures [70], the diagnosis remains challenging. Eyewitness history and especially video-EEG monitoring is very useful to distinguish epileptic attacks from functional seizures.

Restless Legs Syndrome

Functional jerky movements are usually worse when patients are not distracted and therefore many patients report more symptoms when lying in bed. In these patients, the differential diagnosis of restless legs syndrome should be considered. Restless legs syndrome is a circadian disorder with an urge to move the legs, which is often, but not always, accompanied by uncomfortable and unpleasant sensations in the legs. This urge begins or worsens during periods of rest or inactivity such as lying down or sitting, and is relieved by deliberate movements [71]. As in tics, the presence of this urge distinguishes restless legs from FMD. In functional jerky movements, the movements are not deliberate. Neurological examination in restless legs syndrome is mostly normal [71], while functional jerks are often observed in clinic. The diagnosis of restless legs syndrome is made based on clinical criteria [72].

Primary Paroxysmal Dyskinesias

Primary paroxysmal dyskinesias (PxD) are a rare group of movement disorders (0.76% of all movement disorders) characterized by paroxysmal involuntary movements of brief duration [73, 74], that are often misdiagnosed as FMD given their paroxysmal nature. Inherited forms of primary paroxysmal dyskinesias include paroxysmal kinesigenic dyskinesia (PKD), paroxysmal non-kinesigenic dyskinesia (PNKD) and paroxysmal exercise-induced dyskinesia (PED) [74, 75], with the kinesigenic form by far the most common one. All three forms usually start in the first or second decade of life and are caused by different gene mutations. The most well-known are the PRRT-2, MR-1, and GLUT-1 genes, but recently more genes have been detected and there appears to be a large clinical and genetic overlap [76]. They are usually familial, in contrast to functional jerky movements. The main clinical feature discriminating functional jerky movements from PxD's are that the attacks of dystonia, chorea or ballism or a mixture of those in PxD show a consistent pattern and have a consistent trigger, especially the kinesiogenic form.

However, coexistence of functional jerky movements with paroxysmal movement disorders is described in a substantial proportion of patients [13, 17], and should be kept in mind.

Premonitory sensations are reported in the majority of PxD patients and have been described as "butterflies in the stomach", "electricity in the head" or numbness or a tingling sensation in the limbs [77]. Attacks tend to decrease with age. Video-recordings can be very helpful in making the diagnosis, as they can show the consistent pattern of attacks.

Management

An individualized treatment plan including physical, occupational and/or psychotherapeutic interventions can be helpful in treating patients with functional jerky movements. A thorough description of these different therapeutic modalities is found in Part III of this textbook.

Conclusion

Functional jerky movement disorders (or functional myoclonus) are a common manifestation of FMD. The diagnosis can be made based on clinical signs with the help of additional neurophysiological testing; EEG-EMG with back-averaging in order to demonstrate a RP is especially useful. Since functional jerks are heterogeneous in nature, the differential diagnosis is broad and dependent of the phenomenology of each specific patient.

Summary

- Functional jerky movements (functional myoclonus) are a heterogeneous group of involuntary abrupt movements that are mostly paroxysmal with preferential involvement of the trunk, although the movements can also occur in the limbs or neck.
- The diagnosis is based on clinical signs and symptoms that can be supported by clinical neurophysiological tests.
- Clinical signs that contribute to the diagnosis include acute onset, variability of the movements and of symptom severity, and presence of co-morbid functional neurological symptoms.
- Neurological examination often shows variability in duration, localization, amplitude and/or direction of the movements; influence of distraction on the severity of the movements and entrainment can also be appreciated.
- Functional jerky movements typically display a relatively long burst duration and variable muscle recruitment pattern in neurophysiological testing. Back-averaging of the electro-encephalography (EEG-EMG co-registration) can detect a Readiness Potential (RP).
- The differential diagnosis for functional jerky movements includes tics, myoclonus, epilepsy, paroxysmal dyskinesias and restless legs syndrome.

References

1. Factor SA, Podskalny GD, Molho ES. Psychogenic movement disorders: frequency, clinical profile, and characteristics. J Neurol Neurosurg Psychiatry. 1995;59(4):406–12.
2. Hinson VK, Haren WB. Psychogenic movement disorders. Lancet Neurol. 2006;5(8):695–700.
3. Lang A. General overview of psychogenic movement disorders: epidemiology, diagnosis and prognosis. In: Psychogenic movement disorders-neurology and neuropsychiatry. Philadelphia: Lippincott Williams & Wilkins; 2006. p. 35–41.

4. Gelauff JM, Rosmalen JGM, Gardien J, Stone J, Tijssen MAJ. Shared demographics and comorbidities in different functional motor disorders. Parkinsonism Relat Disord. 2020;70:1–6.

5. Zutt R, Elting JW, van der Hoeven JH, Lange F, Tijssen MAJ. Myoclonus subtypes in tertiary referral center. Cortical myoclonus and functional jerks are common. Clin Neurophysiol. 2017;128(1):253–9.

6. van der Salm SM, de Haan RJ, Cath DC, van Rootselaar AF, Tijssen MA. The eye of the beholder: inter-rater agreement among experts on psychogenic jerky movement disorders. J Neurol Neurosurg Psychiatry. 2013;84(7):742–7.

7. Fahn S, Williams DT. Psychogenic dystonia. Adv Neurol. 1988;50:431–55.

8. Shill H, Gerber P. Evaluation of clinical diagnostic criteria for psychogenic movement disorders. Mov Disord. 2006;21(8):1163–8.

9. Gupta A, Lang AE. Psychogenic movement disorders. Curr Opin Neurol. 2009;22(4):430–6.

10. Monday K, Jankovic J. Psychogenic myoclonus. Neurology. 1993;43(2):349–52.

11. Parees I, Kojovic M, Pires C, Rubio-Agusti I, Saifee TA, Sadnicka A, et al. Physical precipitating factors in functional movement disorders. J Neurol Sci. 2014;338(1–2):174–7.

12. van Poppelen D, Saifee TA, Schwingenschuh P, Katschnig P, Bhatia KP, Tijssen MA, et al. Attention to self in psychogenic tremor. Mov Disord. 2011;26(14):2575–6.

13. Ranawaya R, Riley D, Lang A. Psychogenic dyskinesias in patients with organic movement disorders. Mov Disord. 1990;5(2):127–33.

14. Onofrj M, Bonanni L, Manzoli L, Thomas A. Cohort study on somatoform disorders in Parkinson disease and dementia with Lewy bodies. Neurology. 2010;74(20):1598–606.

15. Parees I, Saifee TA, Kojovic M, Kassavetis P, Rubio-Agusti I, Sadnicka A, et al. Functional (psychogenic) symptoms in Parkinson's disease. Mov Disord. 2013;28(12):1622–7.

16. van der Salm SM, Erro R, Cordivari C, Edwards MJ, Koelman JH, van den Ende T, et al. Propriospinal myoclonus: clinical reappraisal and review of literature. Neurology. 2014;83(20):1862–70.

17. Ganos C, Aguirregomozcorta M, Batla A, Stamelou M, Schwingenschuh P, Munchau A, et al. Psychogenic paroxysmal movement disorders--clinical features and diagnostic clues. Parkinsonism Relat Disord. 2014;20(1):41–6.

18. Gelauff JM, Kingma EM, Kalkman JS, Bezemer R, van Engelen BGM, Stone J, et al. Fatigue, not self-rated motor symptom severity, affects quality of life in functional motor disorders. J Neurol. 2018;265(8):1803–9.

19. Gelauff JM, Carson A, Ludwig L, Tijssen MAJ, Stone J. The prognosis of functional limb weakness: a 14-year case-control study. Brain. 2019;142(7):2137–48.

20. Thomas M, Vuong KD, Jankovic J. Long-term prognosis of patients with psychogenic movement disorders. Parkinsonism Relat Disord. 2006;12(6):382–7.

21. Ertan S, Uluduz D, Ozekmekci S, Kiziltan G, Ertan T, Yalcinkaya C, et al. Clinical characteristics of 49 patients with psychogenic movement disorders in a tertiary clinic in Turkey. Mov Disord. 2009;24(5):759–62.

22. Feinstein A, Stergiopoulos V, Fine J, Lang AE. Psychiatric outcome in patients with a psychogenic movement disorder: a prospective study. Neuropsychiatry Neuropsychol Behav Neurol. 2001;14(3):169–76.

23. Kranick S, Ekanayake V, Martinez V, Ameli R, Hallett M, Voon V. Psychopathology and psychogenic movement disorders. Mov Disord. 2011;26(10):1844–50.

24. Tomic A, Petrovic I, Pesic D, Voncina MM, Svetel M, Miskovic ND, et al. Is there a specific psychiatric background or personality profile in functional dystonia? J Psychosom Res. 2017;97:58–62.

25. Dreissen YEM, Boeree T, Koelman J, Tijssen MAJ. Startle responses in functional jerky movement disorders are increased but have a normal pattern. Parkinsonism Relat Disord. 2017;40:27–32.

26. Williams DT, Ford B, Fahn S. Phenomenology and psychopathology related to psychogenic movement disorders. Adv Neurol. 1995;65:231–57.

27. Thompson PD, Colebatch JG, Brown P, Rothwell JC, Day BL, Obeso JA, et al. Voluntary stimulus-sensitive jerks and jumps mimicking myoclonus or pathological startle syndromes. Mov Disord. 1992;7(3):257–62.

28. Edwards MJ, Bhatia KP. Functional (psychogenic) movement disorders: merging mind and brain. Lancet Neurol. 2012;11(3):250–60.

29. Apartis E. Clinical neurophysiology of psychogenic movement disorders: how to diagnose psychogenic tremor and myoclonus. Neurophysiol Clin. 2014;44(4):417–24.

30. Shibasaki H, Hallett M. What is the Bereitschaftspotential? Clin Neurophysiol. 2006;117(11):2341–56.

31. van der Salm SM, Tijssen MA, Koelman JH, van Rootselaar AF. The bereitschaftspotential in jerky movement disorders. J Neurol Neurosurg Psychiatry. 2012;83(12):1162–7.

32. Beudel M, Zutt R, Meppelink AM, Little S, Elting JW, Stelten BML, et al. Improving neurophysiological biomarkers for functional myoclonic movements. Parkinsonism Relat Disord. 2018;51:3–8.

33. Brown P, Rothwell JC, Thompson PD, Britton TC, Day BL, Marsden CD. New observations on the normal auditory startle reflex in man. Brain. 1991;114(Pt 4):1891–902.

34. Bakker MJ, Boer F, van der Meer JN, Koelman JH, Boeree T, Bour L, et al. Quantification of the auditory startle reflex in children. Clin Neurophysiol. 2009;120(2):424–30.

35. Gogan P. The startle and orienting reactions in man. A study of their characteristics and habituation. Brain Res. 1970;18(1):117–35.

36. Cath DC, Hedderly T, Ludolph AG, Stern JS, Murphy T, Hartmann A, et al. European clinical guidelines for Tourette syndrome and other tic disorders. Part I: assessment. Eur Child Adolesc Psychiatry. 2011;20(4):155–71.

37. American Psychiatric Association. Diagnostic and statistical manual of mental disorders. 5th ed. Arlington: American Psychiatric Publishing; 2013.

38. Barry S, Baird G, Lascelles K, Bunton P, Hedderly T. Neurodevelopmental movement disorders – an update on childhood motor stereotypies. Dev Med Child Neurol. 2011;53(11):979–85.

39. Ganos C, Martino D, Espay AJ, Lang AE, Bhatia KP, Edwards MJ. Tics and functional tic-like movements: can we tell them apart? Neurology. 2019;93(17):750–8.

40. Voon V, Gallea C, Hattori N, Bruno M, Ekanayake V, Hallett M. The involuntary nature of conversion disorder. Neurology. 2010;74(3):223–8.

41. van der Salm SM, Koelman JH, Henneke S, van Rootselaar AF, Tijssen MA. Axial jerks: a clinical spectrum ranging from propriospinal to psychogenic myoclonus. J Neurol. 2010;257(8):1349–55.

42. Anderson KE, Gruber-Baldini AL, Vaughan CG, Reich SG, Fishman PS, Weiner WJ, et al. Impact of psychogenic movement disorders versus Parkinson's on disability, quality of life, and psychopathology. Mov Disord. 2007;22(15):2204–9.

43. Parees I, Kassavetis P, Saifee TA, Sadnicka A, Davare M, Bhatia KP, et al. Failure of explicit movement control in patients with functional motor symptoms. Mov Disord. 2013;28(4):517–23.

44. Demartini B, Ricciardi L, Parees I, Ganos C, Bhatia KP, Edwards MJ. A positive diagnosis of functional (psychogenic) tics. Eur J Neurol. 2015;22(3):527–e36.

45. Baizabal-Carvallo JF, Jankovic J. The clinical features of psychogenic movement disorders resembling tics. J Neurol Neurosurg Psychiatry. 2014;85(5):573–5.

46. Obeso JA, Rothwell JC, Marsden CD. Simple tics in Gilles de la Tourette's syndrome are not prefaced by a normal premovement EEG potential. J Neurol Neurosurg Psychiatry. 1981;44(8):735–8.

47. Vial F, Attaripour S, Hallett M. Differentiating tics from functional (psychogenic) movements with electrophysiological tools. Clin Neurophysiol Pract. 2019;4:143–7.

48. van de Griendt JM, Verdellen CW, van Dijk MK, Verbraak MJ. Behavioural treatment of tics: habit reversal and exposure with response prevention. Neurosci Biobehav Rev. 2013;37(6):1172–7.

49. McGuire JF, Nyirabahizi E, Kircanski K, Piacentini J, Peterson AL, Woods DW, et al. A cluster analysis of tic symptoms in children and adults with Tourette syndrome: clinical correlates and treatment outcome. Psychiatry Res. 2013;210(3):1198–204.

50. Weisman H, Qureshi IA, Leckman JF, Scahill L, Bloch MH. Systematic review: pharmacological treatment of tic disorders--efficacy of antipsychotic and alpha-2 adrenergic agonist agents. Neurosci Biobehav Rev. 2013;37(6):1162–71.

51. Fahn S, Marsden CD, Van Woert MH. Definition and classification of myoclonus. Adv Neurol. 1986;43:1–5.

52. Zutt R, van Egmond ME, Elting JW, van Laar PJ, Brouwer OF, Sival DA, et al. A novel diagnostic approach to patients with myoclonus. Nat Rev Neurol. 2015;11(12):687–97.

53. van der Veen S, Zutt R, Klein C, Marras C, Berkovic SF, Caviness JN, et al. Nomenclature of genetically determined myoclonus syndromes: recommendations of the International Parkinson and Movement Disorder Society Task Force. Mov Disord. 2019;34(11):1602–13.

54. Zutt R, Elting JW, van Zijl JC, van der Hoeven JH, Roosendaal CM, Gelauff JM, et al. Electrophysiologic testing aids diagnosis and subtyping of myoclonus. Neurology. 2018;90(8):e647–e57.

55. Dijk JM, Tijssen MA. Management of patients with myoclonus: available therapies and the need for an evidence-based approach. Lancet Neurol. 2010;9(10):1028–36.

56. Lozsadi D. Myoclonus: a pragmatic approach. Pract Neurol. 2012;12(4):215–24.

57. Brown P, Thompson PD. Electrophysiological aids to the diagnosis of psychogenic jerks, spasms, and tremor. Mov Disord. 2001;16(4):595–9.

58. Shibasaki H, Hallett M. Electrophysiological studies of myoclonus. Muscle Nerve. 2005;31(2):157–74.

59. Foncke EM, Gerrits MC, van Ruissen F, Baas F, Hedrich K, Tijssen CC, et al. Distal myoclonus and late onset in a large Dutch family with myoclonus-dystonia. Neurology. 2006;67(9):1677–80.

60. van Tricht MJ, Dreissen YE, Cath D, Dijk JM, Contarino MF, van der Salm SM, et al. Cognition and psychopathology in myoclonus-dystonia. J Neurol Neurosurg Psychiatry. 2012;83(8):814–20.

61. Peall KJ, Kurian MA, Wardle M, Waite AJ, Hedderly T, Lin JP, et al. SGCE and myoclonus dystonia: motor characteristics, diagnostic criteria and clinical predictors of genotype. J Neurol. 2014;261(12):2296–304.

62. Dreissen YE, Tijssen MA. The startle syndromes: physiology and treatment. Epilepsia. 2012;53(Suppl 7):3–11.

63. Hallett M. Physiology of human posthypoxic myoclonus. Mov Disord. 2000;15(Suppl 1):8–13.

64. Beudel M, Elting JWJ, Uyttenboogaart M, van den Broek MWC, Tijssen MAJ. Reticular myoclonus: it really comes from the brainstem! Mov Disord Clin Pract. 2014;1(3):258–60.

65. Bakker MJ, van Dijk JG, van den Maagdenberg AM, Tijssen MA. Startle syndromes. Lancet Neurol. 2006;5(6):513–24.

66. Kang SY, Sohn YH. Electromyography patterns of propriospinal myoclonus can be mimicked voluntarily. Mov Disord. 2006;21(8):1241–4.

67. Erro R, Bhatia KP, Edwards MJ, Farmer SF, Cordivari C. Clinical diagnosis of propriospinal myoclonus is unreliable: an electrophysiologic study. Mov Disord. 2013;28(13):1868–73.

68. Driver-Dunckley E, Stonnington CM, Locke DE, Noe K. Comparison of psychogenic movement disorders and psychogenic nonepileptic seizures: is phenotype clinically important? Psychosomatics. 2011;52(4):337–45.
69. Benbadis SR, Agrawal V, Tatum WOt. How many patients with psychogenic nonepileptic seizures also have epilepsy? Neurology. 2001;57(5):915–7.
70. Dhiman V, Sinha S, Rawat VS, Harish T, Chaturvedi SK, Satishchandra P. Semiological characteristics of adults with psychogenic nonepileptic seizures (PNESs): an attempt towards a new classification. Epilepsy Behav. 2013;27(3):427–32.
71. Wijemanne S, Ondo W. Restless Legs Syndrome: clinical features, diagnosis and a practical approach to management. Pract Neurol. 2017;17(6):444–52.
72. Allen RP. Restless legs syndrome/Willis Ekbom disease: evaluation and treatment. Int Rev Psychiatry. 2014;26(2):248–62.
73. Bhatia KP. Paroxysmal dyskinesias. Mov Disord. 2011;26(6):1157–65.
74. Erro R, Sheerin UM, Bhatia KP. Paroxysmal dyskinesias revisited: a review of 500 genetically proven cases and a new classification. Mov Disord. 2014;29(9):1108–16.
75. Bhatia KP. Familial (idiopathic) paroxysmal dyskinesias: an update. Semin Neurol. 2001;21(1):69–74.
76. Erro R, Bhatia KP. Unravelling of the paroxysmal dyskinesias. J Neurol Neurosurg Psychiatry. 2019;90(2):227–34.
77. Bruno MK, Hallett M, Gwinn-Hardy K, Sorensen B, Considine E, Tucker S, et al. Clinical evaluation of idiopathic paroxysmal kinesigenic dyskinesia: new diagnostic criteria. Neurology. 2004;63(12):2280–7.

Functional Facial Disorders

10

Mohammad Rohani and Alfonso Fasano

Mrs. G. is a 73-year-old woman referred for oromandibular dystonia versus hemifacial spasm. About a year before, she developed sudden onset of pulling of the left corner of her mouth, with forceful sidewise deviation. She went to the Emergency Department where she was evaluated for possible stroke. She did not complain of any other symptoms, such as weakness or dysarthria, and she could tell that this symptom was different from the right facial droop that she had experienced during a previous stroke, from which she had fully recovered. An urgent brain MRI ruled out an acute ischemic lesion and she was then referred to our clinic.

The mouth pulling has persisted since the day of presentation, with episodic worsening on a daily basis, each time lasting minutes. She denies contractions around her eyes or involvement of the muscles in her forehead or neck area. She thinks that these episodes can be triggered by talking, chewing and swallowing although sometimes they occur without any recognizable precipitant.

Introduction

Many systemic and neurological conditions may involve the face, and functional movement disorder (FMD) is not an exception. While eye disorders have historically received more attention, FMD affecting the eyelids, tongue and other facial muscles are often under-recognized. Nevertheless, facial involvement – occurring either alone or in combination with other FMD symptoms – are more common than previously thought [1].

Facial FMD has been already described in the early literature of the nineteenth century. The first description was probably formulated by Charcot in 1887 as 'unilateral hysterical facial spasm' [2]. One year later, Gowers described the 'hysterical' tonic contracture of the facial muscles and mentioned the wrong way tongue deviation as a clue to diagnosis [3]. Tourette described *blepharospasm hysterique* in 1889 with a photograph of a case with unilateral ptosis and dropped eyebrow

Supplementary Information The online version contains supplementary material available at [https://doi.org/10.1007/978-3-030-86495-8_10].

M. Rohani
Division of Neurology, Rasool Akram Hospital, School of Medicine, Iran University of Medical Sciences, Tehran, Iran

A. Fasano (✉)
Edmond J. Safra Program in Parkinson's Disease, Morton and Gloria Shulman Movement Disorders Clinic, Toronto Western Hospital, UHN, Toronto, ON, Canada

Division of Neurology, University of Toronto, Toronto, ON, Canada

Krembil Brain Institute, Toronto, ON, Canada
e-mail: alfonso.fasano@uhn.ca

on the same side who improved with hypnosis [4] and few years later Wood considered blepharospasm a characteristic sign of hysteria [5]. These entities entered subsequent textbooks as 'glossolabial hemispasm' [6] and their description was enriched by important features, such as the variable involvement of other facial muscles, eyelids and platysma in particular. During the same years, the terms 'hook-like appearance' [6] or 'hysterical spasm' [7] were used to describe the tongue of patients with FMD.

After these early descriptions, facial FMD has been largely neglected for almost a century. Functional unilateral spasm of the eyelid has been initially described as 'psychogenic pseudoptosis' [8] and subsequently as 'psychogenic' hemifacial spasm (HFS) [9]. A similar entity has been described by other authors in a few other patients [10, 11]. Over the last two decades, the increased awareness of facial FMD has contributed to a reappraisal of prior literature [1]. For example, some atypical facial disorders have been anecdotally reported as representing rare phenotypes of focal dystonia [9, 12–14]. However, we have recently proposed that these disorders may be better classified as FMD given their inconsistency, incongruence with other known neurological conditions, associated features and response to treatment [1].

Epidemiology

Functional blepharospasm has been reported in 0.3% [15] to 7% [16] of all types of FMD, in 20% of the total population of blepharospasm followed by a single center [17] and in 22% of a consecutive series of 50 patients in a botulinum neurotoxin (BoNT) clinic [18]. Functional HFS was initially described by Tan & Jankovic in 5 of 210 consecutive patients (2.4%) referred for the evaluation of HFS [9]; a subsequent updated retrospective chart review performed in the same center found that 7.4% of all the cases referred for HFS had a functional neurological etiology [19]. The same center more recently reported that functional HFS represents 9.8% of their patients

with FMD, with a female-to-male ratio of 3.5:1 [20].

After tremor, functional HFS and orofacial dyskinesia were respectively the second and third most common FMD in a more recent Indian study on 33 adult patients [21]. Interestingly, all the patients with HFS were female and these phenotypes were much rarer among the 25 children also enrolled in this series, with only one case of facial FMD characterized by excessive blinking resembling tics [21]. In another Indian study facial dystonia was found in 6.8% of 73 cases with FMD [22]. Regarding functional oculomotor disorders, a prevalence of 6% was found among all FMD followed by a tertiary center focused on movement disorders [23], whereas the figure was 4% in a neuro-otology clinic [24].

In conclusion, although no study has specifically addressed the epidemiology of facial FMD, we can conclude that this condition is much more common than previously recognized, as highlighted by a 2012 large series of FMD patients followed in seven tertiary movement disorders centers. This series reported that facial involvement was seen in 16.3% of all FMD cases evaluated during the examined period [1].

Mrs. G.'s neurological exam is unremarkable with the exception of a brief mouth deviation to the left secondary to risorius contraction during speech and a positive Hoffman sign on the right. In particular, there is no weakness seen in the frontalis, orbicularis oculi or perioral muscles. There is no deviation of the tongue at rest or during protrusion. The soft palate elevates symmetrically.

Clinical Features

Like many other FMD subtypes, facial involvement is generally characterized by an abrupt onset, highly variable course, inconsistency of presentation over time, higher prevalence in women and young-adult population, and association with multiple conditions (atypical facial pain, migraine) as well as other FMD signs. There may be speech problems (Video 10.1) or – more frequently – weakness (see Chap. 5) or dystonia (see Chap. 7), generally ipsilateral to the most affected hemiface [1, 25].

In the largest series of facial FMD published so far, a total of 61 patients (92% females; mean age at onset of 37 ± 11.3 years and mean disease duration of 6.7 ± 6.9 years) were further characterized and a common clinical picture emerged, affecting predominantly young women (9:1 female-to-male ratio) [1]. Phasic or tonic muscular spasms resembling dystonia were documented in all patients, most commonly involving the lips (60.7%), followed by eyelids (50.8%), perinasal region (16.4%) and forehead (9.8%). Symptom onset was abrupt in most cases (80.3%) with at least one precipitating psychological stress or trauma identified in 57.4%. The most common type of facial FMD in this series involved muscle overactivity, and three basic patterns could be recognized: (1) bilateral contraction of orbicularis oculi resembling blepharospasm or – less commonly – eyelid opening apraxia; (2) unilateral contraction of orbicularis oculi and/or orbicularis oris, resembling HFS; (3) variable association of unilateral and bilateral signs also involving orbicularis oris and resembling oromandibular dystonia.

More recently, Stone et al. [26] reported 41 cases of facial FMD and described additional phenomena, such as limb weakness, convergence spasm, dysphonia and functional seizures. In addition, these facial FMD cases were often triggered by eye movements or by asking the patient to contract the facial muscles. Compared with the series by Fasano et al. [1], Stone et al. found that facial paroxysmal spasm was more common whereas tongue and jaw deviation were less [26].

Functional weakness or inability to move facial muscles is extremely rare and it is typically characterized by unilateral or bilateral eyelid ptosis, which is variable or improves in response to unusual stimuli, features already recognized more than a century ago [7, 27].

Bilateral Involvement of the Eyelids

A recent series of eight patients (five women, mean age of 42.5 years) with isolated functional blepharospasm has been published. A spontaneous remission took place in four patients, whereas remaining patients experienced prolonged symptomatic relief from administration of placebo (saline injection) [17]. Other clinical features described in functional blepharospasm are: (1) a sustained asymmetry (only described in the initial phases of non-functional blepharospasm); (2) changes in pattern and side of predominant eye closure; (3) association with other ocular symptoms not seen in non-functional blepharospasm (sudden visual loss, oculogyric crisis or convergence spasm) [28]; (4) sudden onset of spasms, in contrast with blepharospasm usually preceded by an increased blinking at rest [29]. Although the improvement/resolution of symptoms during distracting maneuvers (e.g. while performing arithmetic calculations aloud) may help the diagnosis of FMD, this feature should be cautiously interpreted in functional blepharospasm because talking aloud usually decreases the severity/frequency of spasms in non-functional blepharospasm as well [29]. Indeed, the presence of a *geste antagoniste* (or sensory trick) has also been reported in functional dystonias (Fig. 10.1) [25]. In our experience, three cases with functional blepharospasm reported a *geste antagoniste*, one at the second visit, after having received information on the phenomenon during the first visit [1].

Although it represents a rarer phenotype, functional patients can also present the inability to open their eyes, thus resembling an eyelid opening apraxia [30]. In the case of functional eyelid opening apraxia, the strength of patients' eye closure may be noted to vary depending on the force exerted against the eyelids by the examiner, which can be a very useful diagnostic clue.

Unilateral Involvement of the Eyelid and/or Lower Face

Pseudoptosis is the term originally used to describe this condition [8] but it is no longer used as an actual ptosis in the absence of spasm around the eye is usually not present [31]. The few other cases of 'pseudoptosis' reported share common features, such as the acute onset, the

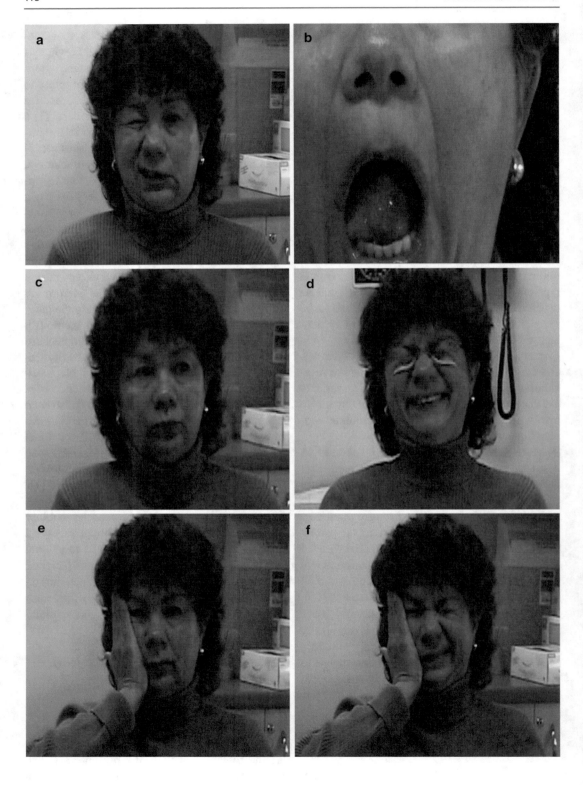

young age, the common involvement of the left side, and response to placebo [32–34]. When spasms are tonic without any phasic component, the picture may resemble a 'unilateral blepharospasm', which was already considered functional in 1898 [35].

Sometimes unilateral orbicularis oris contraction is also present, thus resembling HFS. Almost all patients were women (15 of 16) in a recent series of functional HFS, mean age at onset and disease duration of symptoms were 37.4 ± 19.5 and 1.7 ± 2.2 years, respectively [19]. These patients presented findings incongruent with HFS or facial dystonia, such as acute onset of symptoms, non-progressive course, fluctuations in symptom severity, and spontaneous resolution. Facial spasms may be characterized by upward or lateral deviation of the corner of the mouth [9, 19]. The platysma is also commonly contracted, contributing to the downward deviation of one corner of the mouth. The involvement of the lower lip with downward deviation at the angle of the mouth combined with ipsilateral platysma co-contraction have been previously termed 'smirk' [10]. The corner of the mouth may sometimes be elevated compared to the other side; in this situation the orbicularis oculis is nearly always contracted as well (Fig. 10.1a).

The most common pattern of facial FMD consists of tonic, sustained, lateral, and/or downward protrusion of one side of the lower lip with ipsilateral jaw deviation, as found in 84.3% of the largest series published so far [1]. In this series, spasms of the ipsi- or contralateral orbicularis oculis and excessive platysma contraction occurred in isolation or combined with fixed lip dystonia (60.7%). Paroxysmal (65%)

or fixed (26%) eyelid involvement occurred mostly unilateral with alternating sides (65%). The right side was affected twice as often as the left [1].

In summary, the unilateral downward contraction of orbicularis oris with deviation of the ipsilateral cheek and a possible ipsilateral involvement of the platysma is a very common phenomenology of FMD. Accordingly, the 'lip pulling test' is now seen as a common sign of functional dystonia [36].

Bilateral Involvement of the Lower Face

Bilateral involvement of orbicularis oris is rare, and was documented in a minority (15.7%) of patients belonging to a series of facial FMD; alternating sides was even rarer (3.3%) [1]. Bilateral involvement has been observed in 7 of 16 patients with a reported diagnosis of functional HFS [19]. In general, the phenomenology is the one of fixed dystonia, often associated with tongue involvement (see below). Fixed dystonia of the oromandibular region has been reported to result from peripheral facial injury [37] and may develop within hours to months after a dental procedure [38]. Such onset is in keeping with observations in patients with limb FMD, in whom local traumas are often precipitating factors [39]. Functional jaw opening dystonia was first reported in three women with paroxysmal episodes caused by variable stressors and alleviated by placebo [40]. One of them had additional limb dystonia and another one had limb, trunk and tongue dystonia.

Fig. 10.1 The involvement of the lower lip with downward deviation at the angle of the mouth combined with ipsilateral platysma co-contraction is a very common pattern of facial FMD. This patient shows a different pattern: ipsilateral upward deviation with eye closure, i.e. functional HFS. Note also the absence of Babinski's 'other' sign (**a**). Spasms subside when patient is asked to open the mouth (which triggers tongue deviation) (**b**) or when distracted (**c**). Phenomenology is highly variable, also including episodic bilateral spasms of the upper and lower face (**d**), sensory trick (**e**), which improves the ipsilateral HFS but triggers a contralateral one (**f**). This woman also complains of low mood, generalized pain and episodic spasms of either upper limb. (*Pictures courtesy of Dr. Anthony E. Lang, Toronto Western Hospital, Toronto, ON, Canada*)

Involvement of the Tongue

A variety of FMD can involve the tongue, although these are rarer than other facial disorders and generally seen in the context of involvement of other body parts. As a consequence, little has been written on functional orolingual dystonia.

Tongue deviation caused by a tonic contraction is the most common condition, almost always associated with other – generally ipsilateral – FMD (Fig. 10.1b). A tongue deviation towards the side of the facial spasm has been originally described by Gowers as 'wrong way' tongue deviation [3]. A recent work has evaluated the clinical features of tongue dyskinesias in patients with FMD resembling tics [41]: the coexistence of other functional neurological conditions (e.g., functional seizures) and the lack of benefit from medical treatment (tetrabenazine and haloperidol) supported the diagnosis.

Functional tongue tremor represents another rare condition, usually seen in the context of palatal involvement (see below) [42]. In some cases, a good response to placebo has been reported [43]. Speech can be variably affected by tongue disorders and in some cases stuttering has been described [44].

Involvement of the Palate

Palatal tremor (once called palatal myoclonus) is a movement disorder defined by rhythmic movements of soft palate with a frequency of 0.5–3 Hz. There are two types of palatal tremor: primary (essential) and secondary (symptomatic), the latter being caused by a lesion in the Guillain-Mollaret triangle and often accompanied by MRI evidence of 'pseudohypertrophy' of the inferior olive [45]. In their review of the nosology of essential palatal tremor, Zadikoff et al. emphasized several subcategories of what they preferred to call 'isolated palatal tremors' (emphasizing the absence of imaging abnormalities and other neurological deficits), and one subcategory was 'psychogenic'. These patients occasionally demonstrate extra-palatal movement involving the jaw, tongue and floor of the mouth [42]. Nowadays, essential palatal tremor is mainly considered to be functional in origin and ear click is the common complaint of these patients, in contrast with the pendular nystagmus and cerebellar signs seen with symptomatic forms [46].

Other rarer causes of essential palatal tremor are 'special skill' or tics [47]. In a series of 17 patients with essential palatal tremor a diagnosis of a functional neurological disorder could be formulated in ten cases. Clues to the functional nature were the variability in frequency, amplitude and direction of the tremor. In addition, tremor was entrainable and distractible. Most patients were females and younger than non-functional cases (35 vs. 54 years old). Finally, the functional group had a precipitating trigger (e.g. sore throat) and concurrent functional movements of the head, neck, face and eye [47].

Involvement of the Eyes

Functional eye movements are more difficult to assess as a thorough ophthalmologic examination is often needed. Several terminologies and descriptions are available [46, 48, 49].

Functional Convergence Spasm

Convergence eye movements are used to shift the gaze from a far object to a near one. Abnormal persistence of convergence when a patient is not fixating on a near object is called convergence spasm. Functional convergence spasm is the most frequent functional eye movement disorder. For example, 8 of 15 patients with functional eye movement disorders had convergence spasm in the series by Kaski et al. [24], although no case of convergence spasm was reported in another series of 11 patients [23].

Patients with convergence spasm usually present intermittent diplopia and blurred vision, especially when looking far after near fixation. In these patients one or both eyes remain adducted with forceful medial rectus contraction, and patients may be incorrectly diagnosed with unilateral or bilateral sixth nerve palsy.

Functional Convergence Paralysis

Functional convergence paralysis or insufficiency is a rare condition characterized by the complete or partial failure of ocular convergence. In this situation diplopia occurs at near fixation and the patient is not able to converge when a target is moved towards the patient's face. These patients typically complain of reading difficulties. On examination single eye adduction might be normal (e.g. during pursuit) although differentiating this situation from non-functional cases is more challenging than convergence spasm (see below).

Functional Gaze Limitation

Functional limitation of gaze is usually found on examination rather than being a patient's complaint. Patients usually show eyelid contraction, effortful facial movements or grimacing on eye movement examination. Sometimes they complain of pain while moving the eyes, especially when asked to look upward. Patients might not be able to move their eyes vertically or horizontally when they are asked, but they may show full range of eye movements on optokinetic stimulation or passive head motions.

Functional Ocular Oscillations and Nystagmus

Voluntary nystagmus is a form of special skill more common in children and refers to a high frequency (~10 Hz) low amplitude (~4°) eye oscillation that can be started and terminated voluntarily. Functional nystagmus refers to the same event when it happens involuntarily and it is usually associated with oscillopsia (unstable, or blurred vision with vibrating images), the most common presenting symptom. Like many other functional eye movements, eye movement examination can trigger functional nystagmus, which is usually preceded by a convergent effort [46, 48].

Baizabal-Carvallo and Jankovic have argued that these eye movement should be called 'functional saccadic oscillations' in view of the absence of slow phases that characterizes nystagmus [48]. Although this is a valid semiological argument, we would agree with Kaski et al. that it is of limited clinical utility to challenge a terminology that is well established in the neurological and neuro-ophthalmological literature [49].

Functional Opsoclonus

Opsoclonus is defined as conjugate multidirectional saccadic eye movements without intersaccadic intervals which occur in unpredictable directions with variable amplitudes. Functional opsoclonus has been reported in 5 of 11 patients with ocular FMD, also accompanied by oculogyric crisis in two and ocular flutter in one [23]. Others have described functional opsoclonus in patients with functional head tremor, associated with voluntary nystagmus and functional limitation of gaze [24].

Functional Oculogyric Crisis

Oculogyric crisis describes a tonic eye deviation mostly upward which lasts for a few seconds to several hours. A functional neurological etiology is suspected when the oculogyric crisis has a temporal association with other FMD symptoms, disappears with distraction, and patients are unable to transiently stop it voluntarily, which is common in the non-functional counterpart. Functional oculogyric crisis are brief but longer episodes are also possible and usually associated with photophobia, eyelid closure and functional blindness [46].

Functional Diplopia

Binocular functional diplopia is common in other FMD presentations involving the eyes, convergence spasm in particular. Monocular diplopia is suggestive of a functional neurological disorder in the appropriate clinical setting, although it can rarely happen with other conditions (see below).

During the visit Mrs. G informed us that she has experienced many other sensory symptoms over the past few years, even before the facial pulling started. These include sharp pain involving the neck and head, numbness around the left lip, tightness in the neck, burning in the nose and pain during swallowing. She has been evaluated by multiple physicians – including ENT, orthodontists, and pain specialists – and states that a definite cause for her symptoms was never found. She also underwent multiple treatments, including surgeries of the temporo-mandibular joint and sinus as well as occipital nerve blocks, none of which was effective in relieving the pain.

Her previous medical history includes: stroke causing dysphagia and weakness of the right face and arm, from which she fully recovered; ischemic retinopathy; ulcerative colitis necessitating a colostomy; abdominal hernia repair; peripheral vascular disease; and chronic hip pain. She is a previous smoker of 20 pack-years and regularly drinks one glass of wine a day. Mrs. G. lives with her husband and thinks she's having a lot of stress lately as he has cancer and cognitive impairment. She is his only caregiver and he is verbally abusive towards her.

Associated Conditions

In a series of 61 patients with facial FMD, associated body regions involved included upper limbs (29.5%), neck (16.4%), lower limbs (16.4%), and trunk (4.9%) [1]. Functional dystonia was the most frequent phenotype of extra-facial sites (58%), followed by functional tremor (14%) and functional jerks (10%). When present, limb involvement was ipsilateral to the facial involvement. Along with the motor symptoms, patients complained of a number of comorbidities (Table 10.1). Atypical facial pain as well as depression are very common associated conditions with prevalence much higher than observed in the same age and sex group in the general population [50]. By contrast in the same series, the prevalence of tension-type headache, although very common, was not higher than reported in cohorts without FMD with similar age and sex distribution [51]. Other common comorbidities include fibromyalgia and irritable bowel syndrome.

Mrs. G's symptoms and examination are consistent with a diagnosis of functional facial dystonia. The diagnosis is based on positive signs suggestive of functional facial dystonia (episodic unilateral downward pulling of the corner of the mouth) supported on history by the sudden onset of symptoms and the associated atypical facial pain, which is most likely functional as well. In

Table 10.1 Common comorbid conditions and other features associated with facial FMD [1]

(A) Medical conditions associated with facial FMD[a]	**%**
Depression	38.0
Tension headache	26.4
Migraine	25.9
Anxiety	18.0
Fatigue	17.6
Fibromyalgia	9.8
Hypertension	4.9
Temporo-mandibular joint dysfunction	3.9
Irritable bowel syndrome	3.8
Hearing loss	3.7
(B) Other features associated with facial FMD	**%**
Historical information:	
Employed in allied health professions	28.0
History of minor trauma	26.8
Exposure to a disease model	18.5
History of physical abuse	4.3
History of sexual abuse	2.1
Clinical course:	
Rapid onset	96.7
Non-progressive course	85.2
Remissions	21.3
Suggestibility:	
Movements decrease with distraction	89.6
Placebo effect[b]	89.5
Movements increase with attention	86.0
Resolution when the patient feels unobserved	61.1
Ability to trigger or relieve the abnormal movements[c]	36.4
Disability:	
Functional disability out of proportion to exam findings	47.2
Selective disability[d]	28.1
Secondary gain[e]	20.3
Accompanying features:	
Other somatizations[b]	49.2
False sensory complaints[f]	34.4
Deliberate slowness of movements	27.9
False (give-away) weakness[b]	18.0
Delayed and excessive startle response to a stimulus	1.6
Self-inflicted injuries	0.0

[a]Other, less common (1 case each), conditions were: breast cancer, hypothyroidism, ovary dermoid cyst, otosclerosis, miscarriage, spina bifida occulta, thoracic outlet syndrome, cervical cancer treated with radiation, gastroesophageal reflux disease, osteoarthritis, morbid obesity, intestinal malabsorption
[b]See text for details
[c]By using non-physiological interventions (e.g. trigger points on the body, tuning fork)

(continued)

Table 10.1 (continued)

[d]Defined as disability limited only to specific activities of daily living

[e]Defined as ongoing or pending litigation, disability benefits, release from personal/legal/social/employment responsibilities, and/or increased personal attention

[f]For example, blurred vision, pain, numbness or sense of swelling not following anatomy (whole or half body, ipsilateral hand and foot). Data derived from a cohort of patients published by Fasano et al. [1]

terms of differential diagnosis, she lacks features of other conditions. Oromandibular dystonia is a symmetrical disorder while hemifacial spasm involves other ipsilateral muscles innervated by the facial nerve and involves shorter spasms. Finally, facial central weakness can present with an asymmetric deviation of the mouth but signs are not episodic and weakness can be appreciated during other voluntary actions (e.g. posing a smile).

Diagnosis

Like most FMD subtypes, functional facial disorders have no definitive test or biomarker; however, rather than ruling out non-functional conditions with similar presentations, the diagnosis can be reliably made applying 'positive' diagnostic clinical criteria [52]. In fact, a prompt diagnosis based on phenomenology will avoid the extensive diagnostic work-up characteristic of a diagnosis-of-exclusion approach, prevent unnecessary costly investigations, and permit the institution of appropriate physical, psychological, and medical therapy [53].

In the largest series of facial FMD published so far, the vast majority of these cases received a 'positive' diagnosis rather than a diagnosis based on the exclusion of other diseases. Diagnosis of FMD was made according to the criteria of Fahn and Williams [15] and Gupta and Lang [53], with acknowledgement of the weakness of these diagnostic criteria [54].

The diagnosis of FMD is based on the inconsistency and incongruity of the observed phenomenology. The former refers to the variability over time, which can be spontaneous or triggered

by suggestibility maneuvers (Fig. 10.1c, d). These are not sensitive but highly specific: a non-physiologic or placebo maneuver (most often a vibrating tuning fork or a pen torch) improved 16% and worsened 10% of 19 facial FMD to whom it was applied [1].

Although a facial FMD diagnosis is based upon the presence of positive signs on physical exam, incongruity – i.e. a presentation not fulfilling any of the known medical conditions, can be helpful. Examples include the unilateral isolated spasm of platysma (rarely seen and only in HFS and some tics), the tongue deviation in absence of weakness or an alternating involvement of hemiface, although possible in the rare patients with bilateral HFS [55]. Furthermore, the diagnosis is usually facilitated by the occurrence of more than one functional neurological symptom. A typical example is when the patient has motor symptoms in the upper and lower halves of the face combined with the involvement of the ipsilateral arm and/or leg. Several clinical signs can assist the physician in confirming the diagnosis on clinical grounds (see below) [9, 15, 16, 53, 56–61].

Comorbidities, and particularly psychiatric conditions, may support a functional neurological etiology but their role is limited and sometime confusing. In fact, psychiatric disorders may be absent in patients with FMD; these diagnoses are also commonly present in other movement disorders. Accordingly, the diagnosis of FMD does not require comorbid psychiatric disease or the presence of an identifiable stressor [62], although these conditions and risk factors are still important to look for as they may identify precipitants or inform personalized management.

Electrophysiological studies can be used to provide a laboratory-supported diagnosis of a facial FMD [53], although it should be acknowledged that these studies might also disclose abnormal findings in patients with FMD (see Chap. 7) [63, 64]. A normal blink reflex has been reported in nine patients with 'presumed psychogenic' blepharospasm, in contrast to patients with non-functional blepharospasm, who had an abnormal R2 index [18]. These findings have been confirmed in another series of ten patients with facial FMD [1]. In addition, sensorimotor plasticity has been found normal in functional blepharospasm in contrast to the non-functional counterparts [65].

EMG and a motion capture system using facial markers are helpful in order to document the effects of distractibility maneuvers, placebo or spontaneous inconsistency, as recently described in a case of functional eyelid opening apraxia (Fig. 10.2) [66].

Finally, electrophysiology may also help distinguish HFS from other abnormal facial movements by demonstrating ephaptic impulse transmission between different facial nerve branches [67]. Indeed, a neurophysiological hallmark of HFS is the spread of the blink reflex responses elicited by supraorbital nerve stimulation to muscles other than the orbicularis oculis.

Differential Diagnosis

Many systemic and neurological conditions may involve the facial musculature. Table 10.2 indicates the commonest causes and the clini-

cal features that help distinguish them from functional neurological disorder. From tetanus to blepharospasm, the majority of them are characterized by muscular spasms [63]. While some of them are easily recognizable, sometimes the differential diagnosis can be challenging. For example, diagnosing dystonia following minor peripheral injury remains a major source of controversy in this field as many experts now believe that this condition has a functional etiology [68].

Bilateral Involvement of the Eyelids

Sometimes contraction of the orbicularis oculis is mistaken for ptosis, especially by non-neurologists, who may formulate a diagnosis of myasthenia gravis, also given the asymmetry and variability of presentation. Contraction of corrugator and procerus muscles in the absence of orbicularis oculis' spasms may be seen in patients with FMD (Fig. 10.3a). Narrowing of eyelid fissure and depression of the eyebrows in the presence of eyelid spasms is seen in blepharospasm and is referred to as the 'Charcot sign' (Fig. 10.3b).

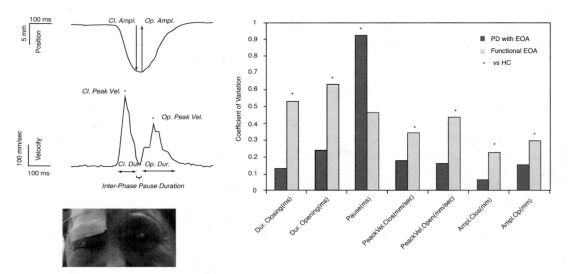

Fig. 10.2 Laboratory-supported diagnosis of functional eyelid movements. EMG and an optokinetic motion capture system using facial markers are helpful in order to capture the different phases of spontaneous and voluntary eyelid closure (left panel, *courtesy of Drs. Alfredo Berardelli and Matteo Bologna, Sapienza University, Rome, Italy*). Measuring the coefficient of variation of a series of voluntary eyelid closures can easily document performance of inconsistency in functional EOA (right panel) [66]. Abbreviations: Ampl: amplitude, Cl. or Clos: closing, Dur.: duration, EOA: eyelid opening apraxia, HC: healthy controls, Op.: opening, PD: Parkinson's disease, Vel.: velocity

The presence of a *geste antagoniste* (or sensory trick) is not particularly helpful in this context; like the non-functional counterpart [29], functional blepharospasm may subside while reading a text and performing arithmetic calculations aloud.

Patients with non-functional eyelid opening apraxia activate many facial muscles, particularly the frontalis muscle, in order to facilitate the function of the levator palpebrae or overcome the excessive activity of the orbicularis oculis. The same accessory movements – although less commonly and less vigorously observed– can be seen in patients with functional eyelid opening apraxia, thus not helping the differential diagnosis (personal observation). Eyelid opening

Table 10.2 Other facial movement disorders and distinguishing features from functional syndromes

Face site	Diagnosis	Clinical and differentiating features vs. functional neurological disorder
Bilateral and symmetric conditions		
Eyes	Non-functional convergence spasm	Diencephalic-mesencephalic junction diseases (thalamic esotropia), Wernicke-Korsakoff syndrome, epilepsy, posterior fossa lesions and phenytoin toxicity.
	Non-functional convergence paralysis	Consistently absent and can't be elicited with a near object or using fusional prisms. Associated with aging and neurodegenerative diseases.
	Supranuclear gaze palsy	Generally associated with slow vertical saccades and eyebrows elevation while following an object. 'Round the house sign' is a typically compensatory sign.
	Nystagmus	The slow-phase eye movement is usually present. It can be also vertical or torsional.
	Ocular flutter	Persistent and associated with cerebellar or brainstem oculomotor signs.
	Opsoclonus	Not distractible and persistent during eyelid closure or sleep. Caused by paraneoplastic, autoimmune, infectious, metabolic, and toxic disorders.
	Oculogyric crises	Tonic eye deviation mostly upward which lasts for a few seconds to several hours. Patients are able to transiently stop it voluntarily. Caused by encephalitis or exposure to antidopaminergic medications, usually in the context of an acute dystonic reaction.
	Binocular diplopia	One of the two images is blurrier and varies depending on the distance and direction of visual target. It resolves with the closure of either eye.
Eyelids	Blepharospasm	Isolated dystonia, bilaterally affecting the eyelids and surrounding muscles; it might be slightly asymmetric (especially at onset) and it's generally preceded by an increased blink rate.
	Eyelid opening apraxia	Isolated dystonia, bilaterally affecting the eyelids that can't be lifted while attempting to open the eyes. Patients may activate many facial muscles, particularly the frontalis muscle, in order to facilitate the function of the levator palpebrae or overcome the excessive activity of the orbicularis oculis.
	Ocular tics	Eyelid movements are bilateral, very fast without forceful closure of the eyes and can be voluntary suppressed, although this is associated with an urge to close the eyes or general discomfort.
	Catatonia	Patients are not responsive and voluntarily close their eyes, also exerting resistance if the examiner tries to open them passively.
Peribuccal muscles	Parkinson's disease tremor	Jaw, lip and tongue tremor (5 Hz) accompanied by the other signs of the disease.
	'Rabbit syndrome'	High frequency tremor of the lips and perioral muscles due to chronic neuroleptic treatment.
	Dyskinesias	Classic non-functional examples are: facial chorea (in the context of generalized signs of chorea), tardive dyskinesias (caused by dopaminergic receptors blockers and often associated with lingual movements), involuntary movements seen during anti-NMDA encephalitis.

(continued)

Table 10.2 (continued)

Face site	Diagnosis	Clinical and differentiating features vs. functional neurological disorder
Tongue	Essential tremor of the tongue	Tremor has the same frequency (4–8 Hz) of hand tremor (when present), with therapeutic benefit from ethanol, propranolol or other drugs used for essential tremor.
	Isolated tremor of the tongue	It may present as an initial finding of essential tremor. Transient tongue tremor has been reported to occur as an isolated side effect of neuroleptics, brain tumors, metabolic conditions (such as liver cirrhosis, Wilson's disease), infections (e.g. in neurosyphilis the so called 'trombone tongue') or head injury (e.g. the 'galloping tongue', in which there is a peculiar episodic slow 3 Hz tremor beginning as posterior midline focal tongue contractions).
	Primary lingual dystonia	Represents an isolated task-induced dystonia induced by speaking and characterized by protrusion. It might be associated with the involvement of other body sites, such as larynx.
	Lingual protrusion dystonia	Tongue protrusion sometimes associated with feeding dystonia is frequently seen in heredodegenerative diseases, including pantothenate kinase-associated neurodegeneration, Lesch Nyhan syndrome, Wilson's disease and – especially – chorea-acanthocytosis, in which represents a disease hallmark. It may be also seen in post-anoxic and tardive dystonia.
	Lingual myoclonus	It is a very rare entity that has been associated with an underlying abnormality, such as Arnold-Chiari malformation, craniovertebral junction abnormalities, brainstem ischemia or systemic lupus erythematosus.
Peribuccal muscles and jaw	Oromandibular dystonia	Bilateral and associated with masticatory and speech dystonia. Gradual onset, slow progression. Very rare and bilateral involvement of platysma. Pain absent.
	Oculomasticatory myorhythmia	A rare condition characterized by relatively fast and continuous slow-frequency muscle twitches associated with cerebral Whipple's disease.
	Geniospasm	Isolated and benign contractions of mentalis muscle with an onset in childhood; it is usually hereditary.
Asymmetric conditions		
Eye	Abducens nerve palsy	Eye abduction is not possible with doll's eye maneuver or optokinetic stimuli. Diplopia does not improve with crinkling the eyelids and it is constant especially when the target moves laterally.
	Monocular diplopia	Very rare and caused by ophthalmological disorders (retinal diseases, refractory disturbances of the lens or cornea) or lesions of the visual cortex.
Hemi-face (upper and lower portion)	Hemifacial spasm	Contractions are normally synchronous and shock-like. The affect one hemi-face, usually eyelid and surrounding muscles, the corner of the mouth and the forehead are commonly involved (see text for the 'other Babinski sign'). It may persist during sleep.
	Facial nerve palsy with synkinetic aberrant reinnervation	Involuntary movements also triggered by voluntary movements involving movements adjacent to previously weak muscles.
	Faciobrachial dystonic seizures	Very brief spasms synchronously affecting the hemi-face and the ipsilateral upper limb (arm and wrist flexion). Seen in anti-LGI1 encephalitis.
Hemi-face (lower portion)	Hemi-masticatory spasm	Involves muscles of mastication only. Only one side of the face is affected, which can also appear atrophic.
Variable distribution		
Facial tic		Brief movements associated with premonitory sensations, urge to move in a patterned response. Other tics are usually present
Facial myoclonus in focal seizures		Very fast muscular twitching, EEG evidence of cortical discharge.
Facial myokymia		Occasional eye or face twitching is common in the general population and made worse with fatigue or caffeine. It may also occur in brainstem lesions (e.g. multiple sclerosis) and other neurological diseases affecting the nerve excitability.

Adapted from Refs. [19, 44]

Abbreviations: *EEG* electroencephalogram, *FMD* functional movement disorder

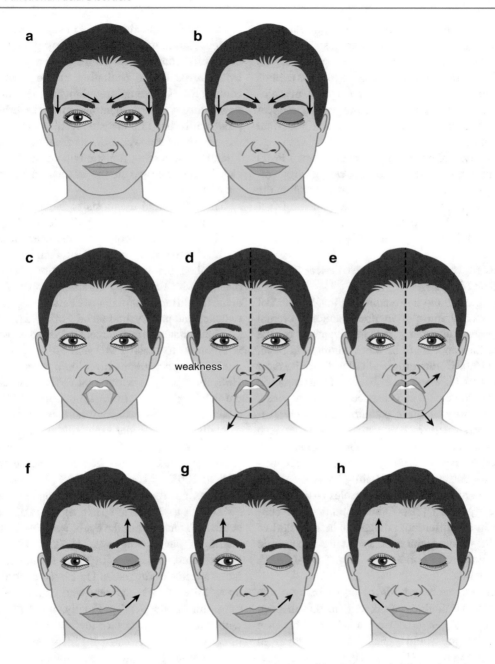

Fig. 10.3 Positive signs useful for the differential diagnosis of facial FMD. (**a**) The narrowing of eyelid fissure and frowning of the eyebrows due to the contraction of corrugator and procerus muscles in the absence of spasm of the orbicularis oculis is seen in patients with FMD whereas patients with blepharospasm (**b**) also have eyelid spasms ('Charcot sign'). (**c**) Normal symmetric face with protruded tongue. (**d**) In case of unilateral facial weakness (on the right side in this example), the contralateral side of the face is pulling due to the tonic contraction of the spared hemiface; in this context, patients may have ipsilateral tongue weakness, meaning that the tongue deviates on the same side when protruded due to the active contraction of the spared hemitongue. (**e**) In case of unilateral facial functional spasm (on the left side in this example), patient's tongue may deviate on the same side ('wrong way' tongue). (**f**) The unilateral involvement of facial muscles is common to HFS and facial FMD (**g** and **h**). However, in HFS there may be elevation of frontalis on the same side as the orbicularis oculis (Babinski's 'other' sign, panel **f**). This sign is not found in patients with FMD with asymmetric spasm of the orbicularis oculis, who, rather, had the eyebrow rising contralateral to the closing eye (panel **g** and **h**)

apraxia should be differentiated from catatonia because patients are otherwise responsive and actually complain about the ocular problem.

Many other conditions may affect the eyelids (myotonia, neuromyotonia and eyelid myoclonus in absence seizure) but the overall clinical picture is usually enough to reach the final diagnosis.

Finally, patients with paroxysmal facial FMD resembling tics usually do not acknowledge voluntary control, urge, or relief of urge after the movements [1]. Moreover, these patients never display rapid movements and spasms are more sustained than those observed in dystonic tics.

Bilateral Involvement of the Lower Face and/or Tongue

In contrast to the more common involvement of upper facial muscles in non-functional cranial movement disorders, the involvement of the lower face appears to be more common in facial FMD [69]. Unlike oromandibular dystonia, most subjects with lower face FMD had asymmetric facial involvement and absence of sensory tricks. The majority of these patients had no involvement of speech, in contrast to frequent speech involvement in oromandibular dystonia [52]. Moreover, FMD affecting the lower face are usually present at rest, contrasting to task-specific dystonia affecting perioral muscles (e.g. embouchure dystonia) [70]. Other conditions to consider in the differential diagnosis include tardive dyskinesia and facial chorea seen in some genetic and acquired conditions, e.g. anti-NMDA encephalitis.

The tongue may be involved by many disorders and particularly weakness; in this respect, 'wrong way' tongue deviation is helpful because a weak tongue would typically deviate away from the affected side [71] (Fig. 10.3c–e). The spectrum of functional and non-functional orolingual tremors has been reviewed by Silverdale and colleagues, who also proposed a classification system helping the differential diagnosis [44] (Table 10.2).

Unilateral Involvement of the Eyelid and Lower Face

In the vast majority of facial FMD, patients display a variable degree of facial asymmetry, as some muscles pull sideways. However, the same clinical picture may be actually caused by weakness of the contralateral hemiface, as pointed out by Babinski at the beginning of the twentieth century [6]. For example, eyebrows can be pulled down during an over-contraction of the orbicularis oculis but clinicians may also wonder if there is unilateral weakness of frontalis muscle. Therefore, assessing the strength of facial muscles is the first step in the evaluation of these patients.

The differential diagnosis of unilateral facial movement disorder is wide (Table 10.2) [19]. Most non-functional conditions are characterized by brief myoclonic twitches of facial muscles rather than the sustained contractions seen in patients with FMD. The duration of spasm also helps the differential diagnosis between epileptic twitches and paroxysmal facial FMD [72].

The unilateral involvement of facial muscles is common to facial FMD and HFS. However, unlike the synchronous myoclonic jerks seen in HFS, most patients with facial FMD show asynchronous, generally tonic contractions [73]. In addition, in HFS there may be elevation of the frontalis muscle on the same side of orbicularis oculis' involvement; this is called Babinski's 'other' sign and has a specificity ranging from 76% to 100% in identifying HFS [74–76]. This sign was not found in any of the patients with FMD with asymmetric spasm of the orbicularis oculis, who had rather the eyebrow rising contralateral to the closing eye [1] (Fig. 10.3f–h). Furthermore, patients with FMD do not report facial spasms during sleep [1, 19], in contrast to up to 80% of HFS patients who exhibit symptoms during sleep [77]. Finally, most patients with FMD have lower face involvement at onset, in contrast to the isolated lid involvement typically present at symptom onset in HFS.

While functional facial movements can often be triggered by examination of eye movements or by asking the patients to sustain muscular contraction of the face [26], it is important to note that this is not specific to FMD. While contraction of orbicularis oculis in facial FMD can sometimes be triggered or increased by asking the patient to elevate the eyebrows or look up, this phenomenon can also be seen in patients with HFS. Clinicians should bear in mind that voluntary facial movement may exacerbate HFS in up to 39% of patients [77], and may also exacerbate the synkinetic movements seen after facial palsy (secondary HFS).

'Unilateral dystonia of the jaw' is uncommon and was first reported in 1986 by Thompson and colleagues in a small series [63]. In retrospect, at least one of these patients was subsequently diagnosed as having a functional etiology [1]. Indeed, few references to unilateral jaw spasms are found in the literature and several of these have clinical features that might support their reclassification as facial FMD [12–14, 63, 78]. Important nonfunctional causes of unilateral contraction of the lower face to keep in mind include hemimasticatory spasm and faciobrachial dystonic seizures seen in anti-LGI1 encephalitis. While the former is easily recognizable, for example due to the association with facial hemiatrophy [79], the latter may be difficult to diagnose especially at onset because it might share features seen in the functional counterpart: ipsilateral involvement of the upper limb, negative EEG, lack of accompanying signs and abrupt onset.

Finally, other entities not to overlook include non-neurological conditions. Examples include local/mechanical disorders of the mandible or temporo-mandibular joint or ophthalmic conditions that can trigger the ipsilateral contraction of corrugator, procerus and orbicularis oculis muscle. The occurrence of local pain and functional impairment (e.g., difficulties with chewing) helps the differential diagnosis.

Involvement of the Eyes

Presence of miosis and ability to induce abduction with doll's eye maneuver or optokinetic stimuli can differentiate convergence spasm from an abducens nerve palsy. In contrast with an oculomotor palsy, blurred vision typically improves with crinkling the eyelids and symptoms tend to last only for a few seconds, although sometimes they can be continuous. Although rare, other etiologies of convergence spasm should be ruled out, including diencephalic-mesencephalic junction diseases (thalamic esotropia), Wernicke-Korsakoff syndrome, epilepsy, posterior fossa lesions and phenytoin toxicity [24, 46].

Functional convergence paralysis might be seen during examination when the patient is pre-

sented with a near object or using fusional prisms, features generally absent with the non-functional counterpart if associated with aging or neurodegenerative diseases [24, 46]. Most cases of nonfunctional supranuclear gaze palsy also feature slow saccades and eyebrow elevation while following an object.

Opsoclonus, ocular flutter, vestibular paroxysmia and superior oblique myokymia are the main differential diagnoses of functional nystagmus. The slow-phase eye movement which is an essential part of nystagmus is missing in voluntary and functional neurological forms. In addition, voluntary nystagmus is only horizontal, can be associated with head tremor and eyelid flutter, decreases in amplitude and duration with time, and does not persist for more than 25 seconds, usually lasting less than 2–5 seconds. Ocular flutter is persistent and associated with cerebellar or brainstem oculomotor signs. Opsoclonus has an extensive differential diagnosis that includes paraneoplastic, autoimmune, infectious, metabolic, and toxic disorders [80]. Functional opsoclonus is usually distractible and disappears during eyelid closure and sleep, in contrast to the other forms.

Oculogyric crises can be seen after encephalitis or exposure to antidopaminergic medications, usually in the context of an acute dystonic reaction.

Non-functional diplopia is typically binocular due to disconjugate gaze caused by the dysfunction of one or more ocular muscles. Asking the patient to look to the direction of the paralyzed muscle increases the severity of diplopia, a feature that might be absent in functional neurological forms. Another feature supporting the functional etiology is the complaint of two separate, clearly defined and equal images. Ophthalmological disorders (retinal diseases, refractory disturbances of the lens or cornea) or lesions of the visual cortex are rare conditions associated with monocular diplopia.

Mrs. G. was educated about the nature of her diagnosis. She was reassured that no other testing was needed and that there was no reason to consider treatments such as BoNT injection or other invasive approaches. We also recommended that she educate herself further on the diagnosis of a facial FMD at the website www.neurosymp-

toms.org. Finally, we referred her to our multidisciplinary program for FMD, which involves the integrated use of physiotherapy, cognitive, behavioral and psychological therapy.

That fall, Mrs. G. underwent an integrated assessment with a neurologist and a neuropsychiatrist, who conducted an extensive assessment and provided her with comprehensive education about the diagnosis of FMD and recommended physiotherapy to help with her pain. She became upset given her symptoms worsened and she also manifested sudden episodes of whispered voice. Nevertheless, she agreed to proceed with the plan.

Several months later, Mrs. G. was evaluated by the neurologist leading the multidisciplinary program for FMD. The patient continued to express confusion about the diagnosis, stating that she had no idea what functional dystonia is. She perceived that she had seen a number of different physicians and from whom she had been receiving conflicting messages. She expressed considerable frustration relating to the persistent pain in her head, neck and face. She also endorsed significant stabbing left ear pain and dizziness, which also caused balance and walking issues. She described progressing numbness in the left face, left shoulder spasms, and losing her voice periodically. Finally, she endorsed depressive symptoms.

Most of the visit was spent educating Mrs. G. on functional neurological symptoms. The neurologist stressed that her symptoms are very common and not 'made up'. The patient admitted that her facial spasms actually resolved and were not occurring anymore. Her clinical picture was now dominated by low mood, pain, headache, and fatigue. She was provided with a handout explaining functional pain and was prescribed an antidepressant. Close follow-up to monitor the situation and the response to the drug was scheduled.

Management

Like other FMD subtypes, the treatment of facial FMD starts with providing the patient with a positive clinical diagnosis and thorough

explanation. Showing the patient the positive motor signs present on their physical examination can form an important part of the explanation of the diagnosis. This step alone can have major therapeutic benefit, and may in some patients be the only treatment necessary [25]. For others, treatment needs to be individualized within an integrated approach consisting of education, specialist physical therapy and psychological therapies, such as cognitive behavioral therapy. Detailed information on communicating the diagnosis and establishing a positive relationship with the patient can be found in Part III of this book.

The management of facial FMD can be challenging and disappointing at times. Sharma et al. reported good results with psychodynamic therapy in 30 patients with FMD, including a patient with abnormal facial movements and one with voice stuttering, who were among the patients with the greatest response [81].

The general rules of management of FMD also applies to functional eye movement disorders. Showing patients videos or pictures of themselves with normal eye movements when they are distracted can be helpful. Although not systemically studied, recognizing and attending to environmental and psychologic stressors is important and should be addressed accordingly. For example, treating anxiety in a teenager with oscillopsia can be very helpful. Some patients can benefit from ocular exercises under the supervision of an optometrist. In refractory cases, cycloplegic agents can be helpful in patients with convergence spasm.

Several months later, Mrs. G returned reporting the resolution of her abnormal facial movements, dizziness and voice issues. Fatigue, mood and pain were slowly improving and she was confident that she was on the right track towards recovery. The medical team caring for her was pleased with her progress. No change of treatment was recommended.

Later that fall, Mrs. G. returned reporting much more severe left facial pain, numbness and pulling as well as severe sinus pain, chest pain, and trouble breathing. She wanted to seek a second opinion and saw an ENT who told her 'noth-

ing was wrong' and it was 'referred pain'. Given the rapid change of the clinical picture and the presence of chest pain and shortness of breath she was sent to the ER to get a chest X-ray, basic labs and ECG. She was grateful and agreed with the plan.

Outcome and Prognosis

Little is known about the treatment response of patients with facial FMD. In a series of 55 patients with facial FMD, medical and/or non-pharmacological treatments caused no improvement (56%) or even worsening (20%); only 20% of these patients improved after treatment (BoNT at therapeutic doses was effective in five cases, antidepressants in three, antiepileptics in two and psychotherapy in one) [1].

Even less is known about the natural history of facial FMD. In the aforementioned series, the course was stable (53%) or variable (33%), with diurnal fluctuations in one fifth of the patients. Spontaneous remissions were reported in 13 subjects (21%), with recurrence in 2 after 2 weeks and 10 years [1].

In conclusion, FMD involving the face are relatively less characterized and no studies specifically focused on their treatment are available. The general recommendations adopted for FMD are certainly a valid starting point. These include educating the patient, recommending rehabilitation if appropriate, avoiding unnecessary tests or treatments, and treating psychological stressors or psychiatric comorbidities with psychotherapy and medications in more refractory cases. Other strategies can – once again – be inspired by successful trials in other FMD subtypes. For example, Garcin et al. used transcranial magnetic stimulation with a frequency of 0.25 Hz over the motor cortex contralateral to the symptoms in 24 cases of FMD involving the limbs. The authors were able to demonstrate positive and sustainable effects, with improvements ranging from 50% to 75% and lasting for an average of 19.8 months [82]. The role of this approach in facial FMD has not been studied but it might be a logical and safe next step for cases refractory to first-line strategies.

Detailed information on treatment approaches can be found in Part III of this book.

Summary
- Facial FMD is more common than previously thought and shares features recognized for other FMD subtypes, including sudden onset with maximal severity at time of onset, inconsistency over time, associated somatizations or non-physiologic sensory or motor findings, distractibility, response to suggestion or psychotherapy, and spontaneous remissions.
- Common associated features of facial FMD include female gender, and comorbidities including depression, headache, facial pain, fibromyalgia, and irritable bowel syndrome.
- Facial FMD can be classified according to the following categories: bilateral involvement of the eyelids (including functional blepharospasm and functional eyelid opening apraxia); unilateral involvement of the eyelid and/or lower face (including functional hemifacial spasm and functional unilateral blepharospasm); bilateral involvement of the lower face; involvement of the tongue; involvement of the palate; and involvement of the eyes (usually bilaterally).
- The most common pattern of facial FMD consists of tonic, sustained, lateral, and/or downward protrusion of one side of the lower lip with ipsilateral jaw deviation and variable involvement of the ipsilateral platysma. The upward deviation of the mouth may be associated with ipsilateral eye spasms.
- The diagnosis of a facial FMD can be reliably made by applying 'positive' diagnostic clinical criteria based on inconsistency and incongruity of the observed phenomenology.

- The treatment of facial FMD starts with providing a positive clinical diagnosis and explanation to the patient. This step alone can have major therapeutic benefit, and may in some patients be the only treatment necessary. Treatment has to be individualized within an integrated approach consisting of education, physical and cognitive behavioral therapy. The presence of associated facial pain is a negative prognostic factor.

Acknowledgments Authors are grateful to: Dr. Sarah C. Lidstone (Toronto Western Hospital, Toronto, ON, Canada) for providing an update on the condition of Mrs. G, Dr. Anthony E. Lang (Toronto Western Hospital, Toronto, ON, Canada) for the pictures used for Fig. 10.1 and Video 10.1, and to Drs. Alfredo Berardelli and Matteo Bologna (Sapienza University, Rome, Italy) for Fig. 10.2.

References

1. Fasano A, Valadas A, Bhatia KP, Prashanth LK, Lang AE, Munhoz RP, Morgante F, Tarsy D, Duker AP, Girlanda P, Bentivoglio AR, Espay AJ. Psychogenic facial movement disorders: clinical features and associated conditions. Mov Disord. 2012;27(12):1544–51. https://doi.org/10.1002/mds.25190.
2. Charcot JM. Leçons sur les Maladies du Système Nerveux faites à la Salpêtrière. Paris: A. Delahaye; 1887.
3. Gowers WR. A manual of diseases of the nervous system. London: J & A Churchill; 1888.
4. Tourette G. De la superposition des troubles de la sensibilité et des spasmes de la face et du cou chez les hystériques. Nouv Iconogr Salpêtrière. 1889;2:107–20.
5. Wood C. The methods employed in examining the eyes for the detection of hysteria. J Am Med Assoc. 1898;31:1136–8.
6. Babinski JJFF. Hysteria or pithiatism. London: University of London Press; 1918.
7. Hurst A. The psychology of the special senses and their functional disorders. London: Oxford University Press; 1920.
8. Hop JW, Frijns CJ, van Gijn J. Psychogenic pseudoptosis. J Neurol. 1997;244(10):623–4.
9. Tan EK, Jankovic J. Psychogenic hemifacial spasm. J Neuropsychiatry Clin Neurosci. 2001;13(3):380–4.
10. Tarsy D, Dengenhardt A, Zadikoff C. Psychogenic facial spasm (the smirk) presenting as hemifacial spasm. In: Hallett M, Fahn S, Jankovic J, Lang AE, Cloninger CR, Yudofsky SC, editors. Psychogenic movement disorders. Philadelphia: Lippincott Williams & Williams; 2006. p. 341–3.
11. Stone J, Carson A. Psychogenic/dissociative/functional facial symptoms—a case report. J Neurol Neurosurg Psychiatry. 2010;81:e8–9. https://doi.org/10.1136/jnnp.2010.217554.20.
12. Kleopa KA, Kyriakides T. A novel movement disorder of the lower lip. Mov Disord. 2004;19(6):663–6.
13. Wohlgemuth M, Pasman JW, de Swart BJ, Horstink MW. Movement disorder of the lower lip. Mov Disord. 2005;20(8):1085–6. https://doi.org/10.1002/mds.20578.
14. de Entrambasaguas M, Plaza-Costa A, Casal J, Parra S. Labial dystonia after facial and trigeminal neuropathy controlled with a maxillary splint. Mov Disord. 2007;22(9):1355–8.
15. Williams DT, Ford B, Fahn S. Phenomenology and psychopathology related to psychogenic movement disorders. Adv Neurol. 1995;65:231–57.
16. Factor SA, Podskalny GD, Molho ES. Psychogenic movement disorders: frequency, clinical profile, and characteristics. J Neurol Neurosurg Psychiatry. 1995;59(4):406–12.
17. Gazulla J, Garcia-Rubio S, Ruiz-Gazulla C, Modrego P. Clinical categorization of psychogenic blepharospasm. Parkinsonism Relat Disord. 2015;21(3):325–6. https://doi.org/10.1016/j.parkreldis.2014.12.005.
18. Schwingenschuh P, Katschnig P, Edwards MJ, Teo JT, Korlipara LV, Rothwell JC, Bhatia KP. The blink reflex recovery cycle differs between essential and presumed psychogenic blepharospasm. Neurology. 2011;76(7):610–4. https://doi.org/10.1212/WNL.0b013e31820c3074.
19. Yaltho TC, Jankovic J. The many faces of hemifacial spasm: differential diagnosis of unilateral facial spasms. Mov Disord. 2011;26(9):1582–92.
20. Baizabal-Carvallo JF, Jankovic J. Distinguishing features of psychogenic (functional) versus organic hemifacial spasm. J Neurol. 2017;264(2):359–63. https://doi.org/10.1007/s00415-016-8356-0.
21. Pandey S, Koul A. Psychogenic movement disorders in adults and children: a clinical and video profile of 58 Indian patients. Mov Disord Clin Pract. 2017;4(5):763–7. https://doi.org/10.1002/mdc3.12516.
22. Kamble N, Prashantha DK, Jha M, Netravathi M, Reddy YC, Pal PK. Gender and age determinants of psychogenic movement disorders: a clinical profile of 73 patients. Can J Neurol Sci. 2016;43(2):268–77. https://doi.org/10.1017/cjn.2015.365.
23. Baizabal-Carvallo JF, Jankovic J. Psychogenic ophthalmologic movement disorders. J Neuropsychiatry Clin Neurosci. 2016;28(3):195–8. https://doi.org/10.1176/appi.neuropsych.15050104.
24. Kaski D, Pradhan V, Bronstein AM. Clinical features of functional (psychogenic) eye movement disorders. J Neurol Neurosurg Psychiatry. 2016;87(12):1389–92. https://doi.org/10.1136/jnnp-2016-313608.
25. Morgante F, Edwards MJ, Espay AJ. Psychogenic movement disorders. Continuum (Minneap Minn).

2013;19(5 Movement Disorders):1383–96. https://doi.org/10.1212/01.CON.0000436160.41071.79.

26. Stone J, Hoeritzauer I, Tesolin L, Carson A. Functional movement disorders of the face: a historical review and case series. J Neurol Sci. 2018;395:35–40. https://doi.org/10.1016/j.jns.2018.09.031.

27. Preston G. Hysteria and certain allied conditions. Philadelphia: P.Blakiston, Son & Co; 1897.

28. Fekete R, Baizabal-Carvallo JF, Ha AD, Davidson A, Jankovic J. Convergence spasm in conversion disorders: prevalence in psychogenic and other movement disorders compared with controls. J Neurol Neurosurg Psychiatry. 2012;83(2):202–4. https://doi.org/10.1136/jnnp-2011-300733.

29. Bentivoglio AR, Daniele A, Albanese A, Tonali PA, Fasano A. Analysis of blink rate in patients with blepharospasm. Mov Disord. 2006;21(8):1225–9. https://doi.org/10.1002/mds.20889.

30. Kerty E, Eidal K. Apraxia of eyelid opening: clinical features and therapy. Eur J Ophthalmol. 2006;16(2):204–8.

31. Stone J. Pseudo-ptosis. Pract Neurol. 2002;2:364–5.

32. Bagheri A, Abbasnia E, Pakravan M, Roshani M, Tavakoli M. Psychogenic unilateral pseudoptosis. Ophthal Plast Reconstr Surg. 2015;31(3):e55–7. https://doi.org/10.1097/IOP.0000000000000069.

33. Matsumoto H, Shimizu T, Igeta Y, Hashida H. Psychogenic unilateral ptosis with ipsilateral muscle spasm of orbicular oculi. Acta Med Indones. 2012;44(3):243–5.

34. Peer Mohamed BA, Patil SG. Psychogenic unilateral pseudoptosis. Pediatr Neurol. 2009;41(5):364–6. https://doi.org/10.1016/j.pediatrneurol.2009.06.006.

35. Wood C. The methods employed in examining the eyes for the detection of hysteria. JAMA. 1898;31:1136–8.

36. Galli S, Bereau M, Magnin E, Moulin T, Aybek S. Functional movement disorders. Rev Neurol (Paris). 2020;176(4):244–51. https://doi.org/10.1016/j.neurol.2019.08.007.

37. Sankhla C, Lai EC, Jankovic J. Peripherally induced oromandibular dystonia. J Neurol Neurosurg Psychiatry. 1998;65(5):722–8.

38. Schrag A, Bhatia KP, Quinn NP, Marsden CD. Atypical and typical cranial dystonia following dental procedures. Mov Disord. 1999;14(3):492–6.

39. Parees I, Kojovic M, Pires C, Rubio-Agusti I, Saifee TA, Sadnicka A, Kassavetis P, Macerollo A, Bhatia KP, Carson A, Stone J, Edwards MJ. Physical precipitating factors in functional movement disorders. J Neurol Sci. 2014;338(1–2):174–7. https://doi.org/10.1016/j.jns.2013.12.046.

40. Yoon WT, Oh ES. Psychogenic (functional) jaw-opening dystonia: three case reports and a comparison of symptomatic jaw-opening dystonia associated with organic causes in the literature. J Neurol Disord. 2017;5(5):1000365.

41. Baizabal-Carvallo JF, Jankovic J. The clinical features of psychogenic movement disorders resembling tics. J Neurol Neurosurg Psychiatry. 2014;85(5):573–5. https://doi.org/10.1136/jnnp-2013-305594.

42. Zadikoff C, Lang AE, Klein C. The 'essentials' of essential palatal tremor: a reappraisal of the nosology. Brain. 2006;129(Pt 4):832–40. https://doi.org/10.1093/brain/awh684.

43. Baik JS, Lyoo CH, Lee JH, Lee MS. Drug-induced and psychogenic resting suprahyoid neck and tongue tremors. Mov Disord. 2008;23(5):746–8. https://doi.org/10.1002/mds.21928.

44. Silverdale MA, Schneider SA, Bhatia KP, Lang AE. The spectrum of orolingual tremor--a proposed classification system. Mov Disord. 2008;23(2):159–67. https://doi.org/10.1002/mds.21776.

45. Ure RJ, Dhanju S, Lang AE, Fasano A. Unusual tremor syndromes: know in order to recognise. J Neurol Neurosurg Psychiatry. 2016;87(11):1191–203. https://doi.org/10.1136/jnnp-2015-311693.

46. Kaski D, Bronstein AM, Edwards MJ, Stone J. Cranial functional (psychogenic) movement disorders. Lancet Neurol. 2015;14(12):1196–205. https://doi.org/10.1016/S1474-4422(15)00226-4.

47. Stamelou M, Saifee TA, Edwards MJ, Bhatia KP. Psychogenic palatal tremor may be underrecognized: reappraisal of a large series of cases. Mov Disord. 2012;27(9):1164–8. https://doi.org/10.1002/mds.24948.

48. Baizabal-Carvallo JF, Jankovic J. Functional (psychogenic) saccadic oscillations and oculogyric crises. Lancet Neurol. 2016;15(8):791. https://doi.org/10.1016/S1474-4422(16)00126-5.

49. Kaski D, Bronstein AM. Functional (psychogenic) saccadic oscillations and oculogyric crises – authors' reply. Lancet Neurol. 2016;15(8):791–2. https://doi.org/10.1016/S1474-4422(16)00121-6.

50. Olsen LR, Mortensen EL, Bech P. Prevalence of major depression and stress indicators in the Danish general population. Acta Psychiatr Scand. 2004;109(2):96–103. https://doi.org/10.1046/j.0001-690x.2003.00231.x.

51. Schwartz BS, Stewart WF, Simon D, Lipton RB. Epidemiology of tension-type headache. JAMA. 1998;279(5):381–3. https://doi.org/10.1001/jama.279.5.381.

52. Hallett M, Lang AE, Jankovic J, Fahn S, Halligan PW, Voon V, Cloninger CR. Psychogenic movement disorders & other conversion disorders. Cambridge, UK: Cambridge University Press; 2012.

53. Gupta A, Lang AE. Psychogenic movement disorders. Curr Opin Neurol. 2009;22(4):430–6. https://doi.org/10.1097/WCO.0b013e32832dc169.

54. Morgante F, Edwards MJ, Espay AJ, Fasano A, Mir P, Martino D. Diagnostic agreement in patients with psychogenic movement disorders. Mov Disord. 2012;27(4):548–52.

55. Holds JB, Anderson RL, Jordan DR, Patrinely JR. Bilateral hemifacial spasm. J Clin Neuroophthalmol. 1990;10(2):153–4.

56. Monday K, Jankovic J. Psychogenic myoclonus. Neurology. 1993;43(2):349–52.

57. Lang AE, Koller WC, Fahn S. Psychogenic parkinsonism. Arch Neurol. 1995;52(8):802–10.

58. Kim YJ, Pakiam AS, Lang AE. Historical and clinical features of psychogenic tremor: a review of 70 cases. Can J Neurol Sci. 1999;26(3):190–5.

59. Hinson VK, Haren WB. Psychogenic movement disorders. Lancet Neurol. 2006;5(8):695–700. https://doi.org/10.1016/S1474-4422(06)70523-3.

60. Shill H, Gerber P. Evaluation of clinical diagnostic criteria for psychogenic movement disorders. Mov Disord. 2006;21(8):1163–8. https://doi.org/10.1002/mds.20921.

61. Stone J, Carson A. Functional neurologic symptoms: assessment and management. Neurol Clin. 2011;29(1):1–18, vii. https://doi.org/10.1016/j.ncl.2010.10.011.

62. Ludwig L, Pasman JA, Nicholson T, Aybek S, David AS, Tuck S, Kanaan RA, Roelofs K, Carson A, Stone J. Stressful life events and maltreatment in conversion (functional neurological) disorder: systematic review and meta-analysis of case-control studies. Lancet Psychiatry. 2018;5(4):307–20. https://doi.org/10.1016/S2215-0366(18)30051-8.

63. Thompson PD, Obeso JA, Delgado G, Gallego J, Marsden CD. Focal dystonia of the jaw and the differential diagnosis of unilateral jaw and masticatory spasm. J Neurol Neurosurg Psychiatry. 1986;49(6):651–6.

64. Kang SY, Sohn YH. Electromyography patterns of propriospinal myoclonus can be mimicked voluntarily. Mov Disord. 2006;21(8):1241–4. https://doi.org/10.1002/mds.20927.

65. Quartarone A, Rizzo V, Terranova C, Morgante F, Schneider S, Ibrahim N, Girlanda P, Bhatia KP, Rothwell JC. Abnormal sensorimotor plasticity in organic but not in psychogenic dystonia. Brain. 2009;132(Pt 10):2871–7. https://doi.org/10.1093/brain/awp213.

66. Hopfing L, Bologna M, Berardelli A, Fasano A. Functional eyelid opening apraxia: a kinematic study. Eur J Neurol. 2018;25(8):e95–7. https://doi.org/10.1111/ene.13682.

67. Valls-Sole J. Facial palsy, postparalytic facial syndrome, and hemifacial spasm. Mov Disord. 2002;17(Suppl 2):S49–52. https://doi.org/10.1002/mds.10059.

68. Lang AE, Chen R. Dystonia in complex regional pain syndrome type I. Ann Neurol. 2010;67(3):412–4. https://doi.org/10.1002/ana.21830.

69. Fabbrini G, Defazio G, Colosimo C, Thompson PD, Berardelli A. Cranial movement disorders: clinical features, pathophysiology, differential diagnosis and treatment. Nat Clin Pract Neurol. 2009;5(2):93–105. https://doi.org/10.1038/ncpneuro1006.

70. Frucht SJ, Fahn S, Greene PE, O'Brien C, Gelb M, Truong DD, Welsh J, Factor S, Ford B. The natural history of embouchure dystonia. Mov Disord. 2001;16(5):899–906.

71. Keane JR. Wrong-way deviation of the tongue with hysterical hemiparesis. Neurology. 1986;36(10):1406–7.

72. Stone J, Carson AJ. The unbearable lightheadedness of seizing: wilful submission to dissociative (non-epileptic) seizures. J Neurol Neurosurg Psychiatry. 2013;84(7):822–4. https://doi.org/10.1136/jnnp-2012-304842.

73. Tan EK, Jankovic J. Bilateral hemifacial spasm: a report of five cases and a literature review. Mov Disord. 1999;14(2):345–9.

74. Varanda S, Rocha S, Rodrigues M, Machado A, Carneiro G. Role of the 'other Babinski sign' in hyperkinetic facial disorders. J Neurol Sci. 2017;378:36–7. https://doi.org/10.1016/j.jns.2017.04.036.

75. Devoize JL. Neurological picture. Hemifacial spasm in antique sculpture: interest in the 'other Babinski sign'. J Neurol NeurosurgPsychiatry. 2011;82(1):26. https://doi.org/10.1136/jnnp.2010.208363.

76. Stamey W, Jankovic J. The other Babinski sign in hemifacial spasm. Neurology. 2007;69(4):402–4. https://doi.org/10.1212/01.wnl.0000266389.52843.3b.

77. Wang A, Jankovic J. Hemifacial spasm: clinical findings and treatment. Muscle Nerve. 1998;21(12):1740–7. https://doi.org/10.1002/(SICI)1097-4598(199812)21:12<1740::AID-MUS17>3.0.CO;2-V.

78. Jacome DE. Dracula's teeth syndrome. Headache. 2001;41(9):892–4.

79. Esteban A, Traba A, Prieto J, Grandas F. Long term follow up of a hemimasticatory spasm. Acta Neurol Scand. 2002;105(1):67–72. https://doi.org/10.1034/j.1600-0404.2002.00119.x.

80. Lemos J, Eggenberger E. Saccadic intrusions: review and update. Curr Opin Neurol. 2013;26(1):59–66. https://doi.org/10.1097/WCO.0b013e32835c5e1d.

81. Sharma VD, Jones R, Factor SA. Psychodynamic psychotherapy for functional (psychogenic) movement disorders. J Mov Disord. 2017;10(1):40–4. https://doi.org/10.14802/jmd.16038.

82. Garcin B, Roze E, Mesrati F, Cognat E, Fournier E, Vidailhet M, Degos B. Transcranial magnetic stimulation as an efficient treatment for psychogenic movement disorders. J Neurol Neurosurg Psychiatry. 2013;84(9):1043–6. https://doi.org/10.1136/jnnp-2012-304062.

Functional Gait Disorder

11

Benedetta Demartini

Clinical Vignette

Description

A 41-year-old woman with history of type 2 diabetes presented to our clinic with abnormal gait and voice disturbance. She reported two previous episodes of transient neurological symptoms that were classified at the time as "medically unexplained symptoms". In March 2018 the patient abruptly developed intermittent stuttering and disturbances in prosody. Her symptoms were distractible and worsened noticeably during explicit examination of speech. In January 2019 she abruptly developed facial deviation of the right labial commissure, along with dysphagia to solids and liquids. At that time she was hospitalized in a general neurology ward. During the 7-day admission the patient's abnormal facial movement completely recovered, while her speech disturbance and dysphagia persisted. Her work-up including MRI brain was unremarkable and she was discharged with the diagnosis of functional neurological disorder; however, the diagnosis was not explained to the patient and no specific referrals or treatment indications were provided. During the following months, the patient's dysphagia gradually improved, although her speech disturbance persisted.

In October 2019, the patient suddenly developed a gait disorder, which had a highly variable pattern and improved with distraction maneuvers. Specifically, standing from a sitting position was possible without help but she showed trunk oscillations during the stabilization phase. The patient complained of poor balance, but did not fall despite side-to-side truncal oscillations, suggesting an intact balance system. Gait was characterized by lower limb dystonia, predominantly on the right leg and foot; the patient demonstrated marked "effort" with this dystonic posture, present with both walking forwards and backwards. She also had occasional scissoring of her gait (see Video 11.1). No significant psychological or physical stressors preceded the onset of the gait disorder. The patient also complained of chronic fatigue, but was not bothered by pain. The gait disorder significantly impacted the patient's quality of life, including her work, social and family functioning. She stopped working, and required help for many of her daily activities. She was referred by her general practitioner to a neu-

Supplementary Information The online version contains supplementary material available at [https://doi.org/10.1007/978-3-030-86495-8_11].

B. Demartini (✉)
Department of Health Sciences, "Aldo Ravelli" Research Center for Neurotechnology and Experimental Brain Therapeutics, Università degli Studi di Milano, ASST Santi Paolo e Carlo, Milan, Italy
e-mail: benedetta.demartini@unimi.it

rologist with expertise in functional neurological disorder. On the basis of the patient's positive clinical features and on the investigations performed, she was diagnosed with a functional movement disorder (FMD), with symptoms of functional gait as well as functional speech. The diagnosis was explained by the neurologist such that the patient understood and agreed with the diagnosis. The patient was referred to psychiatry, psychotherapy, and physical therapy.

The psychiatrist did not formulate any additional diagnosis and did not prescribe any medications, and agreed with the referrals to tailored psychotherapy, speech and physical therapy. The patient began both specific cognitive-behavioral therapy and physical therapy once a week, with a rapid, although incomplete, improvement in her speech and gait. The patient continued to exhibit functional gait and speech at the time of her most recent visit.

Brief Discussion

This is the case of a young woman presenting with a functional gait disorder in the context of a mixed functional neurological disorder, with comorbid functional speech disturbance and functional dystonia, and a history remarkable for two previous episodes of transient neurological symptoms that had been previously classified as "medically unexplained symptoms". Specific features of the case are noted below. Each of these points will be covered at length in this chapter.

- Clinical characteristics of the gait disorder: abrupt onset, subjective complaint of poor balance with an objectively intact balance system, variable pattern, and improvement with distraction maneuvers
- Comorbidity with another functional neurological disorder (ie. functional speech disorder)
- Previous history of other functional neurological symptoms (sensory loss of the upper and lower limbs and visual loss)
- Absence of specific psychological or physical precipitating events

- Comorbidity with chronic fatigue
- Appropriate communication and explanation of the diagnosis by the neurologist expert in functional neurological disorder
- Efficacy of a multidisciplinary treatment approach, including cognitive-behavioral therapy and physiotherapy

Introduction

Functional gait disorder is part of the wide spectrum of functional neurological disorder, disturbances characterized by the presence of neurological symptoms that cannot be explained by other neurological or medical conditions, that are nonetheless genuine in nature and contribute to clinically significant discomfort or impairment in social and/or occupational functioning [1]. Specifically, functional gait disorder is defined as a disorder of ambulatory dysfunction with characteristics that are inconsistent and incongruous with other causes of abnormal gait [2] and represents one of the most frequent phenotypes of FMD seen by neurologists in general movement disorders clinics [3]. Functional gait disorder is diagnosed on the basis of positive physical signs. It might present with an impairment of both equilibrium and locomotion, the two components of normal gait. According to previous data, functional gait disorder accounted for 1.5–26% of patients evaluated in a neurology clinic [4, 5]. Although functional gait disorder has high prevalence in the general population and a significant impact on patients' quality of life, its pathophysiology remains poorly understood.

This chapter will review the main aspects of functional gait disorder, with a particular emphasis on the diagnostic process, including history, clinical signs and differential diagnosis, with the aim of providing helpful clues to clinicians facing this condition. The classification, pathophysiology, management and treatment of functional gait disorder will also be discussed.

Classification

Over the last two decades several classification schemes for functional gait disorder have been proposed; the majority of these classification schemes are based upon clinical presentations (Table 11.1). Since the first systematic report of 60 patients with functional gait disorder in 1989 [6] there has been a general consensus in classifying functional gait disorder as a primary or secondary disorder: in primary functional gait disorder, the gait disturbance is an isolated phenomenon, while in secondary functional gait disorder the gait disturbance is the consequence of another subtype of FMD (e.g. tremor, dystonia, weakness, parkinsonism), which interferes with normal gait [6, 7]. In primary functional gait disorder, the gait disturbance may also be accompanied by other FMD subtypes, albeit considered as two independent phenomena [7, 8].

Over the last few years functional gait disorder has been increasingly classified according to its clinical phenomenology. Studies have identified common patterns of functional gait disorder, including severe limping on one leg, often with dragging of the foot, walking with small, slow steps with both legs as if walking on ice, and truncal ataxia/imbalance [5, 7–9]. However, it is worth to mention that while some of these signs are highly specific for the diagnosis of functional gait disorder (e.g. dragging of the foot), others are not (walking on ice and truncal ataxia).

Recently Baizabal-Carvallo et al. [8] proposed the following categories of functional gait disorder: (i) slow hesitant gait; (ii) astasia-abasia, characterized by the inability to stand and walk requiring the patient to hold onto an object or another person to avoid falls; (iii) bouncing gait, characterized by knee buckling; (iv) scissoring, characterized by leg-crossing during casual gait; (v) wide-based gait; (vi) limping, characterized by asymmetric leg flexion; and (vii) lower limb dystonia, characterized by leg or foot stiffness.

Fung recently proposed a stepwise approach to analyze the phenomenology of functional gait disorder and to classify functional gait disorder into four syndromes: movement disorders mimics (such as dystonic, parkinsonian or ataxic), neurologic mimics (such as hemiparetic, myopathic or neuropathic), musculoskeletal or biomechanical mimics (such as antalgic or hip instability) and isolated disequilibrium or balance disorders (such as tightrope walking). This stepwise approach may be helpful for clinicians when deciding which clinical investigations to pursue when making the diagnosis of a functional gait disorder [10].

Table 11.1 Phenomenological classification schema for functional gait disorder

1	Presenting modality	Primary	The gait disturbance is an isolated phenomenon
		Secondary	The gait disturbance is the consequence of another subtype of functional movement disorder
2	Clinical phenomenology	Slow hesitant gait	
		Astasia-abasia	Significant difficulty standing and walking; requiring the patient to hold an object or another person to avoid falls
		Bouncing	Knee buckling
		Scissoring	Leg-crossing during casual gait
		Wide-based gait	
		Limping	Asymmetric leg flexion
		Lower limb dystonia	Leg or foot stiffness
3	Syndromic description	Movement disorders mimics	Dystonic, parkinsonian or ataxic
		Neurologic (non movement disorders) mimics	Hemiparetic, myopathic or neuropathic
		Musculoskeletal or biomechanical mimics	Antalgic or hip instability
		Isolated disequilibrium or balance disorders	Tightrope walking

Prior studies [7, 9] have shown that 42.3% and 39.2%, respectively, of patients with FMD presented with a primary functional gait disorder; less than 10% of the patients in these studies presented with an isolated functional gait disorder in the absence of other functional neurological symptoms. Among patients with secondary functional gait disorder slowing of gait seems to be the most common gait pattern, while among patients with primary functional gait disorder buckling of the knee seems to be the most common gait pattern [7, 8].

Diagnosis

Given the high prevalence of functional gait disorder, it is fundamental for clinicians to have familiarity with valid diagnostic tools in order to accurately diagnose this condition and to differentiate it from other causes of abnormal gait. Providing patients with the diagnosis of FMD early and in an appropriate manner has been shown to avoid unnecessary investigations, to speed the initiation of a tailored treatment program, and to improve patients' overall progno-

sis [11]. The diagnosis of functional gait disorder should not be a diagnosis of exclusion, but should be based on positive signs, as recommended by the diagnostic criteria of the most recent version of the Diagnostic and Statistical Manual of Mental Disorders (DSM-5) [1], in which emphasis is placed on the presence of positive physical signs, and the requirement for psychological stressors was removed [12]. While Fahn and Williams [13] and Gupta and Lang criteria [14] may serve as valuable instruments to support clinicians during the diagnostic process, it has been recently suggested that the use of phenotype-specific clinically definite FMD diagnostic criteria will increase inter-rater reliability and reduce misdiagnoses (Espay and Lang criteria) [15]. This process involves tailoring the assessment towards phenotype-specific core clinical features instead of supportive but insufficiently sensitive historical and psychiatric examination features [15]. Below, the diagnostic process for a patient with a suspected functional gait disorder is summarized, with particular attention to the clinical interview, clinical features and differential diagnosis (Fig. 11.1).

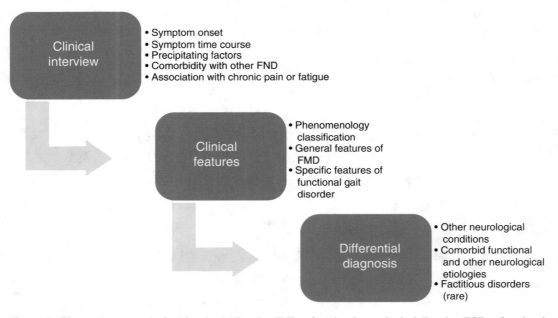

Fig. 11.1 Diagnostic process in functional gait disorder. FND = functional neurological disorder; FGD = functional gait disorder; FMD = functional movement disorder

Clinical Interview

A thorough clinical history is critical, and should direct specific attention to the following aspects:

- Symptom onset, which is generally quite abrupt in functional gait disorder.
- Symptom time course, which may wax and wane in functional gait disorder.
- Presence of any psychological or physical precipitating factors. Functional gait disorder is more commonly preceded by physical precipitating events (e.g. injuries, physical diseases) than by psychological event [3]. Although physical events might also have psychological components (e.g. a car crash, even if relatively minor), it is important to keep in mind that precipitating events are unable to be identified in a good proportion of cases [16].
- Comorbidity with other functional neurological disorder subtypes. The presence of other functional neurological symptoms has been shown to be a good diagnostic clue for functional gait disorder. Previous studies have suggested that the majority of patients with functional gait disorder also present with other functional symptoms, including neuro-ophthalmological symptoms, weakness, and sensory loss. Keane reported that 43% of patients with functional gait disorder had associated functional visual findings, including visual field abnormalities, decreased visual acuity, and eye movement limitation [6]. Association with chronic pain or fatigue has been found to be very common (up to 75% and 82%, respectively), especially in patients with functional weakness [17].
- Past medical and psychiatric history. Concerning psychiatric history, inquiry on mental health problems and past traumatic events, which are not always easily identified [16], should be very carefully handled, and might benefit from the assistance of a psychiatrist or a psychologist, who are generally more experienced and have more time to broach and explore these sensitive areas.

Clinical Features

There has been debate concerning the utility of functional gait disorder classification schema in facilitating the diagnosis. On the one hand, Lempert and colleagues [5] have stated that a strict classification into characteristic subtypes is not useful because predominant features widely vary from patient to patient and occur in various combinations. On the other hand, it has been suggested that clustering related patterns of functional gait disorder into broader, yet well-described categories, such as the ones proposed by Jordbru et al. [9], might help clinicians in organizing their diagnostic process. Here I suggest that the stepwise approach proposed by Fung to analyze functional gait disorder phenomenology and to classify functional gait disorder into four (sometimes overlapping) syndromes might be a useful tool for clinicians when formulating a positive diagnosis of functional gait disorder [10]. In particular, categorizing the suspected functional gait disorder into one or more of the previously mentioned categories (e.g. movement disorders mimics, neurologic mimics, biomechanical mimics, balance disorders) can help the clinician identify the necessary clinical investigations to look for positive evidence of functional neurological etiology and to exclude potential non-functional pathology.

Features of FMD that can be seen in patients with functional gait disorder include the following: abrupt onset; inconsistent and incongruent pattern of the disorder; worsening with attention or improvement with distraction; inconsistency between performance while patient is examined and while he/she is not examined; functional disability out of proportion to clinical examination; and suggestibility/response to placebo.

There are several positive signs on physical examination that specifically support the diagnosis of a functional gait disorder [18]:

- The "huffing and puffing" sign, defined as an excessive demonstration of effort during gait which is out of proportion to clinical examination, generally manifests with the presence of huffing, grunting, grimacing and breath holding. This sign, although not sensitive (sensitivity range from 10.5% to 57%), was found to be highly specific for functional gait disorder (specificity ranged from 89% to 100%), increasing the odds of a gait disorder being functional in nature by 13 times [8–19].

- The "psychogenic toe sign" is defined as a resistance to manipulation of an extended first toe, which can be flexed only at the expense of associated pain or by extending toes two through five. This sign has been only anecdotally observed in a single pediatric case report of a 13-year-old boy affected by functional dystonia and weakness [20], but may warrant further attention in adult patients with functional gait disorder.
- The "fixed plantar flexion sign" is accompanied by subsequent inversion of one foot or both feet, and cannot be overcome with passive manipulation. This sign has been largely investigated in functional dystonia [21], but may warrant attention also in the context of functional gait disorder, since a functional dystonic posture often introduces a secondary functional gait disorder.
- The "swivel chair sign" is a sign of inconsistency in which patients with functional gait disorder seem to be able to use their legs to propel themselves forwards and backwards when seated on an office chair with wheels, but not when walking [22].

In their commentary authors acknowledge that these signs have not undergone proper quantitative analysis and therefore should not be considered diagnostic tools; however, they might be helpful in making a diagnosis [18]. Other clinical signs frequently observed, although not validated, in patients with functional gait disorder but not in patients with other gait disorders include frequent falls onto the knees or repeated lurching towards the examiner but not towards open spaces.

Differential Diagnosis

There are several clinical features of functional gait disorder that aid clinicians in formulating a proper diagnosis. However, there are several conditions where differentiating between a FMD and another gait disorder may be quite challenging. First, isolated dystonic gait may be confused with functional gait disorder because the task-specificity characteristic of dystonia may be misinterpreted as inconsistency [23]. Moreover, in isolated dystonic gait, patient's compensatory posturing might influence dystonic gait [24]; however, in this case, unlike functional gait disorder, underlying balance and locomotive function are preserved. Dystonic gait combined with another movement disorder which is random in nature, such as tic, chorea or cerebellar ataxia [25], may also be challenging to diagnose. In this situation, the gait might appear inconsistent and bizarre, such as in functional gait disorder. However, unlike FMD, an underlying stereotyped pattern of abnormal posturing can be observed. Frontal ataxia is a condition in which the pattern of gait disturbance may widely vary over time, rendering any attempt to distinguish it from functional gait disorder difficult [26]. In this case the differential diagnosis relies on the presence of other clinical signs or on neuroimaging investigations. Recently the examination of a cognitive dual task walking condition was found to further support a proper differential diagnosis in this setting. Patients with functional gait disorder were found to present a paradoxical improvement of their gait disorder under cognitive distraction, while use of this task in patients with ataxia resulted in a decline in gait [27]. Factitious disorder, in which symptoms are deliberately and consciously produced by patients to satisfy a psychological need, is also in the differential diagnosis [28]. However, factitious disorder is thought to be infrequent. Finally, it is important to mention that patients might present with multiple different etiologies for their gait disorder, both functional and non-functional, rendering the diagnostic process even more complex [29].

Pathophysiology

Despite the evidence that patients affected by functional gait disorder have levels of disability, distress and health care utilization that equal, and in some cases surpass, patients with other neurological conditions such as Parkinson's disease [30], the pathophysiology of these disorders remains unclear.

The last two decades have seen a surge of research interest in the pathophysiology of functional neurological disorder. One major outcome has been a downgrading of the importance of historically psychoanalytic theories according to which psychological stressors must always play a major causative role in the development and maintenance of FMD. Several studies have shown that such psychological stressors, although clearly important in some cases, might not always play a unique role in the etiology of FMD [16]. In terms of diagnostic criteria, in the DSM-5, the presence of a causative psychological stressor has been removed from the diagnostic criteria [1]. This demonstrates how the perspective on FMD has changed. New etiopathological hypotheses based on the integration between psychology and neurobiology have been formulated, under the frame of a biopsychosocial model of FMD, and there has been a significant increase in experimental studies focusing on the neurobiology of functional neurological disorder [31]. In particular, neuroimaging studies have made efforts to elucidate the neurobiological mechanisms underlying FMD. The studies specifically conducted on patients with functional gait disorder are summarized below.

Functional Neuroimaging Studies

A pioneering study was conducted in 1998 by Yazici and Kostakoglu in which they assessed cerebral blood flow changes using Single-Photon Emission Computed Tomography (SPECT) in five patients with functional astasia-abasia. They noticed a decreased perfusion in the left parietal region in one patient and in the left temporal region in four patients. This study was limited by the small sample size and by the lack of a control group [32]. During the following years numerous studies were conducted in patients with different subtypes of FMD. It is important to note that functional gait disorder was not the primary functional phenomenology in these studies. Nevertheless, a generalization of the findings might be appropriate, because of the small amount of studies conducted specifically on functional gait disorder. Although results are quite contradictory, potentially due to the different techniques and tasks used in the different studies, these studies showed several functional alterations at the level of different areas of the brain and, more specifically, hypoactivation of the contralateral primary motor cortex [33], decreased activity in the parietal lobe [34], aberrant activation of the amygdala [35], altered temporo-parietal junction activity [36, 37] and hyperactivation of insular regions [38].

Connectomic Studies

Findings from connectomic studies, although not always consistent, seem to underline an aberrant functional connectivity between the supplementary motor areas and areas of the limbic system, mainly the amygdala [39]. This finding has led to the hypothesis that impaired motor conceptualization or preparation and inhibition of motor execution, along with an abnormal limbic-motor or limbic-sensory interaction, might be one of the mechanisms underlying functional gait disorder.

Moreover, a recent study by Diez et al. found, in patients with motor functional neurological disorder, when compared to healthy controls, that early-life physical abuse severity and physical neglect correlated with corticolimbic weighted-degree functional connectivity. Connectivity profiles influenced by physical abuse occurred in limbic (amygdalar–hippocampal), paralimbic (cingulo-insular and ventromedial prefrontal), and cognitive control (ventrolateral prefrontal) areas, as well as in sensorimotor and visual cortices [40].

Treatment Plan

The first step for a successful management of functional gait disorder involves clear communication and explanation of the diagnosis. Neurologists should carefully explain the diagnosis, how the diagnosis was made (i.e. on the basis of positive clinical signs) and the tailored treatment options that are available [41]. It is important for the patient to know that the medical team believes that his/her symptoms are genuine and not "made up" or "all in their head". Communicating the diagnosis to patients in a clear and simple way has been shown to improve functional neurological symptoms, and indeed is thought to represent the first form of treatment for these disorders [42]. Subsequently a tailored treatment program should be proposed to patients. Although no official guidelines for the treatment of FMD have been developed, there is an overall consensus in defining a program which is tailored to the individual patient and which may involve different health specialists in the context of a multidisciplinary team [43]. In the specific case of functional gait disorder, physiotherapy has been shown to be a promising treatment: Jordbru and colleagues conducted a randomized trial specifically on patients with functional gait disorder [44]. A total of 60 patients were recruited and were randomly assigned to immediate treatment or treatment after 4 weeks. Treatment consisted of adapted physical activity within a cognitive behavioral framework, and focused on offering an alternative explanation of symptoms, positively

reinforcing normal gait and not reinforcing dysfunction. Results showed that patients significantly improved their ability to walk and their quality of life after inpatient rehabilitation compared with the untreated control group. The improvements in gait were sustained at 1-month and 1-year follow-up. This is the only study to date conducted specifically on patients with functional gait disorder. However, several studies conducted on patients with FMD that included patients with primary functional gait disorder confirm that specific physiotherapy is a promising treatment for FMD, that can be performed in-person as well as via telemedicine [45–47]. Moreover, Maggio et al. showed that in a subset of individuals with available gait speed data, post-treatment 10-meter gait speed times improved compared with baseline measurements [48]. In particular, according to Nielsen et al. consensus recommendations, gait retraining can be performed in several ways, including facilitating (hands on) support in lieu of walking aids, changing walking speed, building up a normal gait pattern from simple achievable components that progressively approximate normal walking (e.g. side to side weight shifting, continuing weight shift allowing feet to "automatically" advance forward small amounts, progressively increasing this step length with the focus on maintaining rhythmical weight shift rather than the action of stepping), walking carrying small weights in each hand, walking backwards or sideways, walking to a set rhythm (e.g. in time to music) or walking up or down stairs. Gait retraining can be approached in progressively more challenging environments such as outdoors, on uneven surfaces and in crowded environments [49].

Finally, it is important to mention that novel interventions or treatment adjuncts such as transcranial magnetic simulation (TMS), botulinum toxin, therapeutic sedation, hypnosis and electromyographic biofeedback have been recently considered in the management of FMD [50]. In particular there is an accumulating evidence base to support TMS as a safe, well-tolerated and possibly effective treatment for a wide range of functional neurological disorder subtypes [51]. Up to date, there have been five small feasibility randomized controlled trials with encouraging results on TMS, but no studies powered to detect differences between groups [52–56] (for more details see Chap. 28). Possible mechanisms of action of TMS in patients with functional neurological symptoms are placebo response and/or neuromodulation.

Conclusions

Functional gait disorder, which can present as an isolated phenomena or along with other FMD subtypes, is common and can be quite disabling. The diagnostic process, which is not always easy, should include careful inquiry about onset of symptoms and comorbid medical and psychiatric history, as well as detailed examination of gait. Differential diagnosis should consider alternative causes of gait disorders. Successful management of patients with functional gait disorder should start with clear communication and explanation of the diagnosis, followed by a tailored multidisciplinary intervention, which might include psychotherapy and specific physiotherapy.

Summary

1. Functional gait disorder is common in the general population, representing one of the most prevalent clinical presentations of FMD seen by neurologists in general movement disorders clinics.
2. Functional gait disorder may be characterized as primary, where the gait disturbance is an isolated phenomenon, or, more frequently, as secondary, where the gait disturbance is the consequence of another subtype of FMD (e.g. tremor, dystonia, weakness, parkinsonism) which interferes with gait.
3. Although functional gait disorder might present with different phenotypes (slow hesitant gait, astasia-abasia, bouncing, scissoring, wide-based gait, limping gait, and lower limb dystonia) common features include the presence of an inconsistent, incongruent and variable pattern, along with some specific signs, such as the "huffing and puffing" sign, defined as an excessive demonstration of effort during gait which is out of proportion to clinical examination.
4. Recent functional neuroimaging and neurophysiological studies have shown that patients with functional gait disorder have abnormal activation of specific areas of the brain, along with an abnormal functional connectivity between frontal and limbic regions, suggesting a neurobiological substrate of the disorder.
5. The first step in the management of functional gait disorder is a clear communication and explanation of the diagnosis, which is associated with better prognosis.
6. In the context of a multidisciplinary treatment approach to FMD, a tailored program of specific physiotherapy has recently emerged as a promising treatment for functional gait disorder.

References

1. American Psychiatric Association. Diagnostic and statistical manual of mental disorders. 5th ed. Arlington: American Psychiatric Association; 2013.
2. Lang AE. Phenotype-specific diagnosis of functional (psychogenic) movement disorders. Curr Neurol Neurosci Rep. 2015;15(6):32.
3. Edwards M. Functional psychogenic gait disorder: diagnosis and management. Handb Clin Neurol. 2018;159:417–23.
4. Bhatia KP. Psychogenic gait disorders. Adv Neurol. 2001;87:252–4.
5. Lempert T, Brandt T, Dieterich M, Huppert D. How to identify psychogenic disorders of stance and gait. A video study in 37 patients. J Neurol. 1991;238:140–6.
6. Keane JR. Hysterical gait disorders: 60 cases. Neurology. 1989;39:586–9.
7. Baik JS, Lang AE. Gait abnormalities in psychogenic movement disorders. Mov Disord. 2007;22:395–9.

8. Baizabal-Carvallo JF, Alonso-Juarez M, Jankovic J. Functional gait disorders, clinical phenomenology, and classification. Neurol Sci. 2020;4:911–5.

9. Jordbru AA, Smedstad LM, Moen VP, Martinsen EW. Identifying patterns of psychogenic gait by video-recording. J Rehabil Med. 2012;44:31–5.

10. Fung VSC. Functional gait disorder. Handb Clin Neurol. 2016;139:263–70.

11. Thenganatt MA, Jankovic J. Psychogenic (functional) movement disorders. Continuum (Minneap Minn). 2019;25:1121–40.

12. Demartini B, D'Agostino A, Gambini O. From conversion disorder (DSM-IV-TR) to functional neurological symptom disorder (DSM-5): when a label changes the perspective for the neurologist, the psychiatrist and the patient. J Neurol Sci. 2016;360:55–6.

13. Williams DT, Ford B, Fahn S. Phenomenology and psychopathology related to psychogenic movement disorders. In: Weiner WJ, Lang AE, editors. Behavioral neurology in movement disorders. New York: Raven; 1994. p. 231–57.

14. Gupta A, Lang AE. Psychogenic movement disorders. Curr Opin Neurol. 2009;22:430–6.

15. Espay AJ, Lang AE. Phenotype-specific diagnosis of functional (psychogenic) movement disorders. Curr Neurol Neurosci Rep. 2015;15:32.

16. Ludgwig L, Pasman JA, Nicholson T, Aybek S, David AS, Tuck S, et al. Stressful life events and maltreatment in conversion (functional neurological) disorder: systematic review and meta-analysis of case-control studies. Lancet Psychiatry. 2018;5:307–20.

17. Stone J, Warlow C, Sharpe M. The symptom of functional weakness: a controlled study of 107 patients. Brain. 2010;133:1537–51.

18. Sokol LL, Espay AJ. Clinical signs in functional (psychogenic) gait disorders: a brief survey. J Clin Mov Disord. 2016;12(3):3.

19. Laub HN, Dwivedi AK, Revilla FJ, Duker AP, Pecina-Jacob C, Espay AJ. Diagnostic performance of the "Huffing and Puffing" sign in functional (psychogenic) movement disorders. Mov Disord Clin Pract. 2015;2:29–32.

20. Espay AJ, Lang AE. The psychogenic toe signs. Neurology. 2011;77:508–9.

21. Schrag A, Trimble M, Quinn N, Bhatia K. The syndrome of fixed dystonia: an evaluation of 103 patients. Brain. 2004;127:2360–72.

22. Okun MS, Rodriguez RL, Foote KD, Fernandez HH. The "chair test" to aid in the diagnosis of psychogenic gait disorders. Neurologist. 2007;13:87–91.

23. Albanese A. The clinical expression of primary dystonia. J Neurol. 2003;250:1145–51.

24. Trinh B, Ha AD, Mahant N, Kim SD, Owler B, Fung VS. Dramatic improvement of truncal tardive dystonia following globus pallidus pars interna deep brain stimulation. J Clin Neurosci. 2014;2:515–7.

25. Kim SD, Fung VS. Unusual gait disorders. In: Galvez-Jimenez N, Tuite P, Bhatia K, editors. Uncommon causes of movement disorders. Cambridge: Cambridge University Press; 2011.

26. Thompson PD. Frontal lobe ataxia. Handb Clin Neurol. 2012;103:619–22.

27. Schniepp R, Möhwald K, Wuehr M. Clinical and automated gait analysis in patients with vestibular, cerebellar, and functional gait disorders: perspectives and limitations. J Neurol. 2019;266:118–22.

28. Hallett M, Fahn S, Jankovic J, et al., editors. Psychogenic movement disorders. Neurology and neuropsychiatry. Philadelphia: AAN Press, Lippincott Williams & Wilkins; 2006.

29. Stone J, Carson A, Duncan R. Who is referred to neurology clinics? The diagnosis made in 3781 new patients. Clin Neurol Neurosurg. 2010;112:747–51.

30. Carson A, Stone J, Hibberd C, Murray G, Duncan R, Coleman R, et al. Disability, distress and unemployment in neurology outpatients with symptoms "unexplained by organic disease". J Neurol Neurosurg Psychiatry. 2011;82:810–3.

31. Edwards MJ, Adams RA, Brown H, Parees I, Friston KJ. A Bayesian account of "hysteria". Brain. 2012;135:3495–512.

32. Yazici KM, Kostakoglu L. Cerebral blood flow changes in patients with conversion disorder. Psychiatry Res Neuroimaging. 1998;83:163–8.

33. Schrag AE, Mehta AR, Bhatia KP, Brown RJ, Frackowiak RS, Trimble MR, et al. The functional neuroimaging correlates of psychogenic versus organic dystonia. Brain. 2013;136(3):770–81.

34. Espay AJ, Maloney T, Vannest J, Norris MM, Eliassen JC, Neefus E, et al. Dysfunction in emotion processing underlies functional (psychogenic) dystonia. Mov Disord. 2018;33(1):136–45.

35. Hassa T, Sebastian A, Liepert J, Weiller C, Schmidt R, Tüscher O. Symptom-specific amygdala hyperactivity modulates motor control network in conversion disorder. Neuroimage Clin. 2017;15:143–50.

36. Aybek S, Nicholson TR, Zelaya F, O'Daly OG, Craig TJ, David AS, et al. Neural correlates of recall of life events in conversion disorder. JAMA Psychiat. 2014;71(1):52–60.

37. Maurer CW, LaFaver K, Ameli R, Epstein SA, Hallet M, Horovitz SG. Impaired self-agency in functional movement disorders: a resting-state fMRI study. Neurology. 2016;87(6):564–70.

38. Saj A, Raz N, Levin N, Ben-Hur T, Arzy S. Disturbed mental imagery of affected body-parts in patients with hysterical conversion paraplegia correlates with pathological limbic activity. Brain Sci. 2014;4(2):396–404.

39. Wegrzyk J, Kebets V, Richiardi J, Galli S, Van de Ville D, Aybek S. Identifying motor functional neurological disorder using resting-state functional connectivity. Neuroimage Clin. 2018;17:163–8.

40. Diez I, Larson AG, Nakhate V, Dunn EC, Fricchione GL, Nicholson TR, et al. Early-life trauma endophenotypes and brain circuit–gene expression relationships in functional neurological (conversion) disorder. Mol Psychiatry. 2021;26:3817–28.

41. Stone J, Carson A, Hallett M. Explanation as treatment for functional neurologic disorders. Handb Clin Neurol. 2016;139:543–53.

42. Stone J. Functional neurological disorders: the neurological assessment as treatment. Pract Neurol. 2016;16:7–17.
43. Lidstone SC, MacGillivray L, Lang AE. Integrated therapy for functional movement disorders: time for a change. Mov Disord Clin Pract. 2020;7:169–74.
44. Jordbru AA, Smedstad LM, Klungsoyr O, Martinsen EW. Psychogenic gait disorder: a randomized controlled trial of physical rehabilitation with one-year follow-up. J Rehabil Med. 2014;46:181–7.
45. Nielsen G, Ricciardi L, Demartini B, Hunter R, Joyce E, Edwards MJ. Outcomes of a 5-day physiotherapy programme for functional (psychogenic) motor disorders. J Neurol. 2015;262:674–81.
46. Nielsen G, Buszewicz M, Stevenson F, Hunter R, Holt K, Dudziec M, et al. Randomised feasibility study of physiotherapy for patients with functional motor symptoms. J Neurol Neurosurg Psychiatry. 2017;88:484–90.
47. Demartini B, Bombieri F, Goeta D, Gambini O, Ricciardi L, Tinazzi M. A physical therapy programme for functional motor symptoms: a telemedicine pilot study. Parkinsonism Relat Disord. 2020;76:108–11.
48. Maggio JB, Ospina JP, Callahan J, Hunt AL, Stephen CD, Perez DL. Outpatient physical therapy for functional neurological disorder: a preliminary feasibility and naturalistic outcome study in a U.S. cohort. J Neuropsychiatry Clin Neurosci. 2020;32:85–9.
49. Nielsen G, Stone J, Matthews A, Brown M, Sparkes C, Farmer R, et al. Physiotherapy for functional motor disorders: a consensus recommendation. J Neurol Neurosurg Psychiatry. 2015;86:1113–9.
50. Gilmour GS, Nielsen G, Teodoro T, Yogarajah M, Coebergh JA, Dilley MD, et al. Management of functional neurological disorder. J Neurol. 2020;267(7):2164–72.
51. Nicholson TRJ, Voon V. Transcranial magnetic stimulation and sedation as treatment for functional neurologic disorders. In: Hallett M, Stone J, Carson A, editors. Handbook of clinical neurology, functional neurologic disorder, vol. 139. Elsevier; 2016.
52. Broersma M, Koops EA, Vrooman PC, Van der Hoeven JH. Can repetitive transcranial magnetic stimulation increase muscle strength in functional neurological paresis? A proof-of-principle study. Eur J Neurol. 2015;22:866–73.
53. Pick S, Hodsoll BS, Eskander A, Stavropoulos I, Samra K, Bottini J, et al. Trial Of Neurostimulation In Conversion Symptoms (TONICS): a feasibility randomised controlled trial of transcranial magnetic stimulation for functional limb weakness. BMJ Open. 2020;10:e037198.
54. Garcin B, Mesrati F, Hubsch C, Mauras T, Iliescu I, Naccache L, et al. Impact of transcranial magnetic stimulation on functional movement disorders: cortical modulation or a behavioral effect? Front Neurol. 2017;8:338.
55. Taib S, Ory-Magne F, Brefel-Courbon C, Moreau Y, Thalamas C, Arbus C, et al. Repetitive transcranial magnetic stimulation for functional tremor: a randomized, double-blind, controlled study. Mov Disord. 2019;34(8):1210–9.
56. McWhirter L, Ludwig L, Carson A, McIntosh RD, Stone J, et al. Transcranial magnetic stimulation as a treatment for functional (psychogenic) upper limb weakness. J Psychosom Res. 2016;89:102–6.

Functional Tics

12

Tina Mainka and Christos Ganos

Clinical Vignette

A 21-year-old student presented to our clinic with repetitive motor and vocal behaviors that started abruptly 7 months prior to presentation. Initial symptoms developed following an argument with her roommates, after which she felt tired and dizzy, became tearful, and experienced whole body shaking with flailing arm movements and jerks. Over the ensuing days, the repetitive whole-body and arm movements persisted, albeit diminished in intensity and frequency. Several weeks later, during a long car ride, she experienced repetitive vocalizations, consisting primarily of shouting. By the time of presentation, the pattern of motor and vocal behaviors had changed such that she exhibited sudden simple repetitive movements including blinking, head turning, and stomping with one leg, in addition to more com-plex movements such as clapping her hands, hitting her head with her hand, and pulling her leg towards her body while sitting. Repetitive vocalizations included shouts of single words or names of friends, as well as sentences with derogatory and/or coprolalic content (e.g., "I hate you.", "Shut up, bitch."). Further, she described that unexpected loud noises now startled her, causing her whole body to jerk. She was unable to identify alleviating factors; she endorsed increase in repetitive behaviors and onset of whole body shaking when lying supine. Although she described the movements and vocalizations as involuntary and unable to be voluntarily suppressed, she sometimes recognized a mounting feeling of tension in her abdomen which was relieved by their subsequent occurrence. There was no relevant past medical history, and she denied prior history of tics or other abnormal movements. Family history was equally unremarkable. She had previously been treated with a 4 month period of psychoanalytic psychotherapy and risperidone at a dose of 1 mg/day, with no clear effects on the repetitive behaviors.

Neurological examination was unremarkable with the exception of frequent, repetitive and very variable simple (e.g., head turning, foot stomping, whistling, shouting) and complex movements (e.g., standing up from a chair, slapping her face) and vocalizations, including echolalia and coprolalia. There was clear interference of these behaviors with the execution of voluntary actions.

Supplementary Information The online version contains supplementary material available at [https://doi.org/10.1007/978-3-030-86495-8_12].

T. Mainka
Department of Neurology, Charité University Medicine Berlin, Berlin, Germany

Berlin Institute of Health, Berlin, Germany

C. Ganos (✉)
Department of Neurology, Charité University Medicine Berlin, Berlin, Germany
e-mail: christos.ganos@charite.de

Context-dependency was also noted; for example, the patient suddenly moved backwards after the examiner presented her with a pen, and gave the time in a foreign language after checking her watch. Irregular shaking, exaggeration of motor behaviors during examination of deep tendon reflexes, and unusual behaviors, such as "the need to hug the examiner" were also observed (see Video 12.1).

The wide range of repetitive motor and vocal behaviors, which were very variable in presentation, alongside their phenomenological complexity and context-dependency, including explicit coprolalic sentences, were atypical for tic behaviors seen in primary tic disorders. In addition, characteristics such as the sudden adult-onset, the inconsistent description of sensory antecedents for her repetitive behaviors and the lack of suppressibility further underscored the distinct quality of these behaviors. The diagnosis of functional tics (or functional tic-like disorder) was made and treatment options were openly discussed. The patient pursued multimodal inward therapy consisting of intensive physiotherapy, behavioral and occupational therapy, which was not tolerated well and was prematurely stopped. At follow-up 6 months later, the patient had started outpatient behavioral therapy and reported a significant improvement in her repetitive behaviors. The patient also participated in a psychiatric inpatient therapeutic program based on dialectic behavioral and acceptance-commitment therapies. At last follow-up, 1 year since first presentation, no repetitive behaviors were noted. The patient reported improvement in anxiety and distress and a near disappearance of her abnormal repetitive behaviors. She continued to visit a behavioral therapist and was focused on resuming her university studies.

Clinical Characteristics of Functional Tics

Due to overlap of phenomenological features with functional movement disorder (FMD) there has been a long debate as to the etiological origin of tics, and psychological processes ("hysterical tics") were often viewed as the underlying cause. The resemblance of tics to voluntary actions, their often socially bizarre qualities, sensitivity to attention, suppressibility and the behavioral associations of tic disorders, particularly the presence of comorbid attention-deficit hyperactivity and obsessive-compulsive disorder, have all contributed to their etiological misattribution as functional. It was only recently and after decades of research in the clinical characteristics of primary (neurodevelopmental) tic disorders, including Tourette syndrome, that it was possible to distil specific features aiding the distinction between primary tics and tics of functional neurological etiology. For a review of the essential clinical characteristics of primary tic disorders, including Tourette syndrome please see Ref. [1].

The first two studies which directly addressed this issue contrast the characteristics of primary tics with those of functional etiology (also labelled as "psychogenic movements resembling tics", $n = 20$) and identify several distinguishing factors [2, 3]. Firstly, all but two participants with functional tics in these two studies had an adult age at onset of abnormal behaviors, which differs from the classic childhood onset of primary tics [2, 3]. Although cases with adult-onset tics have been previously reported in literature, they usually reflect different etiologies, including neurodegenerative and FMD, and many of the cases labelled as primary adult-onset tics in fact reflect re-emergent tics from childhood [4]. Functional tics, in most cases, also lacked the characteristic waxing and waning that typifies primary tics, and differed phenomenologically. Indeed, in one of the two studies [2], functional tics consisted of more complex motor behaviors, which interfered with the execution of voluntary actions. They also showed a different somatotopic pattern than the classic rostrocaudal gradient of primary tics, which primarily affect the face and neck (see Video 12.1) [5].

In contrast to patients with primary tic disorder, patients in these studies did not report sensory antecedents to their functional tics. They experienced the tics, therefore, as completely involuntary and sometimes surprising events, and did not feel capable of exerting volitional inhibitory control over them [2, 3]. No paliphe-nomena or echophenomena were noted, and there was no relevant family history for tic disorders. Moreover, the profiles of associated neuropsychiatric comorbidities differed. For example, there were no cases with functional tics reported with a comorbid diagnosis of either obsessive-compulsive behavior/disorder and/or attention-deficit hyperactive disorder, despite the common prevalence of these neuropsychiatric comorbidities in people with primary tic disorders [2, 3]. Finally, there was no response to classic anti-tic medications.

In addition to these features, we would also like to highlight that we commonly observe characteristic context-dependency for several functional tics, as described in the case vignette. For example, assessment of the patellar reflex induced intense stomping of the ipsilateral leg, and demonstration of repetitive hand movements by the examiner was followed by a reaching movement towards the examiner's hand (see Video 12.1). Indeed, exacerbation of FMD during neurological examination is well described [6]. Additional FMD subtypes, such as tremor and gait disturbances have also been documented in cases with functional tics [2]. We further note that functional tics are highly variable, both in terms of individual movements (e.g., changes in directionality of movement and amplitude, see Video 12.1b), as well as the number of different repetitive behaviors [7]. Please refer to Fig. 12.1 for further comparison of classic primary tic disorders and functional tics.

Phenomenological Overlap Between Primary and Functional Tics

Despite the clear distinguishing features between the two types of behaviors, some patients may present clinical signs compatible with both primary and functional tics (see Fig. 12.1). For example, in a study of 13 cases with the common presenting feature of repetitive swearing, on the basis of which a misdiagnosis of Tourette syndrome was given, six patients had onset of func-tional tic behaviors in childhood [7]. Of note, repetitive swearing, as in functional coprolalia, differs from coprolalic behaviors encountered in primary tic disorders such as Tourette syndrome. Functional coprolalia consists of loud utterances of many different (compound) words and sentences with obscene content. In contrast, coprola-lia in Tourette syndrome typically involves short words (e.g. 4-letter words in English), embedded in ongoing conversation, but uttered with different pitch and often imprecisely to mask their content.

The same study also described cases where sensory antecedents of abnormal behaviors were reported, although these qualitatively differed from classic descriptions of premonitory urges [8]. Patients with functional tics may describe the need to release increasing "whole-body energy" or a "sudden energy pulse" around the heart or belly. In some cases we have encountered, that these abnormal sensations were continuously experienced and caused major distress (e.g., "water and lymph are overwhelming facial skin" or "body being impaled"). Importantly, in functional tics there appears to be a weaker link between the sensory experience and the subsequent motor and vocal behavior, contrasting to the experience of premonitory urges in primary tics, where sensory experiences trigger specific tic behaviors, typically in the same body part (e.g., muscle tension around the wrist triggers hand tics) [9]. Of note, abnormal sensory experiences are also reported in other functional neurological disorder subtypes (e.g., functional seizures) and in people with anxiety disorders [10]. We have also observed an insidious onset, rostrocaudal distribution and the ability to voli-tionally inhibit functional tics in some of our cases.

Taken together, it becomes apparent that beyond classic cases, in many occasions the distinction between primary and functional tics solely on the basis of clinical signs may be difficult, if not impossible. In these cases, other specific clues or even a combination of clinical characteristics might point to the diagnosis of a FMD. For example, some individuals capable of voluntarily suppressing functional tics may com-

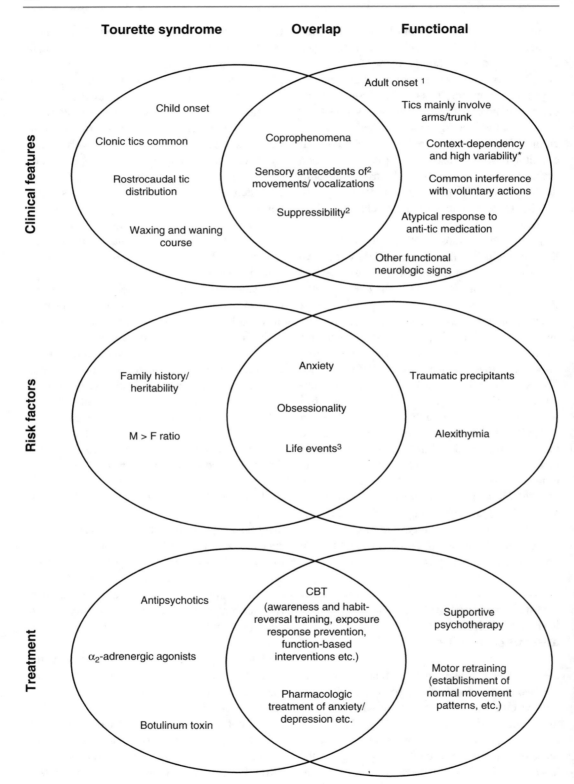

plain of experiencing pain, nausea, or a general feeling of being unwell during effortful suppression [9]. One case from our clinic reported "double-vision" and light-headedness "as if about to faint", which is not typically seen during classic voluntary inhibition of primary tics. Moreover, context-sensitivity may also be useful, for example in cases where waxing and waning is present (e.g., completely tic-free periods over months during holiday with sudden reappearance of tic behaviors upon re-entering their flat or starting their first day at work). We also reported severe cases with exquisite response to cannabinoids (also see section below on "Treatment") [7]. Indeed, although treatment of primary tics with cannabinoids may be helpful [11], complete disappearance of tics of otherwise severe cases should prompt the consideration of a functional tic disorder. However, it should be noted that in some cases the co-existence of both primary and functional tics should be considered. Overlap between FMD and other neurological disorders is indeed quite common, and occurs in up to 22% of patients [12]. Unfortunately, the current state of medical literature does not yet clarify how to confidently clinically distinguish between the different etiologies of overlapping tic phenomena.

Objective Measures to Aid Diagnosis – the Role of Neurophysiology

In addition to the aforementioned clinical characteristics, neurophysiological tools may also be able to aid in differentiating between functional and primary tics. Two early studies investigated the presence of the movement-related cortical potential, first described as the Bereitschaftspotential (BP), in association with motor tics in primary tic disorders. The BP describes a slow negative electroencephalographic (EEG) activity beginning about 2 seconds before movement onset associated with voluntary, self-generated actions. In the first study by Obeso and colleagues there were no BPs preceding tics in five out of the six participants with primary tics due to Tourette syndrome. In one case, only a late BP component was identified, whose morphology differed from the classic morphological characteristics of the BP preceding voluntary actions [13]. The second study by Karp and colleagues somewhat replicated these findings by again demonstrating the presence of a late BP component preceding tic movements in two of five adults with primary tics [14]. Although information on the tic characteristics of the adults in whom a BP was found was not provided (e.g., simple vs. complex tics, tics preceded by premonitory urges vs. not), it was suggested that the detected differences might reflect the level of awareness associated with tic movements. Indeed, this view was also supported by Duggal and colleagues, who described the presence of a BP in all three subjects with tics – and premonitory urges – they examined [15]. Premonitory urges facilitate awareness of tic behaviors, and may also drive the appearance of a BP in these cases.

More recently, van der Salm and colleagues evaluated for the presence of a BP in patients with functional jerky movements (n = 29), including cases which could be labelled as functional tics, and contrasted them to patients with primary tics diagnosed with Tourette syn-

Fig. 12.1 Differences and overlap in primary and functional tics. Schematic Venn diagram of clinical features, risk factors and treatment characteristics that are more prevalent as part of tics in Tourette syndrome (left nonoverlapping section), more prevalent as part of functional tics (right nonoverlapping section), and those that often overlap with features common to both. *Commonly observed in functional tic behaviors. [1]Functional tics may also begin in childhood/adolescence. [2]Qualitative characteristics may differ between primary and functional tics. [3]Life events may precipitate onset of functional tics and typically worsen both primary and functional tics. CBT = Cognitive Behavioral Therapy. (Adapted with permission from Ref. [9])

drome [16]. Functional jerky movements were preceded by a BP in 86% of patients with FMD, thereby differing from primary tics, where a BP preceded abnormal movements in only 43% of patients. Crucially, as in the earlier studies mentioned above [13–15], the morphological features of the BP preceding primary tics differed from that documented in functional movements. Although these studies support the assessment of BP as a helpful neurophysiological tool aiding diagnostic distinction, it should be noted that many factors still remain undetermined. For example, it is unclear whether the prevalence and morphology of the BP differs between different types of tic behaviors, and specifically, whether previous data are based on recordings of simple clonic rather than more complex tics. Compared to simple tics, complex tic movements typically have a longer duration and involve more muscle groups, and patients may more often be aware of their occurrence. Accordingly, it is likely that a complex tic would also be more commonly preceded by a BP. It would, therefore, be very difficult to draw firm etiological conclusions when studying complex tic behaviors with this method. Moreover, the study by van der Salm and colleagues also assessed the presence of BPs prior to self-paced wrist extensions and detected BPs in 93% of patients with Tourette syndrome and all healthy control participants. In contrast, BPs were found only in 41% of patients with FMD, further complicating the interpretation of neurophysiological findings among the different types of movements in patients with primary tics and functional jerky movements [16].

Surface electromyography (EMG) has also been proposed to aid the diagnostic distinction between primary and functional tics and indeed, in some cases with complex motor behaviors, surface EMG might support the clinical observation of great variability in muscle activation patterns [17]. However, given the wide range of motor and vocal behaviors that may present as tics, we find its current use less helpful and do not recommend its routine application to inform diagnosis.

Risk Factors

Although research in the field of functional tics is recent and these patients are historically rare, several risk factors have been suggested to drive the manifestation of abnormal behaviors. Most patients with functional tics experience an abrupt symptom onset (88%), with a clear precipitant in 86% [2, 7]. This precipitant may include physical illness (21%), psychological stressors (33%, e.g., following a conflict with friends or family as in the case presented here) and bodily trauma (29%, e.g., shoulder or back injury, motor vehicle accident) [2, 7]. It has been proposed that the experience of anxiety and panic following such events could precipitate the onset of functional tics [6, 9, 18]. Indeed, anxiety and depression are common comorbidities in patients with functional tics [2]. These comorbidities are also often seen in patients with primary tics [19]. However, in primary tics there has been no association between major psychosocial stressors and onset of the tic disorder [20]. In fact, primary tics typically begin in early childhood (around age 4–6), before anxiety and depression typically manifest in these patients.

Two additional contributing risk factors include alexithymia and obsessionality. Although the three case series mentioned above did not systematically assess the presence of these neuropsychiatric traits in patients with functional tics [2, 3, 7], there is some evidence that alexithymia (the inability to appropriately recognize and verbalize one's own emotional experiences) and obsessionality (cognitive inflexibility due to increased rumination and mental checking) may be associated with the development of functional neurological symptoms [21] such as functional tics. Indeed, a large number of patients with functional tics we see in clinic share these features. Of note, obsessive-compulsive behaviors are also commonly encountered in patients with primary tics, with typical onset several years after the first occurrence of tics [19].

It has often been noted that female sex is more commonly associated with functional neurological symptoms at a ratio of approximately 2–3:1 [22]. However, several case series [2, 3, 7,

23], have failed to demonstrate a clear association between female sex and presence of functional tics. Family history may be present in both primary tic disorders [23] as well as FMD [24] and, therefore, it should not be used to preclude the diagnosis of a functional tic disorder (see Fig. 12.1).

During the COVID-19 pandemic, a significant increase in the proportion of patients with functional tic-like behaviors was noted in specialized tic centers around the world [25]. Although the exact causes of this increase remain understudied, it has been proposed that the social isolation imposed from the COVID-19 pandemic, and a rise in the exposure to tic-like behaviors on social media platforms such as TikTok may be contributing risk factors [25–28].

Treatment

The treatment of functional tics is based on the same therapeutic principles that apply for other FMD [29]. Specifically, as in the case we presented here, a multidisciplinary therapeutic approach is recommended. It should also be noted that the prognosis of patients with functional tics may be more favorable than that of patients with FMD who exhibit non-paroxysmal clinical presentations (e.g., fixed dystonia) [6]. Although the physiotherapy-based multidisciplinary model is a useful tool to teach patients to regain voluntary motor control over their bodies [29], we suggest that for this particular patient population, specific focus should be given on behavioral therapies.

Function-based interventions that allow patients to recognize the environmental contingencies associated with their abnormal behaviors and provide them with coping resources and awareness training methods are key therapeutic tools. Indeed, such methods are being successfully applied in patients with primary tics as therapeutic components of comprehensive packages, such as the comprehensive behavioral intervention for tics (CBIT). In CBIT, patients with primary tics learn to become better aware of bodily

signals preceding tics and develop competing strategies to counter unwanted tic behaviors [30]. Psychoeducation and relaxation training are additional important components [31], which may have an effect on the impact of common comorbidities, including anxiety and increased levels of arousal [32].

Another behavioral therapy used in primary tic disorders is exposure and response prevention (ERP). Tics are viewed as conditioned responses to negatively reinforcing unwanted bodily stimuli, and a dissociation between the two phenomena is the main goal of this treatment [31]. In essence, with therapeutic guidance, patients with tics learn to increase their tolerance towards aversive bodily experiences ("exposure"), whilst preventing the conditioned motor response ("response prevention") [33]. Although patients with functional tics typically do not report premonitory urges, we feel that components of ERP could be helpful, particularly in cases where overwhelming physical experiences related to anxiety and panic might occur.

As with other FMD subtypes, there is no evidence to support pharmacotherapy specifically targeting functional tics, and previous reports document either absent or atypical responses to classic anti-tic medication (e.g., antipsychotics or α_2-receptor-agonists) [2, 3, 7]. Surprisingly, medical cannabis led to dramatic symptom relief in some patients with functional tics [34], although the mechanisms underlying this effect remain unclear and might include placebo responses. Pharmacotherapies aimed at comorbid neuropsychiatric symptoms, such as anxiety and depression, may be required. Of note, some patients may present with both primary and functional tics [9, 35] and in these cases, pharmacotherapy may improve certain behaviors, but not others, which may be deemed as treatment-refractory. In the absence of a well-defined concept of treatment-refractoriness in tic disorders [36] and clear markers to distinguish between primary and functional tics, it is important to consider the possibility of comorbid functional tics prior to referral for invasive surgical procedures, such as deep brain stimulation.

Summary

- Thorough observation, history taking and clinical context are necessary for the diagnosis of functional tics.
- Sudden onset in adulthood, significant variability of symptoms, context-dependency, presence of additional FMD symptoms, and interference of involuntary motor and vocal behaviors with voluntary actions might point to the diagnosis of functional tics.
- Patients with primary tics may also develop functional tics.
- The recognition of functional tics is crucial to guide therapeutic decisions and avoid potentially harmful, invasive procedures in cases that have been deemed "treatment-refractory".
- The treatment of functional tics involves a multidisciplinary approach, including behavioral therapy, tailored to the individual needs of each patient.

References

1. Ganos C, Münchau A, Bhatia KP. The semiology of tics, Tourette's, and their associations. Mov Disord Clin Pract. 2014;1(3):145–53.
2. Demartini B, Ricciardi L, Parees I, Ganos C, Bhatia KP, Edwards MJ. A positive diagnosis of functional (psychogenic) tics. Eur J Neurol. 2015;22(3):527–e36.
3. Baizabal-Carvallo JF, Jankovic J. The clinical features of psychogenic movement disorders resembling tics. J Neurol Neurosurg Psychiatry. 2014;85(5):573–5.
4. Jankovic J, Gelineau-Kattner R, Davidson A. Tourette's syndrome in adults. Mov Disord. 2010;25(13):2171–5.
5. Ganos C, Bongert J, Asmuss L, Martino D, Haggard P, Münchau A. The somatotopy of tic inhibition: where and how much? Mov Disord. 2015;30(9):1184–9.
6. Ganos C, Aguirregomozcorta M, Batla A, Stamelou M, Schwingenschuh P, Münchau A, et al. Psychogenic paroxysmal movement disorders – clinical features and diagnostic clues. Parkinsonism Relat Disord. 2014;20(1):41–6.
7. Ganos C, Edwards MJ, Müller-Vahl K. "I swear it is Tourette's!": on functional coprolalia and other tic-like vocalizations. Psychiatry Res. 2016;30(246):821–6.
8. Leckman JF, Walker DE, Cohen DJ. Premonitory urges in Tourette's syndrome. Am J Psychiatry. 1993;150(1):98–102.
9. Ganos C, Martino D, Espay AJ, Lang AE, Bhatia KP, Edwards MJ. Tics and functional tic-like movements: can we tell them apart? Neurology. 2019;93(17):750–8.
10. Van Hulle CA, Schmidt NL, Goldsmith HH. Is sensory over-responsivity distinguishable from childhood behavior problems? A phenotypic and genetic analysis. J Child Psychol Psychiatry. 2012;53(1):64–72.
11. Artukoglu BB, Bloch MH. The potential of cannabinoid-based treatments in Tourette syndrome. CNS Drugs. 2019;33(5):417–30.
12. Tinazzi M, Geroin C, Erro R, Marcuzzo E, Cuoco S, Ceravolo R, et al. Functional motor disorders associated with other neurological diseases: beyond the boundaries of "organic" neurology. Eur J Neurol. 2021;28(5):1752–8.
13. Obeso JA, Rothwell JC, Marsden CD. Simple tics in Gilles de la Tourette's syndrome are not prefaced by a normal premovement EEG potential. J Neurol Neurosurg Psychiatry. 1981;44(8):735–8.
14. Karp BI, Porter S, Toro C, Hallett M. Simple motor tics may be preceded by a premotor potential. J Neurol Neurosurg Psychiatry. 1996;61(1):103–6.
15. Duggal HS, Nizamie SH. Bereitschaftspotential in tic disorders: a preliminary observation. Neurol India. 2002;50(4):487–9.
16. van der Salm SMA, Tijssen MAJ, Koelman JHTM, van Rootselaar A-F. The bereitschaftspotential in jerky movement disorders. J Neurol Neurosurg Psychiatry. 2012;83(12):1162–7.
17. Vial F, Attaripour S, Hallett M. Differentiating tics from functional (psychogenic) movements with electrophysiological tools. Clin Neurophysiol Pract. 2019;4:143–7.
18. Stone J, Carson A, Aditya H, Prescott R, Zaubi M, Warlow C, et al. The role of physical injury in motor and sensory conversion symptoms: a systematic and narrative review. J Psychosom Res. 2009;66(5):383–90.
19. Hirschtritt ME, Lee PC, Pauls DL, Dion Y, Grados MA, Illmann C, et al. Lifetime prevalence, age of risk, and genetic relationships of comorbid psychiatric disorders in Tourette syndrome. JAMA Psychiat. 2015;72(4):325–33.
20. Steinberg T, Shmuel-Baruch S, Horesh N, Apter A. Life events and Tourette syndrome. Compr Psychiatry. 2013;54(5):467–73.
21. Demartini B, Petrochilos P, Ricciardi L, Price G, Edwards MJ, Joyce E. The role of alexithymia in the development of functional motor symptoms (conversion disorder). J Neurol Neurosurg Psychiatry. 2014;85(10):1132–7.
22. Espay AJ, Aybek S, Carson A, Edwards MJ, Goldstein LH, Hallett M, et al. Current concepts in diagnosis and treatment of functional neurological disorders. JAMA Neurol. 2018;75(9):1132.

23. Nee LE, Caine ED, Polinsky RJ, Eldridge R, Ebert MH. Gilles de la Tourette syndrome: clinical and family study of 50 cases. Ann Neurol. 1980;7(1):41–9.

24. Charcot J-M. Lectures on the diseases of the nervous system delivered at La Salpetriere. London: New Sydenham Society; 1877.

25. Pringsheim T, Ganos C, McGuire JF, Hedderly T, Woods D, Gilbert DL, et al. Rapid Onset Functional Tic-Like Behaviors in Young Females During the COVID-19 Pandemic. Movement Disorders. 2021;36(12):2707–13.

26. Ganos C. Tics and Tic-like Phenomena - Old Questions on a Grand New Scale. Movement Disorders Clinical Practice. 2021;8(8):1198–99.

27. Olvera C, Stebbins GT, Goetz CG, Kompoliti K. TikTok Tics: A Pandemic Within a Pandemic. Movement Disorders Clinical Practice. 2021;8(8):1200–05.

28. Hull M, Parnes M. Tics and TikTok: Functional Tics Spread Through Social Media. Movement Disorders Clinical Practice. 2021;8(8):1248–52.

29. Nielsen G, Stone J, Matthews A, Brown M, Sparkes C, Farmer R, et al. Physiotherapy for functional motor disorders: a consensus recommendation. J Neurol Neurosurg Psychiatry. 2015;86(10):1113–9.

30. Piacentini J, Woods DW, Scahill L, Wilhelm S, Peterson AL, Chang S, et al. Behavior therapy for children with Tourette disorder: a randomized controlled trial. JAMA. 2010;303(19):1929–37.

31. Fründt O, Woods D, Ganos C. Behavioral therapy for Tourette syndrome and chronic tic disorders. Neurol Clin Pract. 2017;7(2):148–56.

32. Sukhodolsky DG, Woods DW, Piacentini J, Wilhelm S, Peterson AL, Katsovich L, et al. Moderators and predictors of response to behavior therapy for tics in Tourette syndrome. Neurology. 2017;88(11):1029–36.

33. Verdellen CWJ, Hoogduin CAL, Kato BS, Keijsers GPJ, Cath DC, Hoijtink HB. Habituation of premonitory sensations during exposure and response prevention treatment in Tourette's syndrome. Behav Modif. 2008;32(2):215–27.

34. Ganos C, Müller-Vahl K. Cannabinoids in functional tic-like movements. Parkinsonism Relat Disord. 2019;60:179–81.

35. Kurlan R, Deeley C, Como PG. Psychogenic movement disorder (pseudo-tics) in a patient with Tourette's syndrome. J Neuropsychiatry Clin Neurosci. 1992;4(3):347–8.

36. Kious BM, Jimenez-Shahed J, Shprecher DR. Treatment-refractory Tourette syndrome. Prog Neuro-Psychopharmacol Biol Psychiatry. 2016;03(70):227–36.

Functional Speech and Voice Disorders

13

Carine W. Maurer and Joseph R. Duffy

Clinical Vignette

A 56-year-old female presented to a neurology clinic with a 2-year history of speech and voice difficulties, widespread body pain, gait abnormalities, vision trouble, and abnormal jaw and lip posturing. Previous workups had considered the diagnoses of multiple sclerosis and systemic lupus erythematosus; magnetic resonance imaging (MRI) of the brain, electromyography (EMG) electroencephalography (EEG), and cerebrospinal fluid (CSF) studies had all been unrevealing.

The patient was referred by her neurologist for formal speech and language evaluation. During the patient's speech consultation she reported a 2-year history of initially intermittent but now constant stuttering, voice difficulty, occasional use of incorrect words or word order, and pulling of the left side of her mouth during

Supplementary Information The online version contains supplementary material available at [https://doi.org/10.1007/978-3-030-86495-8_13].

C. W. Maurer
Department of Neurology, Renaissance School of Medicine at Stony Brook University,
Stony Brook, NY, USA

J. R. Duffy (✉)
Department of Neurology, Mayo Clinic,
Rochester, MN, USA
e-mail: jduffy@mayo.edu

speech. All of her symptoms had worsened to a point where she and her husband had to close a small restaurant in which she cooked and managed the finances.

Her speech during examination was characterized by numerous abnormalities in articulation and prosody. She exhibited frequent sound prolongations, sound and syllable repetitions, and variably abnormal vocal pitch and prosody. She occasionally spoke on inhalation and her speaking rate varied unpredictably from slow-and-drawn-out to rapid. Most of her statements were produced with effort and exaggerated face and neck movements. Occasionally during casual conversation not obviously related to the formal examination, she made brief statements without obvious effort or any appreciable abnormality. Speech alternating motion rates (i.e., rapid repetitive production of syllables such as "puh", "tuh", or "kuh", analogous to rapid alternating movement tasks such as finger tapping task used by neurologists to judge speed, amplitude and regularity of movement excursions) were bizarrely irregular.

She was told that her speech difficulty was consistent with a functional speech disorder and not consistent with speech patterns that reflect structural damage to speech areas of the nervous system. After discussing the nature of a functional speech disorder she was reassured that many people with such problems who are motivated to modify their speech frequently improve rapidly. She was receptive to the diagnosis and expressed motivation to work on her speech difficulties.

During 20–30 min of speech therapy, initially emphasizing a slow, drawn-out pattern of speaking without extraneous movements, all aspects of her speech improved, to a degree that she and the clinician judged to be about 80% normal. She maintained the improvement after her husband joined her. The diagnosis was again reviewed in the presence of her husband, and she was praised for her hard work and success. The clinician conveyed optimism about her potential for normal speech. She was encouraged to talk as much as she wished over the next day and that, if she sensed any regression, she should immediately reset her speech by using one of the strategies that were used during therapy.

She returned the next day for scheduled follow-up, noting that her speech was now 95% normal. Her husband concurred; her daughter and father had remarked on her dramatic progress during a phone call. She had one brief episode of regression but was able to reset her speech as previously recommended. Her speech during the session was near normal and seemingly effortless; she concurred. During discussion of possible causes of her speech symptoms, it was acknowledged that a precise cause might never be known but that it had clearly responded to treatment.

There was no need for ongoing speech therapy though she was encouraged to schedule a follow-up appointment with her neurologist to have a point of contact. She expressed optimism about the future regarding all of her symptoms. As requested, she contacted the clinician by phone 2 weeks later, speaking normally and reporting that her speech had remained normal and that other symptoms were improving with physical therapy.

Introduction

Changes in speech can often be the initial symptom of neurological disease. Being able to appropriately identify the pattern of a patient's speech impairment is critical in guiding management

and treatment. Functional speech and voice disorders, a subtype of functional movement disorder (FMD), are common among patients with FMD and can be challenging to diagnose. This chapter focuses upon the general approach to the diagnosis of functional speech/voice disorders, as well as the characteristics of specific functional speech/voice disorders. While some outcomes of therapy are referred to in this chapter, a more thorough discussion of speech therapy for patients with functional speech/voice disorders can be found in Chap. 25.

Functional speech/voice disorders can be quite heterogeneous, and can affect multiple aspects of speech and voice production. While some healthcare professionals make a distinction between functional speech disorders and functional voice disorders (functional dysphonias), there is significant overlap, and many patients present with abnormalities in both speech and voice. FMD affecting either speech or voice are included under the umbrella term of functional speech/voice disorders in this chapter.

Epidemiology of Functional Speech and Voice Disorders

Although the incidence and prevalence of functional speech/voice disorders have yet to be formally established, numerous studies suggest that they are common diagnoses in neurology and speech-language pathology clinical practices. Within subspecialty movement disorders practices, approximately one-quarter to one-half of patients with FMD have functional speech abnormalities as one of their symptoms [1–3]. In the Mayo Clinic speech pathology practice, a division within Mayo Clinic's Department of Neurology, 4.9% of patients with acquired speech disorders seen during an 8-year period were given the diagnosis of a functional speech disorder [4]. This number does not include patients with isolated functional dysphonias, and may therefore represent an underestimate of the incidence of functional speech/voice disorders in that setting.

Functional speech/voice disorders can be seen comorbid with other functional neurological symptoms, as well as with other neurological conditions such as multiple sclerosis. In a cohort of 92 patients with functional speech/voice disorders seen in the Mayo Clinic speech pathology practice, at least 48% were noted to have additional functional neurological symptoms, including functional seizures (also known as psychogenic non-epileptic or dissociative seizures), other FMD presentations and/or functional sensory symptoms. 14% of patients in the cohort were noted to have other neurological conditions, including four patients with stroke and two patients with multiple sclerosis [4]. The possibility of comorbid disease, whether functional or otherwise, emphasizes the importance of performing a thorough, careful assessment in all patients.

The distribution of specific types of functional speech/voice disorders is not well established, although some clues may be gleaned from the distribution of functional speech/voice disorders within speech-language pathology practices. At the Mayo Clinic, isolated voice disorders have represented the largest category of functional speech/voice disorders when patients seen by speech-language pathologists in neurology and ENT practices are combined. Stuttering-like dysfluencies represented the second most common single category of functional speech/voice disorders. It is important to note that mixed abnormalities, in which two or more speech abnormalities occur in combination, are quite common, and in some cohorts represent the most common presentation of functional speech/voice disorders [3, 4].

Approach to Diagnosis

Differentiating between functional speech/voice disorders and neurogenic motor speech disorders can often be quite challenging, and relies upon clinical experience with a variety of both motor speech disorders and functional speech/voice disorders. As with diagnosis of other FMD subtypes, a careful approach to history and physical examination is required in order to avoid diagnostic errors.

Approach to Diagnosis: Clues from the History

Patients with functional speech/voice disorders frequently describe a history of sudden, intense onset of symptoms. They may report having a cold or similar non-neurologic illness prior to, during, or after symptom onset. Precipitants including physically or psychologically traumatic events may also be endorsed. Patients may report injury or surgery to the head, face, or neck, or complain of pain in the neck, throat or chest. However, while physical or psychosocial stressors may potentially precipitate the patient's speech disorder, it is important not to overly rely on "life stress" in the diagnostic process. Evidence of significant life stress does not establish a functional diagnosis for a given patient's speech deficit, just as its absence does not establish another neurological condition. It is important to maintain diagnostic vigilance when evaluating these patients in order to reach an accurate diagnosis.

In addition to a history of sudden onset and precipitating factors, patients with functional speech/voice disorders may report an episodic quality of their symptoms, with periods of spontaneous remission. Given that both neurogenic motor speech disorders and functional speech/voice disorders can present episodically, it is important to probe for factors that can worsen (trigger) or improve symptoms. Symptoms that fluctuate based upon setting, specific listeners, or environmental stimuli (i.e., particular auditory or olfactory stimuli) should raise suspicions for a functional speech/voice disorder.

Approach to Diagnosis: Positive Signs on Physical Examination

Examination of the Jaw, Face and Tongue

The examination of the oral mechanism, which includes the jaw, tongue and face, should address the following questions (also summarized in Table 13.1).

Table 13.1 Examination signs supporting a diagnosis of functional speech/voice disorder

Speech pattern or non-speech oral mechanism findings do not fit with known patterns associated with neurogenic motor speech disorders or known structural lesion locus

Give-way jaw, face, or tongue weakness

Wrong-way tongue deviation

Paradoxical increased muscle contraction with fatigue

Excessive symptom variability during speech examination

Suggestibility – including symptom amplification during explicit examiner attention to symptoms, or upon suggestion that a task may be difficult

Distractibility – improvement or normalization of voice/speech during informal casual conversation

Indifference or denial of symptoms

Modifiability – rapid resolution or dramatic improvement with behavioral therapy

[a]Recognize that, with the exception of rapid symptom modifiability with therapy, most of these distinctions, especially if considered individually, are not foolproof. A single red flag for a functional speech/voice disorder should be interpreted with caution [3–6]

Is there a predictable relationship between the oral mechanism and the speech abnormality? In motor speech disorders, findings on examination of speech and oral mechanism tend to have a predictable relationship, with the presence of facial asymmetry, lingual atrophy, pathological oral reflexes, or involuntary movements being congruent with other known speech abnormalities. In contrast, in functional speech/voice disorders the abnormalities on examination of the oral mechanism can be grossly disproportionate to the severity of the speech deficit. Patients with functional speech/voice disorders may also exhibit wrong-way tongue deviation on tongue protrusion [7], or give-way weakness of the jaw or tongue.

Is there presence of exaggerated facial posturing? Patients with functional speech/voice disorders may exhibit "struggle behavior" manifesting as marked facial grimacing, lip pursing, eye blinking, or contraction of the periorbital muscles, lower facial muscles, or platysma. Patients may present with an isolated downward retraction of the lower lip, superficially simulat-

ing a central facial weakness. This "paradoxical focal dystonia" is typically present at rest, and may improve or disappear completely with activity, including speech; this pattern of expression at rest and improvement with activity is contrary to the typical action-induced expression of other focal dystonias [8]. Alternatively, patients complaining of weakness may paradoxically present with exaggerated facial posturing that is inconsistent with their complaint of weakness.

Examination of Speech

The examination of speech should address several critical questions, highlighted below as well as in Table 13.1.

Is the pattern of speech abnormality consistent? Motor speech disorders tend to present consistently across speech tasks and speech content. The speech of patients with functional speech/voice disorders, on the other hand, may fluctuate considerably, with variable severity across different examination activities (i.e., casual conversation vs. reading vs. repetition vs. conversation on a sensitive topic). There may be slowness or irregularities present during formal assessment of speech that are no longer noticeable during casual conversation. This worsening of symptoms with attention is consistent with the critical role that abnormally directed attention is thought to play in the underlying pathophysiology of FMD.

Is the speech abnormality suggestible? Worsening of symptoms when the examiner suggests that an otherwise simple task will be difficult would be consistent with the diagnosis of a functional speech/voice disorder.

Is the speech abnormality distractible? Patients with functional speech/voice disorders can often be observed to exhibit improvement in symptoms during casual conversation, as compared to formal speech assessment. This would not be consistent with motor speech disorders such as dysarthria or apraxia of speech and would be suggestive of a functional speech/voice disorder.

How does speech fatigue? With the exception of myasthenia gravis, motor speech disorders typically do not exhibit significant fatigue over the course of a speech assessment. In the case of myasthenia gravis, speech fatigues in a predictable way reflecting increasing weakness, with hypernasality, increasing voice breathiness, and increasingly imprecise articulation potentially observed. Individuals with functional speech/voice disorders, on the other hand, may exhibit a paradoxical fatigability, in which there is an increase rather than a decrease in muscle activity associated with prolonged speech assessment. For example, patients may exhibit increasingly strained voice quality or an increase of abnormal oromotor movements during speech.

Is the speech abnormality reversible? Rapid modifiability of speech abnormalities, such that there is near-normalization of speech within the diagnostic session or one or two therapy sessions, as illustrated in the chapter's clinical vignette and several of the audio clips that accompany this chapter, is highly suggestive of functional speech/voice disorders (Audio clips 13.1, 13.2, 13.3, 13.4, 13.5, 13.6, and 13.7). At the Mayo Clinic, 50% of treated patients improve to normal or near-normal within one to two treatment sessions. It is important to note, however, that while symptoms have the potential to be rapidly reversible, the absence of a treatment response should not rule out the diagnosis of a functional speech/voice disorder. A considerable fraction of patients with functional speech/voice disorders do not respond well to treatment for reasons that remain incompletely understood.

What company does the speech abnormality keep? Functional speech/voice disorders can be accompanied by abnormalities in language as well, such as "broken English" grammar (e.g., "Me go library") in the absence of symptoms of a neurological cause of aphasia.

Characteristics of Specific Functional Speech/Voice Disorders & Approach to Their Diagnosis

Functional speech/voice disorders encompass a wide variety of heterogeneous clinical features and underlying movement dynamics that can be divided into sometimes distinctive but quite frequently co-occurring subtypes [3–5, 9]. In some cases, their individual features can be difficult to distinguish from those associated with motor speech disorders such as dysarthrias and apraxia of speech. The following sections address the primary clinical features of each functional speech/voice disorder subtype and clues to their distinction from motor speech disorders. The key points are summarized in Table 13.2.

Acquired Functional Stuttering

Functional stuttering is probably the most common functional speech/voice disorder that does not primarily involve voice. It raises concerns about neurogenic etiology and co-occurs with confirmed CNS disease such as Parkinson's disease and stroke more often than isolated functional voice disorders [4].

Clinical characteristics Dysfluencies are heterogeneous across patients but generally include sound, syllable, word, or short phrase repetitions, sound prolongations, and silent or audible blocking that abruptly interrupt speech. They are often associated with secondary "struggle behaviors" such as facial grimacing or sustained or clonic neck, torso, or limb movements. Unlike adults with persistent developmental stuttering, acquired functional stuttering often does not improve with choral reading or singing.

Distinction from acquired neurogenic stuttering Functional and acquired neurogenic stuttering can be difficult to distinguish on the basis of dysfluencies alone, but the company kept by them can be very helpful. Acquired neurogenic stuttering is very often accompanied by aphasia

Table 13.2 Clinical characteristics distinguishing specific functional speech and voice disorders from non-functional speech/voice conditions

Primary abnormality	Clinical features	Distinction from other neurological motor speech disorders
Functional stuttering	Sound, syllable, word repetitions, prolongations, or blocks Tends not to improve with singing or choral reading	No evidence of aphasia, dysarthria, or apraxia of speech No clear temporal link to possible neurological causes (e.g., TBI) Speech-associated struggle behavior Excessively stereotypic or variable dysfluencies Pseudo-agrammatism
Functional articulation	Single or multiple speech sound distortions or substitutions, sometimes mimicking developmental articulation errors May be accompanied by visibly abnormal jaw, face and tongue movements	No demonstrable weakness to explain articulatory errors Errors may be more complex or require more force or control than target sounds Slow or irregular speech alternating motion rates in absence of such abnormalities in conversation Abnormal speech errors or structure movements may be inconsistent, excessively predictable, or amplified by examiner attention No sensory tricks
Functional resonance	Hypernasality	Absence of dysphagia and voice abnormalities Prolonged persistence following uncomplicated oral, palatal, or sinus surgeries Inconsistent presence No palatal asymmetry or reduced movement during "ah" or gag
Functional prosody (including foreign accent syndrome)	May generate perception of an accent or infantile speech Difficult-to-characterize fluctuations in rate, pitch, loudness and duration	Pseudo-agrammatism Indifference or unawareness of prosodic abnormality Ability to imitate another accent Incongruent abnormal speech alternating motion rates Functional weakness of jaw, face, or tongue
Functional mutism	No attempt to speak May mouth words without voice or whispering Silent struggle to speak occasionally evident	Absence of aphasia, dysarthria, apraxia of speech Absence of dysphagia Normal oral mechanism or incongruent oromotor abnormalities Willingness and normal ability to write/type Minimal distress over muteness
Functional voice Muscle tension dysphonia	Hoarseness/harshness Abnormal pitch Pitch/voice breaks Intervals of strained whisper Normal structural laryngeal examination	Narrow thyrohyoid space + discomfort with digital pressure Severity similar during singing, speech with voiced and voiceless consonants, and vowel prolongation Uncommon regular voice breaks Improved voice after periods of reduced voice use
Functional aphonia or dysphonia	Tight, strained whisper Occasional traces of normal or high-pitched voice Normal structural laryngeal examination Other features similar to muscle tension dysphonia	Strained, aphonic whisper + sharp cough Paradoxical emergence of strained voice with fatigue Previous periods of unexplained voice loss Iatrogenic and inertial influences

TBI traumatic brain injury

or motor speech disorders (most commonly, hypokinetic dysarthria), or a recent history of those difficulties. Functional stuttering may or may not be tightly temporally linked to a sus-pected structural cause as, for example, when it emerges months following a traumatic brain injury (TBI). In contrast to acquired neurogenic stuttering, functional stuttering is often accompanied by struggle behaviors. It may decrease with distraction (e.g., casual social conversation versus focused, formal speech assessment) and can be excessively stereotypic and severe (e.g., multiple repetitions of every syllable), highly variable from utterance to utterance, specific to a specific environment or task, or spell-like. Sentence structure can be pseudo-agrammatic or "broken English" in character ("Me ha ha ha have trouble talk"). Similar to functional voice disorders, it frequently responds rapidly to behavioral treatment.

Articulation Abnormalities

Isolated functional articulation abnormalities sometimes emerge in the aftermath of dental, oral or maxillofacial surgeries; anterior approach cervical spine procedures; carotid endarterectomy; or head/neck trauma. They often co-occur with other functional speech features, such as dysphonia, stuttering, or prosodic abnormalities.

Clinical characteristics The articulatory abnormalities are typically characterized by distortions or substitutions of single or multiple phonemes. They can resemble developmental articulation errors, such as distortions of "r", "l", and "s" or substitutions for them (e.g., w/r; w/l; th/s). They occasionally are accompanied by dyskinetic or dystonic-like tongue, jaw, or perioral posturing during speech.

Distinction from dysarthrias Isolated functional articulation abnormalities can raise concerns about underlying weakness (flaccid dysarthria) or an involuntary movement disorder (hyperkinetic dysarthria). When functional, there may be no demonstrable weakness in the jaw, face, or tongue to explain the articulatory errors and any apparent weakness may be give-way or wrong-way in character. Or, when weakness is present it may not explain specific articulation errors; for example, when there is no demonstrable weakness of the tongue, functional weakness of the lower face may be associated with articulation errors on sounds requiring tongue, but not facial, movements. Speech alternating motion

rates may be slow or irregular in the absence of slowness or irregularity during conversational speech. Occasionally, articulation is overly precise, emphatic or forceful, the opposite of what would be expected if explanatory weakness is present.

In contrast to hyperkinetic dysarthria associated with involuntary movements, abnormal jaw, face or tongue movements of functional neurological origin during speech may be distractible, inconsistent, excessively predictable, or amplified by obvious examiner attention to them. People with articulation problems secondary to dystonia may have discovered a beneficial sensory trick on their own, such as chewing gum to inhibit lingual dystonia; this is uncommon in patients with functional dystonic-like movements that affect speech. Again, functional articulation disturbances are often rapidly responsive to symptomatic speech therapy, whereas flaccid and hyperkinetic dysarthria are not.

Resonance Abnormalities

Disturbed resonance is an uncommon feature of functional speech/voice disorders. When resonance abnormalities are present, they can raise concerns about flaccid dysarthria secondary to involvement of the pharyngeal branch of the vagus nerve. If intermittent or associated with fatigue, it may justifiably trigger a workup for myasthenia gravis.

Clinical characteristics Hypernasality is the most common feature of functional resonance abnormalities. It can be constantly present or blossom with continuous speaking or fatigue. It sometimes emerges following oral or sinus surgeries, uvulectomy for sleep apnea, or other orofacial trauma. Such associations may reflect somatic compliance, which is the tendency for functional neurological problems to develop in a body structure affected by medical disease (e.g., functional hypernasality that emerges following sinus surgery, or functional seizures that emerge in the presence of confirmed epilepsy).

Distinction from dysarthria Hypernasality due to neurologic weakness is often associated with voice abnormalities and dysphagia, including nasal regurgitation, whereas functional hypernasality is not. Persistent hypernasality following otherwise uncomplicated oral, palatal, or sinus surgeries rarely occurs as a result of intrinsic surgical complications. When functional, hypernasality may vary from moment-to-moment, or be distractible. The gag reflex and palatal movement during vowel prolongation may be normal, whereas with lesion associated disturbances weakness of palatal movement may be reduced or asymmetric.

Prosodic Disturbances

Prosody (variations in pitch, loudness and duration that convey emotional and linguistic emphasis and meaning) can be disturbed in highly variable ways, independent of, or along with, functional disturbances of voice, fluency and articulation. They can be challenging diagnostically because nearly all major motor speech disorders are associated with a variety of prosodic abnormalities.

Clinical characteristics Prosodic abnormalities are sometimes perceived as an accent, sometimes as infantile or child-like, or sometimes as speech that is very rapid or very slow in rate. There also may be highly variable fluctuations in pitch, loudness or rate that cannot otherwise be easily characterized. When perceived as a foreign or regional accent, it can be very difficult to distinguish a functional neurological etiology from the foreign accent syndrome that can occur with neurologic disease, most often due to stroke or TBI [4, 10]. It is important to recognize, however, that functional prosodic disturbances can also occur in the aftermath of stroke or TBI [11]. The specific language or regional dialect associated with the foreign accent is highly variable across patients regardless of underlying etiology, and often cannot be reliably identified as tied to a specific language or dialect.

Distinctions from neurologic prosodic deficits Functional prosodic deficits can be distractible whereas prosodic abnormalities associated with other motor speech disorders or lesion-based foreign accent syndrome are not. Functional prosodic disturbances, particularly foreign accent, can also be accompanied by abnormal grammar (e.g. "Me have trouble talk") which can be distractible, inconsistent, and unaccompanied by other "neighborhood signs" suggesting another neurological cause of aphasia. Some individuals with functional foreign accent may additionally develop behavioral features stereotypically associated with their accent, including gestures and interpersonal behavior [11]. Some people with functional foreign accent or infantile prosody may be indifferent to or even deny the abnormality. Sometimes they can easily imitate another accent on request or adopt a different foreign accent over time, which should be difficult for those with any lesion-associated neurologic prosodic disturbance. Functional weakness can be evident when the jaw, face or tongue are examined, representing an incongruity when the prosodic disturbance is unaccompanied by other voice or speech deficits. The rhythm and amplitude of speech alternating motion rates may be incongruently irregular in people with an isolated functional foreign accent.

Functional Mutism

Mutism can be functional or neurogenic. The mere absence of speech does not distinguish its cause so the clinical milieu must be relied upon.

Clinical features People with functional muteness often make no attempt to speak. Sometimes they mouth words without voice or whisper. Silent struggle to speak may be evident in some cases.

Distinction from other neurological causes of mutism Neurogenic mutism is often associated with clear evidence of one or more of the following: severe aphasia; severe motor speech impairment (i.e., anarthria with dysphagia or severe apraxia of speech); severe motor impairments elsewhere in the body; disorders of responsiveness (e.g., akinetic mutism) or global cognition. The absence of any such impairments should raise concerns about a possible functional neurological cause. Patients with functional mutism may silently-but-accurately mouth words or write willingly and normally to communicate. Some may show no affective distress over their inability to speak, often coupled with family members/caregivers being significantly more distressed about the inability to speak than the patient themselves. Oral mechanism examination is typically normal at rest and without structural abnormalities, but struggle, wrong way tongue deviation, and other oral movement incongruities may be evident. As is the case for functional speech/voice disorders in general, functional mutism sometimes responds rapidly to behavioral speech intervention.

Functional Voice Disorders

Voice abnormalities likely represent the most frequent functional speech/voice disorder. When voice is the only abnormality, affected people more often present to otorhinolaryngologists (ENT) rather than neurologists, and it is usually essential that ENT examination first rules out possible explanatory structural laryngeal pathology such as vocal fold nodules, cancerous growths, or vocal fold paralysis. Referral to neurology following ENT consultation is not uncommon if laryngeal structural abnormalities are not identified or if voice features raise concerns about another neurologic etiology. Direct presentation to neurology occurs more frequently when voice abnormalities are accompanied by other abnormal speech features (e.g. stuttering, abnormal articulation, prosodic abnormalities). Functional voice disorders can be somewhat arbitrarily, and not without some debate, subdivided into muscle tension dysphonia and functional aphonia/dysphonia. The voice characteristics and clues to distinguishing each of them from neurogenic voice

abnormalities are addressed in the following subsections.[1]

Muscle Tension Dysphonia

Muscle tension dysphonia often represents effects of prolonged excessive contraction of laryngeal muscles during speech, often in people for whom speaking is a primary occupational tool (e.g., teachers) or who have ongoing psychological stress, predisposing personality traits, or physiological susceptibility. In some cases, persistent laryngeal muscle tension leads to the development of vocal fold nodules, polyps, or contact ulcers; when this is the case, they do not generally raise concerns about neurologic etiology because even severe strained voice associated with laryngeal spasticity or dystonia do not generally lead to structural laryngeal lesions. Challenges to differential diagnosis exist for patients without structural laryngeal abnormalities, particularly if voice difficulty is the sole presenting symptom, or if additional symptoms suggestive of neurologic disease, such as weakness or abnormal movements elsewhere in the body, are present; they are the focus here.

Clinical characteristics Laryngeal muscle hypercontraction can lead to hoarseness or harshness, and alterations in pitch, sometimes with pitch or voice breaks, as well as intervals of strained whisper. The overall perceptual gestalt is one of strain or effort rather than weakness.

Distinction from neurogenic voice disorders Muscle tension dysphonia can be difficult to distinguish from neurogenic spasmodic dysphonia, which most often reflects a speech-induced laryngeal dystonia or dystonic tremor. Voice breaks, particularly if they occur at relatively regular intervals, are more common in spasmodic dysphonia than muscle tension dys-

---

[1] See Baker [9] for a more detailed discussion of the distinctions between muscle tension dysphonias associated with laryngeal structural lesions and those that are not, and the distinctions between muscle tension dysphonia and functional aphonia/dysphonia.

phonia. Spasmodic dysphonia tends to be more conspicuous during connected speech than during vowel prolongation, whereas in muscle tension dysphonia the two tasks are relatively equivalent. In the adductor form of spasmodic dysphonia voice strain is more evident during production of words with voiced consonants (e.g., "b" or "d") than voiceless consonants (e.g., "p" or "t"), whereas little difference is evident in muscle tension dysphonia. Individuals with spasmodic dysphonia may have evidence of dystonia or tremor elsewhere in the body. Singing is sometimes relatively normal in spasmodic dysphonia but usually not in muscle tension dysphonia. In muscle tension dysphonia there is often narrowing of the thyrohyoid space and pain and discomfort in response to digital palpation in that area. Affected people may note voice improvement during extended intervals when voice demands are not heavy (e.g., summer break for teachers); voice usually does not markedly improve in those with spasmodic dysphonia. In muscle tension dysphonia, the history often provides clear evidence of heavy speaking demands or considerable psychological stress; this is generally less apparent in spasmodic dysphonia although the onset of symptoms at a time of heightened psychological stress is not uncommon.

Functional Aphonia and Dysphonia

Some individuals may be aphonic (i.e., without voice) or dysphonic without clear evidence of musculoskeletal tension or structural laryngeal pathology. Such presentations often raise concerns about underlying vocal fold or laryngeal weakness and not infrequently trigger a workup for peripheral or central nervous system (CNS) causes (e.g., myasthenia gravis, multiple sclerosis, dystonia). Functional aphonia has long been recognized as a symptom of functional neurological disorder.

Clinical characteristics The aphonic voice is often a tight whisper that can be harsh or strained, sometimes with high-pitched or squeaky traces of phonation; brief intervals of normal phonation are sometimes evident. Functional dysphonia without musculoskeletal tension can be highly variable in its specific voice characteristics, sometimes very similar to muscle tension dysphonia but in other cases breathy, hoarse, high in pitch with falsetto pitch breaks, or intermittently aphonic. Structural laryngeal examination is typically normal.

Distinction from neurogenic voice disorders The strained character of the aphonic whisper in functional aphonia and the strained and high-pitched components of functional dysphonia differ from the breathy ("airy"), hoarse quality associated with frank vocal fold weakness. In addition, in functional aphonia/dysphonia, the cough is usually sharp, which demonstrates capacity for vocal fold approximation. The voice may become paradoxically strained with fatigue. Previous episodes of voice loss or difficulty occur more frequently in functional aphonia/dysphonia than vocal fold paresis or any lesion-associated CNS voice abnormality. Functional aphonia/dysphonia is sometimes iatrogenic. For example, some patients who are unnecessarily placed on voice rest for mild voice difficulty worsen or develop chronic difficulty because of fear that speaking will do harm. The problem also may be inertial, such as when aphonia following traumatic frontal lobe injury persists longer than the structural trauma can directly explain, sometimes proven by rapid return of voice during a few minutes of symptomatic voice therapy. In general, a major distinguishing feature is that functional aphonia/dysphonia often resolves rapidly with symptomatic voice therapy.

Summary

- Functional speech and voice disorders commonly co-occur in the setting of other functional movement disorder presentations.
- Clinical clues in the history of a patient with a functional speech/voice disorder include sudden onset, and symptoms that fluctuate based upon environmental stimuli, setting, or listener.
- The examination of a patient with a functional speech/voice disorder should address consistency of speech abnormality as well as distractibility and suggestibility.
- Patients with isolated functional voice disorders more commonly present to otorhinolaryngologists than neurologists, whereas other functional speech/voice disorders present more commonly to neurologists.
- Functional voice disorders, stuttering, and disturbances of prosody, including foreign accent, are the most common manifestations of functional speech/voice disorders, but mutism and abnormalities of articulation and resonance also occur.
- Incongruence between voice/speech characteristics and findings during non-speech oral mechanism examination can aid diagnosis.
- Unlike most motor (neurogenic) speech disorders, functional speech/voice disorders, regardless of their specific manifestations, have the potential for rapid reversibility.

References

1. Hinson VK, Cubo E, Comella CL, Goetz CG, Leurgans S. Rating scale for psychogenic movement disorders: scale development and clinimetric testing. Mov Disord. 2005;20(12):1592–7.
2. Baizabal-Carvallo JF, Jankovic J. Speech and voice disorders in patients with psychogenic movement disorders. J Neurol. 2015;262(11):2420–4.
3. Chung DS, Wettroth C, Hallett M, Maurer CW. Functional speech and voice disorders: case series and literature review. Mov Disord Clin Pract. 2018;5(3):312–6.
4. Duffy JR. Motor speech disorders: substrates, differential diagnosis, and management. 4th ed. St. Louis: Elsevier; 2020.
5. Duffy JR. Functional speech disorders: clinical manifestations, diagnosis, and management. Handb Clin Neurol. 2016;139:379–88.
6. Perez DL, Hunt A, Sharma N, Flaherty A, Caplan D, Schmahmann JD. Cautionary notes on diagnosing functional neurologic disorder as a neurologist-in-training. Neurol Clin Pract. 2020;10(6):484–7. https://doi.org/10.1212/CPJ.0000000000000779.
7. Keane JR. Wrong-way deviation of the tongue with hysterical hemiparesis. Neurology. 1986;36(10):1406–7.
8. Fasano A, Valadas A, Bhatia KP, Prashanth LK, Lang AE, Munhoz RP, et al. Psychogenic facial movement disorders: clinical features and associated conditions. Mov Disord. 2012;27(12):1544–51.
9. Baker J. Functional voice disorders: clinical presentations and differential diagnosis. Handb Clin Neurol. 2016;139:389–405.
10. Lee O, Ludwig L, Davenport R, Stone J. Functional foreign accent syndrome. Pract Neurol. 2016;16(5):409–11.
11. McWhirter L, Miller N, Campbell C, Hoeritzauer I, Lawton A, Carson A, et al. Understanding foreign accent syndrome. J Neurol Neurosurg Psychiatry. 2019;90(11):1265–9.

Beyond Functional Movements: The Spectrum of Functional Neurological and Somatic Symptoms

14

Caitlin Adams and David L. Perez

Case Vignette

35-year-old man, married, on leave from work as a science teacher, with a medical history notable for irritable bowel syndrome, and no formal past psychiatric history presents for a neurological consultation complaining of headache, sound and light sensitivity, arm tremors, balance difficulties, whole-body shaking events, clouded thinking and insomnia. The patient reports that symptoms began 3 months ago when he was hit in the head with a basketball while covering gym class. He did not lose consciousness but reported feeling dazed and developed a headache. He excused himself from work, was evaluated by the school nurse, turned down the suggestion to go to a local emergency room, and went home. Thereafter, he experienced photophobia, phonophobia, headache, and trouble sleeping. He was eager to return to work to ensure that his students' activities were well coordinated but by mid-morning the next day he again had to go home.

His primary care physician evaluated him that afternoon and suspected that the patient had a concussion and ordered a brain MRI that returned unremarkable. The patient's symptoms continued and he was frustrated by his lack of improvement. He continued to coordinate school activities with the covering teacher from home, but also felt that his thinking was clouded. By the weekend, he noticed a tremor that came and went mostly in his right arm. Two days later, he had an event of whole body shaking while awake that lasted 5 min. His wife noticed rapid breathing and a "disconnected" look in his eyes preceding the event. He went to a local emergency department, where his vital signs, basic laboratory tests, and elemental neurological examination were normal (while asymptomatic). He was discharged from the emergency department with a referral for an outpatient routine electroencephalography (EEG) and a neurology appointment. He was also asked to video record any additional events. His routine EEG while asymptomatic was unremarkable.

At the neurology visit, he reported continued symptoms, including 3 additional events with whole-body shaking that were followed by less intense but noticeable arm tremors, stuttering speech, balance difficulties, and widespread body pain that lasted for an entire day afterwards. He showed the neurologist a video of a typical event captured on his phone that demonstrated side-to-side head shaking, high amplitude limb shaking with variable frequency, and preserved ability to speak but with

C. Adams
Department of Psychiatry, North Shore Medical Center, Salem, MA, USA

D. L. Perez (✉)
Departments of Neurology and Psychiatry, Massachusetts General Hospital, Harvard Medical School, Boston, MA, USA
e-mail: dlperez@nmr.mgh.harvard.edu

© Springer Nature Switzerland AG 2022
K. LaFaver et al. (eds.), *Functional Movement Disorder*, Current Clinical Neurology,
https://doi.org/10.1007/978-3-030-86495-8_14

a waxing and waning stuttering speech. He discussed his medical history well, but reported ongoing difficulties in thinking clearly. He felt fatigued and indicated problems with falling and staying asleep at night. On bedside examination, the patient showed a variable and distractible postural tremor that was also entrainable to different frequencies. On tandem gait testing, he displayed non-economical compensatory movements. The diagnoses of a functional movement disorder (FMD), post-concussion syndrome, and suspected additional functional neurological symptoms, most notably functional seizures, were discussed with the patient. He was offered and agreed to an ambulatory EEG for additional work-up. Education about the diagnosis was provided, as well as referrals to physical therapy, occupational therapy and cognitive behavioral therapy. He was prescribed a tricyclic antidepressant for management of insomnia and headache.

Introduction

As outlined in the vignette, FMD presentations commonly co-occur with other functional neurological disorder (FND) symptoms (e.g., functional seizures) as well as other distressing bodily symptoms (e.g., pain, fatigue) and related functional somatic disorders (e.g., fibromyalgia, irritable bowel syndrome). In a retrospective study of 100 patients referred to a subspecialty FND clinic, 1 in 4 patients showed mixed features across hyperkinetic FMD, functional limb weakness and functional seizure diagnoses [1]. As such, this chapter provides a transdiagnostic perspective across the sensorimotor spectrum of FND [1–3]. While not formally part of DSM-5 diagnostic criteria for FND, we will also discuss important themes related to functional cognitive symptoms and persistent postural perceptual dizziness (3PD) among other content. In the schematic diagram of symptom domains for FND shown in Fig. 14.1 by Nicholson and colleagues

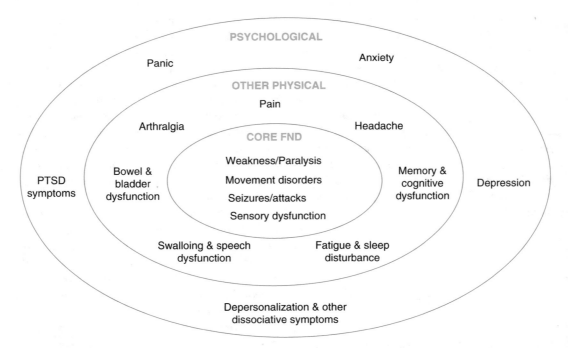

Fig. 14.1 Graphic depiction of core sensorimotor, other physical and psychological symptom domains in patients with functional neurological disorder (FND). (Adopted with permission from Nicholson et al. [4])

[4], this chapter focuses primarily on the "core" and "other physical" domains. Psychological aspects (apart from illness anxiety disorder) are covered elsewhere (Chaps. 3 and 22).

Functional Seizures

The phenotype of paroxysmal FMD can overlap with functional seizures [3, 5]. Similar to the emphasis on physical examination features to guide a diagnosis of FMD across subtypes, certain semiological features can be used to differentiate between functional seizures compared to epileptic seizures (See Table 14.1) [6, 7]. Semiological features favoring functional seizures include: (1) forced eye closure at event onset, (2) ictal crying, (3) memory recall during a full body convulsive event, (4) asynchronous, side-to-side head or body movements, (5) a fluctuating course, (6) pelvic thrusting, and (7) long event duration. Long duration events may also be seen in status epilepticus and pelvic thrusting may not reliably differentiate functional seizures from frontal lobe epilepsy. Approximately twenty percent of individuals with functional seizures have comorbid epileptic seizures, highlighting the need to carefully evaluate each type of event reported [8]. To address a common misconception, tongue biting and urinary incontinence do not differentiate between functional seizures and epileptic seizures [9], although tip of the tongue biting events may be more common in functional seizures while lateral tongue lacerations are more commonly described in epileptic seizures.

Levels of diagnostic certainty for functional seizures include consideration of clinical history, semiology and video-EEG data [10, 11]. Assuming that the clinical history is suggestive of a seizure (either epileptic or nonepileptic), the semiological features should guide the index of suspicion for functional seizures. Available EEG data, with or without video can be subsequently used to further quantify diagnostic certainty. For example, in the clinical vignette, available video data suggests that by semiology there is an index of suspicion for functional seizures. Coupled with a normal routine inter-ictal EEG, such a case would meet LaFrance et al., 2013 criteria for "probable" functional seizures [10]. If during the clinical evaluation the patient has an ambulatory 72-h EEG (without video) at home capturing a typical event without electrographic correlate, the patient would meet "clinically-established" diagnostic criteria for functional seizures (assuming the semiological features of a similar event had also been reviewed and suggestive of functional seizures as well). The highest level of diagnostic certainty can be obtained by concurrently obtaining video and EEG data during typical seizure events, usually done in the inpatient epilepsy monitoring unit (although ambulatory EEGs are increasingly allowing for home video). If a patient has a typical event captured on video and

Table 14.1 Semiologic features supporting the diagnosis of functional seizures vs. epileptic seizures

Signs favoring functional seizures	Signs favoring epileptic seizures	Indeterminate signs
Long duration	Occurrence from physiologic sleep	Gradual onset
Fluctuating course	Postictal confusion	Non-stereotyped events
Asynchronous movements[a]	Stertorous breathing	Flailing or thrashing movements
Pelvic thrusting[a]		Opisthotonus
Side-to-side head or Body movements[b]		Tongue biting
Forced eye closure		Urinary incontinence
Ictal crying		
Memory recall		

Adopted with permission from Perez and LaFrance [6]
[a]Indicates that sign may not reliably differentiate between functional seizures and frontal lobe epilepsy
[b]Indicates that sign may only be helpful in distinguishing convulsive functional seizures and epileptic seizures

EEG concurrently with semiological features suggestive of functional seizures and the EEG does not show any electrographic abnormalities, the highest level of diagnostic certainty – "documented" functional seizures – would be met. See Table 14.2 for additional details regarding levels of diagnostic certainty in patients suspected of functional seizures.

Based on our clinical experience, if patients are having at least weekly events, obtaining either an ambulatory EEG or inpatient video-EEG to capture a typical event and add diagnostic certainty should be considered. In some patients, however, clinical and logistical challenges (e.g., low event frequency; lack of available ambulatory and/or inpatient video-EEG assessments) limit the ability to capture a typical event on EEG. In these cases, it is particularly important to carefully review patient-provided videos to ensure semiological features are indeed suggestive of functional seizures. Some individuals may have distinct seizure types, and efforts should be made to characterize all distinct event types using the above outlined approach. Additionally, clinicians should be mindful of the broader differential diagnosis for paroxysmal movement disorders that should also be considered, particularly if semiological features are not highly supportive of a functional seizure presentation [12].

Functional Somatosensory Deficits

Functional somatosensory deficits are a non-motor form of FND [13], and diagnosis is based on physical examination signs. Sensory symptoms, however, are inherently difficult to describe and are prone to assessment bias, relying on patient – provider interactions. Many of the signs used to assess for functional somatosensory deficits are not highly reliable and generally perform poorly on standardized testing compared to those used to diagnosis FMD or other FND subtypes. Isolated functional somatosensory deficits, while common, are also not generally disabling in and of themselves. By far the more common presentation is that functional somatosensory deficits co-exists with other functional motor symptoms. If functional somatosensory deficits symptoms present in isolation, particularly with hemibody numbness, alternative diagnoses such as possible thalamic infarct should be considered.

Common functional somatosensory presentations include hemi-body numbness (with direct splitting of the midline) and numbness affecting limbs [14]. See Fig. 14.2 for common non-dermatomal functional sensory loss patterns, as well as the typical peripheral nerve dermatomal distributions seen in other neurological conditions. Sensory loss that is non-dermatomal in dis-

Table 14.2 Diagnostic levels of certainty for functional seizures

Diagnostic level	History	Witnessed event	EEG
Possible	+	By witness or self-report/description	No epileptiform activity in routine or sleep-deprived interictal EEG
Probable	+	By clinician who reviewed video recording or in person, showing semiology typical or functional seizures	No epileptiform activity in routine or sleep-deprived interictal EEG
Clinically established	+	By clinician experienced in diagnosis of seizure disorders (on video or in person), showing semiology typical of functional seizures, while not on EEG	No epileptiform activity in routine EEG or ambulatory ictal EEG, capturing a typical ictus[a]
Documented	+	By clinician experienced in diagnosis of seizure disorders, showing semiology typical of functional seizures, while on video EEG	No epileptiform activity immediately before, during or after ictus captured on ictal video EEG with typical functional seizure semiology

Modified with permission from Perez and LaFrance [6]
+ Indicates clinical history consistent with functional seizures, *ES* epileptic seizures, *EEG* electroencephalogram
[a]Captured event should not resemble types of ES that may not show an ictal epileptiform correlate on EEG (e.g., simple partial epileptic seizures)

tribution, such as a circumferential limb sensory deficit ending abruptly at the level of the shoulder (in keeping with the idea of the actual limb), is suggestive of functional sensory loss. A comparison of the interrater reliability of clinical signs found midline somatosensory splitting and splitting of vibration sense (e.g., changes in tactile sensation or vibratory sense directly 1 cm to the right or left of midline) to be highly specific and reasonably sensitive, suggesting that these signs can be used to support a functional somatosensory loss diagnosis [15, 16].

Inconsistency and non-reproducibility can suggest a FND diagnosis in the right clinical context. If, for example, a patient demonstrates markedly poor joint position sense, but performs Romberg and tandem walk without any deficit, this would suggest a functional sign based on internal inconsistency. Caution should be taken to not over-interpret sensory testing inconsistencies based on subjective experience, as parietal lesions for example can present with inconsistencies in sensory testing [13]. Additionally, non-dermatomal sensory deficits are also common in chronic pain disorders [17]. Lastly, sensory processing difficulties, abnormal tactile temporal discrimination and higher-order sensory processing impairments (potentially linked to attentional mechanisms) have also been described in FMD populations [18–20].

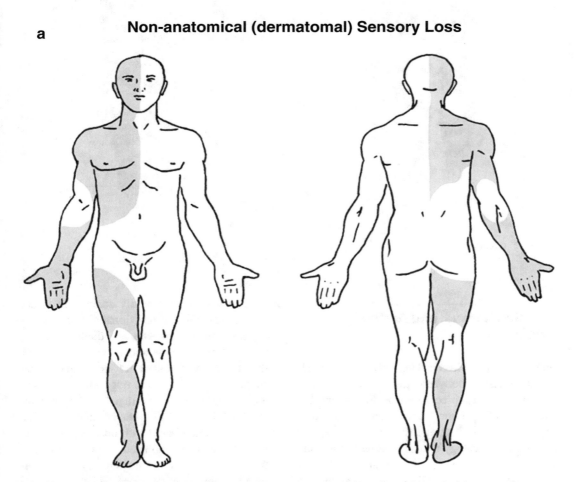

Non-anatomical (dermatomal) Sensory Loss

a

Fig. 14.2 Panel (**a**): nondermatomal patterns in functional somatosensory loss. Panel (**b**): typical dermatomal patterns. (Panel **a** image used with permission from Anderson et al. [14])

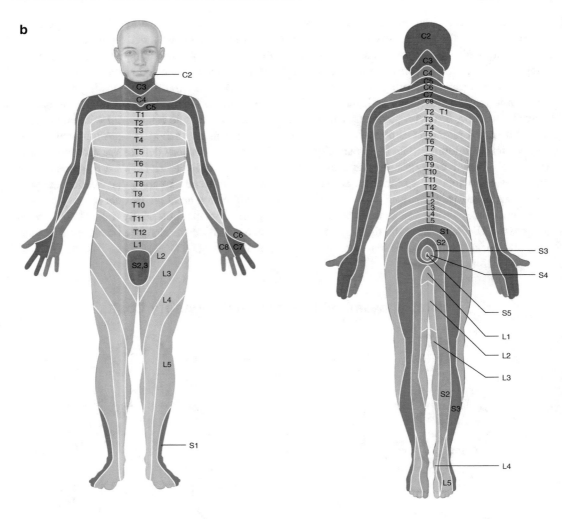

Fig. 14.2 (continued)

Functional Visual and Auditory Symptoms

Functional vision loss is diagnosed when there is incompatibility between the reported visual impairment and appreciable neurological or medical illness [21]. Functional vision loss accounts for as many as 12% of referrals to ophthalmology and 5% of neurology clinics, although it is noteworthy that 16–53% of patients with this condition also have underlying visual system pathology [22]. As such, thorough assessment is critical to identify potentially concurrent visual pathology and signs of functional vision loss.

Patients may complain of double, blurry, diminished or complete loss of vision in one or both eyes. The visual system follows anatomical principles that typically are not common knowledge, which can be leveraged to objectively assess the integrity of the visual system [22]. The assessment should begin with observation of the patient in the waiting room. For example, a patient's ability to navigate the novel environment of a new waiting room while simultaneously complaining of bilateral visual loss suggests a functional vision process. Functional visual disturbances are a "rule-in" diagnosis based on the presence of specific examination signs [21, 22]: (1) tubular visual field loss – the area of identified visual field loss remains unchanged despite moving away from the patient (the established visual field should normally expand when moving further away from the patient); (2) unchanging visual acuity – the visual acuity at 20 feet and 10 feet are equivalent (despite the expectation that visual acuity would improve); (3) optokinetic nystagmus drum test – for patients reporting either binocular or monocular complete vision loss, testing each eye one at a time, and if each eye shows fast and slow phases of nystagmus than visual acuity of at least 20/200 is established; (4) colored lens test – ask patient to wear glasses with one red and one green lens (colored lenses will only allow similarly colored light to pass through), then ask patient to read a chart with alternating red/green letters, allowing eyes to be individually tested without the patient's explicit knowledge; (5) pocket card test – contains objects of progressively decreasing size, but minimum visual acuity needed to see largest object is the same as required for smallest object (those with functional vision loss may be unable to identify the smaller objects on the card); (6) prism test – ask patient to look at eye chart, then place a prism vertically over the "good" eye and the patient is asked if they can see two objects (if they are able to see two objects, vision is confirmed in the "bad" eye as a patient with monocular visual loss would not be able to see two objects through a prism); (7) mirror test – for those reporting complete vision loss, a large mirror is held in front of the patient, slowly rotated back and forth in the vertical axis (preserved vision is confirmed if the patient is seen tracking their reflection in the mirror).

Compared to other functional sensory deficits, clinical descriptions of functional auditory symptoms are sparse, but include a range of presentations such as hearing loss (in the absence of objective confirmation), tinnitus, and auditory hallucinations [23]. The reader is directed to a chapter by Baguley and colleagues for a comprehensive description [23].

Functional Cognitive Symptoms

The presence of cognitive complaints and/or "clouded thinking" are frequently reported by patients with FMD and those with other FND subtypes [24–26]. The spectrum of isolated functional cognitive disorder without prominent additional sensorimotor complaints is also being operationalized [27, 28]. While cognitive difficulties may be attributable to medical and psychiatric comorbidities and/or medication side effects, a subset of patients with FMD may report memory, attentional, language, executive and/or processing speed difficulties consistent with functional cognitive symptoms [26]. As outlined in a systematic review by McWhirter and colleagues, diagnostic features of a functional cognitive disorder with or without another FND syndrome include: (1) symptoms of impaired cognition, (2) evidence of internal inconsistency with observed or measured function, or across distinct situations, (3) symptoms are not better explained by another medical, neurological or psychiatric disorder (or medication side effects), and (4) the cognitive symptoms impair social and/or occupational functioning [27]. With regards to internal inconsistency in cognitive performance, this may be a "rule-in" sign similar to other physical examination signs aiding an FMD diagnosis. Such individuals may complain of poor memory and general cognitive difficulties but also drive unaccompanied to the clinic, recount recent events well with a high level of detail during clinical interview, and express their concerns in an articulate manner. Conversely, when attention is drawn towards their cognition, such as during bedside cognitive testing, impairments in cognitive domains not previously apparent (such as language difficulties) may subsequently emerge.

At the Massachusetts General Hospital FND Program, patients with disabling cognitive symptoms are at times referred for formal neuropsychological testing [26]. While there can be some limitations to obtaining neuropsychological testing (e.g., availability of trained neuropsychologists, time commitment, insurance coverage issues etc.), we have found that some patients

Table 14.3 Suggestions for a neuropsychological test battery in patients with functional movement disorder and prominent cognitive symptoms

Domain	Neuropsychological & psychometric test
Premorbid intelligence (IQ)	Test of Premorbid Functioning
Performance validity	Test of Memory Malingering
	Medical Symptom Validity Test OR Word Memory Test
Symptom validity	Structured Inventory of Malingered Symptomatology
Attention	Wechsler Adult Intelligence Scale—IV Digit Span[a] OR
	Conners Continuous Performance Test—III
	Wechsler Memory Scale—III Spatial Span
Memory	California Verbal Learning Test—III[a]
	Brief Visuospatial Memory Test—Revised
Language	Boston Naming Test
	Controlled oral Word Association Test
Visuospatial	Judgment of Line Orientation
	Beery-Buktenica Test of Visuomotor Integration VI
Executive function	Wechsler Adult Intelligence Scale—IV Similarities, Coding
	Delis-Kaplan Executive Function System Color-Word Interference Test OR
	Stroop Color and Word Test
	Trail Making Test
Motor	Grooved Pegboard Test OR Finger Tapping Test
Personality and psychopathology	Beck Depression Inventory—II OR Patient Health Questionnaire-9
	State-Trait Anxiety Inventory OR Beck Anxiety Inventory
	Personality Assessment Inventory[b] OR Minnesota Multiphasic Personality Inventory—2—RF[b]

This battery includes many common neuropsychological measures that are generally available in neuropsychology testing centers. However, if select tests are not available, alternative tests that similarly interrogate a given cognitive domain may be substituted

[a]Tests include embedded performance validity measures

[b]Tests include embedded symptom validity measures (Modified from Alluri et al. [26]). Also, while failure of performance validity measures should be used to interpret neuropsychological test scores with caution, failure of performance validity measures in isolation should not be used to make a diagnosis of functional cognitive disorder [30]

who go on to perform normally in a neuropsychological testing battery find this reassuring when concurrently framed with validation of their cognitive concerns. Future research could investigate if quantifying a mis-match between subjective cognitive complaints and objective cognitive performance may serve as another "rule-in" marker of a functional cognitive disorder. See Table 14.3 for a preliminary neuropsychological testing battery that is used in our clinical program on an as needed basis. Note, performance validity measures, including embedded measures, are generally encouraged for all neuropsychological testing batteries [29]. While the validity of patients' cognitive complaints are not in question in a workup for suspected functional cognitive disorder, if individuals fail performance validity measures, caution should be taken to not over-interpret neuropsychological

testing results [28]. Instead, primary emphasis should shift to highlighting intact cognitive domains. Additionally, there are a range of disorders where a proportion of patients fail performance validity measures, and as such, failure of performance validity measures alone should not be used as the sole basis for a diagnosis of functional cognitive disorder [30].

Persistent Postural Perceptual Dizziness

Dizziness is a common symptom in neurological and medical practices that is often difficult to describe and can be due to many etiologies including medication side effects. Historically, functional forms of dizziness have received various diagnostic labels including phobic postural vertigo, space-motion discomfort, visual vertigo, and chronic subjective dizziness, among others [31]. In an effort to develop a consensus on a unifying diagnosis, the Barany Society developed criteria for a diagnosis of Persistent Postural Perceptual Dizziness (abbreviated as "3PD" or "triple PD") [32].

3PD is characterized by non-spinning vertigo and unsteadiness that is exacerbated by upright posture, visually stimulating environments, or motion [31, 32]. Following a vestibular insult (e.g., an episode of vestibular neuritis), normal compensatory mechanisms activate, which rely on non-vestibular systems for balance. Once the initial vestibular insult resolves, the system typically returns to normal function. If, however, these compensatory mechanisms persist when no longer needed, functional dizziness and the specific 3PD syndrome may result.

Patients with 3PD describe a sense of imbalance and symptoms may wax and wane. Relief may occur in moments of distraction, however, many patients describe symptoms as constant. Onset is most often acute, and the diagnosis is suggested by presence of visual hypersensitivity to complex stimuli while seated [33]. Involuntary use of high demand postural control strategies and an over-reliance on visual stimuli for spatial organization are features of 3PD. Routine tests of posture and gait can be normal or patients may show minimal difficulty due to an overabundance of caution. Some may demonstrate increased body sway or amplified compensatory arm movements. Improvements with distraction techniques, such as asking patients to identify written letters on their backs, provide positive evidence that unsteadiness has a functional basis [34]. Some patients develop a concurrent functional gait disorder such as fear of falling type gait patterns.

Pain, Fatigue and Other Physical Symptoms

In addition to core sensorimotor symptoms that define FND, many patients have other physical symptoms including chronic pain, fatigue, gas-trointestinal complaints, and urinary difficulties among other concerns [4]. While there are numerous classification systems through which to conceptualize these non-sensorimotor difficulties, the section below focuses on the DSM-5 diagnostic category of somatic symptom disorder (SSD) [35, 36].

Somatoform disorders were first described in the DSM-III. The DSM-IV introduced distinct somatoform disorder diagnostic categories (somatoform pain disorder, undifferentiated somatoform disorder, somatization disorder, hypochondriasis). The literature supports that many patients with FND have comorbid DSM-IV somatoform disorders [11, 37–39], with some studies reporting as high as a 50% comorbidity [38, 40, 41]. Prior to the diagnostic reconfiguration in DSM-5, a somatoform disorder diagnosis was based on the medically unexplained symptoms (MUS) concept, which was problematic given that other diagnoses are not defined based on the absence of specific criteria. The MUS framing also carries the potential implication that symptoms are somehow inauthentic, impeding rapport building between patient and healthcare professionals.

SSD, introduced in the DSM-5, is diagnosed when patients experience one or more somatic symptoms persistent over 6 months that are distressing or result in significant disruption of daily life and are accompanied by excessive unhelpful feelings, thoughts, and behaviors around physical symptoms [36]. The qualifier of "with predominant pain" may also be considered for those with pain as the predominant distressing physical symptom. The SSD diagnosis does not require exclusion of medical comorbidity; additionally, rather than psychological stress being framed as the cause of the symptoms, SSD focuses on how psychological (cognitive-behavioral-affective) factors amplify and/or perpetuate physical symptoms. It should also be pointed out that the diagnostic criteria for SSD continue to be debated amongst leaders in the field, with a lack of consensus regarding its application to individuals with a known medical/neurological causes for distressing bodily symptoms, as well as the utility (or lack thereof) regarding the psychological "rule-in" criteria of the SSD diagnosis [42, 43]. As a rule of thumb when considering the intersection of FND and SSD, FND requires physical examination signs (or semiological features) that are abnormal to guide diagnosis, while patients with SSD (without comorbid neurological conditions) will generally have a normal neurological examination. Although more research is needed, it is generally thought that most patients previously meeting DSM-IV criteria for somatoform pain and undifferentiated somatoform disorders will meet criteria for DSM-5 somatic symptom disorder. Recently, given the ongoing debate regarding the SSD diagnosis, a preliminary revision to the DSM-5 criteria for FND was proposed to allow for an etiologically neutral qualifier of FND "with prominent pain"; similar formulations were also suggested to allow for FND "with prominent fatigue" and FND "with prominent mixed somatic symptoms" [44]. See Fig. 14.3 for additional details regarding this preliminary proposal that could aid the characterization of sensorimotor FND with prominent additional distressing bodily symptoms without requiring the use of a psychological formulation. Additionally, from a medical and neurological perspective, it is important to work-up symptoms such as pain and fatigue with standard medical evaluations to ensure that reversible causes are adequately considered and treated concurrently if present (e.g., consideration of small fiber neuropathy that can be diagnosed by skin biopsy) [45]. However, the above comment does not imply that an exhaustive medical workup is commonly required given the overlap between FND and other prominent physical symptoms. Furthermore, fatigue often goes along with associated sleep problems that should be carefully addressed, and some patients may benefit from a referral to a sleep specialist.

In addition to considering the concurrent presence of a SSD with predominant pain, there is a range of other chronic pain disorder formulations. This includes the diagnosis of fibromyalgia and the intersection of complex regional pain syndrome and functional dystonia, as well as secondary pain related to disuse and maladaptive use of joints and muscles [46]. While generally beyond the scope of the neurological consultation, collaboration with other medical specialties can be helpful to evaluate the broader spectrum of symptoms indicative of functional somatic disorders such as irritable bowel syndrome, other functional gastrointestinal disorders, non-cardiac chest pain and shortness of breath, interstitial cystitis, and others. For patients with chronic pain, assessment by a physiatrist and/or chronic pain specialist can be helpful to effectively address comorbidities and precipitating/perpetuating factors for FMD symptoms.

Illness Anxiety Disorder

Illness Anxiety Disorder (IAD) in the DSM-5 replaced the diagnostic category of hypochondriasis [47]. Patients with IAD place an intense scrutiny on mild or ambiguous symptoms with the goal of identifying the warning signs of a serious illness. Diagnosis is based on a chronic (> 6 months) preoccupation with having or acquiring a serious illness. Somatic symptoms are either not present, or mild in severity, distinguishing it from SSD. Patients demonstrate high levels of anxiety and unhelpful health behaviors, some excessively seek additional diagnostic testing or reassurance, while others avoid medical settings out of fear they may be diagnosed with a serious illness.

Assessment for IAD should also include evaluation for possible depression, anxiety, mania, psychosis, obsessive-compulsive disorder, and post-traumatic stress disorder. Depression and anxiety in particular often co-occur with IAD. Anxiety disorders share similar cognitive patterns with IAD, including bias toward anticipating negative outcomes, increased attribution of negative valence to environmental stimuli, and failure to reappraise the risk of negative outcomes by integration of new information.

Proposed DSM-5 Functional Neurological (Symptom) Disorder Diagnostic Criteria Revision

A) One or more symptoms of altered voluntary motor or sensory function.
B) Clinical findings provide evidence of incompatibility between the symptom and recognized neurological or medical conditions.
C) The symptom or deficit is not better explained by another medical or mental disorder.
D) The symptom or deficit causes clinically significant distress or impairment in social, occupational, or other important areas of functioning or warrants medical evaluation

Specify symptom type:
With weakness or paralysis
With abnormal movement (e.g., tremor, dystonic movement, myoclonus, gait disorder)
With swallowing symptoms
With speech symptom (e.g., dysphonia, slurred speech)
With attacks or seizures
With anesthesia or sensory loss
With special sensory symptom (e.g., visual, olfactory, or hearning disturbance),
With mixed symptoms

Specify If:
    Acute episode: Symptoms present for less than 6 moths
    Persistent: Symptoms occurring for 6 months or more
Specify If:
    With psychological stressor (specify stressor)
    Without psychological stressor
Specify if:
    With prominent pain
    With prominent fatigue
    With prominent mixed somatic symptoms
        Optional secondary specifiers:
        With symptom-related cognitive-behavioral (psychological) features
        With a contributing comorbidity associated with the somatic symptom(s) of concern

Fig. 14.3 Preliminary proposal for a revision to the Diagnostic and Statistical Manual of Mental Disorders – 5th Edition (DSM-5) for Functional Neurological (Symptom) Disorder (FND). Three new FND diagnostic specifiers were suggested by Maggio and colleagues [44]: "with prominent pain"; "with prominent fatigue"; and "with prominent mixed somatic symptoms". Patients must first meet complete criteria for FND (criterion A–D). Additionally, pain, fatigue and/or mixed somatic symptoms should themselves be impairing to social and/or occupational functioning and present for at least 6 months. The above three specifiers are etiologically neutral, which acknowledges the biopsychosocial heterogeneity present in the development and maintenance of these somatic symptoms. To provide additional clarification, two optional secondary specifiers were also proposed: (1) with symptom related cognitive-behavioral (psychological) features; and (2) with a contributing comorbidity associ-

ated with the somatic symptom(s) of concern. The former optional specifier allows the identification of individuals displaying psychological constructs either amplifying or perpetuating pain that can have clinical utility (e.g., cognitive behavioral therapy treatment targets). The latter optional specifier encourages an appropriate (not necessarily exhaustive) medical workup for the identified somatic symptoms, as well as aids the characterization of relevant medical and neurological comorbidities (including functional somatic disorders). If a relevant comorbidity is present, this should be noted when using this optional specifier. Regardless of whether or not this latter optional specifier is used, clinicians should be mindful to evaluate pain, fatigue and other somatic symptoms without "rule-in" physical examination features in FND patients as they would in other populations (to prevent premature diagnostic anchoring)

Conclusion

In summary, when assessing and developing a treatment plan for patients with FMD, it is important to evaluate for the presence of addi-

tional functional neurological symptoms and other physical symptoms that require consideration in a patient-centered treatment plan. In particular, chronic pain, fatigue and cognitive symptoms are very common comorbidities that impact quality of life negatively and may serve as perpetuating factors for FMD if not adequately addressed.

Summary

- FMD commonly presents with other functional neurological and somatic symptoms (e.g., functional seizures, pain, fatigue, cognitive symptoms) that should be evaluated during the clinical assessment, and taken into consideration in the development of patient-centered treatment plans.
- Semiological features help guide the diagnosis of functional seizures.
- Consider persistent postural perceptual dizziness in patients with chronic complaints of dizziness.
- Functional cognitive symptoms can be assessed by evaluating for evidence of internal inconsistency; failure of performance validity measures is not synonymous with a functional cognitive disorder – as a range of conditions can fail performance validity measures.
- Illness anxiety disorder is the DSM-5 framing for the prior diagnostic category of hypochondriasis.

References

1. Matin N, Young SS, Williams B, LaFrance WCJ, King JN, Caplan D, et al. Neuropsychiatric associations with gender, illness duration, work disability and motor subtype in a US functional neurological disorders clinic population. J Neuropsychiatry Clin Neurosci. 2017;29(4):375–82.
2. Perez DL, Dworetzky BA, Dickerson BC, Leung L, Cohn R, Baslet G, et al. An integrative neurocircuit perspective on psychogenic nonepileptic seizures and functional movement disorders: neural functional unawareness. Clin EEG Neurosci. 2015;46(1):4–15.
3. Mula M. Are psychogenic non-epileptic seizures and psychogenic movement disorders two different entities? When even neurologists stop talking to each other. Epilepsy Behav. 2013;26(1):100–1.
4. Nicholson TR, Carson A, Edwards MJ, Goldstein LH, Hallett M, Mildon B, et al. Outcome measures for functional neurological disorder – a review of the theoretical complexities. J Neuropsychiatry Clin Neurosci. 2020;32(1):33–42.
5. Erro R, Brigo F, Trinka E, Turri G, Edwards MJ, Tinazzi M. Psychogenic nonepileptic seizures and movement disorders: a comparative review. Neurol Clin Pract. 2016;6(2):138–49.
6. Perez DL, LaFrance WC Jr. Nonepileptic seizures: an updated review. CNS Spectr. 2016;21(3):239–46.
7. Avbersek A, Sisodiya S. Does the primary literature provide support for clinical signs used to distinguish psychogenic nonepileptic seizures from epileptic seizures? J Neurol Neurosurg Psychiatry. 2010;81(7):719–25.
8. Kutlubaev MA, Xu Y, Hackett ML, Stone J. Dual diagnosis of epilepsy and psychogenic nonepileptic seizures: systematic review and meta-analysis of frequency, correlates, and outcomes. Epilepsy Behav. 2018;89:70–8.
9. Brigo F, Nardone R, Ausserer H, Storti M, Tezzon F, Manganotti P, et al. The diagnostic value of urinary incontinence in the differential diagnosis of seizures. Seizure. 2013;22(2):85–90.
10. LaFrance WC Jr, Baker GA, Duncan R, Goldstein LH, Reuber M. Minimum requirements for the diagnosis of psychogenic nonepileptic seizures: a staged approach: a report from the International League Against Epilepsy Nonepileptic Seizures Task Force. Epilepsia. 2013;54(11):2005–18.
11. Baslet G, Bajestan SN, Aybek S, Modirrousta M, Price J, Cavanna A, et al. Evidence-based practice for the clinical assessment of psychogenic nonepileptic seizures: a report from the American Neuropsychiatric Association Committee on Research. J Neuropsychiatry Clin Neurosci. 2021;33(1):27–42.
12. Xu Z, Lim CK, Tan LCS, Tan EK. Paroxysmal movement disorders: recent advances. Curr Neurol Neurosci Rep. 2019;19(7):48.
13. Stone J, Vermeulen M. Functional sensory symptoms. Handb Clin Neurol. 2016;139:271–81.
14. Anderson JR, Nakhate V, Stephen CD, Perez DL. Functional (psychogenic) neurological disorders: assessment and acute management in the emergency department. Semin Neurol. 2019;39(1):102–14.
15. Daum C, Hubschmid M, Aybek S. The value of 'positive' clinical signs for weakness, sensory and gait disorders in conversion disorder: a systematic and narrative review. J Neurol Neurosurg Psychiatry. 2014;85(2):180–90.
16. Daum C, Gheorghita F, Spatola M, Stojanova V, Medlin F, Vingerhoets F, et al. Interobserver agreement and validity of bedside 'positive signs' for functional weakness, sensory and gait disorders in conversion disorder: a pilot study. J Neurol Neurosurg Psychiatry. 2015;86(4):425–30.
17. Mailis-Gagnon A, Nicholson K. Nondermatomal somatosensory deficits: overview of unexplainable negative sensory phenomena in chronic pain patients. Curr Opin Anaesthesiol. 2010;23(5):593–7.

18. Ranford J, MacLean J, Alluri PR, Comeau O, Godena E, LaFrance CW Jr, et al. Sensory processing difficulties in functional neurological disorder: a possible predisposing vulnerability? Psychosomatics. 2020;61(4):343–52.

19. Morgante F, Tinazzi M, Squintani G, Martino D, Defazio G, Romito L, et al. Abnormal tactile temporal discrimination in psychogenic dystonia. Neurology. 2011;77(12):1191–7.

20. Sadnicka A, Daum C, Meppelink AM, Manohar S, Edwards M. Reduced drift rate: a biomarker of impaired information processing in functional movement disorders. Brain. 2020;143(2):674–83.

21. Egan RA, LaFrance WC Jr. Functional vision disorder. Semin Neurol. 2015;35(5):557–63.

22. Dattilo M, Biousse V, Bruce BB, Newman NJ. Functional and simulated visual loss. Handb Clin Neurol. 2016;139:329–41.

23. Baguley DM, Cope TE, McFerran DJ. Functional auditory disorders. Handb Clin Neurol. 2016;139:367–78.

24. Pennington C, Newson M, Hayre A, Coulthard E. Functional cognitive disorder: what is it and what to do about it? Pract Neurol. 2015;15(6):436–44.

25. Stone J, Pal S, Blackburn D, Reuber M, Thekkumpurath P, Carson A. Functional (psychogenic) cognitive disorders: a perspective from the neurology clinic. J Alzheimers Dis. 2015;48(Suppl 1):S5–S17.

26. Alluri PR, Solit J, Leveroni CL, Goldberg K, Vehar JV, Pollak LE, et al. Cognitive complaints in motor functional neurological (conversion) disorders: a focused review and clinical perspective. Cogn Behav Neurol. 2020;33(2):77–89.

27. McWhirter L, Ritchie C, Stone J, Carson A. Functional cognitive disorders: a systematic review. Lancet Psychiatry. 2020;7(2):191–207.

28. Ball HA, McWhirter L, Ballard C, Bhome R, Blackburn DJ, Edwards MJ, et al. Functional cognitive disorder: dementia's blind spot. Brain. 2020;143(10):2895–903.

29. Boone KB. The need for continuous and comprehensive sampling of effort/response bias during neuropsychological examinations. Clin Neuropsychol. 2009;23(4):729–41.

30. McWhirter L, Ritchie CW, Stone J, Carson A. Performance validity test failure in clinical populations-a systematic review. J Neurol Neurosurg Psychiatry. 2020;91(9):945–52.

31. Popkirov S, Staab JP, Stone J. Persistent postural-perceptual dizziness (PPPD): a common, characteristic and treatable cause of chronic dizziness. Pract Neurol. 2018;18(1):5–13.

32. Staab JP, Eckhardt-Henn A, Horii A, Jacob R, Strupp M, Brandt T, et al. Diagnostic criteria for persistent postural-perceptual dizziness (PPPD): consensus document of the committee for the Classification of Vestibular Disorders of the Barany Society. J Vestib Res. 2017;27(4):191–208.

33. Seemungal BM, Passamonti L. Persistent postural-perceptual dizziness: a useful new syndrome. Pract Neurol. 2018;18(1):3–4.

34. Staab JP. Persistent postural-perceptual dizziness. Semin Neurol. 2020;40(1):130–7.

35. Rief W, Martin A. How to use the new DSM-5 somatic symptom disorder diagnosis in research and practice: a critical evaluation and a proposal for modifications. Annu Rev Clin Psychol. 2014;10:339–67.

36. Dimsdale JE, Creed F, Escobar J, Sharpe M, Wulsin L, Barsky A, et al. Somatic symptom disorder: an important change in DSM. J Psychosom Res. 2013;75(3):223–8.

37. Perez DL, Aybek S, Popkirov S, Kozlowska K, Stephen CD, Anderson J, et al. A review and expert opinion on the neuropsychiatric assessment of motor functional neurological disorders. J Neuropsychiatry Clin Neurosci. 2021;33(1):14–26.

38. Sar V, Akyuz G, Kundakci T, Kiziltan E, Dogan O. Childhood trauma, dissociation, and psychiatric comorbidity in patients with conversion disorder. Am J Psychiatry. 2004;161(12):2271–6.

39. Stone J, Warlow C, Sharpe M. The symptom of functional weakness: a controlled study of 107 patients. Brain. 2010;133(Pt 5):1537–51.

40. Bowman ES, Markand ON. Psychodynamics and psychiatric diagnoses of pseudoseizure subjects. Am J Psychiatry. 1996;153(1):57–63.

41. Begue I, Adams C, Stone J, Perez DL. Structural alterations in functional neurological disorder and related conditions: a software and hardware problem? Neuroimage Clin. 2019;22:101798.

42. Burton C, Fink P, Henningsen P, Lowe B, Rief W, Group E-S. Functional somatic disorders: discussion paper for a new common classification for research and clinical use. BMC Med. 2020;18(1):34.

43. van der Feltz-Cornelis CM, Elfeddali I, Werneke U, Malt UF, Van den Bergh O, Schaefert R, et al. A European research agenda for somatic symptom disorders, bodily distress disorders, and functional disorders: results of an estimate-talk-estimate Delphi expert study. Front Psych. 2018;9:151.

44. Maggio J, Alluri PR, Paredes-Echeverri S, Larson AG, Sojka P, Price BH, et al. Briquet syndrome revisited: implications for functional neurological disorder. Brain Commun. 2020;2(2):fcaa156.

45. Farhad K. Current diagnosis and treatment of painful small fiber neuropathy. Curr Neurol Neurosci Rep. 2019;19(12):103.

46. Popkirov S, Hoeritzauer I, Colvin L, Carson AJ, Stone J. Complex regional pain syndrome and functional neurological disorders – time for reconciliation. J Neurol Neurosurg Psychiatry. 2019;90(5):608–14.

47. Scarella TM, Boland RJ, Barsky AJ. Illness anxiety disorder: psychopathology, epidemiology, clinical characteristics, and treatment. Psychosom Med. 2019;81(5):398–407.

Functional Movement Disorder in Children

15

Alison Wilkinson-Smith and Jeff L. Waugh

Case Vignette

A 15-year-old boy with a history of mild autism spectrum disorder, developmental delay, and asthma was seen by his pediatrician for concerns about "tightness" in his throat, coughing, and voice changes. These were initially attributed to asthma exacerbated by seasonal allergies. However, his symptoms worsened, soon evolving such that he felt he could not catch his breath. He could not speak above a whisper and his voice was strained. A few days later, he developed abnormal movements consisting of violent flinging of his arms and legs, forceful shoulder jerks, and a feeling that his neck was locked in place. He was evaluated by multiple specialists, including otolaryngology, neurology, and speech pathology. He was seen in the Emergency Department on multiple occasions for breathing concerns, always with normal oxygen saturation. Although a functional neurological etiology was suspected within a month of symptom onset, he continued to undergo workup by multiple specialists over the next 10 months. Multiple diagnoses were suggested, including spasmodic

dysphonia, tic disorder, and myoclonus. His symptoms continued to worsen, especially his large-amplitude flailing movements of the arms, and he developed an abrupt loss of muscle tone in his legs that led to many near-falls. His family, concerned for his safety, switched into a home-school option. Multiple medications were tried, including benzodiazepines and agents targeting tics and increased muscle tone, all with limited and only temporary success.

Ten months after symptom onset, the patient was referred to our Pediatric Functional Neurological Disorder Clinic. A review of records revealed that multiple specialists had suspected a functional neurological disorder, and findings consistent with a functional symptom etiology had been demonstrated on multiple laryngoscopies, but this diagnosis had never been shared with the patient or family. On physical exam, his thought content was normal with a realistic appreciation of the limitations imposed by his symptoms. His speech was strained, low volume but with normal articulation. He described his throat as feeling "clenched" at the level of his larynx. His movements were distractible and entrainable. He and his mother described a rapid onset of symptoms which then remained consistent over months. There was no premonitory urge and he had no sense of relief following the movements. The diagnosis of functional neurological disorder with mixed features was confirmed and explained to the family. They were provided with

A. Wilkinson-Smith
Department of Psychiatry, Children's Medical Center Dallas, Dallas, TX, USA
e-mail: alison.wilkinson-smith@childrens.com

J. L. Waugh (✉)
Department of Pediatrics, University of Texas Southwestern, Dallas, TX, USA
e-mail: jeff.waugh@utsouthwestern.edu

© Springer Nature Switzerland AG 2022
K. LaFaver et al. (eds.), *Functional Movement Disorder*, Current Clinical Neurology,
https://doi.org/10.1007/978-3-030-86495-8_15

educational resources, referred for physical therapy and family counseling, and recommended for close follow-up.

Characteristics of Functional Movement Disorder in the Pediatric Population

Patient Demographics

Functional neurological disorder (FND) can occur through most of the lifespan. While FND is uncommon in young children prior to school age, they have been reported in children as young as 3 years of age [1]. They become more common with increasing age, and prevalence in adolescence approaches adult levels [2, 3]. A population-based study in Australia found a mean age of diagnosis in pediatric patients of 11.8 years [1]. That same study estimated an annual incidence of 2.3/100,000 but acknowledged this may have been an underestimate. In the hospital setting, FND is relatively common. One study found that FND diagnoses accounted for 11% of psychiatry consult-liaison requests in an urban pediatric hospital [2]. Sex ratios are roughly equal before puberty. In adolescence, females begin to outnumber males, for reasons that remain uncertain but are potentially related to the higher rates of emotional, sexual and physical abuse suffered by girls and women [4, 5]. While sex differences in FND have been studied to some degree, research on gender diversity in FND is exceedingly limited, and little attention has been paid to transgender and gender nonconforming patients [2, 3].

Phenomenology

Children are more likely than adults to present with multiple functional symptoms [1, 2, 6], and will frequently manifest both a functional movement disorder (FMD) and additional functional neurological symptoms, such as weakness, sensory loss, and functional seizures. Though patients can manifest any form of movement phenomenology as a functional neurological symptom, in our pediatric FND clinic the most common presentations are (in order of frequency): functional gait (either with buckling of knees or astasia-abasia), myoclonus, and tremor. These three types of FMD account for 91% (20 out of 22) of our pediatric FMD presentations. Intriguingly, two other reports of pediatric FMD found overlapping but distinct patterns of phenomenology. Schwingenschuh et al. [7] reported that dystonia and tremor were the most frequent manifestations. Ferrara and Jankovic [8] found that tremor dominated functional movement presentations in children, followed by dystonia and myoclonus. This range of presentations underscores the wide range of functional phenomenologies possible in children, but may also reflect the local referral and recognition practices that lead a patient to be transferred to tertiary clinics. It is also important to recognize that this range of symptoms extends beyond the scope of FND as well, potentially including other types of functional somatic disorders (e.g., functional abdominal pain).

Comorbidities

Patients with FND of all ages have increased rates of somatic symptom disorder and related functional somatic disorders [9], including chronic pain and fatigue [1]. Hypothesized mechanisms include a shared pathophysiology, primed physiological responsiveness and parental sensitivity to physical symptoms facilitating patient distress by otherwise benign somatosensory information. Parents may inadvertently reinforce this tendency by fretting over the child's symptoms. This may underscore that children may be predisposed to develop FND symptoms through genetic or environmental factors (including child-family member interactions). Physical illness and higher levels of healthcare utilization are risk factors for the development of somatic symptoms. For example, patients with functional seizures comorbid with epilepsy (estimated to occur in 10–20% of patients) [10] had worse outcomes 2 years later compared to functional seizure patients without epilepsy [11]. Other neurological comorbidities, including developmental delay, have not been associated with worse response to inpatient intervention [12, 13].

Pediatric patients with FND also have increased rates of psychiatric comorbidities. Anxiety disorders are highly comorbid with FND in pediatric patients [2]. A study investigating different components of emotional distress in pediatric patients with FND found that sensitivity to cognitive symptoms of anxiety (e.g., worrying about losing control of one's mind) predicted severity of physical symptoms [11, 14]. The authors theorized this was related to catastrophic thinking in response to stress. In the same study, severity of depression was also found to predict severity of physical symptoms, even when controlling for anxiety levels [11, 14]. However, psychiatric comorbidities are not limited to internalizing disorders. About half of an inpatient sample of pediatric patients with FND had a history of a disruptive behavioral disorder, most commonly ADHD [2]. Whether such medical comorbidities are the proximate risk factor for FND, or whether the coexistence of these conditions simply reflects a shared predisposing factor (e.g., adverse childhood events such as neglect and family trauma) [15], remains uncertain. The course of a child's comorbid psychiatric disorder can be intertwined with the course of their FND. Comorbid psychiatric disorders that do not respond to treatment have been associated with worse outcomes for FND in pediatric patients [12, 13]. Thus, a comprehensive approach to managing affective and behavioral functioning is recommended. In our experience, infantile behavior or excessive regression during episodes – that is, beyond the expected developmental regression seen in illness – may indicate the coexistence of a possible factitious disorder (voluntary control of some symptoms with amplification for secondary gain [16]) alongside their FMD. Importantly, these features alone do not indicate that symptoms are factitious in nature; such findings must be weighed with other symptoms to determine an overall consistency with the diagnosis. Such coexistence of factitious disorder and FND in children is uncommon in our experience, making up no more than 10% of our pediatric FND clinic population. The parsing of motivation and deception is challenging and relies heavily on clinical judgement, therefore the relationship between factitious disorder and FND remains unclear and understudied [17].

Predisposing Factors

There are a number of risk factors that increase a child's chances of developing FND. Considering the biopsychosocial model for FMD (see Chap. 3 for details), some predisposing factors are innate to the child, while others are linked to adverse life experiences and other external circumstances. Certain personality and temperamental factors can increase a child's vulnerability to developing FND. Children with FND tend to be more anxious and score higher on measures of perfectionism. They are more likely to internalize negative emotions and use coping skills that are passive and solitary [3, 18]. A sensitive, perfectionistic child who struggles to express their emotions and work through distress will be at higher risk for expressing distress through physical symptoms, particularly if there are other risk factors in their environment.

Certain family characteristics can also predispose a child to developing FND. Malas and colleagues [3] described higher rates of both physical and mental health diagnoses in families of children with prominent somatic symptoms compared to controls. They speculated that this could be due to a combination of factors, including genetic predisposition and social learning of the "sick role". Another study found that parents of children with functional seizures were more likely to also manifest somatic symptoms than parents of children with epilepsy [19]. Children and adolescents with FND rated their families as less supportive than did typically-developing children. These same children rated their friends and significant others as just as supportive as typically-developing children did. This suggests that a child's family is particularly important for emotional support and the development of coping skills [14]. Children and adolescents with FND are more likely to show insecure attachment compared to typically developing children [20].

A child's social environment can also be a source of acute precipitating factors for the development of FND. Family-related stressors are a common antecedent to symptom onset [2]. A retrospective study found that children often experienced family conflict (including domestic violence) and loss (separation from a parent, death of a family member) prior to developing functional symptoms [1]. School-related stressors are also frequent precipitating events, including both academic and peer-related (e.g. bullying) concerns [21].

Adults with FND often have a history of childhood trauma – neglect, abuse (sexual, physical, or emotional), or family disruption. However, a history of trauma is less common in pediatric FND patients [2, 22], with frequency similar to the rates of trauma in the general population. However, patients who have experienced trauma tend to have worse outcomes than those that have not [3]. FND in children is associated with a history of stressful life events. For example, compared to their siblings, youth with functional seizures were more likely to have experienced exposure to domestic or community violence, bullying, or serious medical events. They were not more likely to have experienced physical or sexual abuse [18]. Other common stressful events include loss of a family member, parental divorce, school problems [23], and peer conflict [1]. There are many children, however, for whom the clinician is unable to identify a discrete stressful event prior to developing functional neurological symptoms [22].

Prognosis

Overall, children with FND tend to have a more favorable prognosis compared to adults, with both shorter symptom duration following onset (mean 52 ± 7 days) and greater likelihood of remission 6 months following onset [22]. Other authors have reported FMD series in which children improved more than adults, but by smaller

margins [23]. However, early diagnosis and treatment is key. Children whose FMD symptoms have been of sufficient duration and severity to require care at tertiary centers may have a less favorable outcome than the full population with pediatric FMD (as depicted in the clinical vignette in this chapter) [8]. An investigation of an inpatient family-based mind-body intervention for children with functional seizures found that those patients with recent onset of symptoms (<3 months) responded best. Patients with a chronic course (>12 months) were less responsive. Nonetheless, the majority of patients in that study (73%) had complete resolution of functional seizures 12 months after intervention. Another 11% had improvement in both symptoms and functioning without complete resolution [12]. Similarly, a retrospective study of pediatric patients with functional seizures showed that 55% were symptom free, and an additional 30% were improved after 2 years. Patients with a chronic course (>12 months) prior to diagnosis were more likely to continue showing significant symptoms 2 years later [11].

Diagnostic Assessment of Pediatric FMD

Increasing emphasis on coordinated multidisciplinary care is placed across different healthcare settings, including pediatrics. In our center and others, multidisciplinary care has facilitated successful treatment of pediatric FMD. Coordinated care among different healthcare professionals – such as pediatric neurology, child and adolescent psychiatry, neuropsychology, physical and occupational therapy, and social work – has shown to be effective at both inpatient and outpatient levels of care. A typical team approach to FMD treatment addresses education, psychotherapy, rehabilitation therapies, and medication management [6]. It has become increasingly clear that multidisciplinary teams are also highly useful at the assessment stage of FMD [24, 25]. A specialized team can be a helpful resource to medical providers in other disciplines who worry about missing something in the differential diagnosis of FND, lack training in how to best describe these conditions to families or to elicit sensitive histories. Indeed, the framing of the initial diagnosis is a key factor in improving engagement in future treatment. A multidisciplinary approach allows for normalization of behavioral health services and facilitates communication among healthcare professionals, but also helps families to feel they are receiving coordinated care rather than being handed off from the medical world to the psychological world [3]. The family's "buy-in" to a mind-body conceptualization of FND has been demonstrated as helpful to patient response to treatment [13].

Assessment

Building a collaborative relationship with families begins even before the first encounter. It is common for children with FMD to seek evaluation from multiple specialists before receiving a diagnosis of FMD. Since a prolonged, multidisciplinary assessment is not the norm, clear communication about what an FMD-informed visit will include, who the patient will meet, and how the visit may be different from prior encounters are key to building in trust from the outset. We encourage a "no surprises" model of care. Forming an alliance with the family is important to promote belief in the diagnostic process and engagement in treatment. Increased healthcare utilization is typical for these patients and families; therefore, they may have encountered prior medical staff who were dismissive, equivocal in the diagnosis, or even argumentative. Even well-trained and well-meaning healthcare professionals often lack the specific training needed to diagnose and manage FND. As a result, it is not uncommon for patients and families to experience stigma and become defensive or skeptical of the traditional healthcare system over time. Use of empathy, validation and focus on the physical symptoms can help strengthen the alliance between medical professionals, patients, and caregivers [3].

The first step in the evaluation (aside from any record review) is typically an interview with the patient and family (Table 15.1). In many ways, the interview process is similar to other new patient visits. In our experience, first interviews with FND families require roughly double the length of time needed for a typical pediatric neurology visit. In addition to these longer interviews, we incorporate neuropsychological testing for new FND evaluations and – when necessary – physical therapy assessments. These visits therefore require 2–4 h for patients, though the physician can typically see patients in parallel during other portions of the assessment. For example, the physician and psychologist may spend 60–90 min with the patient during an initial assessment, after which the patient and family complete neuropsychological testing (40–60 min). During testing, the physician can see 1–2 other patients. After the neuropsychologist scores the testing (15–20 min), the team develops a consensus plan of care (10–15 min) and returns to the patient for discussion of the plan (15–30 min). It would be difficult to integrate these intensive visits into a rapid-turn-over clinic session; in our own practice this was only possible in clinic sessions dedicated to pediatric FND. A focus on the neurological symptoms as well as medical comorbidities is recommended [26], as this grounds the conversation in concrete

Table 15.1 Factors we consider in the evaluation of children with a suspected functional movement disorder

Factors to include in clinical interviews for pediatric functional movement disorder
FMD clinical history (duration, distribution, site of onset and spread, triggering factors)
Additional physical symptoms of concern
Additional psychiatric symptoms of concern
School and extracurricular performance
Development History
Explicit investigation of bullying and/or hazing (in-person and on-line)
Psychosocial screen for risk-taking behaviors
Medications/Allergies
Household history of social, educational, and workplace disruptions and conflict
Family history of Medical/Psychiatric disease
Medical/Neurological comorbidities

and demonstrable examples. It is crucial that the patient and family feel understood and have an opportunity to voice all concerns about physical symptoms and their impact on daily activities. The physician should convey their belief that the symptoms are real and troubling to the patient.

As the interviewer begins to inquire about temperament, possible stress factors, and mental health history, it is important to maintain a neutral and open-minded approach. The family should experience these questions as a regular part of the clinical interview, not unfounded probing, or insistence on a purely "psychogenic" or traumatic cause that must be pinpointed. It can be helpful to explain why certain questions are being asked, and a focus on the presenting symptoms is again important. For example, we might say, "Many kids who have these kinds of symptoms also have anxiety or depression. Have you been feeling down or nervous?" [To parent:] "Have you noticed that he has been tense, sad, or cranky?" Many families will find these kinds of questions respectful and reasonable. However, others may be apprehensive of questions asking about mental health and stressful life events, especially if they had prior negative experiences in the healthcare system and felt that symptoms were dismissed. For those families, we recommend maintaining openness and curiosity, and simply explaining again the reasons for the inquiry before moving on. For example, "Not everyone has these kinds of problems, but we ask just in case, since it's common." This is another manifestation of our "no surprises" approach – families should never be left to question why we follow particular lines of inquiry, and the emergence of stress indicators should prompt the interviewer to slow the conversation and explain the need for such questions.

It is recommended that healthcare professionals explore stress within the family system, but also sources of resilience [3]. For example, we may ask, "These symptoms can be very stressful for families. How do you cope with the stress? What kind of supports do you have?" Most families will readily acknowledge the impact of FMD and related conditions on their lives. When sharing sources of strength, we can identify possible ways to leverage those resources to improve coping further. We can also identify ways in which the patient and family are not supported, and begin to explore other sources of stress. It is especially important to identify mismatches in resilience, when the child feels unsupported in a domain that their family regards as a relative strength (e.g., a child struggling with faith in a religious family).

It is unfortunately common that a parent leaves or changes their job in order to care for a child with FMD. This can lead to increased financial stress, but can also cause the other parent (in two-parent homes) to disengage in order to work additional hours. Further, the un- or underemployed parent may identify more strongly with a "caregiver of a sick child" role. Some children in this situation may feel guilty for the increased burden on the family, and some may experience non-conscious secondary gain from additional time spent with a parent or from less time spent with the disengaged parent. All of these can serve to perpetuate the cycle of stress on the family system.

In contrast to those working with adult patients, healthcare professionals working with children will almost always have ready access to a caregiver. This allows for the first-hand observation of the parent-child relationship, and sometimes the marital relationship. It is often helpful to conduct at least part of the diagnostic interview with children and parents separately, especially for adolescents. It is however also very informative to speak with everyone in the same room. Does one person answer for everyone? Do family members openly disagree or argue? Is the child quiet when parents are present, but talkative once they leave? While many families may be on the same page about most things, it is rare to not encounter differences in perspectives. It is also very helpful to observe how different family members respond to discussions of emotions and of the mind-body connection. The astute interviewer can gain insight into family system dynamics by observing interactions, not just through the responses provided. Additionally, for interviews where the parents or other caregivers are largely answering for the patient, it can be helpful to transparently comment that the interviewer wants to specifically hear from the patient; one can also highlight, if necessary, that the kind of information the child is able (and not able) to provide can also have treatment implications which are helpful for the physician to understand. Having a mental health professional as part of the multidisciplinary team can also be particularly helpful to assist in navigating psychiatric and psychosocial factors relevant to the presentation.

Physical Exam

Framing the FMD diagnosis around observable patterns of abnormality on the physical exam is a crucial step in building trust in the process. For example, capturing a video of a functional tremor that demonstrates distractibility and/or entrainment, and then immediately reviewing those findings with the patient and family demonstrates the objective nature of the observation and the skill of the examiner. This is true for all positive features of FMD and other FND symptoms (reviewed by Drs. Carson, Hallett, and Stone [27, 28]). Contrasting a functional neurological symptom with other distinct neurological diagnoses is a very helpful demonstration of confidence in the diagnosis. It should be emphasized that FMD is not a "diagnosis of exclusion," but relies on typical features such as variability and distractibility of symptoms. This approach is in contrast with the outdated, and in our experience, highly ineffective method of saving up exam abnormalities to "catch the patient out" [28, 29] – that is, using FND-supportive physical exam features to prove to the patient that their symptoms are false or inconsistent with "real" neurologic symptoms. In our experience, such an approach is highly damaging to the clinician-patient relationship. We have often heard families ask a version of, "Why couldn't the other doctors see that?" Upon review of prior physician notes, it is our frequent observation that prior providers *did* observe the FMD-specific symptom and made an accurate diagnosis – but failed to communicate it effectively to the patient and family.

An effective physical exam for a child with suspected FMD should include a general neurological exam as well as a standardized movement disorder examination. Given the previously mentioned co-occurrence between functional and other neurologic disorders, it is not surprising that careful assessment may reveal additional neurological diagnoses. We estimate that 10% of our pediatric FND patients have a separate, previously undiagnosed neurological disorder that informs and influences their FMD symptoms, and in other cases we found that another neurological condition was a more accurate diagnosis than FMD. Examples include autoimmune encephalitis, chorea, tic disorders, and autism spectrum disorder. In short, patients with suspected FMD benefit from a thorough neurological examination, punctuated by specific teaching and explanation of physical exam features that support or fail to support the diagnosis of FMD.

Diagnostic Testing

Pediatric patients with FMD do not typically require additional testing such as brain imaging or electrophysiologic tests (e.g., MRI or EMG) to confirm a clinically-established FMD diagnosis. Additional diagnostic studies can sometimes be of help if clinical features are indeterminate or if a neurological comorbidity is suspected. In functional myoclonus, muscle activation occurs in longer-duration bursts (typically >70 ms), has a more variable stimulus-induced latency, and has a preceding Bereitschaftspotential that can be captured on a time-locked EMG-EEG recording [30]. When tremor is indeterminate, surface EMG can help to demonstrate entrainment and variability in frequency. We emphasize that the yield of additional diagnostic tests is low in the presence of positive features for FMD and the absence of other concerning abnormalities on neurological examination. The goal of building trust and reducing anxiety in the patient and family about missed alternative diagnoses can sometimes justify ordering diagnostic studies, however it is useful to set the expectation of normal test result in advance.

Neuropsychological Assessment

Neuropsychologists and child/adolescent psychiatrists can play an important role in the multidisciplinary care of children and adolescents with FMD [31]. Neuropsychologists contribute a unique perspective that encompasses both the neurological and the psychiatric aspects important for understanding and treating this condition. Incorporating neuropsychological assessment into the evaluation process of these patients is useful in identifying predisposing, precipitating and maintaining factors as well as targets for treatment interventions. Child psychiatrists can be important partners in understanding the family dynamic and developmental stresses that may influence a child's FMD presentation and treatment. If a child has known or suspected abuse (emotional, physical or sexual) or neglect, we consider the involvement of child psychiatry to be especially helpful, if available in a timely manner.

Several themes have emerged from research on the neuropsychological functioning of individuals with FND. In adults with FND, overall intelligence, executive functioning, and memory (word retrieval tests) have been found to be modestly impaired [32]. However, IQ does not appear to affect prognosis [33], and when FND patients with pre-existing intellectual disability are excluded, such group-level differences in intellectual function appear to resolve. Similarly, children with FND have demonstrated more difficulties on measures of intellectual ability, academic skills, memory, and executive functioning [3]. Difficulties have been observed in executive functioning and memory as well as processing of emotional stimuli for the children with FND. Taken together, these findings may indicate that information processing resources are being over-utilized in hypervigilance to threat [20]. In our clinic, 17% of patients had estimated IQ below the average range, nearly equal to the expected distribution for IQ, and 18% had problems with verbal memory skills. Interestingly, there was very little overlap between those with below-average IQ and those with limitations in verbal memory.

Assessment of emotional functioning is crucial for children and adolescents with FND. Formal assessment allows for comparison to normative information, which can be helpful to gain information on individual strengths and weaknesses. Assessment of personality variables can also be helpful, especially for adolescents, as most of the commonly-used general personality inventories directly measure somatization tendencies. While concerns regarding the sensitivity and specificity of self-report questionnaires in this population have been raised [26], they can provide helpful information when combined with other sources of data, particularly clinical interviews and parent ratings. In our clinic sample, parents rated their children as more depressed or anxious than normal 46% of the time. For those parents who did not indicate concerns, two-thirds of their children reported emotional problems on self-rated questionnaires. Many of those children subsequently disclosed to their parents during the clinic visit that they had been trying to hide depression and/or anxiety. We recommend keeping the limitations of parent and self-rated questionnaires in mind, and to combine information gained through standardized testing and clinical assessment into a composite patient profile. In our clinic, a majority of patients (62–69%) self-reported a significant number of physical or neurological concerns. A third of patients (33–38%) rated significant emotional distress of some kind. These rates are likely an underestimate given that all patients were experiencing unusual physical symptoms and that anxiety and depression are highly comorbid conditions. However, rating scales can give valuable insight into the state of mind of the patient and parent, including awareness and willingness to disclose information.

Performance validity measures (a marker of internal test consistency) should be incorporated into neuropsychological assessments. Such tests have strong specificity (0.96–0.99) and relatively strong sensitivity (0.68–0.70) in pediatric populations [34]. Performance validity testing must be interpreted in the context of the larger testing battery and clinical assessment – a recent review called into question the ability of such tests to distinguish between FND and other clinical populations [35], though notably, this study did not include pediatric patients. Performance validity tests can also be affected by the presence of pain and fatigue [36, 37], and clinicians should be mindful of non-volitional sources of error. Most of the children in our sample (all but one) were able to pass performance validity tests, although some gave other, more subtle, indications of inconsistency, such as incorrect answers on simple items but correct answers on more difficult items measuring the same skill.

Multiple validated measures of symptom validity can be useful in assessing patients with FMD. The Minnesota Multifactorial Personality Inventory, Adolescent Version (MMPI-A) has the most support among pediatric measures for symptom validity [37]. In our clinic, we use the Revised Form (MMPI-A-RF) for adolescents. About a third of our patients produce completely valid profiles (comparable to sex and age norms), while another third shows signs of over-reporting and the final third shows signs of under-reporting of symptoms. Patients who over-report symptoms will likely benefit from a different approach than those who under-report, both in terms of discussing the diagnosis and when planning treatment. Similarly, we assess symptom validity in parents. Approximately one third (31%) of the parents assessed in our clinic produced invalid profiles in which overt recognitions of stress were under-reported relative to their own indirect measures of stress. These parents' pattern of responding showed a strong unwillingness to acknowledge even benign, everyday parenting dilemmas as compared to a non-clinical normative group. This provides an important insight into the parent-child dynamic, especially when paired with the child's self-report. A family in which everyone under-reports is quite different from one in which a parent under-reports but a child over-reports.

Treatment of FMD in Children and Adolescents

A detailed discussion of treatment in pediatric FMD can be found in Chap. 31. Careful and thorough assessment, especially within a multidisciplinary approach, is helpful to inform the types of treatments selected for each patient and family. Children and adolescents with FMD are best managed within a coordinated team approach, with ongoing follow-up care by a neurologist, rehabilitation and mental health experts.

(i) Psychological interventions

Psychotherapy interventions are commonly recommended for individuals with FMD. Careful consideration should be given to whether individual therapy, family therapy, or both are recommended. Family therapy and cognitive-behavioral therapy (CBT) with a parent training component have shown to be effective in treating somatic symptoms in children [3]. When presenting therapy recommendations to the family, it is helpful to take patient- and parent-report findings and preferences into account. While some patients and families may readily accept a connection between emotional and physical symptoms after the diagnosis has been presented, others may be reluctant to accept mental health interventions. Building a good rapport and establishing the connection between physical symptoms and suggested therapy within the biopsychosocial framework can often be helpful.

(ii) Rehabilitation-focused interventions

Motor retraining is a mainstay treatment for FMD [38–40]. Cultivating a network of physical, occupational and speech therapists with experience in FMD and the willingness to work within a multidisciplinary team model is an essential step in building an effective FMD treatment program. Children with FMD may travel many hours to access specialized care, and experienced therapists are often not available in their local areas. It is sometimes feasible to accomplish the initial assessment and development of a patient-specific treatment plan at specialized FND centers, that can then be carried out by therapists closer to home. A model of combined in-person and tele-medicine physical therapy visits [38] holds promise for clinics that serve rural and remote patients.

(iii) Medication management for comorbid conditions

Anxiety and depression can often serve as triggers or perpetuating factors for functional movement symptoms and other FND presentations. Especially in patients whose symptoms are temporally linked to symptoms of anxiety and depression, we find that antidepressant therapy, often with a selective serotonergic reuptake inhibitor (SSRI) can be a helpful adjunct treatment.

(iv) Educational considerations

In addition to taking the family environment into account when planning FMD treatment, it is also crucial to consider the school environment for children and adolescents with FMD. These children often have prolonged absence from school or leave formal school in favor of home-based options [6]. Approximately 27% of the students in our clinic sample were being educated entirely at home. Absence from school can provide a source of non-conscious secondary gain that reinforces symptoms. Perfectionistic, high-achieving children in particular may find that the sick role offers an opportunity to escape the demands of school. Medical professionals can ease the transition back to school by communicating the diagnosis directly with the school and developing a concrete action plan for managing symptoms that emerge at school [3]. Many students require academic accommodations, such as extended time for test taking and a reduced workload. They may need physical accommodations, such as extra time to transition between classes or help carrying materials. In our clinic, 46% of students were receiving some type of formal support in school. Many schools express a reasonable

concern for liability, especially for children who are perceived as at-risk for falls – for example, children with functional seizures or functional weakness. Educating school staff about the nature of functional neurological symptoms and their generally good prognosis can help alleviate anxiety about keeping the student safe, which can help prevent the loss of social contacts and schedule regularity that school provides.

Case Vignette Revisited

At the beginning of this chapter, we described an adolescent boy with functional speech and movement disorder symptoms. Although FND was diagnosed by a prior neurologist soon after symptom onset, the diagnosis was neither confirmed nor discussed with the patient and his family until approximately 1 year later when he was evaluated in our program. He was followed closely in our clinic, and while his family seemed generally accepting of the diagnosis, he continued to struggle. The patient was never able to participate in neuropsychological testing, as his speech was effortful and his movements near-constant during his clinic visits. As such, data on patient's mental health symptoms remained challenging to gather. Parent questionnaires revealed a tendency towards a defensive profile. His mother endorsed less stress than parents of children in a non-clinical sample, despite caring for a child who had significant functional impairment, needed to be homeschooled because of his symptoms, and had frequent visits to specialists and the Emergency Department. His mother rated him as showing significant somatic symptoms, but no other areas of concern. Again, this made the discussion of the importance of mental health interventions more challenging, as there was no objective evidence of prominent mood or anxiety symptoms while there was objective evidence that his mother was not particularly open to discussions of negative emotions.

The patient participated in physical and speech therapy, although his attendance rate was inconsistent. He established care with a psychiatrist and was prescribed an SSRI. He continued to be home schooled. Though our team and his psychiatrist recommended both individual and family therapy, and reiterated this recommendation at follow-up visits, no formal counseling or therapy was initiated. He began experiencing brief periods of remission but has not had substantial improvement in his quality of life. He continues to have occasional emergency room visits for dyspnea (with normal oxygen saturation) and related difficulties.

As is typical for pediatric FMD, this patient experienced onset of symptoms in adolescence, and his presentation quickly evolved to include multiple symptoms. He had a pre-existing chronic medical condition (asthma) as well as developmental concerns (autism spectrum disorder and mild developmental delays). He did not have a known history of maltreatment or acute stressors, although he experienced some academic and social difficulties given his social and developmental challenges. Unfortunately, although FND was suspected early in his course (per chart review), the family was not educated on the diagnosis nor presented with a dedicated treatment plan until his symptoms had become more chronic. By that time, the family had a high degree of healthcare utilization and the patient had been removed from school and other opportunities for peer socialization. It is possible that his illness beliefs and non-conscious secondary gain provided by withdrawal from school reinforced his functional neurological symptoms. Evaluations from multiple specialists without a clear diagnosis may have contributed to parental hesitancy to fully embrace therapeutic recommendations and failure to establish care with a psychotherapist.

Nonetheless, his willingness to engage in physical and speech therapy, and to receive psychiatric care, provides reason for optimism. He showed some gains in function, such as being able to speak in a soft voice for several minutes at a time, albeit without much improvement toward his prior level of function. With continued close management, we are optimistic that the family's relationship with the treatment team can eventually help with willingness to commit to psychotherapy, and that this may provide additional therapeutic gains.

Summary

- FMD in children can present with many phenomenologies, and single patients often have multiple movement types.
- The most frequent FMD phenotypes in our series and those reported elsewhere are functional gait disorder, functional dystonia, functional myoclonus, and functional tremor.
- FMD in children appear to have a better prognosis than in adults, paralleling the general prognosis of functional neurological disorder in children.
- School and extracurricular stressors are frequent risk factors and proximate triggers in pediatric FMD. While clinicians should assess for a history of abuse, in our experience abuse is not frequently uncovered in pediatric patients with FMD.
- Multidisciplinary care teams are time-intensive for initial visits but provide the opportunity for comprehensive care by a team of experts, facilitating the most appropriate treatments for each patient.
- Neurologists should cultivate an ongoing relationship with patients, even while treatment is being provided by other healthcare professionals including physical and occupational therapists, child psychiatrists, and child psychologists.

References

1. Kozlowska K, Nunn KP, Rose D, Morris A, Ouvrier RA, Varghese J. Conversion disorder in Australian pediatric practice. J Am Acad Child Adolesc Psychiatry. 2007;46(1):68–75.
2. Samuels A, Tuvia T, Patterson D, Briklin O, Shaffer S, Walker A. Characteristics of conversion disorder in an urban academic children's medical center. Clin Pediatr. 2019;58(11-12):1250–4. https://doi.org/10.1177/0009922819857541.
3. Malas N, Ortiz-Aguayo R, Giles L, Ibeziako P. Pediatric somatic symptom disorders. Curr Psychiatry Rep. 2017;19(2):11. https://doi.org/10.1007/s11920-017-0760-3.

4. Ludwig L, Pasman JA, Nicholson T, et al. Stressful life events and maltreatment in conversion (functional neurological) disorder: systematic review and meta-analysis of case-control studies. Lancet Psychiatry. 2018;5(4):307–20.

5. Kletenik I, Sillau SH, Isfahani SA, LaFaver K, Hallett M, Berman BD. Gender as a risk factor for functional movement disorders: the role of sexual abuse. Mov Disord Clin Pract. 2020;7(2):177–81.

6. Bolger A, Collins A, Michels M, Pruitt D. Characteristics and outcomes of children with conversion disorder admitted to a single inpatient rehabilitation unit, a retrospective study. PM R. 2018;10(9):910–6.

7. Schwingenschuh P, Pont-Sunyer C, Surtees R, Edwards MJ, Bhatia KP. Psychogenic movement disorders in children: a report of 15 cases and a review of the literature. Mov Disord. 2008;23(13):1882–8.

8. Ferrara J, Jankovic J. Psychogenic movement disorders in children. Mov Disord. 2008;23(13):1875–81.

9. Bègue I, Adams C, Stone J, Perez DL. Structural alterations in functional neurological disorder and related conditions: a software and hardware problem? Neuroimage Clin. 2019;22:101798.

10. Benbadis SR, Agrawal V, Tatum WO 4th. How many patients with psychogenic nonepileptic seizures also have epilepsy? Neurology. 2001;57(5):915–7.

11. Yadav A, Agarwal R, Park J. Outcome of psychogenic nonepileptic seizures (PNES) in children: a 2-year follow-up study. Epilepsy Behav. 2015;53:168–73.

12. Kozlowska K, Chudleigh C, Cruz C, et al. Psychogenic non-epileptic seizures in children and adolescents: part I – diagnostic formulations. Clin Child Psychol Psychiatry. 2018;23(1):140–59. https://doi.org/10.1177/1359104517732118.

13. Kozlowska K, Chudleigh C, Cruz C, et al. Psychogenic non-epileptic seizures in children and adolescents: part II - explanations to families, treatment, and group outcomes. Clin Child Psychol Psychiatry. 2018;23(1):160–76.

14. Yılmaz S, Bilgiç A, Akça ÖF, Türkoğlu S, Hergüner S. Relationships among depression, anxiety, anxiety sensitivity, and perceived social support in adolescents with conversion disorder. Int J Psychiatry Clin Pract. 2016;20(1):10–8.

15. Hunt TKA, Slack KS, Berger LM. Adverse childhood experiences and behavioral problems in middle childhood. Child Abuse Negl. 2017;67:391–402.

16. Ehrlich S, Pfeiffer E, Salbach H, Lenz K, Lehmkuhl U. Factitious disorder in children and adolescents: a retrospective study. Psychosomatics. 2008;49(5):392–8.

17. Factitious disorders and malingering in relation to functional neurologic disorders. In: Handbook of clinical neurology, vol. 139. Elsevier; 2016. p. 509–20.

18. Plioplys S, Doss J, Siddarth P, et al. A multi-site controlled study of risk factors in pediatric psychogenic nonepileptic seizures. Epilepsia. 2014;55(11):1739–47.

19. Salpekar JA, Plioplys S, Siddarth P, et al. Pediatric psychogenic nonepileptic seizures: a study of assessment tools. Epilepsy Behav. 2010;17(1):50–5.

20. Kozlowska K, Palmer DM, Brown KJ, et al. Conversion disorder in children and adolescents: a disorder of cognitive control. J Neuropsychol. 2015;9(1):87–108.

21. Krishnakumar P, Sumesh P, Mathews L. Temperamental traits associated with conversion disorder. Indian Pediatr. 2006;43(10):895–9.

22. de Gusmão CM, Guerriero RM, Bernson-Leung ME, et al. Functional neurological symptom disorders in a pediatric emergency room: diagnostic accuracy, features, and outcome. Pediatr Neurol. 2014;51(2):233–8.

23. Pandey S, Koul A. Psychogenic movement disorders in adults and children: a clinical and video profile of 58 Indian patients. Mov Disord Clin Pract. 2017;4(5):763–7.

24. Jacob AE, Smith CA, Jablonski ME, et al. Multidisciplinary clinic for functional movement disorders (FMD): 1-year experience from a single centre. J Neurol Neurosurg Psychiatry. 2018;89(9):1011–2.

25. McKee K, Glass S, Adams C, et al. The inpatient assessment and management of motor functional neurological disorders: an interdisciplinary perspective. Psychosomatics. 2018;59(4):358–68.

26. Kozlowska K, Cruz C, Davies F, et al. The utility (or not) of self-report instruments in family assessment for child and adolescent conversion disorders? Aust N Z J Fam Ther. 2016;37(4):480–99. https://doi.org/10.1002/anzf.1187.

27. Hallett M. Functional (psychogenic) movement disorders - clinical presentations. Parkinsonism Relat Disord. 2016;22(Suppl 1):S149–52.

28. Carson A, Hallett M, Stone J. Assessment of patients with functional neurologic disorders. Handb Clin Neurol. 2016;139:169–88.

29. Stone J, Edwards M. Trick or treat? Showing patients with functional (psychogenic) motor symptoms their physical signs. Neurology. 2012;79(3):282–4.

30. Pal PK. Electrophysiologic evaluation of psychogenic movement disorders. J Mov Disord. 2011;4(1):21–32.

31. Perez DL, Aybek S, Popkirov S, et al. A review and expert opinion on the neuropsychiatric assessment of motor functional neurological disorders. J Neuropsychiatry Clin Neurosci. 2021;33(1):14–26.

32. Brown LB, Nicholson TR, Aybek S, Kanaan RA, David AS. Neuropsychological function and memory suppression in conversion disorder. J Neuropsychol. 2014;8(2):171–85.

33. Gelauff J, Stone J, Edwards M, Carson A. The prognosis of functional (psychogenic) motor symptoms: a systematic review. J Neurol Neurosurg Psychiatry. 2014;85(2):220–6.

34. Clark HA, Martin PK, Okut H, Schroeder RW. A systematic review and meta-analysis of the utility of the test of memory malingering in pediatric examinees. Arch Clin Neuropsychol. 2020;35(8):1312–22.

35. McWhirter L, Ritchie CW, Stone J, Carson A. Performance validity test failure in clinical populations-a systematic review. J Neurol Neurosurg Psychiatry. 2020;91(9):945–52.

36. Heilbronner RL, Sweet JJ, Morgan JE, Larrabee GJ, Millis SR, Conference Participants. American Academy of clinical neuropsychology consensus conference statement on the neuropsychological assessment of effort, response bias, and malingering. Clin Neuropsychol. 2009;23(7):1093–129.

37. Emhoff SMMA, Lynch JK, McCaffrey RJ. Performance and symptom validity testing in pediatric assessment: a review of the literature. Dev Neuropsychol. 2018;43(8):671–707.

38. Demartini B, Bombieri F, Goeta D, Gambini O, Ricciardi L, Tinazzi M. A physical therapy programme for functional motor symptoms: a telemedicine pilot study. Parkinsonism Relat Disord. 2020;76:108–11. https://doi.org/10.1016/j.parkreldis.2019.05.004.

39. Gray N, Savage B, Scher S, Kozlowska K. Psychologically informed physical therapy for children and adolescents with functional neurological symptoms: the wellness approach. J Neuropsychiatry Clin Neurosci. 2020;32(4):389–95.

40. LaFaver K. Treatment of functional movement disorders. Neurol Clin. 2020;38(2):469–80.

Functional Movement Disorder in Older Adults

16

Mariana Moscovich, Kathrin LaFaver,
and Walter Maetzler

Clinical Vignette: Part I

Mrs. P. was a 76 year old retired teacher and was brought to the hospital by ambulance with reported paralysis of her left side. While she had been at home and attempted to walk from the dining room table to the living room, she felt weak and let herself down to the floor. When she felt unable to get up again, she called an ambulance after crawling to a nearby phone. In the Emergency Department, she could not walk, had difficulty with her speech output and endorsed severe pain in her lower back. She was noted to have a downward drift without pronation of her left arm and apparent motor inconsistency, being unable to lift her left leg in the air on command but observed to move the leg while repositioning herself in bed. She was admitted to the inpatient stroke service, after an acute stroke protocol was activated in the emergency department. Acute thrombolytic treatment with intravenous tissue plasminogen activator (tPA) was offered but she decided against this due to concerns over bleeding risk. A brain computed tomography (CT) scan and CT angiogram did not show signs of a large vessel occlusion, and a brain magnetic resonance imaging scan only showed mild age related volume loss and mild small vessel cerebrovascular disease, but no imaging changes consistent with acute stroke. Her past medical history was notable for high blood pressure, osteoarthritis and well-controlled diabetes. She also had a serious health scare several years ago, where she had severe pain in her legs and stomach, with scans revealing an abdominal aortic aneurysm. She underwent reparative surgery at that time without obvious complications.

Introduction

Conventionally, geriatrics has been defined as medical care for adults over the age of 65 [1], although most people do not require geriatric expertise until their 70s or even 80s. With increasing life expectancy, the population over the age of 65 represents around 15% in the United States alone, about one in every seven Americans. In addition to chronological age, other factors such as multiple chronic medical conditions, increased vulnerability for occurrence of medical complications and threatened loss of autonomy define the elderly patient.

Categorical definitions of the 'old', 'elderly', 'aged' and 'ageing' are neither straightforward nor universally applicable. Old may be defined in individual-, cultural-, country- and gender-

M. Moscovich (✉) · W. Maetzler
Department of Neurology, University Hospital
Schleswig-Holstein, Campus Kiel, Kiel, Germany
e-mail: w.maetzler@neurologie.uni-kiel.de

K. LaFaver
Movement Disorder Specialist, Saratoga Hospital
Medical Group, Saratoga Springs, NY, USA
e-mail: klafaver@saratogahospital.org

© Springer Nature Switzerland AG 2022
K. LaFaver et al. (eds.), *Functional Movement Disorder*, Current Clinical Neurology,
https://doi.org/10.1007/978-3-030-86495-8_16

World

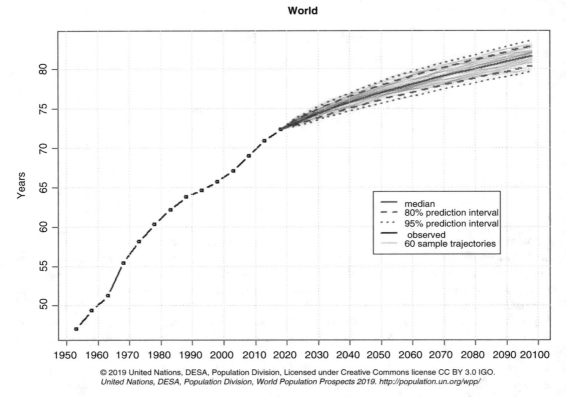

Fig. 16.1 Predicted global life expectancy increase in men and women from 2020 to 2100. (Source: United Nations World Populations Prospect report 2019, https:// population.un.org [May 4, 2021]. Reprinted with the permission of the United Nations)

specific terms. The definitions can differ between the sexes as life-course events contribute to ageing transitions, for example, going through menopause and retirement from work. The United Nations predicts a continued steady increase in global life expectancy in men and in women over the next decades (see Fig. 16.1).

Prevalence of FMD in Older Adults

Although women and younger adults are more commonly affected with functional movement disorder (FMD) [2–4], recent studies have demonstrated that approximately 20% of patients with FMD may have onset of their symptoms after the age of 60 [2, 4–6]. In a recent retrospective study in an academic hospital in Germany, half of FMD diagnoses in patients admitted to an

inpatient neurologic ward were uncovered in patients with previously established neurodegenerative disorders, a level of co-occurrence in the high end of the previously reported range [2]. It is important to note that the age spectrum for first occurrence of FMD can be wide and FMD is likely underdiagnosed in older adults [2, 3, 5]. In an international survey of 519 members of the International Movement Disorder Society in 2008, probing diagnostic and management issues in FMD, it was found that the extremes of age (<6 or >75 years) were "very influential" for steering neurologists towards a diagnosis other than FMD. Similar responses were found in an updated version of the survey 10 years later, emphasizing the need for improved education about FMD for neurologists and other healthcare professionals [7, 8]. Additionally, the lack of reliable prevalence studies for FMD, partly due to use of inconsistent documentation, billing codes and hesitancy by many physicians to make the diagnosis of FMD, make it challenging to provide specific statistics regarding the intersection of older age and FMD presentations.

Missing a diagnosis of FMD in older adults can have serious consequences for patients, such as initiation of unnecessary and potentially dangerous treatments for presumed alternative neurological conditions and missed treatment opportunities (see Clinical Vignette: Part I). A case report by Abrol and LaFaver [9] describes a 66 year-old man with intermittent leg weakness and speech impairment misdiagnosed as myasthenia gravis and chronic inflammatory demyelinating polyradiculoneuropathy (CIDP), who was unnecessarily treated with eight cycles of intravenous immunoglobulin infusions before correctly diagnosed with FMD and achieving a full remission of symptoms after undergoing a multidisciplinary motor retraining program.

Risk Factors for FMD in Older Adults

FMD in older adults frequently presents in the setting of comorbid neurological disorders (this is estimated to be about 10%) [10, 11], after a physical injury, or isolation [5] which occurs frequently in geriatric patients, adding additional challenges to the diagnosis of FMD [11–14].

A diagnosis of FMD can precede the later diagnosis of another neurological condition, such as Parkinson's Disease (PD) or another neurodegenerative condition. In a case-control series of patients with PD and functional neurological symptoms, Wissel et al. [11] reported that FMD preceded or co-occurred with PD in 34% of patients, with FMD occurring nearly always in the most affected body side. Functional neurological symptoms were more common in women with PD, with pre-existing psychiatric disorders and a positive family history of PD as additional risk factors. The authors suggested that functional neurological manifestations may be prodromal to PD in up to one-third of patients. Conversely, functional limb weakness as presented by Gelauff and colleagues [15] was rarely

connected to the later development of another neurological diagnosis but was associated with a higher mortality rate than expected – along with symptom persistence and disability in a large subset. These points argue for the importance of long-term medical follow-up for patients with functional limb weakness, not only to guide treatment, but also to remain vigilant regarding patients' overall health. Also of interest, in 3 of 76 patients in Gelauff's prospective case series, functional limb weakness appeared prodromal to the later development of a neurodegenerative disease (i.e., Huntington's disease, PD, and idiopathic cerebellar degeneration).

Batla et al. [5] performed a retrospective review of patients with FMD who were seen at their center over 5 years. Of 151 patients with FMD, 21% had onset after age of 60 years, defined as elderly. They reported that physical trauma, medical events and surgery were the most common precipitating factors for FMD in the elderly, including road traffic accidents with head injury, accidental falls, and stroke. Psychological triggers were identified in only 9.1% of cases. As an example, one patient developed frequent lip-smacking movement immediately after an MRI investigation for neck pain, during which the patient had experienced severe claustrophobia.

In a recent study on geriatric patients with FMD in an inpatient setting, 22% of patients had a history of physical trauma in close temporal relationship with the onset of functional neurological symptoms in the form of stroke, head injury due to a motor vehicle accident, or accidental falls, while 55% of the patients reported recent familial or financial stressors [2, 5, 6]. Psychological stressors are not always recognized in the initial interaction with the patient and may not be identified because they are not deemed as relevant for the patient's current symptoms, but should always be inquired about.

It is important to note that the new diagnostic criteria in the DSM-5 are applicable to a wide range of potential trigger factors for FMD, such as physical trauma or medical illness in addition to physiological or psychosocial events [3, 16]. Especially in the elderly, changes in relation-

Table 16.1 Examples of common medical and psychosocial concerns in older adults as predisposing (risk) and precipitating (triggering) factors for functional movement disorder

Medical issues	Psychosocial issues
Multiple medical problems and/or multiple medications to manage chronic conditions	Changes in living circumstances, e.g. spouse's illness or death
Increased vulnerability ("frailty")	Loss of independence
Cognitive decline and dementia	Behavioral and mood (neuropsychiatric) changes, including sadness, depression or anxiety
Difficulty performing activities of daily living	Lack of a support network/ loneliness
Weakness from deconditioning	Difficult dynamics with adult children
Balance and gait problems	Fear of dying
Nutritional concerns, including unexplained weight loss	Financial problems

ships, difficult dynamics with adult children, difficulties with identity after retirement, fear of dying [2, 3], familial disputes, financial difficulties, spouse's illness or death [6], and problems originating from loneliness, should be explored as part of the patient's psychosocial history. Batla et al. [5] observed that older adults and younger patients with FMD did not differ significantly in terms of the presence of a stressor or precipitating factors (Table 16.1).

Characteristics of FMD in Older Adults

Acute onset of FMD is common, which can broaden the differential diagnosis to include other acute neurological disorders such as stroke, and poses challenges especially in geriatric patients with multiple medical comorbidities. In addition to differentiating FMD from other acute neurological conditions, the co-occurrence of FMD with other chronic neurological conditions is a common situation as highlighted in the last section.

It is important to evaluate conditions on the differential diagnosis through use of additional diagnostic studies as appropriate. Nonetheless, the most recent suggested diagnostic criteria for FMD [16] highlight the importance of positive clinical signs and replace the view of functional neurological disorder as a "diagnosis of exclusion" [2, 15, 17]. Physicians treating geriatric patients with movement disorders need to be alert regarding the possibility that FMD may be the predominant source of disability [2].

Functional tremor is the most reported phenomenology of FMD, accounting for around 50% [3, 4]. The body parts most commonly affected are the upper limbs, however lower limbs and head can also be affected [6]. Functional gait abnormalities are also reported to be frequently present in older patients and may be even more common than in the younger population [5, 6]. "Fear of falling" presents a typical functional gait manifestation in the elderly, with variable fluctuations of stance and gait, sudden buckling of knees, and, "uneconomic" postures. Please note that not all gait disorders due to fear of falling are functional in nature; some patients present with (pure) phobic and protective gait which has an avoidant, but no demonstrative component. A subset of patients with fear of falling type functional gait will be able to readily report that anxiety and heightened arousal associated with gait tasks (including features such as breath holding) are part of their symptom complex. Also, a "walking-on-ice" gait pattern and exacerbation of other functional movements (particularly dystonia) during walking can be observed. Risk factors for developing these gait patterns can include medical comorbidities such as arthritis and a neuropathy, serving as background vulnerabilities for a fear of falling type gait (potentially with a prior mechanical fall and accompanying anxiety also relevant factors in these clinical presentations). Functional dystonia, choreiform movements and tics can also occur in older patients with FMD; in such instances, providers should work to differentiate alternative diagnoses such as medication-induced chorea (e.g., tardive dyskinesias or levodopa induced dyskinesia) or late onset genetic conditions such as Huntington's disease that can sometimes be found even in the absence of a (known) family history. As with other FMD presentations, symptoms can occur in isolation or in combination [5, 6].

Clinical Vignette: Part II

During her hospital stay, Mrs. P. continued to experience weakness in her left arm and leg. A follow-up neurological examination showed a positive Hoover's sign on the left leg (patient was not able to flex this leg when tested, but the leg exerted a strong downward force when the right leg was flexed in the hip), a new postural tremor in her left arm that was entrainable, and variable and distractible stuttering speech that was particularly evident during bedside language testing. She was diagnosed with FMD, including features of functional limb weakness, functional tremor and functional speech. This was described to her as real, common and treatable, and that one way of understanding this condition is that her "hardware" (brain scan) is generally healthy but her "software" is crashing. She produced a spontaneous laugh with this discussion, in part because she commented that her late husband used to help her with her home computer that was "always crashing". A physical therapist was asked to see the patient for an initial evaluation while in the hospital. The patient initially showed very little movement of her arm and leg and expressed frustration about the severity of her physical symptoms.

She was given educational materials about FMD and a social worker from the geriatrics service was asked to see the patient. Details emerged that she was having difficulties caring for herself in her large two-story home since the passing of her husband from cancer the year prior. There were also ongoing family disagreements related to financial issues, causing an emotional strain between the patient and her two daughters.

Over the course of the next several days, she was able to make considerable progress in physical therapy with the use of distraction techniques and regained use of her leg to a sufficient degree for independent ambulation. The social worker continued to meet with the patient daily to provide emotional support. She was accepted to a sub-acute rehab program and the educational materials gathered by the primary team were *shared with the rehabilitation facility to ensure adequate continued care. The patient's primary care physician was informed of the admission, an outpatient social work appointment was arranged through the primary care's office and neurology follow up was also scheduled. When seen on neurology follow-up a month later, she had recovered back to her baseline function and was planning to relocate to an assisted living facility to simplify her daily life and responsibilities in caring for a large property.*

Special Treatment Considerations for FMD in Older Adults

To date, there is no standard protocol available for treating FMD in elderly and geriatric patients. In several retrospective studies [18, 19] reporting on treatment outcomes in patients with FMD undergoing intensive multidisciplinary treatment programs, age was not found to be a predictive factor. A 1-week physiotherapy program based on the concept of motor reprogramming compared sixty patients ranging from age 17–79 to a control group undergoing standard medical care. Substantial improvement or remission of motor symptoms was reported in 74% of patients, and patient-rated outcomes after 2 years continued to show benefit in 60% compared to 22% in the control group, independent of age [20].

A specific and goal-oriented multidisciplinary geriatric team treatment approach can lead to relevant improvements in outcome parameters in both FMD and comorbidities [2]. Participation of different individualized interventions with input from neurologists, mental health providers and rehabilitation specialists (i.e., speech therapist, occupational therapist, physical therapist) are considered best practice for optimizing treatment outcomes.

As for other age groups, treatment for FMD needs to be individualized and adjusted to a patients' unique sets of predisposing, precipitating and maintaining factors (core components of the biopsychosocial model). Psychoeducation, teaching relaxation and mindfulness, as well as addressing adverse family dynamics can be very helpful as presented in our vignette. According to our clinical experience, a comprehensive assessment by a multidisciplinary geriatric team including a movement disorders neurologist, geriatrician, neuropsychologist (or geriatric/neuropsychiatrist), physiotherapist, occupation therapist, speech therapist and social worker are crucial. With this approach the opportunity to clarify (i) to what extent the patient has an FMD diagnosis, (ii) how this is associated with other medical/neurological diagnoses and which of the diagnoses is most disabling in terms of health-related quality of life, (iii) the level of patient acceptance (or potential acceptance) of the diagnosis, and (iv) to work out the details of a patient-centered treatment plan is higher. Especially point (iii) has to be implemented thoughtfully. Explaining the diagnosis to patients and families should be done in an empathetic manner, validating the patient's symptoms, and explaining how the diagnosis was reached. We often use analogies such as "FMD is like a computer problem where some of the software has been lost or programmed with a part that doesn't belong to the original software" to describe the disorder. "Your brain is stuck in a wrong gear and needs to be retrained on how to get un-stuck" may be another helpful analogy. The explanatory model should be adjusted according to the patient's educational and cultural background. Explaining FMD in terms of temporary brain dysfunction similar to what many of us have experienced during times of high stress or anxiety (e.g. "he was paralyzed with fear") can often help to normalize the diagnosis. Using functional terms and giving hope for a path forward and reversibility of symptoms with treatment are other important strategies. For more details on delivering a diagnosis of FMD, see Chap. 17. When a diagnosis of FMD is presented in this manner, most patients will express interest in further information and treatment for their problems. If there is no interest by of the patient to be referred for FMD treatment services, we nevertheless write the diagnosis in unambiguous terms in the patient's medical chart, inform the patient and the family as well as the referring provider about our assessment of the symptoms, and remain available for further questions and advice.

In patients with cognitive impairment or dementia, the treatment approach may need to be modified and rely on reassurance and behavioural modifications by the patient's partner and other family members rather than insight-oriented or skill-based psychotherapy. Common comorbidities such as chronic pain or insomnia often worsen FMD symptoms and need to be addressed as part of a comprehensive treatment plan.

In light of the increasing recognition of FMD as source of disability in older adults, and the expected rise in affected patients due to increasing life expectancy, further research on understanding and treating FMD in older adults is urgently needed.

Geriatricians, other primary care providers, neurologists, mental health professionals, physical, occupational, and speech therapists should all work together to design both efficient diagnostic approaches and patient-centered treatments for FMD in older adults. As health care professionals gain more awareness of FMD, special considerations towards meeting the needs of older patients should be emphasized.

Summary
- Approximately 20% of patients with FMD may have onset of symptoms after the age of 60 years, and many of those developing FMD earlier in life remain symptomatic as they get older.
- In older patients, FMD is often comorbid with other neurological disorders, and may be precipitated by a physical injury, surgery or stroke.
- Precipitating psychosocial factors for FMD in older adults include changes in relationships, difficult dynamics with adult children, fear of dying, financial problems, spouse's illness or death, loneliness, establishing a new sense of purpose and identity after retirement.

- Tremor and gait disorders are the most commonly encountered symptoms of FMD in older adults.
- Treatment needs to be individualized and is often best delivered in a multidisciplinary approach, addressing relevant comorbidities, precipitating and maintaining factors such as deconditioning, chronic pain and insomnia.
- Older age has not been shown to be a negative predictive factor towards treatment success in FMD, and treatment can often lead to rewarding outcomes for patients and families.

References

1. Orimo H. Reviewing the definition of elderly. Nihon Ronen Igakkai Zasshi. 2006;43(1):27–34.
2. Matzold S, Geritz J, Zeuner KE, Berg D, Paschen S, Hieke J, et al. Functional movement disorders in neurogeriatric inpatients : underdiagnosed, often comorbid to neurodegenerative disorders and treatable. Z Gerontol Geriatr. 2019;52(4):324–9.
3. Thenganatt MA, Jankovic J. Psychogenic (functional) movement disorders. Continuum (Minneap Minn). 2019;25(4):1121–40.
4. Factor SA, Podskalny GD, Molho ES. Psychogenic movement disorders: frequency, clinical profile, and characteristics. J Neurol Neurosurg Psychiatry. 1995;59(4):406–12.
5. Batla A, Stamelou M, Edwards MJ, Parees I, Saifee TA, Fox Z, et al. Functional movement disorders are not uncommon in the elderly. Mov Disord. 2013;28(4):540–3.
6. Chouksey A, Pandey S. Functional movement disorders in elderly. Tremor Other Hyperkinet Mov (N Y). 2019;9.
7. Espay AJ, Goldenhar LM, Voon V, Schrag A, Burton N, Lang AE. Opinions and clinical practices related to diagnosing and managing patients with psychogenic movement disorders: an international survey of movement disorder society members. Mov Disord. 2009;24(9):1366–74.
8. LaFaver K, Lang AE, Stone J, Morgante F, Edwards M, Lidstone S, et al. Opinions and clinical practices related to diagnosing and managing functional (psychogenic) movement disorders: changes in the last decade. Eur J Neurol. 2020;27(6):975–84.
9. Abrol T, LaFaver K. Functional weakness and dysarthria in a 66-year-old man previously diagnosed with CIDP. Pract Neurol. 2017:42–4.
10. Hallett M. Functional (psychogenic) movement disorders – clinical presentations. Parkinsonism Relat Disord. 2016;22(Suppl 1):S149–52.
11. Wissel BD, Dwivedi AK, Merola A, Chin D, Jacob C, Duker AP, et al. Functional neurological disorders in Parkinson disease. J Neurol Neurosurg Psychiatry. 2018;89(6):566–71.
12. Morgante F, Edwards MJ, Espay AJ. Psychogenic movement disorders. Continuum (Minneap Minn). 2013;19(5 Movement Disorders):1383–96.
13. Parees I, Kojovic M, Pires C, Rubio-Agusti I, Saifee TA, Sadnicka A, et al. Physical precipitating factors in functional movement disorders. J Neurol Sci. 2014;338(1–2):174–7.
14. Parees I, Saifee TA, Kojovic M, Kassavetis P, Rubio-Agusti I, Sadnicka A, et al. Functional (psychogenic) symptoms in Parkinson's disease. Mov Disord. 2013;28(12):1622–7.
15. Gelauff JM et al. The prognosis of functional limb weakness: a 14-year case-control study. Brain. 2019;142(7):2137–48.
16. Espay AJ, Aybek S, Carson A, Edwards MJ, Goldstein LH, Hallett M, et al. Current concepts in diagnosis and treatment of functional neurological disorders. JAMA Neurol. 2018;75(9):1132–41.
17. Williams DT, Ford B, Fahn S. Phenomenology and psychopathology related to psychogenic movement disorders. Adv Neurol. 1995;65:231–57.
18. Jacob AE, Kaelin DL, Roach AR, Ziegler CH, LaFaver K. Motor retraining (MoRe) for functional movement disorders: outcomes from a 1-week multidisciplinary rehabilitation program. PM R. 2018;10(11):1164–72.
19. Maggio JB, Ospina JP, Callahan J, Hunt AL, Stephen CD, Perez DL. Outpatient physical therapy for functional neurological disorder: a preliminary feasibility and naturalistic outcome study in a U.S. cohort. J Neuropsychiatry Clin Neurosci. 2020;32(1):85–9.
20. Czarnecki K, Thompson JM, Seime R, Geda YE, Duffy JR, Ahlskog JE. Functional movement disorders: successful treatment with a physical therapy rehabilitation protocol. Parkinsonism Relat Disord. 2012;18(3):247–51.

Part III

Management

"Breaking the News" of a Functional Movement Disorder

Jon Stone, Ingrid Hoeritzauer, and Alan Carson

Clinical Vignette 1

A 30-year-old woman presents with a 9-month history of right sided functional hemiparesis that meant she walked with a cane and was currently no longer at work. At onset there had been a panic attack on an airplane as well as some migraine symptoms. She had been given a diagnosis of stroke during a hospital stay on vacation. At the time of assessment, she was noted to have a previous history of irritable bowel syndrome and chronic pelvic pain. There was also a history of emotional neglect as a child and teenager. Clinical assessment found clear evidence of a functional hemiparesis, with positive Hoover's sign and Hip Abductor sign with no evidence of an additional neurological problem. Neuroimaging was normal.

The doctor explained that the original diagnosis had been wrong as the scans were normal. The diagnosis was that of a 'conversion disorder', or 'psychogenic disorder'. He asked whether she had been sexually or physically abused and explained that it seemed likely that the reason for her right sided weakness related to previous traumatic events in her life. The doctor

explained that he was a neurologist so could only make the diagnosis but would ask one of his colleagues in neuropsychiatry to see her in a few months' time, so they could start the process of assessment and treatment.

In response the patient became upset and angry. She had been told by doctors already that it was a stroke and had shared this diagnosis with her family and employers. She said that the doctors had not done enough tests. She was certain that the abuse as a child was not relevant and she had 'put it behind her'. She put in a formal complaint about the doctor and asked her primary care doctor for another opinion.

Clinical Vignette 2

A 32-year-old man presented with functional hemiparesis combined with dystonia and pain in his right leg beginning with an ankle sprain 2 years earlier. He was in despair and seeking amputation. He had been managed by a chronic pain service as complex regional pain syndrome but had been referred to neurology because weakness, dystonia and sensory loss were more prominent than pain. He had a history of sexual abuse as a child but had good physical and mental health until the accident.

The doctor explained that he had functional neurological disorder (FND) a condition in which the brain and nervous system doesn't function properly. She explained that this is commonly triggered by injuries and leads to a

J. Stone (✉) · I. Hoeritzauer · A. Carson
Centre for Clinical Brain Sciences, University of Edinburgh, Edinburgh, UK
e-mail: Jon.Stone@ed.ac.uk

© Springer Nature Switzerland AG 2022
K. LaFaver et al. (eds.), *Functional Movement Disorder*, Current Clinical Neurology,
https://doi.org/10.1007/978-3-030-86495-8_17

situation where the brain gets 'stuck' in a pattern, as if the injury had just happened. Childhood adversity was discussed as something that may or may not have been relevant to this happening and not a factor in the diagnosis. It was noted he had become depressed and this would have to be incorporated in his multidisciplinary treatment plan rehabilitation team involving a neurologist, neuropsychiatrist and physiotherapist.

The patient cautiously welcomed this explanation which he said was different to what he had heard before and was interested in pursuing further treatment aligned to his functional movement disorder (FMD).

Introduction

The two vignettes above illustrate clinical encounters where 'breaking the news' of FND has had different outcomes in terms of the patient response and subsequent ability to engage with treatment. They also illustrate the difficulty of discussing 'breaking the news' in FND without considering a variety of factors that might affect the outcome of that process including: What is the most appropriate model for understanding the disorder? What are the patient's prior expectations and beliefs about what is wrong and what treatment they should have? Who is giving the diagnosis – a neurologist? a psychiatrist? And what 'back up' or additional team members do they have to help them support and reinforce the explanation given and the treatment associated with it?

In this chapter, we aim to provide a practical overview of the issues involved in explaining the diagnosis of FND and take the reader through various scenarios which can arise. We are keen in doing this not to be prescriptive about what to say, or what language to use. We firmly believe that there is no 'right' way to do this. Clinicians must find a way to communicate that fits with their own communication style, the known data about the condition and the person they are explaining it to. There is no one size fits all. But we will provide some ideas of communication and language based on evidence, where possible and our clinical experience if not. These may be a starting point for

those that have no particular viewpoint or a source of reflection to those that do. We have tried to expand on, rather than just replicate content from our previous articles on this topic [1, 2]. We will refer to FND in this chapter, rather than FMD, as many principles are shared with other symptoms seen in this disorder.

Why Does It Matter How the Diagnosis Is Shared?

To some extent it should always matter, at least a little, how a diagnosis is shared. The treatment of cancer may be the same whether that conversation is handled well or badly, but the person's experience of that treatment could still vary considerably as a consequence.

What is special about FND then, that we need a whole chapter in this book to think through issues around explanation and providing information?

- *A disorder people have not heard of.* FND is typically a condition patients have not heard of from news, TV [3] or social media, although that is gradually changing.
- *A disorder with no laboratory or radiological investigations.* You can't 'see' FND on a scan. The idea of physical symptoms without a structural disease is something alien and misunderstood for many patients and health professionals, although interestingly this isn't so much of a problem for better known conditions like migraine or primary generalised epilepsy.
- *A disorder with a stigmatised past and present.* The history of FND is littered with 'trigger' words that have been shown to equate strongly with 'making it up', 'faking' or 'imagining symptoms' such as psychosomatic, hysteria or non-organic. These issues do not just affect patients' response to explanation, but perhaps more importantly, permeate negative attitudes among health professionals doing the explaining.
- *A disorder where the explanation itself may be an important first step in the treatment itself.* New forms of psychological and physical therapy for FND rely on, and indeed try to

exploit, specific features of the condition such as variability and distractibility, which are also intrinsic to the diagnosis. FMD is a disruption of voluntary movement itself in which therapy is designed to bring movements that are 'out of control', within the patient's control. Without an initial understanding of that, and the important issues of reversibility, our experience is that it is often hard for therapists to approach the disorder in this transparent way. With it, therapists tell us that they can more quickly make progress with trying to alter movement and its associated cognitions.

- *Treatment of FND is an active collaborative, rather than passive process.* The treatment of FND is generally not something that is done *to* someone, it is a rehabilitative process that occurs in collaboration with the patient. This is another reason why the patient's active engagement and agreement with the diagnosis matters.

Some of these themes overlap with the reasons why sharing this diagnosis is often perceived as so difficult, and we discuss further below.

Is There Any Evidence that Sharing the Diagnosis Matters for FND?

This is a surprisingly hard question to answer scientifically. Arguably there are basic standards of respect for an individual and provision of understandable information that form a basic template for any medical encounter and should not be open to question. Nonetheless there are several sources of information that suggest that explanation does matter.

Patients with FND Often Have Poor Experiences of Diagnostic Explanation

A qualitative study of the experiences of 11 patients with functional motor symptoms by Glenn Nielsen and colleagues shows how many patients were on a 'diagnostic odyssey' involving multiple investigations with simply presentations of normal results [4]. Even when FND was diagnosed it was often perceived to have been diagnosed in this exclusionary way:

> 'I just thought, you're putting me in a, you can't find anything specifically wrong with me. My brain MRI is clear... so it has to be a functional neurological disorder. Because we can't find anything else wrong with you", Michael, age 46 [4].

The new conception of FND views psychological factors as important common risk factors but not the sole cause. A number of studies show that patients with FND generally do not perceive themselves to have a condition in which psychological factors may be relevant. Figures for this range between 5% to 33% in neurological settings [1]. This, paradoxically is not the case for people with multiple sclerosis, 56% of whom thought that psychological factors were relevant to the cause of their condition in one study [5]. There have been similar studies showing quite high rates of stress/psychological attribution in cardiovascular disorders and cancer [6]. This was also reflected in Glenn Nielsen's study:

> "Because that's what it feels like, psychological feels like it should mean, it's literally you are making it up. It's all in your head, there's nothing wrong with you at all" Megan, age 22 [4].

Other themes that emerge from this literature in FMD, and of the more extensive literature in functional/dissociative seizures [7], are of patients being made to feel angry, ashamed or blamed for their condition. Some patients also report being made fun of whilst in emergency departments, something that also occurs between health professionals at other times [8].

In March 2020, FND Hope carried out a survey on stigma that had 503 responses (mostly from the UK and US). 82% of respondent reported being treated poorly due to stigma and 61% said they had experienced traumatization as a result of their illness journey. Emergency room physicians came out worst, with general practitioners and neurologists close behind. They also record that a high proportion of patients (around 60%) had concerns that their FND label may adversely have affected past and future care [9].

Studies of prognosis find correlations between patients with poor experiences of diagnosis and outcome [10], although it is hard to assess cause and effect.

The data suggests that in many cases, communication of the diagnosis of FND is failing to meet even a basic standard of clarity and respect for the individual which is surely a pre-requisite for treatment.

Health Professionals Think Diagnostic Explanation of FND Matters

The data we have also suggests that health professionals regard communication of the diagnosis as an important first step in treatment. Members of the Movement Disorders Society considered 'Educating the patient' to be the most important treatment for FND with 90% agreeing that it could be an effective part of treatment [11]. 'Acceptance of the diagnosis' received the greatest endorsement as a positive prognostic factor with 98% agreeing it was important.

Evidence that training health professionals to deliver better communication for FND is less forthcoming. Previous studies which taught health professionals to reattribute physical symptoms as emotional problems have not shown any benefit to patients [12, 13]. In functional seizures, it's been shown across 50 patients and 23 neurologists that a standardised communication package can lead to high acceptability and satisfaction, with the type of negative patient outcome described in the last section rare [14]. In the recent CODES trial, a standardised communication package in 698 patients with functional seizures led to a median score of 'strength in belief in the diagnosis' of 8 out of 10, where 10 is agreeing 'extremely strongly' [15]. This suggests that in research settings it is possible to produce a scenario where patients report being generally satisfied and in agreement with an FND diagnosis, although it remains to be seen whether this process can be influenced to change patient-reported outcomes.

Why Do Doctors Find It Hard to "Break the News" of FND?

Table 17.1 gives a summary of various reasons why health professionals may struggle specifically with telling someone they have FND, even if, in their last consultation they may have been able to skillfully explain to someone that they had multiple sclerosis. Studies among neurologists have shown that the more the symptoms relate to a structural disorder the less 'difficult to help' neurologists find the patient [16]. Neurologists commonly have had little exposure to psychiatry or psychiatric ways of thinking during training and often feel unprepared for this side of their practice [17]. Attempts to combine neurology and psychiatry training are generally welcomed by students but they notice how poorly integrated these areas of practice are by faculty/senior clinicians [18].

Analysis of these factors indicate that most of the difficulties originate from factors related to health professionals and societal bias, rather than issues related to the patient.

Sharing a Diagnosis of FND – Some Solutions

Many of the difficulties that doctors face when sharing a diagnosis of FND, can in our view be overcome, not by treating FND as something different or unusual in neurological practice that requires special training, but by doing precisely the *opposite* - treating it as much as possible, like any other condition in the clinic.

In order to achieve this seemingly simple objective, many clinicians need quite a radical alteration in some core views about FND (see Table 17.1) such as: considering FND to be equal validity as other neurological conditions, worrying as much about missing a diagnosis of FND as any other neurological problem and making time to share a diagnosis with a patient. One senior colleague we worked with, always kind and thorough in his demeanour, was in his late 50s when he confessed to one of us, 'I think it's taken me this long to realise that these patients really do experience the symptoms they report'.

Reaching the point where FND is treated like any other condition in a neurological setting tends to make 'breaking the news' proceed in a much more straightforward way. We have rehearsed before some core elements to this process, many of which are shared with communication for most disorders

Table 17.1 Barriers to communication of the diagnosis of functional neurological disorder (FND)

Societal barriers	Notes	Cognitions for health professionals to help overcome these issues
Stigma about FND	FND is still often considered 'not real', 'imagined' or 'faked' [19].	'I consider a functional neurological disorder just as valid a reason to have symptoms as Parkinson's disease'
Dualism – 'mind and brain are separate things'	Dualism is ingrained in our society – even in the specialities of neurology and psychiatry	'I have realised that separating disorders into those of the brain and mind is scientifically inaccurate and affecting the quality of my work'
Lack of awareness of FND	FND is poorly represented in the media [3] and in teaching	'I will try to make sure that teaching curricula and patient information resources in my service fairly represent functional neurological disorders'
Health professional barriers		
Lack of training	Health professionals often feel that they don't have sufficient training [17, 20] or interest [21] in FND.	'I want to be as skilled in the diagnosis and management of functional neurological disorders as other common areas of my practice'
Concerns about malingering	Health professionals often carry residual concerns that they may be 'duped' by some of their patients [22, 23]	'I recognise that wilful exaggeration does not provide a good explanation for the clinical problems I see in my clinic'
Concerns about misdiagnosis	Health professionals are more worried about missing other neurological conditions vs FND [24]	'I should be equally concerned about missing a diagnosis of FND as a diagnosis of other disorders'
"Root cause" bias	A tendency for clinicians to feel that in FND, as opposed to other disorders like migraine they have to be able to come up with a 'root cause' explanation early on.	'FND is usually multifactorial. I can broach the pathophysiology of the disorder in a similar way to other conditions such as migraine or Parkinson's disease by discussing mechanism first and aetiology second'
"Diagnosis of exclusion" bias	Health professionals may persist with an idea that FND is diagnosed by exclusion	'FND is not a diagnosis of exclusion and I should be careful to frame my language to avoid that impression'
Time	FND is often complex and takes time to explain properly	'I recognise that it may take time for someone to understand a diagnosis of FND'
Patient specific barriers		
Strong views of alternative diagnosis	Some patients carry strong views that their symptom must relate to a cause which is exclusively biological, and which forbids any possibility that symptoms could be improved through rehabilitation alone.	'I recognise the reasons why some people develop these strong views. I will spend time explaining why I hold my perspective, but also recognise the patient's right to hold alternative views, and that there cannot always be agreement.'

1. **Laying the groundwork during clinical assessment.** The process of explanation really begins with the assessment itself [25]. Ideally the assessment will have made the patient feel listened to, and properly understood. Why is the patient in your clinic? Most patients are usually bewildered by their symptoms and want some answers and treatment, but not always – they are sometimes there because a new doctor has encountered someone with an unexplained disability, and they think that they should see a specialist. What do they think might be wrong? If they do not know,

what is their best guess? Or perhaps their family and friends have had some views? Are there particular investigations they have been thinking might be helpful, or treatments they think should have been tried by now? Or others that shouldn't be tried again? Eliciting views like this usually requires a series of questions and may require overcoming some reluctance on the part of the patient to be forthright about what they really think.

2. **Take the problem seriously.** Its preferable if this occurs without having to say, 'I hope it goes without saying that I believe you', but

sometimes that is helpful. Indicating to the patient that what they have is not mysterious, you have seen it many times before and thousands of other people have it in your country can all help.

3. **Make it clear that there is a diagnostic label.** Some clinicians try to explain FND with a formulation but without using a diagnostic label or just indicating that 'nothing is wrong'. They worry about 'medicalising' the problem. We would argue that if someone is in a secondary care setting with a chronic movement disorder then there clearly is 'something wrong'. That patient needs a diagnostic label, to help signpost them to information for treatment, to aid communication between health professionals, and so they have a name to tell their family and employers when they need to explain what is wrong with them. While there are situations, such as transient or mild symptoms, where a formal diagnosis of a 'disorder' is not necessarily desired by the patient or helpful, if the symptoms are longer lasting and requiring treatment, a diagnostic label is likely to be helpful.

4. **Demonstrate the rationale for the diagnosis.** For us, this is one of the key elements of conveying a diagnosis of FND [26]. There ought to be positive evidence of the diagnosis, and sharing that with a patient can be a 'light bulb' moment for them and their families, to see how the diagnosis is being made on positive grounds, and why it is not just about normal investigations. Positive signs in FND do not just provide a diagnosis, they also give insight into the mechanism of the disorder and a window to potential reversibility.

   (a) For paralysis – testing Hoover's sign: 'When you are focusing on your weak leg, you can't keep your heel on the ground. I can easily lift it off. But when you are lifting up your good leg, your weak leg comes back to normal, I can't lift your heel off the ground'. Repeat the test a few times until you are sure that the patient and/or their carer has also seen it.

'What this shows is that there is a problem with voluntary movement, the more you try, I can see the worse it gets. But the automatic movements are normal. So, there is a problem with the function of the nervous system but there isn't damage'

   (b) For tremor: 'When you copy the movements, have a peek over at the other arm/leg. Can you see that the tremor stops/changes to the same rhythm? That is a positive tremor entrainment test and is good evidence this is a functional tremor. The test also shows us that there may be ways using movement therapy that we can help you get better control over the tremor.

   (c) For dystonia: 'Have a look at these photographs of other people with functional dystonia. You have the same pattern of a clenched fist/inward turning foot/platysmal contraction. There are actually very few conditions in medicine where this occurs and, in your case, it is typical of functional dystonia'.

5. **Convey the potential for improvement**

   (a) For any test involving distractibility: "The test also shows us that there may be ways using movement therapy that we can help improve/give you get better control over the tremor/weakness/walking. The test is giving us a window into what may be possible"

   (b) 'It's a bit like a problem with the software of a computer. Nothing is broken in the machine, but the computer is not working (or sometimes it seems to crash). If we can find a way to 'reprogram' the brain, then perhaps we can make it work better?'

   (c) 'But is it psychological or neurological doctor?'. If patients ask this question, our answer is that it's a disorder at the interface of neurology and psychiatry, but in reality, there is a philosophical problem with that question which is similar to asking 'is the colour orange is rough or smooth?'.

6. **Provide information**

Most people forget information from a consultation easily, and so it's worth working harder to improve retention.

Consider sharing your clinical letter with the patient [27]. We prefer to copy the letter that we send to the primary care physician so that they can see what we are saying about them. This is a way of promoting transparency and also acts a reminder of the content of the consultation.

Online sources of information such as our own www.neurosymptoms.org or websites of charities such as www.fndhope.org or www.fndaction.co.uk may be helpful. Preferably, show the patient some pages you would like them to look at, or better still, hand them a prepared factsheet relevant to their condition (Fig. 17.1).

Video is a powerful way of conveying information about FND. An increasing range of short films about FND are now available for patients – for example those found at www.fndaustralia.com (Fig. 17.2).

Do not expect information, on its own, however, to be a treatment. A recent randomised trial showed no difference in primary or secondary outcomes at 6 months in 93 patients who received internet based self-help specifically for patients with functional motor symptoms compared to 93 patients who did not [28]. Helpfully the study also showed that the material was well received by the participants and providing information is not harmful.

What Label Should Be Used?

We have explicitly not tackled here the issue of exactly *what* diagnostic label to provide – e.g. functional, psychogenic, conversion disorder. In our view a diagnostic term needs to be both

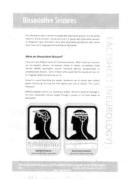

Dissociative Seizures

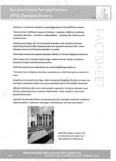

Functional Limb Weakness

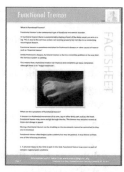

Functional Tremor

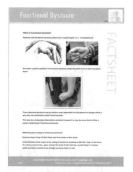

Functional Dystonia

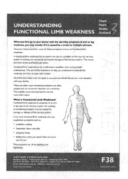

Functional Cognitive Disorder

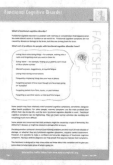

Persistent Postural Perceptual Dizziness

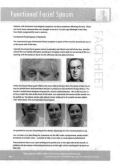

Functional Facial Spasm

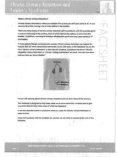

Chronic Urinary Retention

Fig. 17.1 Factsheets from www.neurosymptoms.org (Dissociative seizures from www.codestrial.org). We find it helpful to physically hand these to patients, to ensure that they definitely have the material to read. (By permission from Jon Stone)

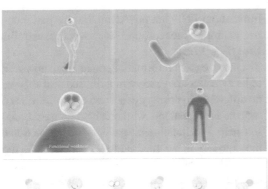
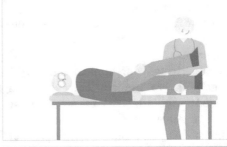
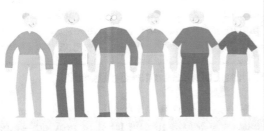
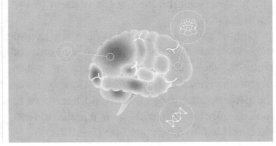
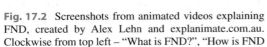

Fig. 17.2 Screenshots from animated videos explaining FND, created by Alex Lehn and explanimate.com.au. Clockwise from top left – "What is FND?", "How is FND diagnosed?", "How is FND treated?" and "What causes FND?". Available at neurosymptoms.org. (With permission from Alex Lehn at www.fndaustralia.com)

compatible with the scientific evidence for the basis of the disorder, focus on mechanism rather than aetiology, be non-dualistic and facilitate treatment [29]. We do feel strongly that it should avoid a 'non-label' such as non-organic, non-organic or medically unexplained which simply indicates a condition that is unknown. The title of this chapter (and book), indicates our personal preference for the 'least worst' term at the current time, 'functional', but we do not think it is perfect and have rehearsed the arguments for and against it, and in relation to other terms, in previous publications [1]. Increasing research in FND continually updates our models of how the disorder occurs. Both our labels and explanations need to be flexible to account for these changes.

An interesting trend recently has been to also consider whether it is reasonable to group those other 'recognised' disorders of the nervous system as 'organic'. We think it is not, which may create a linguistic challenge for some, but one that deserves to be risen to in our view [30].

Breaking the News Some More – Mechanism, Aetiology and Formulation

Being able to agree on a diagnostic label, something of what that means, and developing a relationship of mutual trust is a good start but not the end of imparting diagnostic information. The process of properly understanding FND can sometimes be a goal of treatment rather than something that can be achieved in one or even a few sessions.

Early discussion of the mechanism can be helpful in improving diagnostic confidence and understanding. Depending on the setting and level of assessment, for example, after neuropsychiatric assessment, or perhaps on a second visit to a neurologist, discussion of the formulation of the potential aetiological risk factors involved can be a helpful starting point for treatment. These issues have been explored in an article by Caitlin Adams and colleagues titled 'You've made the diagnosis of FND, what next' which we recommend [31].

Examples of exploring triggering mechanism might be:

- 'It's interesting that you had a high fever at the time this tremor came on. It could be that the shaking started with the fever, but your brain got 'stuck' in that abnormal pattern even though the fever had gone away [32].
- 'I think it's clear that you had migraine with aura that initially triggered the weakness down your right side. We know that migraine is quite a common trigger for functional limb weakness. Normally those symptoms don't last longer than 24 h, but if the experience is new or frightening, that can make the abnormal patterns stay longer and turn in to FND' [33].
- 'Physical injury and pain are common at the onset of a functional movement disorder. Its normal for the brain to activate a 'protect and immobilise' mechanism when this happens. In FND that mechanism becomes overactive and carries on even though the tissues have healed'.
- 'You had a panic attack when this started. That produced some shaking and also that "zoned out/out of body" feeling called dissociation. It was the combination of all these things, and probably all the stress you've told me about before that led to the changes in your brain producing FND. You were having a complete 'out of body' experience but only half of your body came back properly under your control'.

It can also be helpful to find ways to translate neuroscience of FND into explanations that hopefully patients can grasp. Examples of such statements include:

- For many FMD presentations: "We think in FND that the brain is working too hard on movement. Movement is meant to be automatic. In FND the brain has got into a habit of thinking really hard about it. The more the brain tries to actively control it, the worse it gets. It's a bit like trying really hard to go to sleep – the more you try the less you can sleep".
- For many FMD presentations: "The experiences you mentioned in the past and all the stress you've been under may have put your brain in a more vulnerable situation for these kinds of abnormal pathways to get 'stuck'".

- For functional limb weakness: "Have you heard of phantom limb syndrome? That's when someone loses a limb, but their brain still thinks it's there. The map of the limb in the brain is still intact. In FND its often the opposite. The brain thinks the limb has gone, even though it's still there." From a neuroscience perspective, using predictive processing models of the brain, both disorders involve a failure to update 'top down' models of the body with 'bottom up' sensory input.
- For functional dystonia: "To reduce pain or horrible sensations, the brain can try to 'lose' the map of the limb so that it doesn't feel part of the person anymore. The problem is that this doesn't work properly and the patient with FND is left with a limb which they can't move or feel properly but is still really painful."
- For functional dystonia: "When these maps of the arms or legs become distorted the limbs revert to a 'primitive' reflex protective position"
- For functional dystonia: "What position does your ankle feel in when you close your eyes?" If the patient says it feels straight, then 'Your brain thinks this is the normal position now – we are going to have retrain it to learn that it isn't' [34].
- For functional jerks: We recommend exploring whether patients experience a transient 'build up' just before a jerk, a bit like a sneeze. This is often not present and also occurs in straightforward tics. If it is present however, ask if *is it transiently relieved for a second or two by the jerk?* If it is, then you have the beginnings of a mechanistic explanation of why their brain has got into a habit of producing this movement. It's trying to do something useful- just not in a very useful way.
- For tremor: 'Functional tremor happens when your brain gets into a habit of making your limb shake'. You can explore similar ideas of whether something bad 'builds up' if they try to suppress the tremor or hold down the limb, or whether it feels more 'normal' to shake.

Formulation describes the process of synthesising all the available information from the clinical assessment into a framework that seeks to explain not only the causes and mechanism of the symptoms, but also the factors that may need to be focused on to make progress with treatment.

All health professionals, including neurologists, can potentially benefit from incorporating an appropriate degree of formulation into their clinical practice. This is especially important when addressing comorbid symptoms and diagnosis in FND, which are almost universal, for example:

- For pain: "We know now that chronic pain occurs through a similar process of abnormal nervous system functioning. 'Volume knobs' in pain pathways have become turned up throughout the nervous system... have you seen these resources on chronic pain – for example www.tamethebeast.com".
- For memory and concentration symptoms: "I would expect you to have these memory symptoms, given your description of sleep disturbance and fatigue. They are a consequence of your brain's concentration systems not working properly".

A complete diagnostic biopsychosocial formulation can be undertaken by a psychiatrist, psychologist and/or social worker and is an extended form of diagnostic explanation.

Should I Discuss the Potential Role of Psychological Factors in the First Consultation?

Exploring the full range of aetiological factors in someone with FND clearly follows on from these kinds of discussions, and a discussion of all of them is out with the scope of this chapter. The reader will notice that we have not strongly emphasised discussion of adverse experiences, when relevant, in this discussion of an *initial process* of 'breaking the news'.

This is because, in our experience, such discussions can often wait, and indeed are often more fruitful if the topic has been introduced by the patient themself, and at a pace and content

that they are comfortable with. The problem here, is a tendency, especially among health professionals such as the neurologist who may not be trained, or planning to actually explore a formulation with a patient, to want to explain what they perceive to be a 'root cause' as soon as possible, to 'wrap up' up the case. Such 'root cause bias' has been especially encouraged by Freudian conversion disorder theory and provides a simplistic and appealing solution to a problem that is much more complex. "If only the problem could be unlocked then everything will be better". This bias has links back to confessional and religious transactions, with the clinician taking on the role of 'saviour' and the emphasis on past 'sins'.

For a physician, resisting the temptation for some amateur psychiatry can be hard, but can pay dividends. It allows the clinician to keep an open mind about all the possible risk factors and reduces the risk of alienating the patient. A health professional who pushes hard on psychological causes may not realise that as an 'authority' figure attributing blame to adverse experiences, they may be re-enacting feelings of accusation and blame that are actually part of the adverse experience itself, and can be retraumatising. Often making links between traumatic events and FND, when that is relevant, is a goal of therapy, and not something that should be forced on a patient at an initial consultation.

There are patients who clearly present with, and want to discuss, potential psychological risk factors. In that, less common, scenario it is clearly much more straightforward to do so. Even then, it is often important, as in Clinical Vignette 2 at the beginning of this chapter to emphasise that the presence of adverse experience, while important and potentially relevant for treatment, has not been influential in *making the diagnosis*. This distinction is often important for patients who feel repeatedly labelled as 'neurotic' and that their physical symptoms are not eliciting careful enough evaluation as a consequence.

Ultimately stress and psychological factors are of key importance in many patients with FND, but in the same way that smoking is of key importance for many people with heart disease.

It's important but not relevant for everyone, and there are plenty of other reasons for developing FND within the framework of an aetiological model (See **Chap. 3** for additional details).

Using a Follow Up Visit to Assist Triage

A follow up visit, or at least giving the patient some time to digest information, is really helpful, in our view, to learn whether the communication strategies you are using are working in the way you want them to, and often the best time to judge whether to move forward with therapy.

One of the commonest pitfalls in initial management we see is the scenario where a neurologist has explained and documented their diagnosis and then cannot understand why treatment is not proceeding as expected. Management of FND should be collaborative between health professional and patient. We need to find out how receptive the patient and their family is to the diagnosis before we can move forward with referral.

Two key things to find out at the end of the consultation or a follow up visit are:

1. The patient's degree of confidence and agreement with the diagnosis? and
2. The extent to which, now is the right time for change with rehabilitation?

You might start by asking the patient to repeat back some of their understanding of their condition – its name and roughly what has gone wrong. Did they receive a copy of the clinic note/letter? Did they think it was a fair summary? Were there things that were omitted or were not correct? Perhaps they didn't read it?

Sometimes this process allows the doctor to appreciate that a substantial change has occurred in the patient's cognitions. They do feel listened to, and that someone has finally made the correct diagnosis (Fig. 17.3).

On the other hand, it's not easy for patients to say to a doctor, 'you've been very helpful, but I'm really not at all confident that you've made the right diagnosis', or alternatively 'I do think that's right, but I really have too much going on at the moment to contemplate embarking on the kind of treatment you are talking about'. Try asking the patient to rate their scores for the two questions above from 0-10, and to overcome response bias, perhaps suggest an initial low number to make it easier for the patient to express ideas that they may be reluctant to give you.

Be careful in how you interpret responses. If the patient cannot give you a high score that might reflect general confusion about their health, or confidence that treatment can help, rather than confidence in your diagnosis. If they do not feel it is the right time for treatment make sure that this is not just a consequence of phobic avoidance by

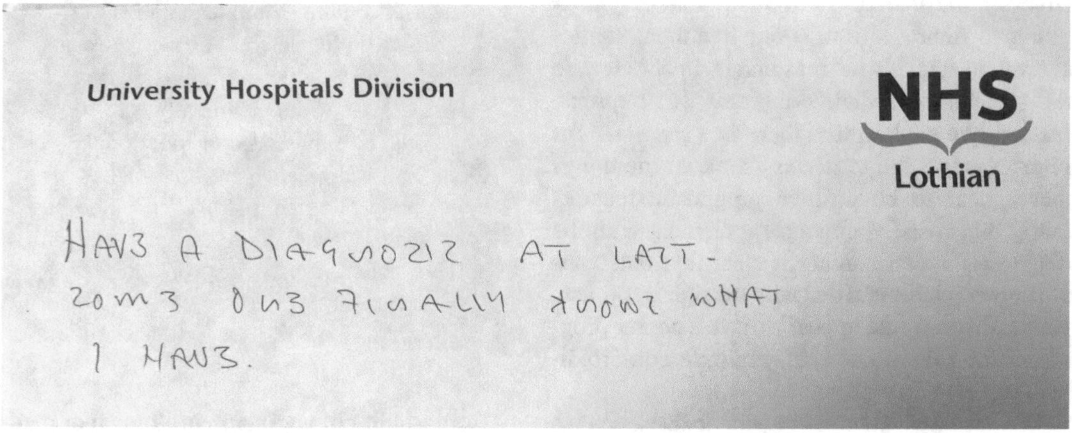

Fig. 17.3 A patient with FND who could not speak and had a functional writing disorder giving feedback at their second appointment. (By permission from Jon Stone)

exploring the reasons why they do not want to embark on it. Avoidance may have become an important comorbidity in their presentation and something that needs to be addressed as part of treatment.

Whilst most patients are keen for treatment, for some it is a relief to have these frank conversations, and it can spare therapist time for patients.

What Should Be Said About Prognosis?

As with any condition, people with FMD want to know what their outlook is. Will they remain disabled? Could things get worse? Studies of prognosis of FMD show that a wide range of outcomes are possible, and also that its hard, even at a group level to predict outcome using baseline variables. A systematic review of prognosis in 10,491 patients across 24 studies found that on average 39% were the same or worse at follow up after 7 years, which, looked at another way, suggests that the majority improved at least a bit [35]. In a 14 year study of 76 patients with functional limb weakness, the symptom had only remitted completely in 20% of patients [36].

Some health professionals present a relentless optimistic prognostic view to patients with FMD on the grounds that a gloomy outlook may adversely affect outcome but again, we would advocate transparency. FMD is not an easy condition to improve from – our treatment studies show that – and it's not reasonable, in our view, to tell a patient that their symptoms *will* improve. Instead, we explain that there is a *potential* for improvement, and to discuss some of the things that appear to be positive prognostic features (early diagnosis, young age, agreement with the diagnosis) whilst making it clear that outcomes are unpredictable and that with the right approach, patients who would appear to have a poorer prognosis (long duration, pain, multiple comorbidities) can also do well.

It's usually helpful in our experience to explain, *in advance*, that FMD is usually a relaps-

ing disorder, and that in people who do improve, that improvement often occurs via a series of relapses, rather than a linear trajectory, with improving self-management over time.

Clinicians should especially avoid blaming people with FMD for not improving. Such outcomes are unfortunately common, even when a patient agrees with the diagnosis and is motivated for change. In that scenario we would 'leave the door open' for change in the future, something that can occur in FMD unlike for example advanced multiple sclerosis.

Difficult Communication Encounters in FND

With all of the barriers to communication described earlier in this chapter it's not surprising that FND has more than its fair share of challenging communication encounters. Here are some with examples:

Case 1: The Patient with a Combination of Another Neurological Condition and FND

A 42-year-old woman presents with Multiple Sclerosis which is clinically definite based on McDonald diagnostic criteria. However, her lesion burden is low and there has been little radiological progression over 10 years. Clinically she has a functional hemiparesis and functional dystonia, and it appears that most of her disability may be arising from FND. She has been really upset at the suggestion from another doctor that her disability was 'psychological'.

Comorbidity of another neurological or medical condition is one the strongest risk factors for FND [37], so it's important to know how to handle dual diagnosis. In fact, it can be discussed straightforwardly. The patient has two conditions – one of which, FND, may be potentially more reversible, or have different treatments compared to the other one, in this case MS. Often patients feel threatened that you want to remove their existing diagnosis, which may have become part of their identity over a long period. Diagnosing FND in MS should be no different to diagnosing migraine or anxiety in MS, also potentially treatable comorbid conditions.

Case 2. The Patient with Fixed Ideas of Alternative Diagnosis

A 35-year-old man presents with fatigue, tremor, jerking and widespread pain. He is convinced that he has chronic Lyme disease. There was no definite tick bite, rash or acute Lyme syndrome and the local serology test for Borrelia was negative, but he sent the sample to a private lab who told him that he had a chronic infection. Another doctor has suggested that he have further long-term antibiotics. He has rejected your diagnosis of FND despite a patient explanation of the rationale.

There are many powerful factors listed in Table 17.1 which might drive patients away from a diagnosis of FND. In addition, there are many places both in standard health services, but perhaps especially in the private sector, where patients can obtain alternative diagnoses which will often be more appealing to them than FND. It is not possible to persuade every patient that their diagnosis is correct. For those running an FND service it is important to know when to 'agree to disagree', respect the right of a patient to hold a different view and move on. At the same time, if a clinician is never 'uncertain' or sometimes wrong in your diagnoses, then there is something wrong there too.

Case 3. The Patient in a Medicolegal Case

A 42-year-old man is seen for a personal injury medicolegal report with a diagnosis of functional hand dystonia. You had been asked to potentially assist with treatment. The solicitor sends a video showing evidence of wilful exaggeration. The patient was able to use his hand normally to play video games at a time when he said he had not been able to do so for 6 months.

Wilful exaggeration does occur throughout medicine and sometimes with FND presentations. It is rare to obtain evidence of lying, or a major discrepancy between reported and observed function, in routine clinical practice. If such evidence does emerge then it may no longer be possible to make a diagnosis. Often this signals the end of treatment, although in some cases, open discussion of falsification, for example in factitious disorder, which should be regarded as a separate diagnosis to FND, may be part of treatment.

Case 4. The Angry Family Member/ Friend

A 37-year-old woman has a diagnosis of FND including hemiparesis and functional seizures. She agrees with the diagnosis and is keen for treatment. Her husband, however, considers the diagnosis to be wrong and insists that she should have a further opinion elsewhere.

In this scenario it may be helpful to take a step back and ask him to expand on why he thinks it is wrong diagnosis, and more importantly what would it take for him to agree it was correct? Has the husband been at key previous consultations and perhaps missed some of that material? This may move the discussion from an antagonistic "you against him", to shared problem of "I've failed to adequately explain the diagnosis to you so help me understand exactly what it would take". In such situations it is seldom the 'medical' answer that is the main issue, for example, proving that the seizure was captured on videotelemetry. In one recent case the solution involved exploring a previous difficult encounter with a health professional and reviewing the husband's own video recordings that had led him to doubt the diagnosis.

Case 5. The FND Patient with Intellectual Disability

A 26-year-old man with moderate intellectual disability presents with functional arm tremor associated with mobility issues. He cannot read or write. His carers accompany him to the clinic appointment.

Explanations can follow along similar lines. Where complexity is an issue for the patient then it can be helpful to enlist the aid of carers so that they understand it, and can reinforce messages later in a way that the patient can understand.

Case 6. The Patient with FND who is Unlikely to Improve

A 62-year-old man presents with a 30-year history of being in a wheelchair after an industrial accident. He had been admitted to hospital with pneumonia and his admitting team thought he should have a neurological assessment. He states that he had a broken back and a stroke but in fact there is evidence for neither and the problem is clinically mainly one of FND with chronic pain. He has carers four times a day and has been noted to have dependent personality traits.

It is not possible to help all patients with FND. After 30 years and with this scenario it is unlikely that treatment is likely to make a substantial difference to this person's independence. Improvements can occur after long periods, even in people where it would seem unlikely. However, those scenarios often involve catching patients at the 'right time' in their life when obstacles to rehabilitation have reduced. So, it would be worth probing a little to see if improvement could be on the cards. There is no reason why explanation of the FND could not proceed in the same way, but it may not be appropriate to spend so long on the potential for reversibility if treatment is not going to be helpful.

Box: Resources for FND Diagnostic Explanation Training

- Carson A, Lehn A, Ludwig L, Stone J. Explaining functional disorders in the neurology clinic: a photo story. Pract Neurol. 2016;16:56–61.
- Stone J, Hoeritzauer I. How Do I Explain the Diagnosis of Functional Movement Disorder to a Patient? Mov Disord Clin Pract. 2019; 6:419–419. This 'video article' goes through some of the principles in this chapter.
- **www.neurosymptoms.org, www.fnd-hope.org, www.fndaction.org.uk** – websites for patients with FND written by the author, and by patients and carers with ideas about how to talk about FND.
- Twitter accounts: @FNDportal, @FNDrecovery – two twitter accounts exemplifying the new 'patient voice' in FND which can help orientate health professionals towards constructive communication.
- FND Society – www.fndsociety.org. Society resources include webinars dealing with communication skills and health professional training.

Summary

- Sharing a diagnosis of FND well appears to be an important prerequisite for treatment and can have some therapeutic benefit itself.
- There are barriers to good communication, but these largely reside with health professional and societal attitudes and are rarely related specifically to the patient.
- Core elements of diagnostic explanation are the same for FND as for any other condition, indeed the process may work better if it is not regarded as 'different' or 'special'.
- Supplementing explanation with written or online information is appreciated by patients and important to do but is probably not a treatment by itself.
- Seeing the patient again allows you to improve communication skills and is a good time to consider triage for treatment.

References

1. Stone J, Carson A, Hallett M. Explanation as treatment for functional neurologic disorders. In: Handbook of Clinical Neurology: Functional Neurologic Disorders; 2016. p. 543–53.
2. Stone J, Hoeritzauer I. How do I explain the diagnosis of functional movement disorder to a patient? Mov Disord Clin Pract. 2019;6:419.
3. Popkirov S, Nicholson TR, Bloem BR, et al. Hiding in plain sight: functional neurological disorders in the news. J Neuropsychiatry Clin Neurosci. 2019;31:361–7.
4. Nielsen G, Buszewicz M, Edwards MJ, Stevenson F. A qualitative study of the experiences and perceptions of patients with functional motor disorder. Disabil Rehabil. 2019;8288:1–6.
5. Stone J, Warlow C, Sharpe M. The symptom of functional weakness: a controlled study of 107 patients. Brain. 2010;133:1537–51.
6. Keynejad RC, Frodl T, Kanaan R, Pariante C, Reuber M, Nicholson TR. Stress and functional neurological disorders: mechanistic insights. J Neurol Neurosurg Psychiatry. 2019;90(7):813–21.
7. Rawlings GH, Reuber M. What patients say about living with psychogenic nonepileptic seizures: a systematic synthesis of qualitative studies. Seizure. 2016;41:100–11.
8. Tolchin B, Baslet G, Dworetzky B. Psychogenic seizures and medical humor: Jokes as a damaging defense. Epilepsy Behav. 2016;64:26–8.
9. Hope F. FND hope stigma survey. 2020. https://fnd-hope.org/fnd-hope-research/. Accessed 22 Sept 2020.
10. Carton S, Thompson PJ, Duncan JS. Non-epileptic seizures: patients' understanding and reaction to the diagnosis and impact on outcome. Seizure. 2003;12:287–94.
11. LaFaver K, Lang AE, Stone J, et al. Opinions and clinical practices related to diagnosing and managing functional (psychogenic) movement disorders: changes in the last decade. Eur J Neurol. 2020;27:975–84.
12. Morriss R, Dowrick C, Salmon P, et al. Cluster randomised controlled trial of training practices in reattribution for medically unexplained symptoms. Br J Psychiatry. 2007;191:536–42.
13. Weiland A, Blankenstein AH, Van Saase JLCM, et al. Training medical specialists in communication about medically unexplained physical symptoms: patient outcomes from a randomized controlled trial. Int J Pers Cent Med. 2016;6:50–60.
14. Hall-Patch L, Brown R, House A, et al. Acceptability and effectiveness of a strategy for the communication of the diagnosis of psychogenic nonepileptic seizures. Epilepsia. 2010;51:70–8.
15. Stone J, Callaghan H, Robinson EJ, et al. Predicting first attendance at psychiatry appointments in patients with dissociative seizures. Seizure. 2020;74:93–8.
16. Carson AJ, Stone J, Warlow C, Sharpe M. Patients whom neurologists find difficult to help. J Neurol Neurosurg Psychiatry. 2004;75:1776.
17. Juul D, Gutmann L, Adams HP, O'Shea SA, Faulkner LR. Training in neurology: feedback from graduates about the psychiatry component of residency training. Neurology. 2021; 96:233–36.
18. Mowchun JJ, Frew JR, Shoop GH. Education research: a qualitative study on student perceptions of neurology and psychiatry clerkship integration. Neurology. 2021;96:472–77.
19. Stone J, Colyer M, Feltbower S, Carson A, Sharpe M. "Psychosomatic": a systematic review of its meaning in newspaper articles. Psychosomatics. 2004;45:287–90.
20. Lehn A, Bullock-Saxton J, Newcombe P, Carson A, Stone J. Survey of the perceptions of health practitioners regarding Functional Neurological Disorders in Australia. J Clin Neurosci. 2019;67:114–23.
21. Evans RW, Evans RE. A survey of neurologists on the likeability of headaches and other neurological disorders. Headache. 2010;50:1126–9.
22. Kanaan R, Armstrong D, Barnes P, Wessely S. In the psychiatrist's chair: how neurologists understand conversion disorder. Brain. 2009;132:2889–96.

23. Ahern L, Stone J, Sharpe MC. Attitudes of neuroscience nurses toward patients with conversion symptoms. Psychosomatics. 2009;50:336–9.

24. Friedman JH, LaFrance WC. Psychogenic disorders: the need to speak plainly. Arch Neurol. 2010;67:753–5.

25. Stone J. Functional neurological disorders: the neurological assessment as treatment. Pract Neurol. 2016;16:7–17.

26. Stone J, Edwards M. Trick or treat? Showing patients with functional (psychogenic) motor symptoms their physical signs. Neurology. 2012;79:282–4.

27. Parry AM, Murray B, Hart Y, Bass C. Audit of resource use in patients with non-organic disorders admitted to a UK neurology unit. J Neurol Neurosurg Psychiatry. 2006;77:1200–1.

28. Gelauff JM, Rosmalen JGM, Carson A, et al. Internet-based self-help randomized trial for motor functional neurologic disorder (SHIFT). Neurology. 2020;95:e1883–96.

29. Creed F, Guthrie E, Fink P, et al. Is there a better term than 'medically unexplained symptoms'? J Psychosom Res. 2010;68:5–8.

30. Stone J, Carson A. 'Organic' and 'non-organic': a tale of two turnips. Pract Neurol. 2017;17:417–8.

31. Adams C, Anderson J, Madva EN, LaFrance WC Jr, Perez DL. You've made the diagnosis of functional neurological disorder: now what? Pract Neurol. 2018;18:323–30.

32. Pareés I, Kojovic M, Pires C, et al. Physical precipitating factors in functional movement disorders. J Neurol Sci. 2014;338:174–7.

33. Stone J, Evans RW. Functional/psychogenic neurological symptoms and headache. Headache J Head Face Pain. 2011;51:781–8.

34. Stone J, Gelauff J, Carson A. A 'twist in the tale': altered perception of ankle position in psychogenic dystonia. Mov Disord. 2012;27:585–6.

35. Gelauff J, Stone J, Edwards M, Carson A. The prognosis of functional (psychogenic) motor symptoms: a systematic review. J Neurol Neurosurg Psychiatry. 2014;85:220–6.

36. Gelauff JM, Carson A, Ludwig L, Tijssen MAJ, Stone J. The prognosis of functional limb weakness: a 14-year case-control study. Brain. 2019;142:2137–48.

37. Wissel BD, Dwivedi AK, Merola A, et al. Functional neurological disorders in Parkinson disease. J Neurol Neurosurg Psychiatry. 2018;89:566–71.

Benjamin Tolchin and Steve Martino

Illustrative Vignette

Ms. C, aged 41, had presented to Dr. Diaz with a progressively worsening dystonic gait and tremor, which rendered her unable to walk without a walker or to work outside her home. Dr. Diaz had diagnosed Ms. C with a functional movement disorder (FMD) and referred her to a combined physical therapy and psychotherapy program at a center specializing in the treatment of FND. At follow-up in Dr. Diaz's office 3 months later, Ms. C had not yet scheduled an appointment with her physical therapist or psychotherapist.

Dr. Diaz again reviewed the diagnosis of FMD and proposed a physical therapy and psychotherapeutic treatment plan. However, Ms. C was unable to concentrate on the neurologist's words. "I've got a terrible headache. I… I… hear glass breaking". She fumbled to retrieve and open a bottle of acetaminophen from her purse. As Dr.

Diaz tried to explain the treatment plan, Ms. C's symptoms persisted, and she remained focused on the bottle of acetaminophen.

Recognizing that Ms. C's difficulty in concentrating might signify ambivalence about the diagnosis of FMD and the treatment plan, Dr. Diaz decided to use motivational interviewing (MI) to explore and resolve this ambivalence and to enhance Ms. C's engagement with physical therapy and psychotherapy. Dr. Diaz offered MI not as treatment for Ms. C's FMD, but rather as an opportunity for Ms. C to discuss the impact of the disorder on her life, to explore her own reasons for seeking treatment, and to take ownership of plans for therapy. Dr. Diaz asked Ms. C how her tremor and gait difficulties affected her life. "Well, my mom and dad have to watch me all the time in case I fall. They're both getting old and my dad is out of breath a lot". Dr. Diaz responded: "Because of your functional movement disorder, your parents have to provide care for you, when you feel that you should be providing care for them in their old age". This was an MI technique of "complex reflection," in which the interviewer explicitly states ideas implied by the patient.

Ms. C became much more actively engaged in the conversation and eagerly explained that her movements left her unable to work or drive, and dependent on her parents for money, shelter, and transportation. She discussed her parents' growing frailty and her own feelings of guilt that she was not caring for them and was burdening them

B. Tolchin (✉)
Comprehensive Epilepsy Center, Department of Neurology, Yale University School of Medicine, New Haven, CT, USA

Epilepsy Center of Excellence, Neurology Service, VA Connecticut Healthcare System, West Haven, CT, USA
e-mail: benjamin.tolchin@yale.edu

S. Martino
Department of Psychiatry, Yale University School of Medicine, New Haven, CT, USA

Psychology Service, VA Connecticut Healthcare System, West Haven, CT, USA in their old age. Dr. Diaz responded, "it sounds like your parents give you a lot of care and attention around the movements, which you greatly appreciate, and you worry that this is burdensome to them at a time when they really need your help". This reflection of the patient's words is "double-sided" in that it emphasizes Ms. C's self-stated reasons for behavior change, while also acknowledging with less emphasis the parental affection and assistance that Ms. C was receiving because of her FMD. Her headache and tinnitus did not manifest during this conversation.

At this juncture, Dr. Diaz summarized Ms. C's expressed need to eliminate the FMD in order to care for her parents and asked her about what steps she might take to meet this need (a "key question" or attempted transition from evoking change talk to planning for change). Ms. C immediately clutched her head and reported again the sound of breaking glass. This response potentially communicated her insufficient readiness to begin planning. Dr. Diaz backtracked and reflected again Ms. C's description of the impact of the FMD on her parents and her life. With this move away from concrete planning, the symptoms of headache and tinnitus again resolved, and Ms. C could re-engage in the conversation. Later in the visit, with Ms. C's permission, Dr. Diaz returned to the planning process, this time focusing on a specific, measurable, achievable, relevant, and time-limited (SMART) goal of trying an initial session of physical therapy and an initial session of psychotherapy within the next 2 weeks. Dr. Diaz introduced this goal using an ask-tell-ask structure, in which Dr. Diaz asked the patient's permission to offer a suggestion, then described the physical therapy and psychotherapy options and potential benefits as reported by other patients with FMD, and then asked for the patient's thoughts on that suggestion. When reframed in this way, Ms. C was able to embrace a time-limited trial of mindfulness-based psychotherapy as her own plan for treatment of her FMD.

Following MI, Ms. C attended both a physical therapy and mindfulness-based psychotherapy session and at that point agreed to participate in weekly sessions of both treatment modalities. In fact, Ms. C canceled, rescheduled, or no-showed nearly half of her weekly sessions. Nonetheless, after 4 months of physical therapy and psychotherapy Ms. C was able to walk reliably without a walker or cane and became a volunteer at an animal shelter – her first work outside the home in 4 years.

Introduction

Patients with functional movement disorder (FMD) and other functional neurological disorder (FND) subtypes can benefit from specific therapies, particularly psychotherapies and physical therapy, but often struggle to engage in and adhere to treatment, especially over long durations [1, 2]. Poor clinician training in FND and communication techniques resulting in suboptimal explanations of FND, intense stigma, and patients' own ambivalence about the diagnosis may all contribute to poor and gradually declining adherence and engagement. Helping patients with FMD to implement and sustain psychotherapy and physical therapy is critical for improving their treatment outcomes and quality of life. While treatment adherence for chronic illness involves many factors, such as patient demographics, treatment complexity and side effects, and availability of social and environmental supports [3], an important strategy to promote adherence is to activate the patients' motivation to self-manage their disorder [4].

This chapter describes an approach for enhancing patients' motivation for change called motivational interviewing (MI). MI increasingly is being used in health care settings to counsel patients with chronic diseases, including FND [5, 6]. The chapter reviews the theoretical reasons and evidence to support the use of MI for improving self-management and treatment adherence among patients with FND, and gives an overview of the basic principles and techniques of MI, concluding with recommendations for learning MI.

Empirical Support

Several systematic reviews and meta-analyses have examined the large body of MI research to determine *if MI works* across a wide range of problem areas (e.g. diet/exercise, treatment adherence/engagement, blood pressure, weight loss, smoking and substance use, and physical activity) [7–10]. A systematic review of 104 narrative reviews and meta-analyses of MI treatment outcome studies suggests that the evidence for beneficial effects of MI is strongest for reducing binge drinking, frequency and quantity of alcohol consumption, smoking and substance abuse and for increasing physical activity in people with chronic health conditions [11]. MI also has shown effectiveness in enhancing treatment attendance [12]. Treatment effects for MI usually occur with brief intervention. For example, a meta-analysis examining the application of MI in primary care found MI to be useful in promoting health-related behavior change in as little as one session [11]. Additionally, Lundhal and colleagues examined 119 studies and found MI to successfully produce behavior change, but in less time, compared to other behavioral interventions [8].

The effectiveness of MI delivery systems outside of face-to-face interactions have also demonstrated effectiveness. Studies have demonstrated the acceptability and feasibility of computer and web-based platforms [13, 14]. There has been some success with computer-based MI interventions for adults related to initiating substance use treatment after a 2-month follow-up, and also related to weekly minutes of moderate and vigorous physical activity [15, 16]. Randomized trials related to postpartum substance use have demonstrated efficacy and acceptability of electronic "screening, brief intervention and referral to treatment" (SBIRT) models that utilize MI [17, 18]. Other studies have also found equivalence between electronic SBIRT and clinician-delivered SBIRT models where both included similar MI components [19].

MI is also effective for changing health behaviors across the developmental lifespan. A meta-analysis focused on adolescent health behaviors (such as risky sexual behavior, physical activity and diet), demonstrated short-term post-intervention effects that were maintained, on average, 8 months after the intervention concluded [20]. Among middle aged and older adults, MI has demonstrated effectiveness in reducing episodes of unprotected sex following a 4 session, telephone-delivered MI intervention [21]. Health promotion and disease prevention efforts among older adults are also benefitted by MI, particularly with increasing fruit and vegetable consumption, physical activity, and glycemic control [22].

Studies examining *how MI works* have supported the underlying theory of MI. Miller and Rose provide a helpful summary of this literature [23]. In brief, these studies have shown that providers who adhered to MI, in contrast to those who did not, were more likely to have patients who became more motivated to change and, in turn, had improved treatment outcomes (e.g., reducing drinking, meeting dietary goals, increasing activity level) [24–27]. A meta-analysis of MI process studies found that when providers use a higher proportion of MI consistent strategies, their actions are likely to result in patients who use proportionally more change than sustain talk [28]. Higher proportion change talk, in turn, was related to reductions in risk behaviors at follow-up. MI inconsistent behaviors were correlated with more sustain talk. Independent of other effects, more sustain talk was associated with worse outcomes. This meta-analysis suggests that MI works well when providers perform it well (i.e., with adherence to its principles and strategies). Getting enough training and supervision to learn MI is imperative (see section on Learning Motivational Interviewing below).

Furthermore, nuances in the frequency and movement in change talk (i.e. towards change, away from change) appear to impact clinical outcomes. One study found that ending treatment sessions when in a "towards change" position resulted in less alcohol consumption per week when compared to sessions that ended with "away from change" [29]. Most notably, Glynn and Moyers employed an applied behavior analysis design to intentionally increase or decrease the amount of change talk, with success [30]. This finding suggested that even within the absence of other MI skills, evoking change talk specifically may be a critical strategy for any behavior change intervention.

Applications in Functional Movement Disorder

Ambivalence, non-adherence, and non-engagement with treatment have been noted as obstacles to treatment in FND, including both FMD and functional seizures (also known as psychogenic nonepileptic seizures) [1, 2]. In patients with functional seizures, non-adherence with psychotherapy is associated with higher functional seizure frequency, worse quality of life, and greater emergency department utilization at 12–24 month follow-up following diagnosis [31]. The benefits of MI for patient populations ambivalent about treatment attendance has informed the clinical use and study of MI in the treatment of patients with FND [11].

Although MI has not yet been studied in the treatment of FMD, there is preliminary evidence it is effective in enhancing adherence with psychotherapy and other treatments among populations with high levels of non-adherence, including among patients with FND. A single center trial randomized 60 participants with functional seizures either to receive a single session of MI from a neurologist in a multidisciplinary FND clinic prior to referral to psychotherapy (29 participants) or to be referred directly to psychotherapy (31 participants) [5]. The two study arms were well matched in terms of demographic characteristics, psychiatric comorbidities, and FND characteristics. In the study, MI targeted a behavior change of increased engagement with subsequent psychotherapy. Participants randomized to receive MI prior to psychotherapy had better adherence with psychotherapy, a greater reduction in functional seizure frequency, and a greater improvement in quality of life at 16-week follow-up. The absolute risk reduction in probability of non-adher-

ence was 34% and the number needed to treat with MI, to convert one participant from non-adherent with psychotherapy to adherent with psychotherapy was 2.9. Participants randomized to receive MI experienced a 76% reduction in functional seizure frequency at 16-week follow-up, as compared to a 35% reduction in functional seizure frequency in the control arm, with a Cohen's d of 0.59 (medium effect size). Participants randomized to receive MI experienced a 7-point improvement on a 40-point quality of life scale, compared to a 2-point improvement on the same scale in the control arm, with a Cohen's d of 0.60 (medium effect size). These findings are consistent with prior studies demonstrating improved treatment adherence and outcomes when MI is used to enhance adherence with psychotherapy and medical therapies in other patient populations [32, 33].

Common obstacles encountered in providing MI to patients with FND include somatic symptoms distracting from clinician-patient communication, patient ambivalence about making concrete plans for treatment, and frequent psychiatric comorbidities [6]. Strategies for overcoming these obstacles include the use of complex reflections to enhance patient engagement, the use of an ask-tell-ask format to convey information, close collaboration between neurology and psychotherapy teams, and specific, measurable, achievable, relevant, and time-limited (SMART) goals to facilitate treatment planning. Further research is needed to examine the efficacy of MI in enhancing adherence and engagement with treatment among patients with FMD and to identify obstacles and facilitators to MI in this specific patient population.

What Is Motivational Interviewing?

Miller and Rollnick define MI as "a collaborative, goal-oriented style of communication with particular attention to the language of change. It is designed to strengthen personal motivation for the commitment to a specific goal by eliciting and exploring the person's own reasons for change within an atmosphere of acceptance and compassion" [34]. The approach is grounded in humanistic psychology, especially the work of Carl Rogers, in that it employs a very empathic, non-judgmental style of interacting with patients and presumes that the potential for change lies within everyone [35]. MI is distinct from nondirective approaches, however, in that providers intentionally attend to and selectively reinforce patients' motives that support change [34]. The elements of (1) partnering with patients, (2) non-judgmentally accepting their stance, (3) showing compassion, and (4) evoking the patients' own arguments for change collectively represent the spirit of MI. Over the course of the interview, providers help patients identify change-oriented motives, elaborate upon them, and resolve ambivalence about change. If successful, patients become more likely to commit to changing their behaviors and initiating a change plan.

MI is best construed as a "conversation about change" that is designed to strengthen personal motivation and commitment to change [34]. In this regard, MI often is discussed within the context of the Stages of Change model by James Prochaska and Carlo DiClemente [36]. The Stages of Change model posits that behavior change occurs sequentially across recurring stages. The earlier stages include precontemplation (patients are unaware or do not believe there is a problem or need to change it), contemplation (patients are ambivalent about recognizing a problem and shy away from changing it), and preparation (patients are ready to work toward behavior change in the near future and develop a plan for change). The later stages include action (patients consistently make specific changes) and maintenance (patients work to maintain and sustain long-lasting change). Tailoring treatment strategies to achieve stage-related tasks is a hallmark of this model (e.g., conducting a cost-benefit analysis for someone contemplating change). MI naturally fits into the Stage of Change model in that it can be used to help move patients from one stage to another, especially in the early stages of the model.

MI emerged out of early efforts to establish brief interventions for alcohol problems [12].

These interventions shared a harm reduction approach in that they aimed to help patients move toward reduced drinking to lower risks rather than to automatically advocate for total abstinence as the only acceptable goal. As applied to the management of FMD, the harm reduction stance of MI implies that the aim of MI is to help patients prepare themselves to make changes in any behaviors that might positively impact their FMD. While patients with FMD do not exercise conscious control over their disordered movements, MI has the potential to enhance engagement with therapeutic interventions, such as psychotherapies and physical therapy. Determining what areas matter most to them (e.g. regaining mobility, being able to care for their children), which areas they believe they can change (e.g. participating in physical therapy, exercising regularly), and what goal to achieve (e.g. walking for 30 min every day for 2 weeks) is more important than pushing them to commit to something they may not want to or feel able to achieve, even if full adherence would have obviously better health outcomes.

Implied in the above discussion is that MI is behaviorally specific and has direction. This means that providers need to be clear about what it is that they are trying to motivate patients to do or to change. Motivation for change in one area does not guarantee motivation for change in another (e.g., a patient may commit to physical exercise, but not be willing to engage in psychotherapy). Each behavior may require a separate motivational enhancement process.

Four MI Processes

There are four processes that comprise MI: (1) engaging; (2) focusing; (3) evoking; and (4) planning, with processes often overlapping with each other (Table 18.1).

Miller and Rollnick define engaging as, "the process of establishing a mutually trusting and respectful helping relationship" [34]. In the engaging process, the provider seeks to establish a partnership by facilitating the patient's story using fundamental MI strategies (e.g., open-

Table 18.1 Processes of motivational interviewing

Process	Description	Clinical examples
Engagement	Establishing an open, empathic, patient-centered relationship	Patient: I'm willing to talk, but I really think the doctors here are making a mistake about this diagnosis of functional movement disorder. Interviewer: You have some serious doubts about the diagnosis you've been given, and you're here to learn more about it.
Focusing	Helping the patient to identify a specific target for behavior change	Interviewer: Tell me about how these problems with walking affect your life.
Evoking	Drawing out the patient's own motivations supporting the target behavior change	Patient: The tremor prevents me from doing anything! I can't work, I can't drive, I can't even watch after my kids! Interviewer: The tremor prevents you from fulfilling your responsibilities. It's stripped you of your independence.
Planning	Eliciting the patient's specific plans for behavior change, and for overcoming obstacles to those plans	Interviewer: Given what you've said about how the tremor undermines your independence, what steps might you take to gain more control over the tremor?

Four overlapping processes comprising MI. Clinical examples include brief interactions that might take place during each process between a patient and a motivational interviewer, rather than the entirety of the process. *MI* motivational interviewing

ended questions and reflections). In doing so, patients can share their perspective, and rapport is cultivated within the clinician-patient dyad.

Focusing is "an ongoing process of seeking and maintaining direction" by identifying areas for exploration in treatment [34]. These areas are determined through a combination of the patient's goals (e.g. regaining mobility), the setting (e.g. the neurologist's office), and the clinical expertise of the provider (e.g., improving anhedonia that is interfering with treatment engagement). Listing agenda items on paper and helping the patient prioritize them is a hallmark strategy used to focus the interview on specific behavior change targets (see section "Other Useful Strategies" below).

Evoking is the third process in which the provider tunes into the patient's language that favors change ('change talk') and applies strategies to generate change talk if not readily offered by the patient. There are several ways for providers to evoke change talk as outlined by Miller and Rollnick including, but not limited to (1) eliciting what the patient knows, providing information, and eliciting the patient's reactions to the information, (2) using open-ended questions and reflections to further change-oriented discourse, (3) assessing and exploring the patient's impor-

tance and confidence related to making changes using a numeric scale, and (4) engaging the patient in a decisional balance activity to explore the benefits of change and the costs of not changing [34]. These strategies can be used in traditionally briefer medical encounters and applied by members of the patient's interdisciplinary care team, making them ideal for multi-specialty settings.

Finally, the last process is planning, where the patient identifies a self-prescriptive behavior change goal. It is described as "developing a specific change plan that the person is willing to implement" [34]. Often, a patient is ready to transition to planning when the frequency of change talk has increased and indicates the patient is ready to prepare for change. This includes expressing commitment to change, activation or readiness around change (e.g., pondering potential options to facilitate change), and taking initial steps to initiate behavior change. During this stage, providers assist patients in setting the change plan which includes anticipating obstacles, identifying supportive others, and reaffirming their commitment to change. If the patient voices ambivalence during the planning process, providers explore it rather than pushing to complete the plan when the patient has backtracked motivationally.

Strategies

While MI is a style of interacting with others rather than merely an application of techniques, it does incorporate several strategies to promote behavior change [34]. These strategies include (1) those that are fundamental to the approach and used throughout the MI processes, such as open questions, affirmations, reflections, and summaries ("OARS") and (2) direct methods for evoking change talk and resolving ambivalence toward change. The continuous interplay of fundamental patient-centered strategies and direct methods to elicit and reinforce change talk and reduce sustain talk is essential to conducting MI proficiently.

Fundamental Strategies: Open Questions, Affirmations, Reflective Summaries – OARS

Fundamental strategies are a mainstay of MI in that they help providers understand the patients' perspective, convey empathy, and build a positive relationship with their patients. As the conversation unfolds, clinicians attend to the balance of statements made by patients that support or thwart behavior change (i.e., change vs. sustain talk) to gauge the patients' level of motivation and adjust their use of MI techniques accordingly.

Open questions encourage patients to talk more and may be used to strategically draw out motivations for change (e.g., "What would be good about participating in physical therapy?"). They stand in contrast to closed questions, in which providers seek specific information (e.g., demographics, history, symptoms), often with questions that can be answered with a "yes" or a "no" response. For example, a patient's positive response to the closed-ended question, "Have you been sticking with the exercise plan we discussed last time?" would provide some useful information. However, he or she would not have fully elaborated on adherence to various aspects of the plan, which an open question (e.g., "What

parts of your exercise plan have you been able to stick with since we last met?") might have elicited.

Affirmations (i.e., acknowledgment of a person's strengths, attitudes, and efforts that promote behavior change) build collaboration between providers and patients and promote self-efficacy. Sometimes this entails reframing a behavior in a manner that helps patients see it in a more positive light. For example, a provider who has a patient who becomes dismayed by a series of missed exercise goals might say, "You've been working hard to get better – setting demanding goals for yourself."

MI also relies heavily on the skilled use of *reflective listening* in which clinicians restate or paraphrase their understanding of what patients have said to express empathy, as well as to bring attention to ambivalence, highlight change talk, and explore and lessen language that supports the status quo. In MI, reflections are "simple" when a provider essentially repeats what the patient has said and "complex" when the provider articulates new meaning implied by the patient's original statements. Complex reflections demonstrate a deeper understanding of the patient's experiences. As an example, a provider asks a patient with FMD, "How have things been going with physical therapy?" The patient responds by saying, "What difference does it make?" A clinician could use a simple reflection to encourage more discussion about the patient's expressed skepticism ("You're not sure physical therapy makes a difference"). A complex reflection would capture the patient's implied demoralization and show more empathy ("You seem pretty discouraged").

Summaries provide opportunities for clinicians to demonstrate fuller understanding of their patients' experiences and help them consider the bigger picture of their motivations for change. Summaries also allow clinicians to collect multiple change talk statements as a strategy to enhance motivation, link discrepant statements that capture ambivalence, and shift focus to other behavioral areas (e.g., move from discussing psychotherapy adherence to exercise).

Direct Methods to Evoke Change Talk

Direct methods for evoking change talk hinge on the capacity of health care providers to recognize how patients talk about change [34]. Change talk is embodied in the acronym DARN-CAT (Table 18.2).

DARN (desire, ability, reasons, and need) is sometimes referred to as preparatory language in that these statements are motivational factors that prepare patients to commit to change [37]. Desire statements indicate a clear wish for change ("I don't want my functional movement disorder to get worse"). Ability statements indicate patients' beliefs that they can change, given their skills and available resources ("I used to swim, and there's a YMCA in my town that I could go to"). Reason statements note the benefits of change and the costs of not changing ("I will feel better" or "If I stop drinking soda, I might get my weight under better control"). Need statements underscore how the problem behavior interferes with important areas of an individual's life and how changing the behavior would likely improve matters ("I don't want to lose my job" or "I want to teach my kids how to live a healthy life to prevent this from happening to them").

CAT (commitment, activation, taking steps) represents statements that suggest patients are mobilizing themselves for change.

Commitment statements convey the stated intention to change ("I'm going to start physical therapy by the end of the month"). Activation statements indicate how patients are getting ready to change ("I'm going to call and schedule my first physical therapy appointment right after I leave here"). Statements about taking steps to change are the strongest demonstration of commitment in that the patients have put their words into action and are reporting these early efforts to the provider ("Instead of going home and watching TV after work, I went to the gym and exercised").

During the interview, providers identify the extent to which patients express motivation in each of these areas, use their fundamental skills to support and develop patients' change talk and have them elaborate further, and in a goal-oriented fashion, directly attempt to evoke motivation for change. MI offers multiple techniques for these purposes. Some options are described below:

1. Evocative questions – directly asking open-ended questions to elicit change talk (e.g., "In what ways do you think you can better manage your functional movement disorder?" [evoking ability to change] "How would things be better for you if you followed the recommended exercise plan?" [evoking reasons to change])

2. Readiness rulers – asking patients to rate themselves from 0–10 about the importance of and their confidence in changing a specific behavior related to their FMD and following up with evocative questions designed to elicit change talk (e.g., "How come you said a 5 rather than a 0?" "What would it take for you to go from a 5 to a 6?")

3. Looking forward – asking patients open-ended questions to look to the future at some time interval (e.g., 1 year from now) and consider where their lives might be headed with and without healthy lifestyle changes (attempting to reveal potential reasons or need to change to enhance the importance of change).

Table 18.2 Change Talk Categories: DARN-CAT

Category	Definition
Desire	Statements that indicate a clear wish for change
Ability	Statements that indicate patients' beliefs that they can change
Reason	Statements that note the benefits of change and the costs of not changing
Need	Statements that underscore how the problem behavior interferes with important areas of a patient's life and how changing the behavior would likely improve matters
Commitment	Statements that convey a patient's intention to change
Activation	Statements that indicate how patients are getting ready to change
Taking Steps	Initial demonstration of behaviors that would support change

4. Exploring goals and values – inquiring about what matters most to patients (e.g., being a good parent or available grandparent, independence) through reflections and open-ended questions and exploration on how the targeted behavior fits with these goals or values (e.g., "The thought of being tethered to a dialysis machine is unacceptable to you. How would being more physically active affect your level of independence?").

5. Past successes – exploring past periods when patients were successful in some areas and how they might import these experiences into their current circumstances ("It's great that you were able to control your tremor in the past. What helped you be successful then? How can those strategies work for you again?")

Other Useful Strategies

The management of FMD typically requires simultaneous attention to several behavioral issues (e.g. exercise, adherence with psychotherapy, adherence with physical therapy, adherence with antidepressants or other medications), and this reality often is overwhelming to patients and clinicians during any one appointment where time is limited. Clinicians can use a simple agenda setting chart in which they record the pertinent behavior change issues on paper and have patients indicate which of them they want to discuss during the interview [37].

Education, advice-giving, and direction are commonplace in the health care settings, particularly because clinicians often have a natural tendency to try to fix patients' problems (referred to as the "righting reflex") [34]. When patients have not solicited professional input, however, they may not be receptive to it. Instead, clinicians should ask permission to provide information or advice and employ an elicit-provide-elicit (or ask-tell-ask) technique in which clinicians (1) elicit from patients what they know about the topic being discussed, (2) provide information as needed, and (3) elicit patients' reactions to the shared information. For example, a clinician may wish to recommend that a patient meets with a physical therapist. Instead of providing the recommendation in an unsolicited manner, the provider would first ask the patient about his or her past experiences with physical therapists and then, with permission, talk about how a physical therapist might be helpful to the patient and conclude by getting the patient's reaction. This technique promotes collaboration and reduces the chance that patients experience clinicians as lecturing or telling them what to do.

Use of a decisional balance activity (i.e., exploring the costs and benefits of changing and not changing) is common in MI [34]. By strategically eliciting more reasons for change and, to the extent possible, resolving reasons to remain the same (e.g., identify some healthy foods that taste good and are affordable), a clinician might help the patient tip the balance toward change. However, it is recommended that the use of decisional balances be applied with caution. Miller and Rose found that that use of decisional balances with clients who were ambivalent ultimately decreased the decision to change [38]. They suggest that the use of decisional balances be reserved for patients who have already decided to change, in whom use of this strategy can strengthen their commitment. They recommend other evocation strategies, like some of the direct methods described above, as potentially more effective in resolving ambivalence.

Another important skill is how to gauge patients' readiness to change and transition from the evoking process to that of planning for change. Providers typically recapitulate what patients have said, especially those statements that suggest how they are now ready to change. Following this summary, providers then pose a key question to solidify commitment to change ("What's your next step?" or "From what you've told me, how do you want to proceed?"). Miller and Rollnick have used the analogy of a person as a skier standing at the summit (assisted up the mountain by the clinician) [34]. The key question provides a supportive nudge that helps the person go down the mountain.

Change planning is a strategy that clinicians use to negotiate a plan with patients about how they will change their behavior [34]. Critical to this process is maintaining a patient-centered stance in which the plan is derived by the patient, with the assistance of the clinician, rather than the clinician becoming prescriptive at this point. Clinicians ask patients to set their targeted behavior change goal ("I am going to walk at least a block once a day"), describe steps they will take to change ("I will walk in the evening before I eat dinner"; "I will record my walking each day in my exercise journal"), identify who might support them and how ("I am going to ask my wife to review my exercise journal at the end of each week"), anticipate obstacles ("it'll be hard to walk outside when it snows"), and reaffirm their commitment to the plan. If during the process of mobilizing their commitment, patients become uncertain again (the cold-feet phenomenon), the clinician reflects this ambivalence rather than trying to press through it and provides another opportunity to revisit the plan in the current meeting or at another time. Being in a hurry to complete the plan when patients are not ready is a common trap into which clinicians fall.

Handling Sustain Talk and Discord

Sustain talk conveys the patient's motivations to not change behavior [34]. The patient may offer reasons for maintaining the behaviors ("using a wheelchair makes getting around so much easier and safer") or the difficulties of trying to change them ("the pain is worse after I do physical therapy"). Sustain talk in this context informs providers about dilemmas faced by individuals, thereby providing opportunities for addressing obstacles to change. Some strategies for skillfully handling sustain talk include: (1) simply reflecting the sustain talk to show empathy and better understand the issue ("you feel unsafe trying to walk without the wheelchair"); (2) amplified reflections to determine the degree of commitment to a discordant statement ("doing physical therapy just isn't worth it"); (3) double-sided reflections to pair the sustain talk with other things said that favor change, thereby introducing some ambivalence back into the conversation ("you want to keep using the wheelchair for now, but you're worried

that if you do you might never get out of it"); and (4) emphasizing personal choice and control to assure the patients that it is they who determine what they will do, not others ("physical therapy is not easy, but it is manageable and you have a few options about how to do it. We will work with you to determine what the best way is to go about starting physical therapy, and ultimately it is your decision").

Miller and Rollnick describe discord as "smoke alarms" or "a change in the air" to alert providers that there has been a shift in the working alliance [34]. They describe patient behaviors such as defending themselves through external blaming or justification, squaring off with a provider (i.e. "You don't care, don't know, have no idea, etc."), interrupting, and disengaging from the conversation as examples of discord. When using MI, a provider avoids a confrontational, authoritative, warning, or threatening tone (all inconsistent with MI), which might cause the patient to become even less engaged in treatment [37]. These behaviors can originate from the patient, well before the visit begins, or discord can arise during the visit (often unintentionally provoked by the provider). Provider behaviors such as using labeling language (e.g. psychogenic, alcoholic, psychotic), disagreement over which behaviors to focus on, over-correction of patient's beliefs and perspectives about change, and prematurely pushing toward planning can generate discord within the interaction. Strategies for navigating discord include affirming patient's strengths and effort, which can attenuate defensiveness. Additionally, shifting the focus of the conversation away from the activating topic can bring patient and provider back in sync on their shared goals for treatment.

Learning Motivational Interviewing

Techniques for training clinicians in MI are evolving. The most popular approach has been the use of multi-day workshops. Research on the effectiveness of MI workshops (expert facilitated didactics and skill-building activities delivered in a group format) shows clinicians consistently improve their attitudes, knowledge, and confidence in MI, but immediate skill gains resulting from the training diminish within a few months. A meta-analysis of MI training studies showed that the addition of approximately monthly post-workshop supervisory feedback and coaching sessions over a 6-month period was sufficient to sustain workshop training effects [39]. Others have found that coaching MI trained clinicians on their skills throughout the intervention results in greater beneficial effects, especially with MI interventions to enhance treatment adherence [40].

Several provider performance rating scales are available that can be used to reliably supervise MI practice in this manner [41–43]. This approach to supervision is particularly important given that providers typically evaluate their performance more positively than when the same sessions are reviewed by their supervisors or independent judges [44]. Moreover, in the absence of supervision in MI, providers may be more prone to initiate informal discussions (i.e., chat) about matters that are unrelated to their patients' treatment [44].

A variety of training resources exist to learn MI. These resources include textbooks, treatment manuals, training videotapes, a supervision toolkit, and an international training group called the Motivational Interviewing Network of Trainers. Many of these resources are accessible at www.motivationinterviewing.org.

Conclusions

MI is a potentially useful adjunctive treatment for addressing behavioral problems for motivating patients with FND, including FMD, to adhere to various aspects of the complex psychological and physical treatment regimens and other healthy lifestyle activities that are important for these patients. There is some emerging evidence to support its efficacy from one RCT in functional seizures, as well as a broad array of randomized trials in other disorders. While the use of MI in FND needs further study, it is likely to be a low cost and safe option for enhancing psychotherapies and physical therapy. MI has a clear set of principles and strategies that guide implementation and substantial training resources to prepare

providers to conduct MI proficiently. The popularity of MI continues to grow and the health care field remains challenged to study if and how it works within its new applications, such as for the management of FMD, and to ensure that providers implement it with integrity to improve treatment outcomes. The FND community should learn how to apply MI techniques in FMD clinics and treatment programs. Carefully done studies will then need to be done to document the impact of MI on a variety of patient outcomes.

Summary
- Motivational interviewing is a patient-centered method of counseling that focuses on eliciting "change talk" (i.e., a patient's reasons for healthy behavioral changes) and resolving "sustain talk" (i.e., expressed motivations to not change).
- Motivational interviewing relies on four overlapping key processes: *engaging* the patient, *focusing* the topic of discussion, *evoking* change talk, and *planning* behavioral changes.
- Motivational interviewing employs fundamental strategies such as open questions, affirmations, reflections, and summaries (OARS) to elicit change talk and resolve sustain talk.
- Patient non-adherence with treatment is a common obstacle to treatment of FND, including FMD, and is associated with worse outcomes.
- Motivational interviewing is effective in enhancing adherence with psychotherapy, physical therapy, and other treatments, as well as associated treatment outcomes, across a wide spectrum of patients and disorders, including FND.
- The combination of a multi-day workshop followed by practice cases with supervisory feedback and coaching is an evidence-based approach for learning and improving motivational interviewing skills.

References

1. Tolchin B, Dworetzky BA, Baslet G. Long-term adherence with psychiatric treatment among patients with psychogenic nonepileptic seizures. Epilepsia. 2018;59:e18–22.
2. Sharma VD, Jones R, Factor SA. Psychodynamic psychotherapy for functional (psychogenic) movement disorders. J Mov Disord. 2017;10:40.
3. Julius RJ, Novitsky MA Jr, Dubin WR. Medication adherence: a review of the literature and implications for clinical practice. J Psychiatr Pract. 2009;15:34–44.
4. Bodenheimer T, Wagner EH, Grumbach K. Improving primary care for patients with chronic illness: the chronic care model, Part 2. JAMA. 2002;288:1909–14.
5. Tolchin B, Baslet G, Suzuki J, et al. Randomized controlled trial of motivational interviewing for psychogenic nonepileptic seizures. Epilepsia. 2019;60:986–95.
6. Tolchin B, Baslet G, Martino S, et al. Motivational interviewing techniques to improve psychotherapy adherence and outcomes for patients with psychogenic nonepileptic seizures. J Neuropsychiatry Clin Neurosci. 2020;32(2):125–31.
7. Hettema J, Steele J, Miller WR. Motivational interviewing. Annu Rev Clin Psychol. 2005;1:91–111.
8. Lundahl B, Kunz C, Brownell C, Tollefson D, Burke B. Meta-analysis of motivational interviewing: twenty five years of empirical studies. Res Soc Work Pract. 2010;20:137–60.
9. Vasilaki EI, Hosier SG, Cox WM. The efficacy of motivational interviewing as a brief intervention for excessive drinking: a meta-analytic review. Alcohol Alcohol. 2006;41:328–35.
10. VanBuskirk KA, Wetherell JL. Motivational interviewing with primary care populations: a systematic review and meta-analysis. J Behav Med. 2014;37:768–80.
11. Frost H, Campbell P, Maxwell M, et al. Effectiveness of motivational interviewing on adult behaviour change in health and social care settings: a systematic review of reviews. PLoS One. 2018;13:e0204890.
12. Lawrence P, Fulbrook P, Somerset S, Schulz P. Motivational interviewing to enhance treatment attendance in mental health settings: a systematic review and meta-analysis. J Psychiatr Ment Health Nurs. 2017;24:699–718.
13. Shafii T, Benson SK, Morrison DM. Brief motivational interviewing delivered by clinician or computer to reduce sexual risk behaviors in adolescents: acceptability study. J Med Internet Res. 2019;21:e13220.
14. Osilla KC, Kennedy DP, Hunter SB, Maksabedian E. Feasibility of a computer-assisted social network motivational interviewing intervention for substance use and HIV risk behaviors for housing first residents. Addict Sci Clin Pract. 2016;11:14.
15. Lerch J, Walters ST, Tang L, Taxman FS. Effectiveness of a computerized motivational intervention on treatment initiation and substance use: results from a randomized trial. J Subst Abus Treat. 2017;80:59–66.
16. Friederichs SA, Oenema A, Bolman C, Guyaux J, van Keulen HM, Lechner L. I Move: systematic development of a web-based computer tailored physical activity intervention, based on motivational interviewing and self-determination theory. BMC Public Health. 2014;14:212.
17. Ondersma SJ, Svikis DS, Thacker LR, Beatty JR, Lockhart N. Computer-delivered screening and brief intervention (e-SBI) for postpartum drug use: a randomized trial. J Subst Abus Treat. 2014;46:52–9.
18. Pollick SA, Beatty JR, Sokol RJ, et al. Acceptability of a computerized brief intervention for alcohol among abstinent but at-risk pregnant women. Subst Abus. 2015;36:13–20.
19. Martino S, Ondersma SJ, Forray A, et al. A randomized controlled trial of screening and brief interventions for substance misuse in reproductive health. Am J Obstet Gynecol. 2018;218:322 e321–12.
20. Cushing CC, Jensen CD, Miller MB, Leffingwell TR. Meta-analysis of motivational interviewing for adolescent health behavior: efficacy beyond substance use. J Consult Clin Psychol. 2014;82:1212.
21. Lovejoy TI, Heckman TG, Suhr JA, Anderson T, Heckman BD, France CR. Telephone-administered motivational interviewing reduces risky sexual behavior in HIV-positive late middle-age and older adults: a pilot randomized controlled trial. AIDS Behav. 2011;15:1623.
22. Purath J, Keck A, Fitzgerald CE. Motivational interviewing for older adults in primary care: a systematic review. Geriatr Nurs. 2014;35:219–24.
23. Miller WR, Rose GS. Toward a theory of motivational interviewing. Am Psychol. 2009;64:527.
24. Magill M, Gaume J, Apodaca TR, et al. The technical hypothesis of motivational interviewing: a meta-analysis of MI's key causal model. J Consult Clin Psychol. 2014;82:973.
25. Apodaca TR, Longabaugh R. Mechanisms of change in motivational interviewing: a review and preliminary evaluation of the evidence. Addiction. 2009;104:705–15.
26. Gaume J, Gmel G, Faouzi M, Daeppen J-B. Counselor skill influences outcomes of brief motivational interventions. J Subst Abus Treat. 2009;37:151–9.
27. Hodgins DC, Ching LE, McEwen J. Strength of commitment language in motivational interviewing and gambling outcomes. Psychol Addict Behav. 2009;23:122.
28. Magill M, Apodaca TR, Borsari B, et al. A meta-analysis of motivational interviewing process: technical, relational, and conditional process models of change. J Consult Clin Psychol. 2018;86:140–57.
29. Bertholet N, Faouzi M, Gmel G, Gaume J, Daeppen JB. Change talk sequence during brief motivational intervention, towards or away from drinking. Addiction. 2010;105:2106–12.

30. Glynn LH, Moyers TB. Chasing change talk: the clinician's role in evoking client language about change. J Subst Abus Treat. 2010;39:65–70.

31. Tolchin B, Dworetzky BA, Martino S, Blumenfeld H, Hirsch LJ, Baslet G. Adherence with psychotherapy and treatment outcomes for psychogenic nonepileptic seizures. Neurology. 2019;92:e675–9.

32. Dean S, Britt E, Bell E, Stanley J, Collings S. Motivational interviewing to enhance adolescent mental health treatment engagement: a randomized clinical trial. Psychol Med. 2016;46:1961–9.

33. Palacio A, Garay D, Langer B, Taylor J, Wood BA, Tamariz L. Motivational interviewing improves medication adherence: a systematic review and meta-analysis. J Gen Intern Med. 2016;31:929–40.

34. Miller WR, Rollnick S. Motivational interviewing: helping people change. 3rd ed. New York: Guilford Press; 2013.

35. Waterman AS. The humanistic psychology–positive psychology divide: contrasts in philosophical foundations. Am Psychol. 2013;68:124.

36. Prochaska JO, DiClemente CC. The transtheoretical approach: crossing traditional boundaries of therapy. Krieger Pub Co; 1994.

37. Rollnick S, Heather N, Bell A. Negotiating behaviour change in medical settings: the development of brief motivational interviewing. J Ment Health. 1992;1:25–37.

38. Miller WR, Rose GS. Motivational interviewing and decisional balance: contrasting responses to client ambivalence. Behav Cogn Psychother. 2015;43:129–41.

39. Schwalbe CS, Oh HY, Zweben A. Sustaining motivational interviewing: a meta-analysis of training studies. Addiction. 2014;109:1287–94.

40. Zomahoun HTV, Guenette L, Gregoire J-P, et al. Effectiveness of motivational interviewing interventions on medication adherence in adults with chronic diseases: a systematic review and meta-analysis. Int J Epidemiol. 2017;46:589–602.

41. Forsberg L, Forsberg LG, Lindqvist H, Helgason AR. Clinician acquisition and retention of motivational interviewing skills: a two-and-a-half-year exploratory study. Subst Abuse Treat Prev Policy. 2010;5:8.

42. Martino S, Ball SA, Nich C, Frankforter TL, Carroll KM. Community program therapist adherence and competence in motivational enhancement therapy. Drug Alcohol Depend. 2008;96:37–48.

43. Moyers TB, Rowell LN, Manuel JK, Ernst D, Houck JM. The motivational interviewing treatment integrity code (MITI 4): rationale, preliminary reliability and validity. J Subst Abus Treat. 2016;65:36–42.

44. Martino S, Ball SA, Nich C, Frankforter TL, Carroll KM. Correspondence of motivational enhancement treatment integrity ratings among therapists, supervisors, and observers. Psychoth Res. 2009;19:181–93.

Gaston Baslet and Barbara A. Dworetzky

Case Vignette #1

A 19 year-old sophomore in college is diagnosed with a functional gait disorder that impacts her ability to participate in competitive sports. She developed her symptoms 6 months prior to her presentation to the neurologist. She reports that 2 months prior to the onset of her gait symptoms, she had a concussion during track practice; she felt dizzy after running, collapsed to the ground and hit her head but did not lose consciousness. She felt back to herself within a few minutes and did not require immediate medical attention. On the days following the injury, she experienced nausea and fatigue that subsided within a few weeks. Afterwards, she began to notice she was swaying sideways when walking and had to grab onto walls fearing she would fall (although in fact she did not experience any falls).

The patient denies any prior psychological distress, diagnosis or treatment. She and her family describe her as "very strong", always "on the go", and "a high achiever". She played competitive sports all her life until the onset of her functional gait disorder. She is convinced that her gait is the result of the concussion she suffered and that she needs to be treated in a brain injury (concussion) clinic. She also complains of increased forgetfulness and attention problems for the last 6 months and has requested special accommodations in school, but eventually decided to take a leave for the rest of the semester.

Her neurological exam shows non-economical compensatory movements during gait testing (astasia-abasia) that improves with distraction. The rest of her neurological exam is unremarkable. Brain MRI is normal. Bedside cognitive examination shows mild difficulties with retrieval and executive tasks, with preserved encoding and attention. She displays a labile affect during the appointment, especially when reporting the impact of symptoms on her life. She denies any safety concerns and reports a euthymic mood.

Based on the history and exam, she is given the diagnosis of "functional gait disorder". The diagnosis is explained as being influenced by many factors, including life events, physical changes she experienced (for instance from her post-concussive symptoms) and psychological/cognitive processing difficulties that perpetuate her functional symptoms. As the clinician provides this explanation, the patient becomes quite angry by the inclusion of "psychological" factors, as the patient firmly believes that the

G. Baslet (✉)
Division of Neuropsychiatry, Brigham and Women's Hospital, Boston, MA, USA

Harvard Medical School, Boston, MA, USA
e-mail: gbaslet@bwh.harvard.edu

B. A. Dworetzky
Division of Epilepsy, Brigham and Women's Hospital, Boston, MA, USA

Harvard Medical School, Boston, MA, USA
e-mail: bdworetzky@bwh.harvard.edu

© Springer Nature Switzerland AG 2022
K. LaFaver et al. (eds.), *Functional Movement Disorder*, Current Clinical Neurology,
https://doi.org/10.1007/978-3-030-86495-8_19

concussion she suffered is the only reason she developed symptoms and demands to be referred to a "concussion clinic." The clinician explains that a skillful physical therapist will be able to help with her gait problems and will adapt the specific exercises based on her symptoms. Ultimately, she declines the referral and attends a "concussion specialty clinic" that refers her to physical therapy. After 2 sessions, she calls the neurologist back to let her know that she received "physical therapy for (her) concussion" and that she is doing better now, but now wants to be evaluated for new-onset headaches.

Introduction

Establishing a connection to patients through open and empathic communication is the basis of good clinical practice [1]. The doctor-patient relationship, if built on trust, is a therapeutic opportunity that can be especially helpful for chronic and difficult to treat disorders [2]. Communication in a medical encounter can improve health outcomes through a number of mechanisms: enhanced therapeutic alliance, increased social support, increased access to care, greater patient knowledge and understanding, higher quality medical decisions, patient agency and empowerment, and better management of emotions [3].

Functional neurological disorder (FND) can be difficult for clinicians to explain to patients [4, 5] for a variety of reasons. For example, a systematic review including 30 studies about functional [psychogenic nonepileptic/dissociative] seizures identified the most common perceptions from approximately 3900 health care providers: uncertainty about the disorder, the belief that symptoms are largely explained by psychiatric factors, mixed views about who is responsible for the patient, the belief that patients are challenging/frustrating, and that the symptoms are volitional and not as severe as other disorders such as epilepsy [6]. In functional movement disorder (FMD), most specialists are concerned about missing another diagnosis [7]. The belief that FMD or functional seizures are not severe disorders is contrary to evidence that qualify of life can be as impaired as in Parkinson disease and epilepsy [8, 9]. As a result, for instance, patients with functional seizures experience confusion and feel that their symptoms are being dismissed or attributed solely to psychiatric factors [10].

Both patients and clinicians arrive at a clinical conversation with backgrounds that need to be considered. On the patient's part, that background is informed by the relationship with the health care system, such as the negative experiences of patients with functional seizures with health care professionals [11]. On the clinician's side, there may be a bias of not thinking about FND as a "legitimate" medical disorder, as is the case with many other "medically unexplained symptoms" [5]. Additionally, where, when and who else is present when a communication takes place can make a substantial impact on the outcome of the communication and the clinical outcome in general.

Despite significant advances in the last decade that have clarified aspects of the underlying pathophysiology of FND [12, 13], we have limited understanding about this condition compared to many other neuropsychiatric disorders. This, in part, is the result of having neglected FMD and other FND subtypes for decades, making this common condition understudied, and therefore challenging to explain.

In this chapter, we discuss the different patient, clinician and health care system factors that contribute to challenges in the communication between clinicians and patients with FMD and other FND phenotypes. Within each section, we will offer some solutions for clinicians on how to overcome the difficulties that impact communication. Most of these recommendations are based on our clinical experience (particularly in working with patients with functional seizures). We will illustrate specific challenges by linking them to case vignettes where appropriate. Given the overlap and similarity between FMD and other subtypes of FND [14], many references are based on published work on FND in general or specific subtypes such as functional seizures.

Patient Factors That Can Make the Communication Challenging

While most of the communication challenges pertain to the initial delivery of the news about an FMD diagnosis [15], clinicians should keep in mind that these communication challenges can present from the time the diagnosis is suspected (but the news not yet delivered) to later when the patient is engaged in treatment.

FMD is not a popularly known diagnosis that patients can relate to. In most cases, patients have not heard about FMD (or other FND subtypes) until they are told about the diagnosis by their clinician. Exposure to the name and the concept of FMD (or FND more generally) is limited, and therefore the disorder is conceptualized in people's minds as a "strange" or rare disease, when in reality FND is amongst the more common disorders in neurology clinics [16]. Patients' perception of clinician's confidence in the diagnosis and treatment has been documented to be a positive prognostic factor in FMD [17]. Reassuring patients about the frequent nature of the disorder and about the clinician's expertise could prove useful in demystifying the diagnosis and helping patients trust the clinician.

Skepticism about the FMD diagnosis may occur for a variety of reasons. A common reason is the inconsistency that patients perceive between their symptoms and the explanation: patients expect to be given the diagnosis of a more commonly recognized movement disorder (e.g., Parkinson's disease) and suddenly they hear an explanation that often suggests some psychological contributions and therefore feel dismissed [10]. Our recommendation is to provide a brain-based explanation of the disorder and to expect and allow skepticism with an open and transparent dialogue. Starting treatment while there is still skepticism can allow patients to gain confidence in the diagnosis; however, embarking in treatment while the skepticism is leading to other medical tests or opinions can be counterproductive and derails attention towards treatment.

Some patients with FMD may seemingly accept the diagnosis and even start a course of treatment, only to bring up skepticism later in the process (which can be due to a variety of reasons: the development of new symptoms, influence of others, including other clinicians). Clinicians should expect these regressions and be prepared to validate patients' concerns, reinforce their confidence in the diagnosis, openly consider other diagnoses if new data justifies it, and clearly communicate with others involved in the patient's care to help solidify the diagnosis, if appropriate.

Skepticism may also be informed by prior negative experiences with the health care system [11]. Many patients with FMD feel they have been ridiculed and their concerns were not taken seriously, leading to ongoing frustration and re-traumatization [18]. It is always good practice to inquire about past experiences with a diagnosis of FMD and make sure to adhere to trauma-informed care, an approach that acknowledges past traumatic experiences and prioritizes physical and emotional safety as a first step in care [19].

Stressful life events, including abuse and neglect, are more common across all FND phenotypes, including FMD, compared to healthy controls [20]. Avoidance is a psychological trait that has been described in FMD [21]. One of the traditional psychological theories for the development of functional neurological symptoms states that avoidance of emotional distress plays an important role [22]. Introduction of a psychological explanation (including a link to past stressful events) can actually create reluctance to accept the diagnosis and may interfere with developing the necessary rapport for successful communication. Initial communication about the diagnosis of FMD does not need to include a psychological explanation, especially when such factors are not clearly present or yet identified. Some patients may in fact disengage from the communication when a psychological explanation is brought up. Psychological factors may rather be presented as one of many potential contributing factors that can lead to the development of symptoms, but may or may not be relevant in a given patient. Some patients may start linking past stressful life events to their functional symptoms over time, when applicable. Timing the content of the communication to the patient's openness to accept such content is more impactful than sharing all the clinician's knowledge about FMD at once, even if conceptually correct. Initial discussions on the diagnosis of FMD are usually focused on "what" the diagnosis is based on rule-in signs. Explanations regarding "why" an individual has a FMD are more nuanced and multifactorial and in many instances the answer(s) may become evident as patients engage in their therapeutic journey [23].

As illustrated in Case Vignette # 1, many patients develop FMD following a sentinel physical event such as a concussion, which may lead to transient distressing symptoms [24, 25]. Psychological and cognitive factors (such as somatic hypervigilance and health expectations) lead to the development and reinforcement of functional neurological symptoms [26]. People normally link events in time as causal, and thus patients develop narratives linking their functional neurological symptoms to the sentinel physical event, which may not actually follow a direct pathophysiological process. In the described patient, the concussion itself does not lead to the development of functional gait directly, but rather through a number of indirect biological, psychological and social processes. The concussion can be identified, however, as a relevant precipitating factor within the context of a biopsychosocial formulation (see Chap. 3 for more details). We believe that explanations that are not physiologically valid should not be reinforced, but also not argued against. In such cases, it is best to put etiological discussions aside and be pragmatic in terms of treatment recommendations. In our case example, the patient only accepted treatment by a "concussion" specialist despite the neurologist's attempts to engage the patient, leading to a very sudden symptom improvement, potentially a placebo (positive expectation) effect. The concern in such cases is the possibility of other functional neurological symptoms (and related functional somatic symptoms) developing over time. For example, the patient's headaches will need further assessment and management.

Patients with FMD commonly present with mixed FND symptoms, other functional somatic symptoms [27] (e.g., pain, fatigue), and symptom change or substitution over time [28]. In the case of patients with multiple functional bodily symptoms, the clinician is presented with the challenge of deciding whether all phenotypic presentations should be jointly explained as part of the same disorder. This depends on each case: if the patient is ready to understand and accept a comprehensive explanation that encompasses multiple symptoms, it will be helpful to provide this integrated view, especially if the treatment for multiple symptoms overlap. However, if the patient is convinced of a given symptom being caused by a different, specific mechanism, forcing a new explanation for that secondary symptom can be perceived negatively and can lead to more resistance to the primary FMD diagnosis. In this case, it would be prudent to time those comprehensive explanations as the patient becomes more open to consider them. For example, this can be important for patients with FMD and fibromyalgia. Additional functional neurological symptoms may also directly impact the process of communication. For instance, patients with functional cognitive symptoms may not recall an important conversation about their diagnosis. In such cases, it is relevant to anticipate this problem and address it proactively by providing written information with a summary of the points discussed during the diagnosis delivery [29].

Some patients may react negatively to a diagnosis of FMD. They may feel dismissed and angry. This is, in fact, well reported in functional seizures and is considered a negative prognostic factor [30]. In such cases, clinicians should validate the patient's feelings of rejection or abandonment by reassuring them about the clinician's ongoing presence and commitment through the process of treatment. In some instances, patients may feel anger to the point that they decide to leave the clinician's care. In such circumstances, patients should be told that they will be welcomed back if eventually they want to reconsider their decision to transition away from clinical care at a given practice.

Pending litigation and pursuing disability benefits can also constitute a source of conflict for patients to accept the diagnosis of FMD, and these factors can be linked to poor prognosis [31]. This may be a challenging topic to discuss with patients who feel disabled by their symptoms. An open discussion of the literature on prognosis can provide a more hopeful outlook if symptoms are viewed and diagnosis presented as potentially transient and treatable rather than causing permanent disability. Temporarily suspending pursuit of litigation or disability claims in favor of engaging in treatment can be a fair compromise for some patients. Additionally, it can be helpful to discuss transparently with patients that the primary focus of the clinical encounters is to work towards clinical improvement, making sure that the ratio of clinical discussions to disability paperwork discussions slants towards treatment. That being said, prognosis in some patients may be poor [32], suggesting that there may be a role for applying for disability in some cases (while ensuring that the overall clinical focus remains on treatment participation).

In addition to tips on how to overcome each specific challenge above, there are other general recommendations on how to improve communication with patients with FMD. We recommend clinicians not to engage into an emotionally-charged debate with patients; this is usually counterproductive. Rather, understand where patients stand in the process of accepting the diagnosis and allow an open discussion on how they feel about the diagnosis. To clarify any misconceptions, it is helpful to ask patients to repeat an explanation back, so corrections can be offered in real-time and clarifications discussed. Sharing handouts or brochures from educational (www.neurosymptoms.org) or patient advocacy websites (e.g. www.fndhope.org), and writing a letter summarizing the discussed points [29] allow patients to rely on written information that is less vulnerable to recollection bias. Reading about FMD also provides patients with the opportunity to continue a dialogue with their clinician as they understand more about their diagnosis and they further engage in their own recovery process. Encouraging patients to view some of the patient testimonials found in the above websites can also help with engagement.

Table 19.1 summarizes many of the patient factors that can make communication challenging with practical suggestions on how to address them.

Table 19.1 Patient barriers that can make communication challenging and practical suggestions for clinicians on how to address them

Patient barriers	Practical suggestions for clinicians
Overall suggestions to improve communication with patients	Understand patient's beliefs and reactions about diagnosis. Ask patient to repeat explanations to clarify misconceptions. Share educational resources. Remain open to ongoing dialogue and questions.
Specific patient barriers	
Diagnosis is new, never-heard of	Educate and reassure patients about how common FMD is. Provide written educational resources &/or websites to review; recommend that patients return to discuss what they have learned.
Skepticism about diagnosis	Expect and allow skepticism. Be clear about your diagnostic certainty, including referencing "rule-in" physical examination signs as the basis for the FMD diagnosis. If starting treatment, postpone other medical testing and opinions to focus on treatment.
Past traumatic experiences with health care system	Validate feelings regarding past experiences. Follow trauma-informed care principles.

(continued)

Table 19.1 (continued)

Patient barriers	Practical suggestions for clinicians
Avoidance of discussion of psychological factors	Explore patient's openness to discuss psychological factors. Present psychological and cognitive processing factors as one of many contributing (predisposing, precipitating and perpetuating) factors that may or may not be present. Use "brain-based" terminology. Follow trauma-informed care principles.
Attachment to purely somatic explanatory narratives	Do not agree with a knowingly incorrect explanation. Be pragmatic and focus on recovery plan. Set aside etiological discussions for the moment (focusing early on the "what" of the diagnosis rather than the "why") Contextualize physical factors as one of many possible contributing factors.
Multiple functional symptoms and/or symptom substitution	Explore patient's readiness to understand the underlying common etiology of multiple functional symptoms. Time comprehensive explanations for multiple symptoms as patient is able to accept them. Anticipate and problem solve other functional symptoms interfering with treatment (i.e., provide written reminders in patients with cognitive complaints).
Negative emotional reactions (anger, dismissive)	Validate feelings. Remain available if patient tells you they plan to leave treatment.
Pending litigation or disability claims	Openly discuss prognostic implications of these factors. Discuss symptoms as transient and treatable for many patients. Suggest temporary suspension of the pending claims while undergoing treatment where appropriate.

Clinician Factors That Can Make Communication Challenging

Case Vignette #2

A patient has a history of weakness after a ceiling tile fell on him at work and struck him in his right leg. Initially, his leg was painful and bruised. As the bruise healed, he developed a limp that made it more challenging for him to climb a ladder, and he became slower on the job. Within 6 weeks, he was dragging his right leg behind him. On testing, he is found to have a positive Hoover's sign of the right leg, along with a dragging monoplegic gait. The neurologist refers him to a physical therapist and a psychiatrist without a discussion about how the diagnosis was made and why the treatments can help. The patient refuses to attend the appointments and feels angry that the neurologist thinks he can return to work and won't write him a letter for disability. He decides to arrange for a new consultation at another institution.

Case Vignette #3

A patient has migraine headaches and has been followed by a neurologist for many years. The patient then presents to the same neurologist with right leg dragging after a work-related injury and the exam reveals a positive Hoover's sign of the right leg. The patient is referred to a neurologist specializing in FMD because the referring neurologist feels the gait disorder is functional. The consultation is completed by the FMD specialist and the patient is offered physical therapy as a treatment and told to follow up with the referring neurologist. The patient indicates that the referring neurologist had previously discharged her from his practice, saying he cannot help her given that the condition is "not neurological." The FMD specialist contacts the referring neurologist to communicate that his help is needed to engage the patient in care, and that he should continue to be involved. The neurologist says that he has no idea what to do with this patient now that the gait disorder is confirmed to be FMD. He will not expect to see this patient back in his office.

Communication is challenging for clinicians who may lack knowledge or understanding about FMD, lack empathy or have negative attitudes or beliefs, and lack training or the skills to explain

FMD so that patients understand and are ready to engage with the recommended treatments. Closely associated healthcare system factors, that may negatively impact clinical care in FMD, are discussed later in this chapter.

Many neurologists and other clinicians lack knowledge and feel uncertain with FMD patients [33], which affects their communication. Using conversational analyses, interactional challenges such as resistance or outright rejection of the diagnosis were found between neurologists and patients with FND [34]. There is a delay in recognizing the disorder [35] which may in part stem from lack of knowledge of how FMD presents in the early stages. Including FMD as a diagnostic possibility early in the first encounter may allow neurologists to practice more open communication, to lessen the need for unnecessary testing and additional consultations, and potentially decrease the duration of worry that each new referral brings. Furthermore, for decades, there has been uncertainty and lack of consensus about what to call the disorder [36, 37]. Other than for FMD and related FND presentations, clinicians are comfortable generating an inclusive differential for clinical symptoms and systematically ruling out the most likely and most worrisome disorders. Given how common functional neurological symptoms are, all clinicians, not just subspecialists, should be trained on how to make and relay the diagnosis of FND. The common practice of trying to eliminate all other possible diagnoses without mentioning the possibility or likelihood of FND [38] can erode the trust in the doctor-patient relationship. This can be especially problematic when the diagnosis of FMD is finally conveyed and the clinician becomes uninterested in following up with their patient.

Uncertainty is also common within the medical system and medical charts. A Veterans Administration study reported that even for patients with confirmed functional seizures, neurologist notes still tended to use ambiguous language such as "thought to be" rather than diagnostic of FND [39]. Even when FND is recognized early, many neurologists may feel uncomfortable [7] communicating the diagnosis and may not know how to do so, despite published recommendations [40, 41]. Case Vignette # 2 illustrates a clinician prescribing treatment without an explanation, a missed opportunity to actually engage the patient in treatment.

There is also the common situation of clinicians not feeling certain in making the diagnosis of FMD [40] or worrying about the legal ramifications if they are wrong. Movement disorder neurologists were queried and 64% preferred to order tests to rule out all possible conditions out of concern for missing a diagnosis [7]. These worries are in contrast to the actual rate of misdiagnosis in FMD, as demonstrated by a longitudinal study of functional limb weakness [32]. Studies have shown that most patients want to understand what is wrong and how to get better, and are less interested than physicians are in testing [42].

Uncertainty is also demonstrated when FMD is not clearly discussed and patients seek other opinions to elucidate what illness is causing their suffering, such as in Case Vignette #2. New possible diagnoses are brought to light with each new clinical encounter and can readily add to the list of disorders that the patient often does not have.

Communication through body language, limiting time with the patient, as well as language in the form of certain commonly used phrases such as the symptoms are "due to stress", "not neurological" or "see a psychiatrist, I can't help you" may send nontherapeutic and confusing messages to patients who experience the symptoms as physical. Analysis of transcripts of neurologists communicating with patients with FND indicates more hesitations in speech, fewer open-ended questions, and language that reveals the discomfort of the clinician [34].

Knowledge about how to discuss patient skepticism is important for clinicians to understand when addressing FMD patients so that they can inform patients about their diagnosis, address concerns, and set expectations for treatment and improvement. Education for clinicians to address some of the above-mentioned barriers is a potential solution to many current communication challenges. There are excellent resources for patients and clinicians on the website of the new Functional Neurological Disorder Society (https://www.fndsociety.org/fnd-education). Building collaborative relationships for consistent messaging from all involved clinicians is extremely helpful to address ongoing patient concerns as they arise to maintain the individual engaged in treatment. It also helps provide ongoing support for the primary clinicians who want to know what they can do to help their patients.

Another common reason that clinicians find communication with FMD patients challenging is that some clinicians harbor negative attitudes and beliefs about the disorder [7]. The attitude of the clinician is of critical importance in fostering a positive therapeutic relationship to provide optimal care for the patient. Physician attitude may be the deciding factor determining whether the patient accepts the diagnosis and engages in treatment or whether they move on to a new clinician in a new health system. Negative beliefs also lead to lack of interest and motivation to obtain training and knowledge on best practices to help patients with FND. Patients can easily tell whether the clinician believes them and wants to help or not. Common misconceptions shared by many neurologists are that FMD symptoms are voluntary and can therefore be stopped at will [5]. Lack of awareness of the clinician's role in FMD can also lead to mismanagement and potentially worse outcomes.

There is also the common belief among neurologists that patients diagnosed with functional neurological symptoms should be discharged from the neurology practice (see Case Vignette # 3). For patients who have been in the clinician's practice with a therapeutic relationship already developed, the realization that a patient has FMD may sometimes lead a clinician to stop following the patient, which can be devastating, especially for those who have experienced prior trauma. When symptoms continue, clinicians may lose patience. Clinicians may inform the patient that "everything is normal", or equate the diagnosis of FMD to "good news"; while these statements may be perceived by the clinician as reassuring, patients may perceive that the clinician does not believe their symptoms, or thinks they are trying to manipulate the system by making up symptoms. The "good news" message is also invalidat-

ing as patients struggle with disabling physical symptoms and a "good news" framing of the condition fails to meet the patient where they are at. This messaging is further complicated by terminology such as "psychogenic" that stigmatizes patients adding to prior negative experiences within health care [37]. The belief that symptoms are all psychological and caused by stress often makes no sense to the patient who may have had far worse stressors in the past without developing symptoms of FMD. The belief that patients with FMD belong in the psychiatrist's or psychotherapist's office may relinquish neurologists of their important task of explaining the diagnosis and helping to catalyze engagement. A poorly executed explanation of the diagnosis can delay treatment and worsen outcomes [30]. Not offering to work with the patient until the disorder is understood and accepted may convey an implicit message that the neurologist does not care about their suffering. Many neurologists will refer patients with FMD to psychiatry and discharge them from their care, despite an awareness that many patients with FMD are unlikely to adhere to the recommendation to see a psychiatrist [43]. Clinicians are ethically minded as a rule, so this lack of empathy may emerge from a belief that there is no underlying 'real' neurological disorder to be concerned about (Cartesian dualism), or that the patient may have a factitious disorder, or be malingering [44]. See Chap. 4 for updated conceptualizations on bridging neurologic and psychiatric perspective in FMD care. Additionally, in any other chronic disorder, clinicians would likely be concerned if there were no follow up scheduled. All of these challenges also speak to the limited education that many well-intentioned neurologists receive during their training (see below).

Another common belief is that all FMD patients are difficult to communicate with or treat [4], leading some clinicians to avoid the usual development of the doctor-patient relationship. Solutions to this challenge include educating clinicians about the impact of negative beliefs (including their recognition and how to address them) while emphasizing the growing evidence supporting that the disorder is not voluntary, but clearly brain-based [45, 46]. Empathy and relationship-building with patients can be taught and may allow both clinicians and patients to feel better about the encounters [47].

Clinicians may lack the necessary skills and training to be able to explain the diagnosis of FMD effectively to patients without stigmatizing them, and may choose to avoid discussions when the explanation makes little sense to the patient or is at odds with the patient's beliefs. The language that the clinician chooses when communicating is important in order to engage rather than offend the patient. Word choice reveals clinician bias and may inadvertently send the wrong message. Offending patients by implying the disorder is not significant or that it is not a true disorder happens outside of the conscious awareness of well-meaning clinicians. In the absence of a neurologist trained to persist in engaging patients in treatments for FMD, patients may continue to search for new subspecialists without having a clinician responsible for coordination of care. Given how commonly FMD presents, this lack of coordination of care is likely responsible for a significant amount of unnecessary health care resources. Taking the patient's complaints seriously, explaining the rationale for the diagnosis, and emphasizing the expectation of improvement or even possibility of reversibility are among the ways to use explanation as a treatment and engagement tool for patients [48]. A team-based approach with clearly defined roles for each health care provider can offer patients a sense of belonging to a care team while setting up realistic expectations about treatment.

Other solutions to widespread lack of skills and training for FND include increasing evidence-based curricula and research support to improve communication skills and decrease the negative attitudes toward patients with FND. This training makes use of the natural abilities of clinicians to engage patients in treatment as well as to set appropriate expectations for improved function which may be slow and require active participation on the part of the patient. Anticipating some of the common concerns that arise during conversations with patients with FND is helpful for clinicians so they can be better prepared and more comfortable with good practices and develop an open channel of communication when new worries arise. If testing is recommended, it is preferable for clinicians to communicate the expected results of these studies, and when the patient should expect to receive results in order to decrease worry. There is an entire society devoted to communication in health care (www.achonline.org) and there is evidence that skills and effective communication can be taught to improve clinical outcomes [49].

Table 19.2 summarizes many of the clinician barriers that interfere with communication, how they interact with patients' reactions and practical solutions to overcome them.

Table 19.2 Clinician barriers that can make communication challenging and practical suggestions on how to address them

Clinician barriers	Associated patient barriers	Practical suggestions for clinicians
Negative attitudes	Perceived stigma	Education to make clinicians aware of their own implicit bias and cognitive errors
Uncertainty regarding FMD diagnosis	Lack of public awareness of FMD and FND more broadly	Further training to develop diagnostic confidence
Lack of knowledge/ training in FMD	Sensitivity to "psychiatric" language	Training and practice in trauma-informed care and what is being communicated
Concern about malingering	Not feeling believed	Communicate to validate that the symptoms are real
		Education on low probability of malingering in FMD
Concern about misdiagnosis (liability?)	Strong alternative views of diagnosis	Transparent and empathic communication
Not providing adequate time	Lack of trust in clinician/health system	Take the time to develop rapport and listen to the patient; be curious

System Factors That Can Make Communication Challenging

The health care system is highly complex and quite difficult for patients to navigate. It is very easy for patients to become confused or lost in the system without a clinical leader taking ownership for the oversight of their care. In the large tertiary/quaternary academic centers where many patients with FMD are referred, there are multitudes of subspecialists focused on getting to the diagnosis by ruling out every possible diagnosis, even those that are quite rare. Functional disorders are extremely common in all fields of medicine. In neurology, symptoms can sometimes be quite severe and disabling, and patients may present to the neurologist without a primary doctor coordinating the patient's care. Communication in busy clinical environments where appointments are too short is oftentimes challenging; while this is compounded when clinicians for the same patient are located in different healthcare systems, it can also be the case when the clinicians reside within the same hospital system. Patients with FMD are too common to be seen only within FMD programs or by FMD specialists, as these programs would become quickly overwhelmed [50]. The incentive to take more time and get the diagnosis correct may not be aligned properly with corporate medicine's incentive to meet the bottom line, and generate more procedures. There may be long waits for certain specialists and patients may spend months getting a work up without receiving a diagnosis. The diagnosis and treatment plan can remain "up in the air" in the "borderland" between specialists; this type of delay is known to worsen prognosis of FMD by prolonging untreated symptoms. All too common is the lack of a primary clinician who is willing to take ownership of the patient's care (which is a product not only of the clinician's potential lack of willingness but also a range of complex systems issues). Clear communication between professionals who are involved in the care of a patient is critical [51] as is creating an integrated treatment team, assigning roles, and maintaining collaborative communication with the patient at the center [18]. Unhelpful advice from one clinician may lead to avoidance on the part of the patient and therefore hinder recovery.

Family members are important allies to consider when communicating with patients. They can doubt reasonable explanations and bring skepticism and/or urge patients to pursue other tests or second (or third or fourth) opinions. Clinicians should bear in mind that patients may seemingly accept a diagnosis; however, if a family member remains skeptical, gains from a seemingly successful communication can be easily lost. Family members need to be educated and trained to engage in therapeutic, helpful behaviors that will reinforce acceptance of the diagnosis and engagement in treatment. It is not reasonable to expect treatment to be effective if the environment that the patient spends most time in questions the diagnosis and/or rationale for treatment. Other examples of unhelpful family behaviors include constant monitoring of symptoms by family members, high arousal states (often associated with panic) in response to patients with paroxysmal FMD (and functional seizures) and drastic changes in lifestyle because of the symptoms. Such environmental and interpersonal changes reinforce symptoms and make new learning from physical therapy and/or psychotherapy challenging, rendering a possible poor prognosis [31].

Some patients may be hesitant to include family members in their communications with their clinician. This attitude may signal skepticism about the diagnosis of FMD, but may also reflect a desire to keep the diagnosis private. Rather than forcing the presence of family members, it is important to understand the reasons behind their inclusion or exclusion, and how this may influence the patient's engagement in treatment.

In addition to family, other people involved in the patient's life need to be considered when discussing the diagnosis and treatment plan. Being economically dependent (for instance, on disability benefits) has been shown to be a negative prognostic factor in FMD [52], although this finding is not consistent across studies [17].

Encouraging participation or re-engagement in work or school should always be favored, if feasible, and discussed early. If the work or school environment is thought to reinforce the symptom, precautions and changes will need to be instituted so that symptoms do not escalate. Involvement of others (school, work) is time-consuming and not accounted for in our health care system. Usually the question "can I go back to work / school?" is presented in the last few minutes of a clinical encounter. We encourage clinicians to bring up this topic early during the clinical encounter so there is plenty of opportunity to discuss a plan of reintegration to work or school. Creating a shared agenda at the start of clinic visits can also prevent important "action items" from being left to the end of encounters. The clinician needs to also consider the task of writing letters that explain the diagnosis (always with the patient's input and permission), outline a gradual work or school re-integration plan and recommend accommodations to account for the patient's physical limitations and to allow treatment participation. Those who interact with patients in school and work settings need to be educated on how to react to and manage symptoms; this may be particularly relevant in paroxysmal FMD that may create confusion and question the need for urgent intervention.

The public knows little about FMD [53] and media frequently publicizes "missed diagnoses", causing patients to worry about rare diagnoses, and clinicians to worry about being sued. Additionally, the diagnosis of FMD carries stigma (despite the terminology change from "psychogenic" to "functional," which aimed to reduce stigma). Some patients may not mind disclosure of an FMD diagnosis when the clinician discusses it with others, while other patients may want the clinician to be as non-specific as possible. Discussions with patients about the content of prospective discussions with others need to take place before the clinician reaches out to anyone who will be enlisted to help the patient. One helpful way to improve communication is to use part of the clinic visit to call a given

provider or family member with the patient present so that discussions are transparent. In many respects, educating others about FMD should include similar content to the original diagnosis discussion with the patient and their immediate family members. Providing and sharing educational resources with interested parties represents another way of expanding awareness about FMD and other FND in general.

Many health care systems lack the infrastructure necessary to support ongoing, collaborative and multidisciplinary work. However, this is exactly what patients with FMD need. As evidence-based treatments become more commonplace and outcomes are shown to improve, interest in early interventions could increase and resources could become properly allocated to satisfy the need for coordination of care and multidisciplinary collaboration. An integrated and stepped model of care (a system where the most effective, yet least resource intensive treatment, is delivered first, only "stepping up" to more intensive services as required) has already been shown to help outcomes in other chronic medical conditions [54]. While this has yet to be fully proven for FMD, there are many factors that suggest that such models of integrated care [55], including a stepped care approach, offer great promise [56].

Communicating the diagnosis of FMD is a therapeutic skill that clinicians must be trained for, in a similar way that we are trained to perform a lumbar puncture or interpret an MRI brain scan. This is an important systems limitation as training programs tend to invest poorly on communication strategies, especially in FMD. This is a larger issue that requires a major shift in priorities in medical training. The Academy of Communication in Healthcare teaches relationship-centered communication and could be an excellent resource for neurologists and psychiatrists to incorporate into their training programs.

Table 19.3 summarizes the many system factors that can make communication challenging with practical suggestions on how to address them.

Table 19.3 System barriers that can make communication challenging and practical suggestions for clinicians on how to address them

System barriers	Practical suggestions for clinicians
Overall suggestions to improve communication with others	Share educational resources. Review with patient any prospective discussions that will take place with others (and try to involve the patient in those discussions when possible).
Specific system barriers	
Skeptical families	Educate families on FMD. Be clear about therapeutic and non-therapeutic family behaviors that can impact outcome. Engage family members as treatment allies.
Disability status at work/school	Proactively bring up this issue. Evaluate reinforcing behaviors in work/school settings. Educate work/school about diagnosis with permission. Prepare a plan that includes accommodations, gradual re-integration and recommendations for management of symptom exacerbation/crisis.
Multiple clinicians involved in the care of the patient	Consider integrated, multidisciplinary care models. Maintain communication among all treatment providers and provide consistent messaging. Ask the patient to identify a "trusted" clinician as the main contact or "leader" in the care system.
Primary clinician uncomfortable with FMD diagnosis and suggesting more testing	Educate as needed and offer open communication and stay connected with the clinicians and the patient.
Limited training in communication	Training programs need to prioritize communication education with ongoing feedback from experts.

Conclusions

Communication with patients with FMD and their support systems should be seen as a longitudinal process rather than as a one-time intervention. Clinical communication with patients should aim to help patients engage, feel validated and become their best self-advocates. While a clinician discusses a diagnosis of FMD, the language, content and pace of delivery will need to be adjusted to each situation and patient to optimize the chances of a successful outcome.

Communication is not only between a patient and a clinician. Other clinicians, family members, and community supports must be considered when discussing a diagnosis and treatment plan. Even if a patient does not want other people involved during a communication encounter, a clinician should always consider and account for the impact of a diagnosis of FMD on those who interact with the patient. When possible and allowed, others should be included as part of a communication strategy as uniform and consistent messaging will help reinforce understanding.

Clinicians should think about communication as an open-ended process that carries a dialogue and changes over time as new information is brought forward. While we hope that change will include more accepting and self-advocacy attitudes over time, one should account for possible regressions and skepticism about the diagnosis, which may be influenced by a number of factors.

Finally, communication is a skill that requires real-time training and should be carefully evaluated as clinicians complete training programs. This requires the support of major stakeholders who need to believe in the power of a therapeutic communication strategy.

Summary

- Communication between patients with FMD and clinicians should aim to provide validation to patients and engage them in their care to become their best self-advocates.
- In addition to patient and clinician, communication should include other clinicians, family members, and community supports.
- Patient-related factors need to be considered when communicating about FMD. These factors include novelty of the diagnosis, skepticism about the diagnosis, previous traumatic experience with the healthcare system, avoidance of psychological explanations, attachment to other medical explanations, and pending litigation.
- Clinician-related factors impacting communication include negative attitude towards patients with FMD, lack of knowledge about the disorder, uncertainty about diagnosis, false brain-mind dichotomies, concern about malingering, concern about misdiagnosis and liability, and not providing an adequate amount of time to patients.
- System factors that impact communication include skeptical families, involvement of multiple providers, a tendency to order tests unnecessarily, and limited emphasis on communication in training programs.
- Communication is a skill that requires training and should be prioritized in clinical education programs on FMD.

References

1. Suchman AL, Matthews DA. What makes the patient-doctor relationship therapeutic? Exploring the connexional dimension of medical care. Ann Intern Med. 1988;108(1):125–30. https://doi.org/10.7326/0003-4819-108-1-125.

2. Windover AK, Boissy A, Rice TW, Gilligan T, Velez VJ, Merlino J. The REDE model of healthcare communication: optimizing relationship as a therapeutic agent. J Patient Exp. 2014;1(1):8–13. https://doi.org/10.1177/237437431400100103.

3. Street RL, Makoul G, Arora NK, Epstein RM. How does communication heal? Pathways linking clinician-patient communication to health outcomes. Patient Educ Couns. 2009;74(3):295–301. https://doi.org/10.1016/j.pec.2008.11.015.

4. Carson AJ, Stone J, Warlow C, Sharpe M. Patients whom neurologists find difficult to help. J Neurol Neurosurg Psychiatry. 2004;75(12):1776–8. https://doi.org/10.1136/jnnp.2003.032169.

5. Pridmore S, Skerritt P, Ahmadi J. Why do doctors dislike treating people with somatoform disorder? Australas Psychiatry. 2004;12(2):134–8. https://doi.org/10.1080/j.1039-8562.2004.02085.x.

6. Rawlings GH, Reuber M. Health care practitioners' perceptions of psychogenic nonepileptic seizures: a systematic review of qualitative and quantitative studies. Epilepsia. 2018;59(6):1109–23. https://doi.org/10.1111/epi.14189.

7. LaFaver K, Lang AE, Stone J, et al. Opinions and clinical practices related to diagnosing and managing functional (psychogenic) movement disorders: changes in the last decade. Eur J Neurol. 2020;27(6):975–84. https://doi.org/10.1111/ene.14200.

8. Anderson KE, Gruber-Baldini AL, Vaughan CG, et al. Impact of psychogenic movement disorders versus Parkinson's on disability, quality of life, and psychopathology. Mov Disord. 2007;22(15):2204–9. https://doi.org/10.1002/mds.21687.

9. Rawlings GH, Brown I, Reuber M. Predictors of health-related quality of life in patients with epilepsy and psychogenic nonepileptic seizures. Epilepsy Behav. 2017;68:153–8. https://doi.org/10.1016/j.yebeh.2016.10.035.

10. Rawlings GH, Reuber M. What patients say about living with psychogenic nonepileptic seizures: a systematic synthesis of qualitative studies. Seizure. 2016;41:100–11. https://doi.org/10.1016/j.seizure.2016.07.014.

11. Robson C, Lian OS. "Blaming, shaming, humiliation": stigmatising medical interactions among people with non-epileptic seizures. Wellcome Open Res. 2017;2:55. https://doi.org/10.12688/wellcomeopenres.12133.2.

12. Baizabal-Carvallo JF, Hallett M, Jankovic J. Pathogenesis and pathophysiology of functional (psychogenic) movement disorders. Neurobiol Dis. 2019;127:32–44. https://doi.org/10.1016/j.nbd.2019.02.013.

13. Voon V, Cavanna AE, Coburn K, Sampson S, Reeve A, LaFrance WC Jr. Functional neuroanatomy and neurophysiology of functional neurological disorders (conversion disorder). J Neuropsychiatry Clin Neurosci. 2016;28(3):168–90. https://doi.org/10.1176/appi.neuropsych.14090217.

14. Erro R, Brigo F, Trinka E, Turri G, Edwards MJ, Tinazzi M. Psychogenic nonepileptic seizures and movement disorders: a comparative review. Neurol Clin Pract. 2016;6(2):138–49.

15. Carson A, Lehn A, Ludwig L, Stone J. Explaining functional disorders in the neurology clinic: a photo story. Pract Neurol. 2016;16(1):56–61. https://doi.org/10.1136/practneurol-2015-001242.

16. Stone J, Carson A, Duncan R, et al. Who is referred to neurology clinics? – the diagnoses made in 3781 new patients. Clin Neurol Neurosurg. 2010;112(9):747–51. https://doi.org/10.1016/j.clineuro.2010.05.011.

17. Thomas M, Vuong KD, Jankovic J. Long-term prognosis of patients with psychogenic movement disorders. Parkinsonism Relat Disord. 2006;12(6):382–7. https://doi.org/10.1016/j.parkreldis.2006.03.005.

18. Baslet G, Dworetzky BA. Toward the integration of care. In: Psychogenic nonepileptic seizures: toward the integration of care. Oxford University Press; 2017. p. 308–14.

19. Raja S, Hasnain M, Hoersch M, Gove-Yin S, Rajagopalan C. Trauma informed care in medicine: current knowledge and future research directions. Fam Community Health. 2015;38(3):216–26. https://doi.org/10.1097/FCH.0000000000000071.

20. Ludwig L, Pasman JA, Nicholson T, et al. Stressful life events and maltreatment in conversion (functional neurological) disorder: systematic review and meta-analysis of case-control studies. Lancet Psychiatry. 2018;5(4):307–20. https://doi.org/10.1016/S2215-0366(18)30051-8.

21. Marotta A, Mirta F, Riello M, et al. Attentional avoidance of emotions in functional movement disorders. J Psychosom Res. 2020;133:110100. https://doi.org/10.1016/j.jpsychores.2020.110100.

22. Goldstein LH, Mellers JD. Ictal symptoms of anxiety, avoidance behaviour, and dissociation in patients with dissociative seizures. J Neurol Neurosurg Psychiatry. 2006;77(5):616–21. https://doi.org/10.1136/jnnp.2005.066878.

23. Stone J. We must tell our patients what is wrong with them even if we don't know why they have symptoms. Pract Neurol. 2011;11(2):98–9. https://doi.org/10.1136/jnnp.2011.241802comm.

24. Perez DL, Aybek S, Popkirov S, et al. A review and expert opinion on the neuropsychiatric assessment of motor functional neurological disorders. J Neuropsychiatry Clin Neurosci. 2021;33(1):14–26. https://doi.org/10.1176/appi.neuropsych.19120357.

25. Baslet G, Bajestan SN, Aybek S, et al. Evidence-based practice for the clinical assessment of psychogenic nonepileptic seizures: a report from the American Neuropsychiatric Association Committee on Research. J Neuropsychiatry Clin Neurosci. 2021;33(1):27–42. https://doi.org/10.1176/appi.neuropsych.19120354.

26. Nielsen G, Ricciardi L, Demartini B, Hunter R, Joyce E, Edwards MJ. Outcomes of a 5-day physiotherapy programme for functional (psychogenic) motor dis-orders. J Neurol. 2015;262(3):674–81. https://doi.org/10.1007/s00415-014-7631-1.

27. Gelauff J, Stone J, Edwards M, Carson A. The prognosis of functional (psychogenic) motor symptoms: a systematic review. J Neurol Neurosurg Psychiatry. 2014;85(2):220–6. https://doi.org/10.1136/jnnp-2013-305321.

28. McKenzie PS, Oto M, Graham CD, Duncan R. Do patients whose psychogenic non-epileptic seizures resolve, "replace" them with other medically unexplained symptoms? Medically unexplained symptoms arising after a diagnosis of psychogenic non-epileptic seizures. J Neurol Neurosurg Psychiatry. 2011;82(9):967–9. https://doi.org/10.1136/jnnp.2010.231886.

29. Reuber M. Dissociative (non-epileptic) seizures: tackling common challenges after the diagnosis. Pract Neurol. 2019;19(4):332–41. https://doi.org/10.1136/practneurol-2018-002177.

30. Carton S, Thompson PJ, Duncan JS. Non-epileptic seizures: patients' understanding and reaction to the diagnosis and impact on outcome. Seizure. 2003;12(5):287–94.

31. Morgante F, Edwards MJ, Espay AJ. Psychogenic movement disorders. Continuum (Minneap Minn). 2013;19(5 Movement Disorders):1383–96. https://doi.org/10.1212/01.CON.0000436160.41071.79.

32. Gelauff JM, Carson A, Ludwig L, Tijssen MAJ, Stone J. The prognosis of functional limb weakness: a 14-year case-control study. Brain. 2019;142(7):2137–48. https://doi.org/10.1093/brain/awz138.

33. Fouché M, Hartwig L, Pretorius C. Management of uncertainty in the diagnosis communication of psychogenic nonepileptic seizures in a South African context. Epilepsy Behav. 2019;98(Pt A):45–52. https://doi.org/10.1016/j.yebeh.2019.06.009.

34. Monzoni CM, Duncan R, Grünewald R, Reuber M. How do neurologists discuss functional symptoms with their patients: a conversation analytic study. J Psychosom Res. 2011;71(6):377–83. https://doi.org/10.1016/j.jpsychores.2011.09.007.

35. Reuber M, Fernández G, Bauer J, Helmstaedter C, Elger CE. Diagnostic delay in psychogenic nonepileptic seizures. Neurology. 2002;58(3):493–5. https://doi.org/10.1212/wnl.58.3.493.

36. Asadi-Pooya AA, Brigo F, Mildon B, Nicholson TR. Terminology for psychogenic nonepileptic seizures: making the case for "functional seizures". Epilepsy Behav. 2020;104(Pt A):106895. https://doi.org/10.1016/j.yebeh.2019.106895.

37. Edwards MJ, Stone J, Lang AE. From psychogenic movement disorder to functional movement disorder: it's time to change the name. Mov Disord. 2014;29(7):849–52. https://doi.org/10.1002/mds.25562.

38. Stone J, Edwards M. Trick or treat? Showing patients with functional (psychogenic) motor symptoms their physical signs. Neurology. 2012;79(3):282–4. https://doi.org/10.1212/WNL.0b013e31825fdf63.

39. Altalib HH, Elzamzamy K, Pugh MJ, et al. Communicating diagnostic certainty of psychogenic nonepileptic seizures - a national study of provider documentation. Epilepsy Behav. 2016;64(Pt A):4–8. https://doi.org/10.1016/j.yebeh.2016.08.032.

40. Morgante F, Edwards MJ, Espay AJ, Fasano A, Mir P, Martino D. Diagnostic agreement in patients with psychogenic movement disorders. Mov Disord. 2012;27(4):548–52. https://doi.org/10.1002/mds.24903.

41. Stone J, Hoeritzauer I. How do I explain the diagnosis of functional movement disorder to a patient? Mov Disord Clin Pract. 2019;6(5):419. https://doi.org/10.1002/mdc3.12785.

42. Salmon P, Humphris GM, Ring A, Davies JC, Dowrick CF. Why do primary care physicians propose medical care to patients with medically unexplained symptoms? A new method of sequence analysis to test theories of patient pressure. Psychosom Med. 2006;68(4):570–7. https://doi.org/10.1097/01.psy.0000227690.95757.64.

43. Tolchin B, Dworetzky BA, Martino S, Blumenfeld H, Hirsch LJ, Baslet G. Adherence with psychotherapy and treatment outcomes for psychogenic nonepileptic seizures. Neurology. 2019;92(7):e675–9. https://doi.org/10.1212/WNL.0000000000006848.

44. Bass C, Halligan P. Factitious disorders and malingering in relation to functional neurologic disorders. Handb Clin Neurol. 2016;139:509–20. https://doi.org/10.1016/B978-0-12-801772-2.00042-4.

45. Voon V, Gallea C, Hattori N, Bruno M, Ekanayake V, Hallett M. The involuntary nature of conversion disorder. Neurology. 2010;74(3):223–8. https://doi.org/10.1212/WNL.0b013e3181ca00e9.

46. Aybek S, Vuilleumier P. Imaging studies of functional neurologic disorders. Handb Clin Neurol. 2016;139:73–84. https://doi.org/10.1016/B978-0-12-801772-2.00007-2.

47. Green B, Norman P, Reuber M. Attachment style, relationship quality, and psychological distress in patients with psychogenic non-epileptic seizures versus epilepsy. Epilepsy Behav. 2017;66:120–6. https://doi.org/10.1016/j.yebeh.2016.10.015.

48. Stone J, Carson A, Hallett M. Explanation as treatment for functional neurologic disorders. Handb Clin Neurol. 2016;139:543–53. https://doi.org/10.1016/B978-0-12-801772-2.00044-8.

49. Ammentorp J, Sabroe S, Kofoed P-E, Mainz J. The effect of training in communication skills on medical doctors' and nurses' self-efficacy. A randomized controlled trial. Patient Educ Couns. 2007;66(3):270–7. https://doi.org/10.1016/j.pec.2006.12.012.

50. Aybek S, Lidstone SC, Nielsen G, et al. What is the role of a specialist assessment clinic for FND? Lessons from three national referral centers. J Neuropsychiatry Clin Neurosci. 2020;32(1):79–84. https://doi.org/10.1176/appi.neuropsych.19040083.

51. Goldstein LH, Mellers JDC. Psychologic treatment of functional neurologic disorders. Handb Clin Neurol. 2016;139:571–83. https://doi.org/10.1016/B978-0-12-801772-2.00046-1.

52. Crimlisk HL, Bhatia K, Cope H, David A, Marsden CD, Ron MA. Slater revisited: 6 year follow up study of patients with medically unexplained motor symptoms. BMJ. 1998;316(7131):582–6. https://doi.org/10.1136/bmj.316.7131.582.

53. Popkirov S, Nicholson TR, Bloem BR, et al. Hiding in plain sight: functional neurological disorders in the news. J Neuropsychiatry Clin Neurosci. 2019;31(4):361–7. https://doi.org/10.1176/appi.neuropsych.19010025.

54. Davy C, Bleasel J, Liu H, Tchan M, Ponniah S, Brown A. Effectiveness of chronic care models: opportunities for improving healthcare practice and health outcomes: a systematic review. BMC Health Serv Res. 2015;15:194. https://doi.org/10.1186/s12913-015-0854-8.

55. O'Neal MA, Baslet G, Polich G, Raynor G, Dworetzky B. Functional neurological disorders: the need for a model of care. Neurol Clin Pract. 2021;11(2):e152–6.

56. Sawchuk T, Buchhalter J, Senft B. Psychogenic non-epileptic seizures in children-Prospective validation of a clinical care pathway & risk factors for treatment outcome. Epilepsy Behav. 2020;105:106971. https://doi.org/10.1016/j.yebeh.2020.106971.

Developing a Treatment Plan for Functional Movement Disorder

20

Mark J. Edwards

Case Vignette

A 33-year-old woman was seen in neurology clinic after a recent onset of acute left sided weakness and sensory disturbance. She presented initially to the emergency department, and was suspected of having a stroke. However, examination at that time revealed a positive left Hoover's sign and brain MRI was normal. She was told that she had not had a stroke. She recalled one of the doctors telling her she might have hemiplegic migraine, despite her lack of a migraine history.

On assessment in clinic she described being previously well, working as a care assistant. She lived with her husband and 2 children (4 and 7). She worked 50–60 h a week. She reported having a flu-like illness 3 weeks previously during which time she had continued to work. She reported feeling fatigued and "spaced out". At the time of symptom onset she had just climbed 3 flights of stairs and described feeling faint, dizzy and was breathing fast. It was at this moment she felt tingling down the left side of the body and then found she could not move it. On further enquiry she described a period of post-viral fatigue at the age of 16 which had lasted about 12 months in total during which time she missed about

6 months of schooling. She had recovered with a paced return to activity and support from a clinical psychologist for concurrent low mood.

Examination revealed a pattern of intermittent recruitment of muscle power in the left arm and leg and a positive left Hoover's sign. Her understanding of the problem was that she probably had hemiplegic migraine. She had done quite a lot of research on the topic and had been prescribed topiramate by her primary care physician. She was worried about the genetic implications of the diagnosis for her children.

The diagnosis of a functional neurological disorder (more specifically a functional movement disorder (FMD)) was explained, including demonstration of the physical signs compatible with that diagnosis. She was perplexed as to why it had happened given that she was well previously and not particularly "stressed". She described being very stressed now as her employer was putting pressure on her to return to work and she was concerned about her financial security and that of her family.

An assessment was arranged with a multidisciplinary team of psychology, physiotherapy and occupational therapy, all with experience of working together with people with FMD. The diagnosis was further explained and a narrative was constructed integrating her past experience of post-viral fatigue and depression, her recent illness, her heavy work and family commitments, and the triggering of symptoms via exertion and

M. J. Edwards (✉)
St George's University of London, London, UK

Atkinson Morley Regional Neuroscience Centre, St George's University Hospital, London, UK
e-mail: medwards@sgul.ac.uk

© Springer Nature Switzerland AG 2022
K. LaFaver et al. (eds.), *Functional Movement Disorder*, Current Clinical Neurology,
https://doi.org/10.1007/978-3-030-86495-8_20

a likely "fight or flight" reaction. Treatment consisted of specific physiotherapy treatment aimed at automatic activation of muscles with attention diverted away from her symptoms, occupational therapy regarding pacing of activity, and psychology for cognitive behavioral therapy regarding depressed and anxious mood. The team helped with negotiations with her employer regarding her need for a break from work during recovery and then a phased return to work, with advice that she should try to reduce her hours of work overall.

Motor symptoms improved rapidly, but fatigue remained a significant problem. Depressed mood became more evident and following psychiatric assessment she was started on an antidepressant medication alongside ongoing psychological therapy.

By 6 months after symptom onset she had returned to work 2 days per week. Over the next 6 months she built up to 4 days a week at work. She was supported to explore alternative employment options, given that the physicality of care work continued to cause a flare-up of symptoms every few weeks.

Introduction

The historical and modern medical literature on functional movement disorder (FMD), and indeed functional neurological disorder (FND) in general, has focused strongly on diagnosis. This reflects a general neurological interest with the process of diagnosis, but of course diagnosis is not an end itself. It should instead be the gateway to management and longitudinal care. Even in the setting of incurable neurological disease without any specific medical remedies, there are basic standards of care that are part of normal clinical practice. These include continued neurological involvement, advocacy for social care and support, symptomatic medical treatment, and physical and psychological supportive treatments. However, for patients with FMD, the diagnostic process often ends in a cliff-edge. This cliff-edge represents the end of neurological and indeed any medical involvement and the

metaphorical pushing of the patient over the edge, because fundamentally the neurological job is done. The clinical diagnostic expertise and the expensive tests have given a conclusive verdict: there is not a neurological problem. This is the uncomfortable end of the road for many patients with FMD, leaving them unable to access either specific treatment or even the basic standards of supportive management and care we would expect for all our other patients with neurological symptoms [1].

Times are changing, slowly, and there is a growing realization and expectation that patients with FMD are within the orbit of responsibility of neurologists [2], and that there are, in addition, specific treatments that can be of benefit [3]. As outlined in Chap. 4 of this textbook, there is a push for a clear framing of FMD and related FNDs as core neuropsychiatric disorders at the intersection of neurology and psychiatry. This reframing acknowledges that physical health and mental health are closely intertwined, and as such the psychologically-informed neurologist is a core component of not only the diagnostic process but longitudinal care as well. These changes bring to the forefront the importance of considering how to plan treatment and services for patients with FMD, in order to offer rational access to useful treatment. Importantly, we also need to consider the wider question of how to best help patients with persistent symptoms despite treatment.

Setting Up a Specialized FMD Service

Healthcare services differ across the world, affecting access to care and the kinds of treatments that might be available. However, there are some basic facts about FMD which are universal. First, it is a common problem, accounting for about half of those with FND (if you include weakness as an FMD which is our framing here), and up to 20% of those attending specialist movement disorder clinics [4]. This means that a specialist service for FMD has to have a way of managing a high volume of patients at one time.

Second, it is a disorder which is fundamentally quite hard to explain and understand. It is easier to explain neurological symptoms on the basis of "brain lesions", such as in stroke, multiple sclerosis or brain tumors, compared to a "network dysfunction" of a system of perception and voluntary action which has a complex relationship with emotions and past and present physical/mental health. It is perfectly possible to create good diagnostic understanding, but it does take time, particularly in patients who have had a long journey through healthcare to receive a diagnosis. This means that a way needs to be found to offer time and space for consultations with patients with FMD to support the development of good diagnostic understanding, an essential pre-requisite of effective treatment. Third, it is a disorder that presents across multiple services. Patients present to primary care physicians, emergency services (including stoke services), general and sub-specialty neurology services (remember that 15% of those with neurological disease also have FND [5]), and other medical and surgical specialties (particularly orthopedics and rheumatology). There is also overlap with patients in chronic pain and post-concussive symptoms treatment programs. To effectively capture patients with FMD across different medical settings, an effective FMD specialist service has to have a long reach so that patients can be diagnosed and triaged into treatment effectively wherever they might present. Lastly, patients are very heterogenous in their symptoms, co-morbidities, severity and outcome with currently available treatments. This means that a service needs to be able to generate an accurate holistic view of the person with FMD and their problems and to triage effectively into relevant treatment(s). It also needs to have a way of continuing to help those who have persistent symptoms in the long term. With our current state of treatment (which is typically poorly available and given if at all after long delays in diagnosis), about 40% of patients with FMD remain with similar or worse symptoms in the long-term, and most of the remainder have some persistently disabling symptoms [6]. The chronic nature of FMD symptoms and co-morbidities

needs to be taken into account when designing services for FMD.

These universal properties of FMD are challenges which an excellent service for patients with FMD has to solve. The solutions to these challenges might therefore be considered as essential structural supports in the building that is an excellent FMD service (Fig. 20.1), acknowledging that there are likely to be many ways to design such a service. By managing patient flow (high volume, presenting across multiple services), creating good diagnostic understanding and trust, facing up to heterogeneity through good diagnostic skills and triage, and managing chronic care of patients with FMD we have the essential supports for an excellent service for FMD (and by extension FND in general). Below I will consider these themes in more detail to indicate how they might be developed practically into a workable clinical service that can create good treatment plans for its patients.

Managing Patient Flow

Keeping Some Patients Outside of Highly Specialized Services

With a common illness such as FMD, it is of great importance to keep a proportion of patients outside of a specialist service, but at the same time to ensure that their management is happening according to good practice recommendations and that patients can easily move into (and then out of) specialist services according to need. This is akin to observations that not all patients with migraine headaches can receive care in specialized headache clinical programs.

People with mild symptoms may not need to be referred into a specialist FMD service. For example, a patient with an episode of functional leg weakness following a bad migraine which resolves over the course of a few days may be referred to neurology clinic following an attendance at the Emergency Department. In this setting, and with appropriate assessment and screening, the patient is likely to be managed very effectively with simple diagnostic explana-

Fig. 20.1 Pillars of an excellent service for functional movement disorder

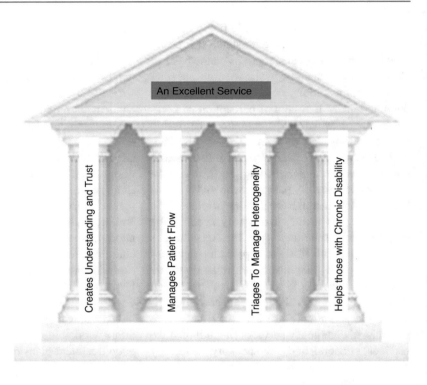

tion and advice and the provision of open follow up if symptoms recur. The key here is for neurologists in general to have support and training in diagnostic assessment and explanation and "red flags" in symptoms and co-morbidities which would suggest the need for onward referral into a specialist FMD service. Indeed, there may be some situations where explicit labelling of the problem as an FMD or FND more broadly is not needed and may be counter-productive. In some patients there is a very clear situational trigger for symptoms which can be best explained in a narrative manner (potentially using a broad mind-body formulation), rather than with diagnostic labelling. For example, a person who has had a severely painful injury who develops shaking of the affected part of the body lasting for an hour or so may not really benefit from being told that they have an FMD. It might be best to explain how severe pain can trigger other responses in the body, perhaps due to activation of autonomic "fight or flight" systems, which then usually go away once the pain improves.

There is a more complex situation with regard to patients with an established diagnosis of FMD who have had access to treatment within a specialist service, but have not had benefit. Such patients may be very anxious not to lose contact with the specialist service even though no active treatment is planned at the current time. This is often because of bad experiences previously within healthcare, and the fear of being abandoned, without any access to advocacy regarding their ongoing health problems. This is a difficult situation, but at the same time, a specialist service can become overwhelmed by closely following up a huge case-load of chronically disabled people, where, in the right circumstances, support could be given within primary care.

The aim of keeping some patients outside of the specialist service is so that the service itself can run in an effective manner without becoming overwhelmed by referrals and therefore progressively less and less responsive to the needs of patients with FMD. We expect a level of competence across neurologists in diagnosing and managing a range of common conditions (e.g. headache) without referring all patients into specialist services. This should also apply to a proportion of patients with FMD.

There are multiple solutions to achieving this in clinical practice. For example, we set up an educational workshop for newly diagnosed patients with FND to which a neurologist who had made and explained the diagnosis could refer patients for further information about FND and its treatment before they saw the patient again for a follow up appointment [7]. The workshop got positive ratings from patients and family members and may have helped neurologists be more confident in delivering the diagnosis, knowing that they had some back-up for generating good diagnostic understanding. Training for neurologists in diagnosis and diagnostic explanation [8], easy availability of an FMD team member for discussion about individual cases, responsiveness when assistance is needed (which builds confidence that if there was a problem the service would step in), and provision of information about community-based services to help support people with chronic symptoms are amongst a range of ways of helping patients to be successfully managed outside of a specialist service. The key component of all of these interventions is the building of confidence, skills and knowledge amongst patients and healthcare professionals to manage symptoms and providing a clear route to specialist advice when needed.

Connection with Other Services

As mentioned above, patients with FMD present across multiple services. This can mean that diagnosis, effective diagnostic explanation and access to treatment are all delayed, and there is the chance for iatrogenic harm from unnecessary treatments or procedures. Some patients with paroxysmal FMD present frequently to emergency services and may well end up in conflict with such services, becoming labelled as drug-seeking (as a range of sedative drugs will often abort attacks of FMD). Such conflicts tend to make diagnostic explanation and instigation of more rehabilitative treatment much harder than if an effective diagnostic explanation was given at the first presentation. Stroke services are another service where patients with FMD present – about

10% of people seen in acute stroke services have FND [9]. Such services are used to rapid turnover of patients and are highly protocolized. Patients with FMD do not fit within these protocols and therefore may not receive an optimal experience, often just discharged from the hospital even though they have persistent severe motor symptoms. A less common, but often dangerous, situation is the presentation of patients with painful fixed functional dystonia to orthopedic services. Indeed this syndrome may be triggered in the first place following an orthopedic operation or injury. If the correct diagnosis is not made, repeated operations, casting and splinting may be tried, sometimes with poor results [10]. Some patients will go on to amputation of the affected limb which can also lead in many cases to worsening symptoms [11].

The solution here is one based on communication and training, meaning that the specialist FMD service needs to be really embedded within other hospital services, offering responsive and effective in-reach in order to assist with diagnosis, diagnostic explanation and management. Once local pathways and protocols are in place, conflict between services and patients is reduced and it is more likely that patients will receive a timely well explained diagnosis and be able to access effective treatment.

Protecting the Service

While it has perhaps always been this way, the rise of care pathways and protocols and the dissolution of medicine and neurology into smaller and smaller sub-specialties, means that patients who do not fit (like patients with FMD) are vulnerable to being passed from service to service without anyone taking responsibility. In neurology, there are a large number of patients who do not have FMD, but also do not fit into other established sub-specialty clinics. They often have chronic psychiatric and social problems, perhaps with a neurological disease as well, but with difficulties driven by non-neurological factors. Another large group have an illness anxiety disorder, for example an intense pre-occupation with the possibility of having amyotrophic lateral sclerosis/motor neuron disease. When one establishes a service for FMD, it can become a place where all patients who do not have a natural "home" are referred. This is difficult, because although the skills of an FMD team might be useful for such patients, there are other services who should have that responsibility (or any FMD service would need to double/triple in scope/capacity/funding to make such an extension of service remotely possible). Paradoxically, by accepting everyone who is complex to manage into an FMD service, regardless of whether they have FMD or not, one may make the overall situation worse, as more appropriate services are not forced to improve and develop. This means that there need to be strong inclusion and exclusion criteria for referral to the service, and clear signposting for unsuitable referrals to a more appropriate service. In my experience this difficulty has been most acute between neurology and mental health services. A patient may have FMD, but the overwhelming disabling problem may be a personality disorder or post-traumatic stress disorder (PTSD). An FMD service is not really the correct service to see and treat such patients (at least not as the primary service guiding overall treatment recommendations). Unfortunately, in some circumstances a service for patients with personality disorder or PTSD may refuse to accept the patient due to their FMD diagnosis. Similar issues may arise with patients with FMD and overwhelming pain or fatigue where a specialist pain or fatigue management service might seem most appropriate, but will not accept the patient due to their FMD diagnosis.

In the end, such issues can only be resolved through good communication, and making sure there is a pathway so that people can flow from the FMD service to other services, particularly mental health services. However, making sure as a team that inclusion and exclusion criteria are agreed and enforced is a good start to running a service that can retain staff and be effective in the long term.

Creating Diagnostic Understanding and Trust

Surveys of doctors and other health professionals suggest that diagnostic explanation is perceived as difficult in patients with FMD/FND. Many have an experience during training of seeing confrontational and angry interactions between physicians and patients with FND, and so there is perhaps no surprise that this produces fear and apprehension about discussing the diagnosis.

Elsewhere in this book and in numerous published papers are approaches to diagnostic explanation in FMD/FND that are usually effective and provide an ideal foundation for considering treatment options [8].

Beyond this advice, there are some specific considerations that are important in developing a service for patients with FMD. The first is that proper assessment, diagnosis and diagnostic explanation for patients with FMD often takes a long time. Many patients have had symptoms for years and may have complex psycho-social backgrounds which are important to explore. In contrast, most neurological outpatient services have set appointment times regardless of the nature of the problem the patient presents with. We would not expect a neurosurgeon to spend the same amount of time decompressing the carpal tunnel as removing a pituitary tumor, and so it is no surprise that it is difficult to do an effective job of assessing a person with FMD in a 20–30 min appointment.

The solution to this will differ depending on the health system that operates in your country. However, there is no way of escaping the need for time to fully consider the patient's problems and to properly explain the diagnosis and how that may interact with other diagnoses and problems. As a rough guide, some clinical programs have set aside 60–90 min for a new consultation in a patient being referred for assessment and management of suspected FMD.

There are possible methods to speed up consultations while maintaining quality. For example, making sure you have understood the full range of symptoms is an essential part of diagnostic assessment. Patients could be asked to complete a symptom list prior to clinic to aid this process. Questionnaires can be used pre-clinic to assess quality of life, to record normal daily activities, medication, mood and so on. However, large numbers of pre-clinic questionnaires, particularly those asking about mood (and especially trauma), may not be popular with patients and may risk placing the consultation on the wrong foot before it has even started. Following the appointment, written information handed out can be useful as well as referral to online sources of support such as www.neurosymptoms.org. However, care is needed here too as a brief labelling of the diagnosis and referral to a website without further explanation is not likely to be an effective way to communicate the diagnosis of FMD (or indeed any diagnosis). Even very well supported referral to online resources after careful diagnostic explanation should not be assumed to be the only intervention needed. Even though this may be appreciated by patients and help to improve knowledge and confidence in the diagnosis, information alone should not be expected to lead to improvement in symptoms on its own for most patients [12].

Scheduling the patient for a follow up appointment, ideally soon after the original appointment, may be an effective way to make sure the diagnosis has been understood and to answer questions that have arisen – particularly in health care setting where the initial consultation time is limited. In cases such as this, the process of diagnostic explanation and treatment planning can be conducted over a series of initial visits (being transparent with the patient about this approach can also be helpful). Follow-up visits may also be a more appropriate time to explore co-morbidities and etiological factors using the biopsychosocial formulation (see Chap. 3 for more details) that may or may not be relevant, including difficult topics such as past trauma. However, this also places extra demands on the service which may

not be possible for all. Group workshops, as discussed above, may be an adjunctive intervention here.

It is important to recognize that there will be some patients with FMD who, despite time and an explanation delivered as competently and sensitively as possible, will not find the explanation convincing. They may remain of the opinion that either the true diagnosis is still unknown, or that there is a specific other diagnosis which is the correct one. In this situation, providing one has made efforts to appropriately try to deal with concerns, perhaps even offering a second opinion from a colleague, it is important to end the clinical relationship in as therapeutic a manner as possible. First, it is not appropriate to refer such patients into treatment for FMD. One should not be in the position of "pushing" FMD treatment onto a patient who has no belief in the diagnosis. Similarly, efforts to "convince" the patient about the diagnosis without some flexibility on the patient's part to be willing to explore a FMD diagnosis as an accurate formulation for their clinical picture can prove fatiguing for the physician and, even more importantly, does not set the appropriate therapeutic stage for potential treatments that are to come (where the patient plays an important role in their own recovery). Second, it is important to communicate your diagnosis clearly in writing to the patient and to other doctors involved in their care. This serves an important protective function, helping to avoid the patient being given inappropriate treatment by others. It also serves as a clear record of your diagnosis and your belief in the reality of the patient's symptoms. This means that there cannot be a claim from the patient or other doctors in the future that "Doctor X told me I had nothing wrong with me…". Lastly, it is important, as far as possible, to terminate contact in a positive manner and with an invitation to come back again. This means that if the patient reconsiders at a future date they will have a route back in which has been given as an open and genuine invitation [13].

Triage

Triage is a short word, but it is a complex process, and one that is essential to developing an effective treatment plan and running an effective service for patients with FMD.

Triage and Symptom Type

FMD covers a very wide range of symptoms from weakness, gait disturbance, tremor to jerks and fixed dystonia. Such symptoms may be present all the time or may be paroxysmal, in some patients overlapping with functional [psychogenic nonepileptic/dissociative] seizures.

These differences in symptoms are important to triage when treatment planning. Persistent functional motor symptoms are often amenable to treatment with specialist physiotherapy. However, different techniques may be useful for different symptom types. For example, fixed dystonia may result in fixed contractures and the presence of very severe pain may limit the use of hands-on rehabilitation. In such patients there may be a necessity for an examination under anesthesia prior to commencing treatment to check for the presence of mechanical contractures, and then a slow rehabilitation program that works first on habitual postures (e.g. sitting position) while gradually building up to standing. Paroxysmal symptoms may be difficult to treat with physiotherapy, especially if symptoms are very intermittent and cannot be induced easily during a treatment session. In this situation, psychological techniques used in treatment of functional seizures may be more applicable. These examples show the need for effective multidisciplinary teams to be involved in treatment planning for patients with FMD so that the patient is not exposed to the counter-therapeutic experience of being referred to treatment only to be told they are not suitable [14, 15]. These examples also show the importance of flexibility within treatment programs for patients with FMD so that a patient may be able to have, for example, treatment intermittently over some months, whereas others may receive a brief intensive treatment.

Triage and Other Functional Symptoms

FMD rarely occurs in isolation: the majority of patients have other functional neurological (e.g., functional seizures) and somatic symptoms [16]. These symptoms confer disability in their own right and can sometimes dramatically alter the kind of treatment that is suitable.

A triumvirate of fatigue, chronic pain and cognitive "fog" is exceedingly common in patients with FMD, and for some are the dominant cause of disability (and may be their chief complaint). Indeed, several studies have now found that the correlation between quality of life and motor symptom severity in patients with FMD is poor, and that in contrast, quality of life relates much more closely to fatigue, pain and mood [17, 18].

When triaging patients into treatment, it is important to draw a distinction between two groups of patients with FMD. On one side are patients who will report pain, fatigue and cognitive fog, sometimes at quite high levels, but at the same time have good levels of activity on a daily basis. Such patients tend not to have to sleep during the day and they can usually perform activities every day such as hobbies, work or education. On the other side are patients who report severe levels of fatigue, pain and cognitive fog, but in addition, the symptoms are very volatile. This means that with activity, sometimes even minimal activity, they may experience a severe flare-up of these symptoms, meaning they will need to be completely inactive, sometimes for several days. As a result they will often report needing to sleep on most days and will have very limited or no ability to do daily activities.

Understanding this situation for an individual is very important. Intensive rehabilitation tends to be ineffective for patients with very volatile fatigue, pain and cognitive function. Such patients often simply cannot tolerate the intensity of treatment and will develop rapidly worsening symptoms. A more appropriate approach would be a slow, paced approach to building resilience to activity, similar to that used within chronic pain and chronic fatigue rehabilitation programs [19]. In fact, involvement in chronic pain or cognitive rehabilitation programs may be the most appropriate option, and careful considerations need to be given to assess for sleep, autonomic and psychiatric disorders amenable to specific treatments. Treatment planning for this group of patients often requires a staged approach as outcome from engagement in traditional FMD rehabilitation programs can be poor. If patients have appropriately engaged but failed to benefit from rehabilitation approaches, consideration needs to be given for offering chronic supportive care rather than active treatment. This is a clear area in need for novel treatment development.

Figure 20.2 gives an example of a randomized study that attempted to recruit 60 patients with FMD into either specialist intensive physiotherapy or standard physiotherapy treatment [20]. In order to find 60 suitable patients, over 200 were screened, with dominant pain and fatigue as well as untreated mood disturbance the key factors leading to exclusion from this treatment. As an example of the success of this triage approach,

the initial cohort study where this treatment was developed where inclusion was much broader found on average a 9-point change in the SF36 physical function scale [21]. The subsequent randomized study with more stringent criteria found on average a 19-point change in the same measure.

Triage and Co-morbidity

Patients with FMD can have a range of other problems including other neurological disorders, general medical disorders and psychiatric disorders. If diagnosis of these disorders is not prioritized at the beginning of the pathway, then treatment that is decided upon may be ineffective, and indeed direct harm can result from a failure to identify and treat a more important medical problem than the FMD.

Overlap between FND and neurological disorders is common, with rates of about 15% reported

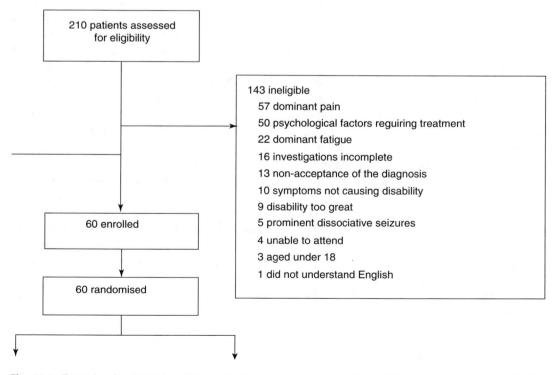

Fig. 20.2 Example of patient triage into specialist physiotherapy for patients with functional movement disorder (Diagram adopted with permission from Nielsen et al. 2017)

in the literature [5]. FND can present as a prodrome for the later development of another disorder (this has been reported in Parkinson's Disease for example [22]), or it may develop alongside an established disorder. Dissecting the relative contributions of each disorder can be difficult, but it is very important, particularly where potentially toxic or invasive treatments might be being considered such as deep brain stimulation surgery for Parkinson's disease or immunomodulatory therapy for multiple sclerosis. Close working relationships between an FMD service and other neurology subspecialties are important here, including the use of a shared language with the patient for discussing the FMD.

Patients with FMD may have other nonneurological diagnoses. A history of complex medical illness in itself a risk factor for development of a FND. Some medical conditions result from the FMD as secondary problems, for example the development of sleep apnea secondary to weight gain caused by medications and loss of mobility. There is no replacement here for careful extensive history taking and keeping an open mind on the cause of symptoms even if they are common in patients with FMD (e.g. fatigue). There is sometimes a fear amongst clinicians in "opening Pandora's box" by re-investigating someone with an established diagnosis of FMD. However, within a good clinical relationship and with a clear explanation of what the purpose of investigations are, this need not result in destabilization of the FMD diagnosis. Conversely, the practice of automatically assuming that any new symptom results from the FMD is a very dangerous one indeed.

Psychiatric co-morbidity is clearly present in many patients with FMD, occurring both as a secondary consequence of the personal impact of symptoms and as pre-existing risk factors for the development of FMD. Diagnosis of such problems can be complex as patients with FMD may be reluctant to discuss such issues, given fears about their symptoms in general being dismissed as "just depression" and only being offered medical and psychological treatments for their mental health. There is also the complex issue of alexithymia in patients with FMD, where they may

have difficulty in recognizing and labelling their emotional state [23]. This may mean that symptoms of underlying depression, anxiety and/or post traumatic stress disorder are relatively underappreciated and will not be identified except with careful interviewing.

Furthermore, there are a number of psychiatric diagnoses where physical symptoms are quite common. For example, physical symptoms are commonly reported in people with schizophrenia, even when prominent psychotic symptoms such as visual and auditory hallucinations are not present; we have encountered patients referred for suspected FMD/FND who were somatically-preoccupied and did not meet criteria for FND but rather were in the prodromal stages of a primary psychotic spectrum illness. Other individuals may have FMD, but there is an additional psychiatric diagnosis that is of much more importance in disability, such as a severe anxiety disorder, or obsessive compulsive disorder. In such cases, the FMD can be seen to be "driven" by the underlying psychiatric diagnosis: this is perhaps most often seen in the context of severe PTSD [24]. In all these situations, psychiatric diagnosis and treatment advice is essential.

This situation indicates the need for proper integration of psychiatric skills within the FMD team, ideally a neuropsychiatrist – although there are far too few "card carrying" neuropsychiatrists to meet the clinical needs. Similar to the above comment of the need for neurologists seeing this population to be psychologically-informed, psychiatrists generally benefit from a component of increased neurological training where possible. It is also essential that this person is a team member and not acting in isolation. Involvement needs to be at the beginning of the process of triage: getting it right, diagnostically, at the beginning makes the process of treatment much more likely to succeed.

Triage and Timing

I have discussed above the importance of recognizing and appropriately managing patients with FMD who do not have any confidence in the diagnosis at this time. There are another group who are also very important to identify in triage: those with severe symptoms who are not likely to benefit from intensive multidisciplinary rehabilitation at this time.

There is sometimes a view amongst health professionals that if a person with FND believes the diagnosis, then there is no reason why they should not get better. This is simply untrue: there are many patients who have excellent diagnostic understanding and excellent commitment to treatment who do not improve at a particular point in time. There is a related view which is also often untrue, which is that if symptoms are really severe, then the only treatment that is worthwhile is a really intensive multidisciplinary program. This is an idea borrowed from medical problems such as infection, where the more severe the symptoms, the more intense the treatment needs to be.

Many people with FMD will remain with symptoms despite a belief in the diagnosis, commitment to treatment and the provision of reasonable treatment. A specialist FMD service needs to be mindful of this. There are likely to be many reasons why people do not improve with treatment, many of which remain unknown at this time. It may be possible to identify major maintaining (perpetuating) factors that are present and may be changeable over time within the context of the biopsychosocial formulation. For example, some patients are in abusive relationships or have severe housing problems which, if improved (perhaps with help and advocacy from the team) might place them in a better situation to benefit from treatment. For some people, illnesses such as personality disorder or treatment resistant depression make FMD recovery more difficult. This topic is explored in more detail in Chap. 30 of this book on overcoming treatment obstacles.

It is important, therefore, that triage takes a holistic view of the patient, their difficulties and their past attempts at treatment, in order to understand what is the best advice to give at this time. I have found that for some patients, a shift of focus from impairment-based to participation-based treatment and support can be very effective. This may mean that even though symptoms are still present at a similar level of severity, people are in less distress and are participating more in pleasurable activities.

Triage: Getting It Right First Time

I have mentioned above how consultations with people with FMD are often longer than those for other conditions, and the need to find a way to set aside sufficient time to get the initial assessment right. Getting triage right is similar – it needs time. Investing heavily in triage (in terms of time, expertise, and therefore healthcare costs) is worthwhile as it prevents patients being directed towards ineffective or inappropriate treatments. In my own practice, the team are moving towards, in a subset of patients who we judge to be more "complex", a period of extended assessment and therapy. This is conducted online or as an outpatient and involves a multidisciplinary team who work with a patient over a few weeks in a combination of extended assessment, exploration of goals/goal setting, and trialing some simple interventions (often related to fatigue management). We have found this approach to be useful in getting a better picture of the patient *and their environment*, something that is hard to achieve even in an extended outpatient appointment. This process can also provide information on diagnosis (for example relating to personality disorder or other psychiatric diagnoses that were not apparent on initial assessment), ability to engage with the rehabilitation process, confidence in the diagnosis, and maintaining factors present in the home and wider social environment, as well as making sure that patients who are suitable for multidisciplinary rehabilitation are primed to get the most out of the time they have in treatment.

Chronic Care

FMD is a chronic condition for many patients. The hope is that with earlier diagnosis, better diagnostic explanation and rapid access to appropriate evidence-based treatments, a majority of patients will achieve long-lasting treatment success. However, we are a long way from this now, and even with the widespread implementation of optimal services for patients with FND, many patients are likely to have chronic symptoms.

It is important that an excellent FMD service recognizes this and makes suitable provision for such patients. Many patients with FMD are very reluctant to be discharged from specialist services. This is entirely understandable as they have often had negative experiences in other services, and are concerned that if they are discharged they will never be able to get support in the future if they need it.

The solution here is for there to be strong relationships between the FMD team and other services, particularly primary care and community mental health and social care services. The optimal outcome is for there to be training and support from the specialist service to allow others to take on the day to day management of patients with FMD. The flip side of this is for the service to be rapidly responsive to a crisis situation (e.g. sudden worsening of symptoms, development of new symptoms) so that these can be rapidly evaluated and advice given for treatment (including going back into the specialist service). This fluid

stepping up and stepping down between services is difficult to achieve in practice, but from the perspective of patient care and experience it is a goal worth striving for.

What Treatment Is Right for Whom? A Broad Overview

In the chapters that follow there are detailed descriptions of specific treatment approaches for people with FMD. Figure 20.3 gives a general scheme for an FND treatment pathway, with clear diagnosis and diagnostic explanation at the beginning, an "easy" triage of a proportion of patients direct into physiotherapy-led treatment or psychiatry/psychology services, and then a more complex group of patients who *may* benefit from specialist intensive multidisciplinary rehabilitation, but where a further period of assessment is needed to make the best decision. The pathway has some provision for chronic care, ideally in close collaboration with community services, where patients can step out of and back into the service depending on need. Within this broad overview there are a large number of unan-

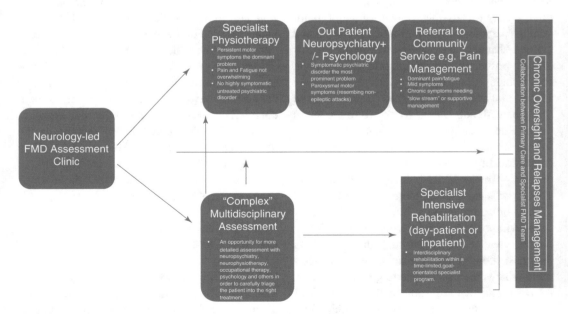

Fig. 20.3 Example of a care pathway for functional movement disorder (FMD)

swered questions. What is the best setting for treatment to take place: home-based, outpatient, day-patient, inpatient? What is the right intensity of treatment? What is the optimal "dose" of treatment? Should treatment continue long term in some form in order to prevent relapse? These and other questions do have answers, and part of the excitement of the FMD field is that so much still is left to be discovered, in partnership with patients, clinicians and researchers.

Conclusions

FMD is a common and complex condition and often associated with several co-morbidities. An effective treatment plan has to encompass all of this complexity and provide a logical approach to what is for many patients a chronic illness.

Summary Box 20.1 gives some pointers for the components of an excellent service for patients with FMD considering pre-service factors, the service itself, and then the process following discharge from the service.

The absolute priority is to get it right at the beginning. In practice this means:

1. Getting the patient into the right service early before diagnostic uncertainty, conflict and unnecessary treatments and investigations have happened.
2. Getting all the diagnoses that are present (across neurology, psychiatry and general medicine) established and explained effectively as early as possible.
3. Optimizing treatment decisions based on this diagnostic knowledge and the available services.

Following this path provides a good opportunity for getting high quality care and positive outcomes for patients with FMD.

Summary Box 20.1 Aspects of an Excellent Service
- **Pre-service**
  - Educates referral services and **supports them to manage mild and chronic patients**
  - Manages expectations of referrers and what patients are told about specialist services
- **Service**
  - Entry criteria, not a dumping ground
  - Provides effective exploration of **all the diagnoses present** and explains them well
  - Moves patients into services that are appropriate for symptoms and that speak the same language based on **robust triage**
  - Manages overlap with other relevant services (pain, fatigue, general psychiatry)
  - Provides a route back to the service for reassessment and refocussing.
  - Has the confidence to say no to specific types of treatment
- **Post Service**
  - Manages discharge effectively through managing patient and referrer expectations
  - Interfaces with community services and supports them
  - Provides a way back in

References

1. Edwards MJ. Functional neurological disorder: an ethical turning point for neuroscience. Brain. 2019;142(7):1855–7.

2. Perez DL, Haller AL, Espay AJ. Should neurologists diagnose and manage functional neurologic disorders? It is complicated. Neurol Clin Pract. 2019;9(2):165–7.

3. Gilmour GS, Nielsen G, Teodoro T, Yogarajah M, Coebergh JA, Dilley MD, Martino D, Edwards MJ. Management of functional neurological disorder. J Neurol. 2020;267(7):2164–72.

4. Hallett M. Psychogenic movement disorders: a crisis for neurology. Curr Neurol Neurosci Rep. 2006;6(4):269–71.

5. Stone J, Carson A, Duncan R, Roberts R, Warlow C, Hibberd C, Coleman R, Cull R, Murray G, Pelosi A, Cavanagh J, Matthews K, Goldbeck R, Smyth R, Walker J, Sharpe M. Who is referred to neurology clinics? – the diagnoses made in 3781 new patients. Clin Neurol Neurosurg. 2010;112(9):747–51.

6. Gelauff J, Stone J, Edwards M, Carson A. The prognosis of functional (psychogenic) motor symptoms: a systematic review. J Neurol Neurosurg Psychiatry. 2014;85(2):220–6.

7. Cope SR, Smith JG, Edwards MJ, Holt K, Agrawal N. Enhancing the communication of functional neurological disorder diagnosis: a multidisciplinary education session. Eur J Neurol. 2021;28(1):40–7. https://doi.org/10.1111/ene.14525.

8. Carson A, Lehn A, Ludwig L, Stone J. Explaining functional disorders in the neurology clinic: a photo story. Pract Neurol. 2016;16(1):56–61.

9. Gargalas S, Weeks R, Khan-Bourne N, Shotbolt P, Simblett S, Ashraf L, Doyle C, Bancroft V, David AS. Incidence and outcome of functional stroke mimics admitted to a hyperacute stroke unit. J Neurol Neurosurg Psychiatry. 2017;88(1):2–6.

10. Schrag A, Trimble M, Quinn N, Bhatia K. The syndrome of fixed dystonia: an evaluation of 103 patients. Brain. 2004;127(Pt 10):2360–72.

11. Edwards MJ, Alonso-Canovas A, Schrag A, Bloem BR, Thompson PD, Bhatia K. Limb amputations in fixed dystonia: a form of body integrity identity disorder? Mov Disord. 2011;26(8):1410–4.

12. Gelauff JM, Rosmalen JGM, Carson A, Dijk JM, Ekkel M, Nielsen G, Stone J, Tijssen MAJ. Internet-based self-help randomized trial for motor functional neurologic disorder (SHIFT). Neurology. 2020;95(13):e1883–96.

13. Adams C, Anderson J, Madva EN, LaFrance WC Jr, Perez DL. You've made the diagnosis of functional neurological disorder: now what? Pract Neurol. 2018;18(4):323–30.

14. Aybek S, Lidstone SC, Nielsen G, MacGillivray L, Bassetti CL, Lang AE, Edwards MJ. What is the role of a specialist assessment clinic for FND? Lessons from three national referral centers. J Neuropsychiatry Clin Neurosci. 2020;32(1):79–84.

15. Jacob AE, Smith CA, Jablonski ME, Roach AR, Paper KM, Kaelin DL, Stretz-Thurmond D, LaFaver K. Multidisciplinary clinic for functional movement disorders (FMD): 1-year experience from a single centre. J Neurol Neurosurg Psychiatry. 2018;89(9):1011–2.

16. Nicholson TR, Carson A, Edwards MJ, Goldstein LH, Hallett M, Mildon B, Nielsen G, Nicholson C, Perez DL, Pick S, Stone J, and the FND-COM (Functional Neurological Disorders Core Outcome Measures) Group. Outcome measures for functional neurological disorder: a review of the theoretical complexities. J Neuropsychiatry Clin Neurosci. 2020;32(1):33–42.

17. Věchetová G, Slovák M, Kemlink D, Hanzlíková Z, Dušek P, Nikolai T, Růžička E, Edwards MJ, Serranová T. The impact of non-motor symptoms on the health-related quality of life in patients with functional movement disorders. J Psychosom Res. 2018;115:32–7.

18. Gelauff JM, Kingma EM, Kalkman JS, Bezemer R, van Engelen BGM, Stone J, Tijssen MAJ, Rosmalen JGM. Fatigue, not self-rated motor symptom severity, affects quality of life in functional motor disorders. J Neurol. 2018;265(8):1803–9.

19. Jimenez XF, Aboussouan A, Johnson J. Functional neurological disorder responds favorably to interdisciplinary rehabilitation models. Psychosomatics. 2019;60(6):556–62.

20. Nielsen G, Buszewicz M, Stevenson F, Hunter R, Holt K, Dudziec M, Ricciardi L, Marsden J, Joyce E, Edwards MJ. Randomised feasibility study of physiotherapy for patients with functional motor symptoms. J Neurol Neurosurg Psychiatry. 2017;88(6):484–90.

21. Nielsen G, Ricciardi L, Demartini B, Hunter R, Joyce E, Edwards MJ. Outcomes of a 5-day physiotherapy programme for functional (psychogenic) motor disorders. J Neurol. 2015;262(3):674–81.

22. Wissel BD, Dwivedi AK, Merola A, Chin D, Jacob C, Duker AP, Vaughan JE, Lovera L, LaFaver K, Levy A, Lang AE, Morgante F, Nirenberg MJ, Stephen C, Sharma N, Romagnolo A, Lopiano L, Balint B, Yu XX, Bhatia KP, Espay AJ. Functional neurological disorders in Parkinson disease. J Neurol Neurosurg Psychiatry. 2018;89(6):566–71.

23. Demartini B, Petrochilos P, Ricciardi L, Price G, Edwards MJ, Joyce E. The role of alexithymia in the development of functional motor symptoms (conversion disorder). J Neurol Neurosurg Psychiatry. 2014;85(10):1132–7.

24. Gray C, Calderbank A, Adewusi J, Hughes R, Reuber M. Symptoms of posttraumatic stress disorder in patients with functional neurological symptom disorder. J Psychosom Res. 2020;129:109907.

Psychological Treatment of Functional Movement Disorder

Joel D. Mack and W. Curt LaFrance Jr.

Introduction

Psychological approaches have a long history in the treatment of functional neurological (conversion) disorder (FND), including functional movement disorder (FMD). How psychological factors are intertwined with FMD conceptual frameworks [1], nomenclature [3], and approach to treatment [4], however, have fluctuated over time. Despite the integral, albeit at times debated, role of psychological approaches in treating FND over the last 150 years, evidence-based guidance for incorporating psychological therapies into "real world" treatment of FMD has been sparse. Recent years have seen increased interest and advancement in the approach to FMD, including further study of psychological interventions as an important element in multi-disciplinary treatment planning, with a goal of offering effective therapeutic options and hope to a group of patients who have often been historically approached by some neurologists and mental health clinicians with a sense of therapeutic nihilism.

Diagnosis of FMD can be categorized based on phenotype-specific findings rooted in neurological examination [5]. While updated DSM-5 diagnostic criteria no longer *require* identifying the presence of psychological disturbance [6], psychological factors remain critically important as contributors to the etiology. The diagnostic formulation involves characterizing predisposing, precipitating, and perpetuating factors in FMD, and mounting evidence supports the use of psychotherapy interventions addressing these factors in the treatment of FMD and other FND subtypes. The authors aim to equip practitioners treating FMD with a practical foundation in the process and content of using psychological treatment to help patients with FMD gain control of their abnormal movements and improve their lives. It is also important to highlight that clinicians not directly involved in delivering psychotherapy to their patients can be informed by psychotherapeutic principles in their longitudinal follow-up with patients to help catalyze treatment [7].

J. D. Mack (✉)
Department of Psychiatry, Veterans Affairs Portland Health Care System, Portland, OR, USA

Northwest Parkinson's Disease Research, Education, and Clinical Center, Department of Neurology, Veterans Affairs Portland Health Care System, Portland, OR, USA

Departments of Psychiatry & Neurology, Oregon Health and Science University, Portland, OR, USA
e-mail: mack@ohsu.edu

W. C. LaFrance Jr.
Brown University, Providence, RI, USA

Providence Veterans Affairs Medical Center, Providence, RI, USA

Departments of Psychiatry and Neurology, Rhode Island Hospital, Providence, RI, USA
e-mail: william_lafrance_jr@brown.edu

© Springer Nature Switzerland AG 2022
K. LaFaver et al. (eds.), *Functional Movement Disorder*, Current Clinical Neurology,
https://doi.org/10.1007/978-3-030-86495-8_21

What Is Psychological Treatment?

Psychological treatments can be loosely defined as healing practices that utilize talk and behavioral techniques for the sake of relieving distress. This definition is initially useful in differentiating psychological interventions from "physical" treatments, such as physiotherapy, or "biological" treatments, such as neuropsychiatric medications or neuromodulation (e.g., transcranial magnetic stimulation). However, psychological treatments have biological correlates: advances in brain science reveal the impact psychological treatments have on the neurobiology of the "plastic" brain, dissolving the traditional dichotomous psychology and biology view and encouraging an integrative approach [8, 9]. At first glance, this definition may also impart blurred boundaries in which one considers psychological treatments to include activities such as coaching, vocational counseling, or patient support groups, but, for the sake of this chapter, we will limit our discussion of psychological treatments to refer specifically to psychotherapy and its practice.

Psychotherapy can be defined as:

An interpersonal treatment that is (1) based on psychological theory and principles; (2) involves a trained therapist and a patient who is seeking help with a particular disorder, problem, or complaint; (3) is intended by the therapist to be helpful for the presenting disorder or problem; and (4) is adapted for the particular patient and his or her disorder, problem, or complaint [10].

Psychological theory guides the process of understanding a patient's problems and developing solutions, providing a "road map" to navigate human functioning and the process of change, as well as a structure for conceptualizing data provided by the patient and guidance for therapeutic action [10]. While there have been hundreds of psychotherapies developed, it is worthwhile to consider a brief introduction to major paradigms in psychological theory that inform current approaches to treating FMD (Table 21.1; also see historical perspectives covered earlier in this text).

Psychotherapeutic Modalities

Psychodynamic (insight-oriented) psychotherapies are rooted in the psychoanalytic theories of Sigmund Freud, who posited the conversion model of "hysterical" physical symptoms. In this model, psychological conflict is considered to be repressed, triggering conversion of tension into physical symptoms, providing relief from anxiety as well as allowing escape from threatening situations [11]. The treatment is based on the premise that insight into the connection between psychological conflict (or traumatic events) and symptoms allows resolution of the conflict and ultimately the physical symptoms. Pierre Janet, a contemporary of Freud, who posited that a singular psychosexual formulation for the development of hysteria was an oversimplification, developed the concept of dissociation to account for "hysterical" symptoms. Janet's dissociative model referred to the process by which a psychological stress or trauma leads to fragmentation of the mind into separate compartments, with dissociative symptoms being due to "compartmentalization," characterized by a loss of voluntary control over apparently intact processes and functions [18]. Janet believed that dissociative symptoms were reversible, but his model was incongruous to Freud's unconscious conversion theory that went on to dominate the psychotherapeutic approach of the time. Nonetheless, Janet's conceptualization of dissociation has remained important to the formulation of FND symptom genesis.

Dissatisfied with the lack of observable evidence offered by the psychoanalytic approach, therapists developed behavioral approaches that began to emerge from learning theory in the early twentieth century as characterized by the work of Pavlov (classical conditioning) and later Skinner (operant conditioning). In the 1960s, Aaron T. Beck combined behavioral approaches with cognitive therapy, which aimed to reverse maladaptive patterns of information processing (automatic thoughts), to synthesize cognitive-behavioral therapy (CBT). While initially developed as a treatment for depression, CBT has been

Table 21.1 Psychotherapy: theoretical approaches to functional neurological disorder

Psychotherapy approach	Theoretical background	Therapeutic stance/ techniques	Goals/outcomes
Psychodynamic (Insight-Oriented) [10, 11]	Psychoanalysis, early attachment, psychosexual stages of development, unconscious motivation, defense mechanisms	Formal, Therapist-Patient Roles	Insight, resolution of unconscious conflicts, ego strength, healthy defenses, integration
Cognitive-Behavioral Therapy (CBT) [10, 12]	Learning Theory, behaviorism: classical and operant conditioning, cognitive theory	Guided discovery, Collaborative-empiricism	Distress Reduction, Symptom Reduction, Adaptive Functioning
Dialectical Behavior Therapy [13]	CBT, mindfulness, *Dialectic*-understanding concepts by examining and appreciating their opposites	Support oriented; collaborative; See CBT & Mindfulness	Establishing safety, emotion regulation, distress tolerance, interpersonal effectiveness
Prolonged Exposure Therapy [14]	CBT, Learning Theory, Trauma Processing	In vivo and imaginal exposure	Decreased fear/anxiety and avoidance related to trauma stimuli
Humanistic-Existential [10]	Humanistic philosophy, self-determination, self-actualization	Authentic, present-focused, client-centered	Authenticity, meaningful existence, freedom, self-actualization
Mindfulness [15, 16]	Adapted from Buddhist meditation, Elements of CBT and psychoeducation in mindfulness-based therapies	Enhanced awareness, Present focused, Emotional acceptance	Increased awareness, Sustained attention, Self-compassion, Enhanced emotional regulation
Integrative (Holistic) [10, 17]	Biopsychosocialspiritual, addressing the whole person in the continuity of their humanity	Patient-led, Therapist guided, addressing how past narrative influences here and now	Utilizing/synthesizing specific elements of various psychotherapies to treat the specific patient and presenting problem; identifying schema, making the implicit explicit, paradoxical surrendering control to gain control

See selected references for additional background

the most studied psychotherapy across a variety of neuropsychiatric conditions, including FND [12, 19–21], and CBT principles have served as the foundation for a myriad of specialized adaptations. Dialectical Behavior Therapy (DBT) is an operationalized form of CBT originally developed with the aim of improving emotion regulation, distress tolerance, and interpersonal effectiveness to treat borderline personality disorder, but it has since been found to be useful in treating a number of neuropsychiatric disorders, including FND [13], a group of patients in which altered emotional processing is thought to be a link between psychosocial risk factors and functional neurological symptoms [22]. Prolonged Exposure Therapy is a form of CBT developed to treat Post Traumatic Stress Disorder (PTSD), utilizing in vivo and imaginal exposure to traumatic stimuli to process trauma and

decrease related anxiety and avoidance. Prolonged exposure therapy techniques may be particularly useful for treatment of patients dually diagnosed with FND and PTSD [14].

A third, parallel wave of humanistic-existential psychotherapies arose following World War II, with a basis in humanistic philosophy and goals grounded in the pursuit of self-actualization and meaning in life, and an increased use of mindfulness-based techniques. Mindfulness has been defined as "the awareness that emerges through paying attention with purpose, in the present moment, and non-judgmentally to the unfolding of experience moment by moment," [15]. It is used in many forms of meditation and specific psychotherapies developed around mindfulness practices (Mindfulness-Based Stress Reduction, Mindfulness-Based Cognitive Therapy), developed in the 1980s, have shown efficacy across a range of psychological problems [23]. It has been proposed that mindfulness exerts its effects via changes in attention regulation, body awareness, emotion regulation, and perspective on the self [16], each of which is thought to be abnormal in FMD [24].

Although differentiation of psychological approaches is useful for a contextual framework and highlighting specific concepts and techniques in each school of psychotherapy, many psychotherapies (and psychotherapists) pull from an eclectic mix of psychological approaches to provide patient-centered treatments. An integrative (holistic) approach uses a biopsychosocial-spiritual framework and utilizes multiple modalities to equip the patient with tools to address the past and present, addressing symptoms and schema, examining self, and interacting with their social-cultural environments and existential concerns.

The State of the Evidence: Psychotherapy in FMD

The use of psychotherapy to treat FMD is supported by an accumulating body of evidence, although studies to date have been limited by open-label, retrospective, or case-based designs and small sample sizes. The range of psychotherapy approaches and techniques used across FMD studies has varied, blurring the generalizability and reproducibility of findings. Despite issues with study design and uniformity of treatment approaches, available data lay a foundation of efficacy for FMD-psychotherapy interventions, and ongoing conceptual refinements in FMD phenotyping and neurobiology are informing more nuanced, integrated, and consistent approaches to psychological treatment of FMD. Study design issues have been addressed, to some degree, in treatment trials of other FND subtypes, specifically functional [psychogenic non-epileptic/dissociative] seizures, with psychotherapy showing promise in pilot randomized, controlled trials using conventional CBT

[25] and manualized treatment of cognitive behavioral therapy-informed psychotherapy (CBT-ip) [20], also referred to as Neuro-Behavioral Therapy [NBT]) [26].

In the follow up to Goldstein et al.'s pilot RCT, the recently published conventional CBT + standardized medical care vs standardized medical care (SMC) alone RCT showed improvement in quality of life with CBT and a reduction in functional seizures at 6 months, but no difference at 12 months compared to SMC [19]. Whether the benefits of psychotherapy for other FND subtypes can be extrapolated to FMD specifically is grounds for further research, although FMD and functional seizures have been shown to have clinical, phenotypic, and neuro-biologic similarities [27], and some psychotherapy treatments have shown promise across FND subtypes [28]. Optimal FMD outcomes will rely on psychotherapy not as a siloed modality of care, but as a tool combined with physical interventions in a multidisciplinary, integrated approach to treating patients with FMD [29].

Cognitive Behavioral Therapy for FMD

CBT-based therapies are the best-established treatment for mind-body disorders generally [30], have a strong evidence base in treating other types of FND (e.g., functional seizures) [31], and have been evaluated in FMD across a range of movement phenomenology. Despite unifying principles underlying the provision of CBT, the multitude of techniques in the CBT "toolbox" can make for variability in the process of therapy, but also allows for tailored interventions for individual patients with FMD or related problems. Manualized CBT interventions address the issue of variability and offer a uniform approach to CBT, and further development of manualized CBT approaches will play an important role in multi-center trials and dissemination of CBT-based FMD treatments to more practitioners.

Espay et al. [9] showed markedly reduced tremor severity in an open-label trial of CBT for

15 patients with functional tremor, with remission or near remission of tremor (>75% reduction in tremor severity) observed in almost three-quarters of subjects in the functional tremor group. The CBT intervention consisted of 12 weekly, one-hour outpatient sessions, with the goal of helping patients identify how thoughts impact emotions that present as physical symptoms or behaviors, and the authors note a focus on thought monitoring, identifying cognitive distortions, and thought restructuring consistent with Aaron Beck's model of cognitive therapy. The investigators used a non-manualized protocol, noting this allowed for tailoring the intervention to individual patients at the potential expense of increased variability. The improvement in functional tremor following CBT was also associated with a significant decrease in anterior cingulate/paracingulate overactivity but no significant change in motor area activity on fMRI, highlighting the role that emotion and attention centers of the brain may play in the generation of functional tremor and providing the first published study utilizing neurobiological imaging correlates to assess outcomes in FMD-psychotherapy research. More work is needed to disentangle neural mechanisms of psychotherapy response, as well as baseline biomarkers predicting treatment response.

While the CBT intervention in Espay et al. [9] was not manualized, it based treatment sessions on a manualized protocol initially developed as CBT-ip used for functional seizures [32]. The 12-session, workbook-based, time-limited Neuro-Behavioral Therapy equips patients to address adverse life experiences, negative core beliefs, cognitive distortions, maladaptive stress responses, and resulting somatic symptoms, with the goal of treatment being positive behavioral change, increased self-efficacy, and ultimately improved seizure control [33]. Extending from a previous open-label, pilot trial [32], the benefit of this therapy was further shown in a four-treatment arm pilot RCT for functional seizures, consisting of: CBT-ip, CBT-ip with antidepressant medication, antidepressant alone, and standard medical care [20]. The two groups treated with CBT-ip demonstrated a significant reduction in seizure frequency, both with antidepressant (59.3%) and CBT-ip alone (51.4%). Patients receiving CBT-ip also showed improvement on measures of depression, anxiety, quality of life, and global functioning. LaFrance and Friedman [28] also demonstrated symptom improvement in a young woman suffering from a 5-year history of functional dystonia, who had complete resolution of abdominal, arm, and facial dystonia following the CBT-ip protocol, and she remained symptom free at 16-month follow up.

An intervention based on Goldstein et al.'s [25] manualized conventional CBT for functional seizures was used to treat a group of 29 patients with FMD (mostly functional tremor) randomized to CBT alone, CBT plus adjunctive exercise (low/moderate intensity walking), or standard medical care [34]. Both treatment groups significantly improved on measures of motor function, depression and anxiety relative to controls, although there were no significant differences on the same measures between the active treatment groups. While the study failed to find beneficial effect of adjunctive exercise on any outcome measure, CBT was shown to be effective across physical and emotional domains.

Sharpe et al. [21] evaluated a CBT-based guided self-help (GSH) intervention in a group of 127 patients with mixed FND, some of whom had FMD. They found that the addition of GSH to usual care improved subjective change in overall health (primary outcome) and presenting symptoms at 3 months compared to usual care alone. While improvement in primary outcome was no longer significant at 6 months follow up, improvements in secondary outcomes including change in presenting symptoms, less belief in symptoms being permanent, greater satisfaction with care, and improved physical functioning were maintained. There was no therapist-provided CBT in this intervention, although there was a maximum of four half-hour "guidance sessions" provided by a clinician trained in CBT. The authors cite the potential simplicity, feasibility, acceptance by patients, and cost-effectiveness of GSH interventions as reasons they are worthwhile to explore for FND treatment.

A retrospective study of 98 patients with motor FND (most commonly weakness, pain, and tremors) found that nearly half of patients showed significant improvement in motor symptoms and significant decreases in depression and psychological distress following a course of CBT [35]. The single predictor of motor symptom improvement in the motor FND group was acceptance of a psychological explanation of functional motor symptoms prior to CBT. CBT was at least as effective in the motor FND group when compared to a group with other neuropsychiatric conditions (for example Tourette's syndrome or multiple sclerosis), highlighting that patients with FMD can get better and providing grounds for clinicians rejecting the "therapeutic nihilism" sometimes associated with FMD.

Psychodynamic Psychotherapy for FMD

Psychodynamic psychotherapy interventions for FMD are also supported in the literature, although negative results have also been published. Sharma et al. [36] retrospectively evaluated the clinical outcomes of 30 patients with FMD treated with psychodynamic psychotherapy (mean number of therapy sessions was 4.9). The psychotherapy led to improvement in 60% of patients, with good outcome (near complete resolution of movement symptoms) in 10 patients. Patients with poor outcomes tended to be less receptive to diagnosis and lacking insight into the functional nature of their symptoms when compared to good responders. Duration of symptoms was longer in poor responders compared to good responders (4.6 years versus 1.3 years).

An earlier study showed significant improvement in Psychogenic Movement Disorders Rating Scale scores (pre-treatment, 71.2 vs post-treatment, 29.0, p = 0.0195), as well as improvement in measures of depression and global

functioning, in 10 patients treated with a 12-week psychodynamic psychotherapy intervention accompanied by adjunctive treatment with psychiatric medication [37]. However, Kompoliti et al. [38] did not see a significant benefit in terms of motor symptoms or mood from immediate or delayed psychodynamic treatment in 15 patients with FMD when compared to neurological observation/support at 3 and 6 months in a randomized cross-over trial, concluding that regular follow up with a neurologist could be as effective as psychodynamic approaches.

Humanistic-Experiential, Mindfulness, and Integrative (Holistic) Approaches

Psychotherapy treatments falling purely into models of Humanistic psychotherapies (person-centered, gestalt, and existential therapies) have not been formally studied in treating FMD, although core elements of these approaches (see Table 21.1) may be interwoven into eclectic models. The Integrative (Holistic) approach has not been used in an RCT of FMD, but case reports using the approach in a patient with functional dystonia [28] and in one of the author's (WCL) Neuropsychiatry and Behavioral Neurology Division has shown improvement in symptoms and functioning in patients with FMD. Other modalities have been tested, including a randomized clinical trial of hypnosis vs wait list control in 44 patients with FMD, which showed improvement in the hypnosis group [39]. Elements of mindfulness have been incorporated into integrative FND-psychological treatments and may offer a framework for future research.

Acceptance and Commitment Therapy (ACT) is a mindfulness-informed, acceptance-based behavior therapy that draws upon elements of humanistic approaches and classic CBT techniques with a goal of increasing psychological flexibility and supporting behaviors that are consistent with a person's overarching values. It has been studied broadly across patient groups and can be adapted to address a range of psychological problems. Graham et al. [40] describe a case of a young woman with functional myoclonus who experienced improvements in psychological flexibility, function, and mood, as well as near complete resolution of motor symptoms following a six-session ACT intervention. Authors utilize the case to demonstrate how unique features of ACT may render it particularly useful in the context of FMD. A follow-up case series by the same group [41] of 8 patients with various FND symptoms including FMD showed "reliable improvements" in symptom-related functional interference and mood in around 50% (but statistically significant change in only 25% of patients).

Integration of Psychotherapy into Multidisciplinary FMD Treatment Models

While integration of neurologic and psychiatric approaches to FMD is covered earlier in the text, it is worth reiterating that psychological interventions should be viewed as an element of an integrated treatment plan with common goals. Functional movement symptoms are the multidisciplinary domain of neurologists, psychiatrists/psychological practitioners, and physiotherapists, occupational and speech therapists, among others, and a transdisciplinary approach allows interdisciplinary learning and skill-building, improved communication, and ultimately modeling of brain-mind-body integration for the patient [29]. Studies to date have not compared effectiveness of psychotherapy *versus* physiotherapy for FMD, but an alternative focus may include complementary or synergistic effects of physical and psychological interventions and which specific components are effective across disciplines.

Nielsen et al. [42] highlight biopsychosocial treatment principles of physiotherapy for FMD including elements such as, "create an expectation of improvement," and "recognize and challenge unhelpful thoughts and behaviors," both of which are based in psychotherapeutic concepts and speak to overlap across disciplines. A randomized, unblinded, study examining an inpatient, "adapted physical activity within a cognitive behavioural framework" intervention to treat 31 patients with functional gait disorder showed improvement in ability to walk and quality of life compared to a group of 29 untreated controls [43]. Benefits were maintained at 12-month follow up. Symptom explanation was provided by a multidisciplinary team accompanied by an explicit expectation of quick recovery, and treatment consisted of daily adapted sports activities with positive reinforcement of function but not of dysfunction. The authors acknowledged that the study design did not allow for deciphering which elements of the intervention accounted for therapeutic effects but pointed to further study of specific effective treatment factors as a future direction.

Psychotherapy for FMD: A Practical Approach

Clinical Vignette, Part 1: History of Present Illness

S. is a 27-year-old, right-handed, single man evaluated in the movement disorders specialty clinic for abnormal jerking movements of 5 years duration and more recent gait disturbance. Jerking movements started at age 22 abruptly in his right arm and trunk while on a 6-month deployment at sea during his naval service. He had suffered a blow to the head on a steel beam during a training exercise the week prior with brief, seconds-long loss of consciousness but recovered quickly and returned to training. Over the following months, jerking movements became more diffuse, and he had two events in which he experienced whole-body shaking and fell to the ground with preserved wakefulness but inability to speak during the event. He was sent for evaluation at the naval medical center where brain MRI and two routine EEGs were normal. Despite the ongoing evaluation, he was medically dis-

charged from the military with a diagnosis of "seizure disorder." He had no prior history of abnormal movements or seizures earlier in life. He also experienced occasional migraine headaches following the head trauma. His mother had bouts of headaches, fatigue and weakness, and thought he had heard "multiple sclerosis" mentioned when he was young; there was no family history of definitive neurological illness to his knowledge.

In the few years following military discharge, he saw neurologists in different locations and had trials of anticonvulsant medications, none of which provided benefit for jerking movements. He was taking topiramate "for the movements and headaches." A psychiatrist diagnosed him with "tic disorder" and prescribed trials of haloperidol, lorazepam and guanfacine, to which the patient admitted poor adherence, due to lack of benefit, although he felt lorazepam provided mild relief from anxiety. He described periods of decreased jerking movements as well as spontaneous remissions for as long as 2 months, specifically noting decreased symptoms during a 1-year romantic relationship with a woman. When the relationship ended (age 26-years-old), he experienced abrupt re-emergence of severe symptoms in multiple areas of his body. One whole-body jerking event resulted in a fall to the ground while drinking alcohol socially with friends. He subsequently developed fear of falling (although without additional falls) and difficulty walking. Ultimately, he was referred to a seizure monitoring unit for video-EEG monitoring, which revealed normal awake EEG rhythms and no epileptiform discharges despite capturing numerous brief head, trunk and limb jerks, noted to be variable in quality, duration, and direction, without alteration of consciousness. His jerking limb movements were also noted to be distractible to mental tasks, would amplify when attention was drawn to them and demonstrated entrainment with volitional movements performed in other body parts. Movements were not present during sleep. Repeat brain MRI was also normal. He

was referred for evaluation in the movement disorders clinic.

In addition to the above neurological observations, evaluation by a movement disorders neurologist revealed a gait that appeared normal upon a short walk into the exam room but was slowed and cautious ("walking on ice") with astasia-abasia (non-economical compensatory movements) when formally examined.

A diagnosis of "functional movement disorder" was explained as a disorder of communication between his brain and body using a "hardware-software" analogy, and core phenomenological features were demonstrated to the patient. While reluctant to fully accept the diagnosis, S. voiced relief at having an explanation for his abnormal movements and to hear news that there would be continued follow-up and helpful treatment options. He accepted recommended online educational resources and agreed to follow up with the neurologist and other members of the multidisciplinary treatment team, including the clinic psychiatrist.

Diagnosis as the Initial Step in Psychotherapy

As discussed in Chap. 17 of this book, delivering the FMD diagnosis is the first step in the therapeutic process, and doing so in an empathic, confident and understandable manner is vital to facilitating subsequent treatment planning. Stone et al. [44] recommend: taking the patient seriously, giving the problem a diagnostic label, explaining the rationale for the diagnosis, some discussion of how symptoms arise (i.e. hardware versus software analogy), emphasis on reversibility, and effective triage for treatment. Despite historical debate about FMD nomenclature, *how* the FMD diagnosis is presented is as important as what you call it, with high patient confidence in the diagnostic explanation being a positive prognostic factor [45]. It is important to have completed relevant neurological/medical workup prior to diagnosis so as not to leave room for unnecessary questioning of the FMD diagnosis, while also allowing for some degree of diagnostic fluidity should evidence for an alternative diagnosis or relevant comorbidity come to light through longitudinal follow-up. An integrated diagnostic approach involving both neurology and psychiatry will serve to bolster patient understanding and confidence, and scheduling follow up with the diagnosing movement disorders specialist is important to display ongoing support and ensuring follow through with treatment plans.

Who Is the "Right" Patient for Psychotherapy?

Pursuing psychotherapy is about sending the right patient for the right treatment for the right indication at the right time [17]. Engaging a patient with FMD to initiate psychotherapy starts with the basics: a clear FMD diagnosis and a patient open to psychological treatment. Referring a patient who is adamantly resistant to psychotherapy as a treatment is akin to prescribing a medication to a patient who states they will not take it. [46].

Acceptance of a psychological explanation for FMD symptoms has been shown to result in better psychotherapy outcomes [35], but a requisite motivation for change may be adequate to begin to engage in the therapy process. The patient needs to have some buy-in that their own work in their recovery is a critical element in the therapeutic process (which is different from just taking a pill). For those who do not fully "buy in" to a psychological explanation, other motivating factors, including a desire to decrease symptoms, improve function, enhance well-being, or foster healthy relationships with oneself and others, can function as a starting point. Assessing locus of control, the belief that one's own actions (internal) versus outside forces (external) impact outcomes in their life, is useful early on, as therapy both relies on

and encourages the patient to view themselves as the agent of change in the therapeutic process, and ultimately increasing this sense of agency in regard to abnormal movements and life circumstances is a goal of therapy.

DSM-5 diagnostic criteria for FND relegated identifying the presence of a stressor as linked to functional neurological symptoms to a clinical note, not a required criterion because patients may not acknowledge (or be aware of) "stress" as a contributing factor prior to psychotherapy, and because some patients may also find it difficult to readily share traumatic information in brief encounters with clinicians [46]. O'Connell et al. [35] defined a "psychological" explanation as "an information-processing account that invokes attentional processes, attribution errors, and behavioral avoidance and that acknowledges the temporal relationships between symptoms and 'stress,' mood, anxiety, or dissociation." Demonstrating positive exam signs encourages patient acknowledgment of aberrant attentional and behavioral aspects of abnormal movements, and this acknowledgement may be adequate to engage in psychotherapy even if a stressor is not initially identified.

Early stages of psychotherapy explore the connections between past and present experiences, and temporal relationships between stressors and symptoms may be realized as the process proceeds. Comorbid problems tend to be common for patients with FMD, and factors such as under-retreated (and under-recognized) mood and anxiety symptoms, maladaptive personality traits (for example, high external locus of control), potential financial gain, cognitive complaints, and current substance use disorder among other factors may be obstacles to the therapeutic process [17]. Those whose schedules are perceived as "too busy" due to life circumstances may have difficulty in therapy as the core therapeutic work lies in assignments (i.e. "homework") completed between sessions. This can be a common predisposing vulnerability and perpetuating factor, prioritizing the needs of many others in one's life while under attending to one's own physical and emotional well-being.

Who Provides Psychotherapy?

Psychotherapists emanate from a wide range of disciplines, typically including psychologists, psychiatrists, social workers, licensed counselors, psychoanalysts, mental health nurses and nurse practitioners. However, with appropriate training both "psychologically-minded neurology practitioners and neurologically-minded psychology practitioners" can obtain the tools to provide psychotherapy [47]. Psychotherapists treating patients with FMD should have an interest in treating this patient group, background in evidence-based approaches, and a knowledge of FMD-specific illness features. There may be benefit in the FMD-psychotherapist being someone other than the prescribing neurologist or psychiatrist to disentangle the psychotherapy process from other aspects of treatment such as medication management that may distract from the therapeutic process.

For those who desire proficiency to adequately deliver psychotherapy for FMD and related conditions, training beyond this chapter will be necessary, but a working understanding of the concepts and process of psychotherapy will prove beneficial to any practitioner involved in diagnosing and treating within a multidisciplinary FMD treatment team. Reading some of the published psychotherapy manuals available for treating the greater spectrum of FND would provide additional educational value [17, 48]. Other treatment modalities, such as physiotherapy, involve elements of psychotherapy technique, and incorporating psychotherapy principles into interactions with patients with FMD is beneficial for maintaining therapeutic rapport across treatment modalities.

Published work on FMD-specific psychotherapy interventions has not included group psychotherapy designs, although a pilot study of 16 patients with functional seizures or "other functional neurological symptoms" treated with a CBT-based group therapy intervention showed promise in regard to feasibility and significant improvements in measures of emotional well-being, as well as positive mean score in the clinician-rated (CGI) improvement scale [49]. Most recent FMD psychotherapy studies have been based on an outpatient model, although the option to hospitalize for intensive treatment, if available, offers the opportunity to engage in efficient treatment with regular access to the full multidisciplinary team while the patient maintains distance from deleterious perpetuating factors outside of the hospital [50].

Initial Assessment and Formulation

Psychotherapy begins with a complete history. In addition to understanding the history and presentation of movement symptoms, it is important to elicit an account of the patient's life story including family-structure, development, educational background, and childhood experiences through to adulthood regarding social, relationship and occupational functioning and spiritual belief system. A review of past psychiatric treatment and substance use, both from the patient and available records, is important. A listening, empathic approach, allowing the patient to tell the story from his or her perspective, will encourage openness and lays the groundwork for establishing rapport. When the therapist inquires about traumatic childhood or adult experiences during the developmental history, direct questioning about such topics, especially early on in treatment, may be met with emotional guarding, anxiety, or suspicion of the therapist's motives. Utilizing open-ended, non-judgmental questions allows the patient to reveal details at a pace comfortable to them.

"What was the atmosphere like in your home growing up? How would you describe your relationship with your parents and siblings when you

were a child? How did everyone get along at home? How did your parents handle disagreements? What was your parents' stance on alcohol use? Would you say you felt safe and secure at home?"

A thorough initial assessment provides content to synthesize a formulation of the patient's illness across the neurological, characterological, behavioral, and life-story perspectives [51]. While it is important to obtain history from childhood experiences through to current symptoms and function, the goal of initial assessment is one of information-gathering. Guiding the patient to "make connections" *is not* the aim at this early stage. Information from the initial assessment is integrated into a theoretical framework from which treatment and psychotherapy will proceed, and case conceptions will be further refined or altered as therapy progresses.

Based on the evidence-base for psychotherapy treatment in FMD and the goal of outlining a practical treatment approach, we will provide a framework for conducting psychotherapy, at times highlighting elements of NBT (CBT-ip treatment) of FMD, which not only includes CBT principles but also utilizes targeted elements of other psychotherapy approaches for known pathologies in this population.

Case, Part 2: Biopsychosocialspiritual History

Upon psychiatric assessment, S. reported being born without known complications. He grew up in a middle-class household including both parents and an older brother. His father was described as "authoritarian," and S. noted, "Nothing was ever good enough for him." His father occasionally used physical punishment ("hit with a belt") and frequently resorted to emotional criticism and physical intimidation, especially when using alcohol. He recalled that his father would ridicule him for displaying emotions. He denied childhood sexual abuse. He was an average student with a few friends and denied significant behavioral issues. He briefly attended

community college but left after one term to work while living with his parents. He was raised attending church "off and on" with his family. He denied adherence to any particular religious faith, but he voiced a belief in "God or some higher power." At age 20, he joined the military, leaving the family home for the first time. He had never been married and had no children, having had two romantic relationships with women, each of approximately 1-year duration.

S. discharged from the military at age 23-years old and returned to his hometown, where his parents had since separated. He again attempted to attend college but found he had difficulty focusing on schoolwork. He worked several jobs but could not hold one for more than 6 months, which he related to his abnormal movements and difficulty being around people. His financial situation led him to move into his father's house. While he hoped to "start fresh" with his father given the arrangement, he soon found that patterns of emotional abuse resurfaced.

S. had used alcohol in a binge fashion during the military and continued to do so on occasion, although he had stopped for a period following onset of his motor symptoms. He smoked small amounts of cannabis at night, which he believed helped with sleep, and occasionally smoked cigarettes.

He described ongoing symptoms of anxiety and depression since leaving the military. He felt "on edge" in crowds and suffered broken sleep and nightmares. He engaged in intermittent mental health treatment with a psychiatrist and was prescribed antidepressants and various sleep aids but admitted to poor adherence after feeling paroxetine caused him to feel "out of it." His most recent psychiatrist suspected post-traumatic stress disorder (PTSD) related to military experiences and referred him to a psychologist, but S. did not follow through with the appointment and discontinued follow up.

Open-ended questioning about S.'s military experience revealed he had been sexually assaulted by a superior officer shortly after deployment to sea. He did not report the incident and described being "stuck on the ship" and having to work closely with the assaulting officer. S. noted that he has declined further assessment for PTSD as he would rather "leave it in the past."

Elements of the patient's history can be considered in terms of predisposing, precipitating, and perpetuating factors [52, 53] for the development and maintenance of FMD and related functional neurological symptoms.

- Predisposing (genetics, adverse childhood experiences, characterological and coping vulnerabilities, symptom modeling):
  - Emotionally and physically abusive father
  - Potential symptom modeling from mother
  - Emotional privation during developmental periods
- Precipitating (physical injury, psychological trauma, life stress):
  - Head trauma on ship
  - Sexually assaulted on ship
- Perpetuating (psychiatric disorders, social benefits, illness beliefs, deconditioning, plastic brain changes)
  - "Stuck" living with abusive father
  - Untreated depression and possible PTSD
  - Unable to hold a job

Placing these elements into a theoretical framework provides the basis from which to proceed with psychotherapy. We demonstrate both CBT and psychodynamic-based formulations (Fig. 21.1a and b), as both may be useful in an NBT approach, and different perspectives may be called upon while abiding with the patient during the treatment. It is vital to have a clear idea of the patient's understanding of their illness, as imposing a model of illness on the patient that they are unable to reconcile will result in resistance and disengagement.

While CBT is generally present-focused, incorporating the understanding of the contributing role of past experiences, traumas, and relationships for the patient can encourage rapport building and individualized treatment planning. Psychodynamic theory historically stemmed from Freud's "conversion" model of hysteria, and, while more recent neurologically-based approaches to FMD diagnosis do not include psychological stressors as necessary criteria, contemporary neuroscience evidence supports the relevance of adverse life events and related psychological concepts in the modern conceptualization of FND [11]. Patients with FND, including FMD, experience higher rates of childhood trauma, including greater emotional and physical abuse/neglect and sexual abuse [54, 55]. Particular FND patient groups may be more likely to have experienced traumatic life events: an association between sexual abuse and FMD may contribute to a preponderance of this condition in women [56], and United States veterans with FND, a predominantly male group with high levels of trauma exposure (as in the case of *S.*), have been shown to have higher rates of psychiatric illness, including PTSD, compared to veterans with other neurological illnesses [57, 58]. A psychodynamic approach exploring early life experiences, the atmosphere surrounding the family of origin, and stresses or traumas over the lifetime may be particularly useful with some patients. Relationships between past experiences and current symptoms are brought to awareness through the therapeutic process allowing resolution of conflicts and related physical symptoms, as well as adaptation of healthy coping mechanisms. Treating patients with FMD using purely Freudian psychoanalytic techniques is less common in present-day psychotherapy practices. The concepts of conversion, however, are useful tools in formulating some patients with FMD and are often included as elements of NBT and other psychotherapy approaches, as laid out in this chapter. As a cautionary note, the conversion disorder formulation may not apply to all patients with FMD and related FND subtypes, which is why a patient-centered formulation leveraging the biopsychosocialspiritual formulation is critical for informing the integrative psychotherapeutic process, addressing specific themes that are relevant for each patient.

Psychoeducation and Treatment Planning

In the early stage of treatment, expectations and goals of therapy are discussed. Initial psychother- apy sessions are used to educate patients about the psychotherapy process and ensure a clear understanding of what can be expected from them and the therapist over the upcoming episode of treatment.

A typical episode of conventional CBT is time-limited, consisting of between 5 and 20 sessions of 40 to 60 min each. Sessions have a set structure, and manualized versions are available for treatment of many psychiatric disorders with

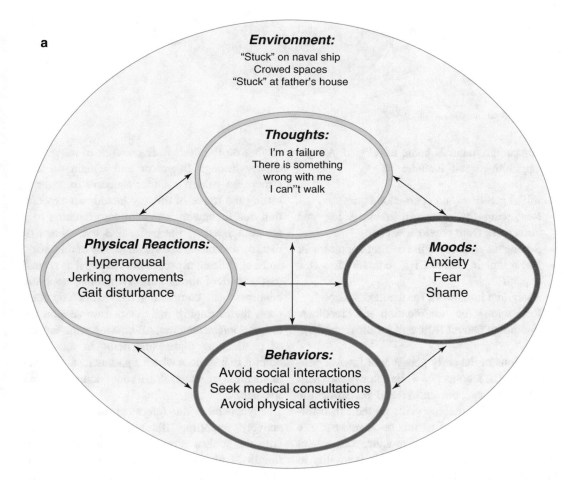

Fig. 21.1 Psychotherapy formulation: the case of S. Panel (**a**) Neuro-behavioral therapy formulation: five aspects of life experiences. (Adapted with permission from Oxford University Press: Reiter et al. [33]). Panel (**b**) Psychodynamic "conversion" formulation. (Formulation diagram modeled from Cretton et al. [11])

Note: while the "conversion" model of functional move- ment disorder and related functional neurological symp- toms continues to apply to many patients, it may not universally apply to all patients. As such, a patient-cen- tered biopsychosocialspiritual formulation should be applied across the spectrum of functional neurological disorder, allowing for considerable individual differences. (*Reprinted with permission from the Journal of Neuropsychiatry and Clinical Neurosciences, (Copyright ©2020). American Psychiatric Association. All Rights Reserved*)

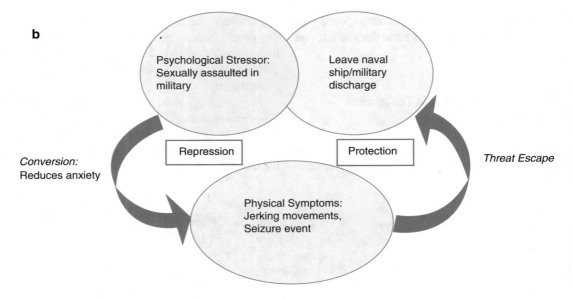

Fig. 21.1 (continued)

FMD-specific manuals being developed. A typical appointment will include:

- Initial greeting (and open-ended question)
- Reviewing the symptom tracking log and homework from previous session
- Setting an agenda for the current appointment
- Engaging in core CBT content for that session
- Assigning homework for the next session
- Reviewing for clarification or feedback (including patient feedback for the therapist).

Sessions in the early phases will involve education on CBT concepts while later phases will focus on relapse prevention and preparing the patient to utilize therapy skills on their own following termination of treatment. A set structure helps therapy stay on track to address treatment goals but there is adequate built-in flexibility to tailor therapy to each individual patient.

In the NBT (CBT-ip) collaborative care model, it is important to learn about and integrate the patient's goals into therapy ("patient-led") while relying on the therapy framework to move efficiently through treatment and remain on task ("therapist-guided"). Other elements to cover in setting the frame of therapy include an expectation that homework and symptom tracking logs are completed by the patient, as the content of therapy sessions are based on review of this work, and a significant aspect of the "therapy" is related to the patient monitoring symptoms, applying concepts, and completing the "work" on their own, then bringing their work into session for discussion/clarification. Addressing some aspects of challenging homework items in session is helpful in instances where a patient needs further explication of material, without "doing the work for them".

Psychoeducation refers to the process of actively imparting illness-related information with the goal of providing patients and/or their families with an understanding of concepts and skills that foster illness self-management, improve treatment adherence, and support relapse-prevention. Psychoeducation is often utilized as a tool in a broader psychotherapy intervention although can be delivered as a therapy on its own.

Two separate studies examining brief psychoeducation interventions in FND have shown promise: a group of patients with functional seizures showed improved function and decreased health care resource utilization (although not decreased seizure frequency) when compared to controls receiving usual treatment [59], and another group showed significant reduction in seizure frequency in over half the patients treated [60] following psychoeducation. In CBT, psychoeducation can be used throughout the therapy process to highlight and clarify information by way of techniques such as providing mini lessons to illustrate illness concepts, using manualized workbooks or handouts, and providing recommended reading. It is useful to incorporate "real-world" examples from a patient's life into psychoeducational lessons to increase relevance and application of the information.

Neuro-Behavioral Therapy (CBT-informed Psychotherapy): Process and Techniques

Initial therapy sessions entail equipping the patient with a foundation in the language and concepts necessary to further explore the interaction of thoughts, emotions, behaviors, situations and physiological reactions (Fig. 21.1a). Patients engage in identifying these elements. A worksheet list of emotions, thoughts, and situations for them to identify may identify challenges with alexithymia or concept enmeshment (for example, consistently mistaking thoughts for situations). Examples from the worksheet include:

Frightened	_Emotion_
Eating at a restaurant	_Situation_
I'm a failure	~~Situation~~ (corrected to _Thought_)

The Antecedents, Behaviors, and Consequences (ABC) model helps to observe and assess the "cause and effect" relationships of their behaviors. Antecedents may be emotions, thoughts, situations, physiological responses, or other behaviors. Consequences can be categorized as positive or negative, depending on whether they increase or decrease the likelihood a behavior will occur again, respectively. Many patients believe that situations give rise to behaviors, discounting the role of their emotions and thoughts. Alexithymia, a failure to identify and describe emotions in oneself and a difficulty in distinguishing and appreciating the emotions of others, has been shown to be a risk factor for FMD [61], and so it may be especially important to promote this ability in this patient group. Journaling, ideally daily, should be encouraged from early in therapy, as this provides a "safe space" for the patient to identify and process these elements on their own.

The symptom tracking log (Box 21.1) provides an opportunity to observe in greater detail how specific emotional, situational, or physical triggers relate to their abnormal movements. It is important that a patient fills out the symptom log accurately each day as a means of tracking abnormal movement frequency and severity, as well as observing relationships between their abnormal movements and other aspects of daily life. Caution should be taken; however, for a subset of patients that may be hypervigilant and obsessional, such that symptom monitoring may perpetuate unhelpful patterns – in such individuals, greater emphasis may be given to distraction and relaxation techniques (see below).

Box 21.1: Abnormal Movements Log

ABNORMAL MOVEMENTS LOG   _____ / _____ / _____ (date)

Frequency/Duration of abnormal movements:_____

Time(s) of day:_____

Body parts affected:_____

Description/Type of movement:_____

Location(s):_____

Severity (1: mild, 2: mod, 3: severe):_____

Trigger(s) (physical, emotional, situational):_____

Precursor(s) / Warning Signs:_____

Improved with:_____

Impact on your day:_____

Impact on others:_____

Use the space below or on back to describe any significant information not covered in this record:

_____

_____

Were you successful in stopping any abnormal movements this week: yes ☐ no ☐

Please mark which movements you stopped with an asterisk (*).

Adapted with permission from Oxford University Press: Based on Reiter et al. [33].

CBT is based in the reciprocal interactions between thoughts, feelings, behaviors, and, in the case of FMD, physical symptoms (Fig. 21.1a). Table 21.2 highlights several specific CBT-based techniques that may be tailored to the individual patient with FMD over the course of therapy.

Cognitive Techniques

Some of the work in CBT involves identifying and changing maladaptive thoughts and beliefs about oneself. Maladaptive cognitive processing occurs in those with psychological disturbance at two main levels: *automatic thoughts* and *core beliefs (or schemas)*, with intermediate beliefs forming a bridge between the two (Box 21.2). Automatic thoughts are cognitions that occur quickly in our minds when we are engaged in or remembering situations. Despite typically being outside of conscious awareness, automatic thoughts have a significant impact on one's emotions. Core beliefs function as a template, providing rules for information processing that aid in assigning meaning to situations. Maladaptive automatic thoughts are real-time manifestations of dysfunctional core beliefs about oneself that the patient experiences as "truth." A significant focus of NBT utilizes a schema-based *Thought Record (TR)*, which provides a structured tool to bring automatic thoughts and core beliefs into conscious awareness in order to challenge negative schemas, allowing dysfunctional thoughts to be replaced with more adaptive thought patterns and ultimately improving emotional well-being. The TR aids in observing and identifying distorted automatic thoughts and emotions related to a particular situation, drilling down to the core belief underlying the automatic thought, examining the evidence for the core belief, and developing more adaptive alternative beliefs accompanied by corresponding positive changes in emotion.

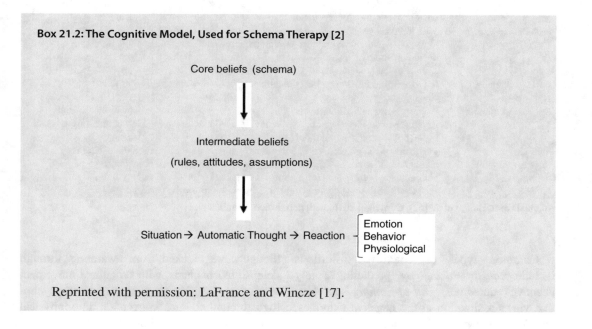

Box 21.2: The Cognitive Model, Used for Schema Therapy [2]

Core beliefs (schema)

Intermediate beliefs

(rules, attitudes, assumptions)

Situation → Automatic Thought → Reaction — Emotion / Behavior / Physiological

Reprinted with permission: LaFrance and Wincze [17].

Table 21.2 Commonly encountered cognitive behavioral techniques

Guided discovery (or Socratic questioning)	Constructing questions in a manner which helps patients clarify their thoughts and beliefs. The aim is to help clients to work out alternative ways of looking at things and to test out the usefulness of new perspectives for themselves.
Behavioral assessment	Gather information about activities engaged in currently and in the past. Want to establish both activities patient is currently engaging in and what they are avoiding.
Activity record	Prospective record compiled by the patient of activities. The patient is often asked to record intensity of symptom experience during each activity. This can help to identify activities associated with improvement or worsening of symptom experience.
Activity scheduling	A basic technique often used early in CBT to program pleasant or satisfying activities and improve mood. It is however a fundamental part of the treatment of Functional Movement Disorders and related conditions, in which avoided activities must be identified and specifically programmed. The consequent increase in positive interactions with the world will itself improve feelings of wellbeing and sense of productivity. In essence pathogenic contingencies of reinforcement are replaced with salutary ones. If fatigue is prominent activities should be planned to gradually increase as stamina improves to prevent precipitating aversive post-exertional fatigue.
Exposure plus response prevention	Exposure to feared/triggering stimuli without escape or avoidance. Through habituation and extinction the exposure loses ability to trigger symptoms.
Graded exposure	Increasing exposure to avoided, anxiety-inducing stimulus in a planned, gradually increasing way. For therapeutic benefit the discomfort associated with a planned level of exposure must be tolerable, or it will simply result in escape/avoidance. Increases in intensity of exposure only occur when the patient has sufficiently de-sensitized to the current level of exposure such that it leads only to modest levels of anxiety.
Behavioral experiment	Planned intervention to gather information about consequences of changing a particular behavior. They are used to test and modify dysfunctional beliefs. An example of how a behavioral experiment may be used could be to test the consequences of not sitting down as soon as they feel dizzy, but instead keep walking for 5 min to see what happens. They note what happens and then reflect on the implications of this for thinking and behavior.
Problem solving	Structured process to identify the problems to be solved and the steps a person might take to try to solve them. It includes outlining the pros and cons of each potential option to help decide on and plan a specific course of action. Most people do not lack problem-solving skills, but they may be avoiding their problems.
Functional analysis	A process for clarifying what is maintaining behaviors which involves looking at their triggers and consequences.
Relaxation training	Approaches which aim to lower physiological arousal. Diaphragmatic breathing and progressive muscle relaxation (sequentially tensing and then relaxing all the muscle groups of the body) are most commonly used.
Symptom monitoring form (or thought record)	Form on which symptoms are monitored together with the situation the patient is in and associated emotions and thoughts. They gather information on potential triggers for symptoms as well as gathering information about (often catastrophic) thoughts and provide the patient with practice in recognizing the emotions they experience.

Adapted from: Hallett et al. [62], Copyright 2016, with permission from Elsevier

Common types of cognitive distortions include *catastrophizing* by predicting solely negative outcomes, *all-or-nothing thinking* that views a situation at the negative extremes, *emotional reasoning* in which negative feelings overrule facts to the contrary, or *magnifying* (the negative)/*minimizing* (the positive). Psychodynamic theory posits that problematic thoughts are blocked from awareness through defense mechanisms, with functional movement symptoms resulting from repression of psychological conflict, and conversion into physical symptoms, thus allowing relief from anxiety associated with the conflict (Fig. 21.1b). CBT and psychodynamic approaches to cognition may be used complementarily in treating FMD.

Behavioral Techniques

Behavioral aspects of CBT are designed to change patterns of avoidance or helplessness, reduce autonomic arousal, modify attentional focus, or build coping skills.

Behavioral activation is a technique aimed at increasing a patient's engagement in activity, allowing for behavioral "successes" and positive reinforcement, and ultimately increasing hope, improving function and decreasing emotional distress. It is frequently used early in the treatment process but may be called upon at any point, for example to re-engage patients in the setting of slowed progress. Behavioral goals should be action-oriented, measurable, and small enough that they are achievable but challenging enough to gain a sense of accomplishment and mastery.

The goal of relaxation techniques is to decrease tension and reach a relaxed (but awake) state to alleviate stress, anxiety, and hyperarousal. Patients with FMD are encouraged to develop a daily practice of intentional relaxation. They should be reminded that they will not become experts straightaway, but with regular practice patients will realize a sense of bodily awareness and control and be able to call upon relaxation skills more easily. Techniques are numerous and may include body scans, progressive muscle relaxation, diaphragmatic breathing and guided-imagery, but other focused activities such as mindfulness meditation, yoga, tai chi, or prayer may also be encouraged. It is best to practice techniques that do not require additional equipment, as to eventually be able to call upon relaxation techniques in stressful situations to decrease hyperarousal and abnormal movements in the presence of triggers. Patients should start by finding a technique that works for them and focusing on proficiency. The therapist should check in with patients about their relaxation practice and elicit feedback on patient progress or difficulties. Adjustments may be required for patients with focal pain symptoms or cardiopulmonary disease. Box 21.3 provides instructional tips for getting started with relaxation training.

Box 21.3: Relaxation Training Tips
- Start with an overview of the rationale for relaxation training.
- Encourage patients to rate their muscle tension and anxiety before and after a session (for example, on a 0-100 scale, where 0 is no tension and 100 is maximum tension).
- Ensure patient comfort (comfortable chair, relaxed position and clothing, dim lights, use restroom beforehand).
- Slow deep breathing, in through the nose and out through the mouth.
- Teach the patient a relaxation method starting with the hands, for example:

Now use your mind to concentrate on the palms of your hands. Let yourself sense your palms so that they tingle and become strongly present with you and your body. When you can clearly sense the palms of your hands, imagine that a wave of warm, calming relaxation is beginning to form at the palms of your hands. … Slowly over the next few minutes, this wave of relaxation will spread throughout your entire body. …

- Use a systematic approach to relax all the major muscle groups. A sequence might be hands, lower and upper arms, shoulders, neck, head, face, chest, back, abdomen, hips and buttocks, upper then lower legs, and feet.
- Encourage the use of pleasant mental imagery or a relaxing phrase/mantra.
- Debrief after each session.
- Encourage regular practice: start with 5–10 min daily.
- Elicit feedback on how personal practice is going.

Coping skills include a wide array of potential skills and activities that function to help deal with life-stresses. External (situational) circumstances, internal (emotional) conflicts, and physical symptoms can all function as stressors, and in turn may be triggers for abnormal movements or other somatic symptoms. Developing coping skills provides patients with a "toolbox" of productive outlets to call upon when faced with stressors. A helpful exercise is to examine with patients which sources of stress they feel might be changed and those which are unlikely to change. For example, S. feels "stuck" in his current situation living at his critical father's house because his financial situation does not allow him to move out right now, leading him to feel helpless and anxious when at home. He does not see how this situation will change soon. Coping skills allow S. to decrease stress levels and mitigate the negative emotional states brought on by living at his father's house. Potential coping skills may include pleasant distracting activities such as going to a movie or recreation, physical exercise, seeking social support, opportunities for self-expression (journaling or music), or learned CBT skills such as relaxation exercises (discussed above) or thought-stopping, a behavioral skill using vivid imagery to "stop" dysfunctional thoughts and replace them with pleasant scenes. Encouraging action directed at the source of stress, such as searching for a job, may help S. see potential to change his situation.

Relationships and Communication

Family and social support is an important element in the therapeutic process of controlling FMD. Psychoeducation for family members can aid them in interacting appropriately with patients and helping with illness management at home. And healthy relationships encourage open communication, expression of feelings, and positive coping skills. Alternatively, relationships can be the source of predisposing, precipitating and perpetuating FMD factors including feelings of rejection, positive re-reinforcement of problematic behaviors and learned helplessness, re-experiencing of abuse, and symptom modeling.

Often patients view relationship conflicts as a source of stress that they have little power to change, for example a marital relationship in which they feel their needs are not being met or a friendship that revolves around unhealthy habits. S. feels anxious and helpless when dealing with his father and has learned to take a *passive* role when faced with his father's *aggressive* communication style. However, stressful relationships can be changed with using healthy communication. Encouraging healthy *assertive* communication, in which one expresses feelings honestly and stands up for oneself while also respecting the other person's feelings and opinions, allows for a "win-win" outcome. Changing one's communication style takes practice, and *role playing* can be a useful tool to explore communication in different scenarios.

Approaching FMD as a disorder of communication is a useful paradigm for treatment. Aberrant communication is evident at many levels, including difficulty recognizing maladaptive thoughts and communicating emotion (alexithymia), in interpersonal relationships, and in the disordered messaging between brain, mind and body that results in functional movement symptoms. Furthermore, empathic, confident communication of FMD diagnosis is an important factor in FMD treatment success. Patients with FMD have been shown to display an impaired sense of agency, the ability to exert and perceive control over one's actions [63], although have also been shown to report high "within our control" frame of reference relative to other movement disorder patients [64]. NBT provides language, skills, and a therapeutic relationship through which to improve communication to facilitate thought and emotional regulation and may offer a process to encourage an internal locus of control and sense of self agency.

Case, Part 3: Psychotherapy

S. commenced engagement in a 12-week, manualized, NBT treatment with a neuropsychiatrist, who had been formally trained in the modality. He initially had difficulty filling in his abnormal movement symptom log consistently, but by practicing with his therapist in session he became more comfortable with the process and recognized its importance in tracking his symptoms. He was able to identify triggers, including situations where he felt a decreased sense of control, which occurred in the setting of interactions with his father as well as other males who he sensed as "threatening." In exploring the relationship between feeling powerless and increased movement symptoms, he believed this was connected not specifically to the sexual assault he experienced but to the sense of being "stuck" on a ship with the perpetrating officer and later a similar feeling in being "stuck" living with his critical father.

Completing thought records allowed him to re-assess core beliefs that he "would never be good enough," and recognize strengths including that he is a caring, thoughtful individual who deserved reciprocal relationships. He found role-playing interpersonal situations particularly helpful, and while he found it difficult to "mend" his relationship with his father he felt less trapped in the situation, and used assertive communication to arrange that his father would lend him money to get his own place while he searched for a job.

Utilizing healthy assertive communication also helped him step back from a friendship that revolved around binge alcohol use, which he recognized through functional analysis of his symptom log led to increased anxiety and abnormal movements. A daily relaxation practice allowed him to decrease hyperarousal in stressful situations and he found this helpful as he attended job interviews. He also began attending yoga weekly with a friend. His gait disturbance had resolved, and jerking movements occurred occasionally but were less severe and generally self-limiting.

At 3 months follow up, post-treatment, S. had maintained benefits in terms of abnormal movements reduction. He had engaged in ongoing therapy for PTSD. He got involved in an equine therapy program for veterans, and ultimately this led to a volunteer position and then a job caring for horses, which he enjoyed and found therapeutic. He experienced less fear and felt his life was "moving the right direction" in terms of his goals.

Wellness Planning and Termination of Treatment

In time limited therapies, end of treatment planning occurs throughout the therapeutic process, with duration of treatment spelled out in the first session. Later sessions in treatment should include wellness planning, in which patients reassess self-derived personal goals and develop a written plan for symptom control and well-being across life domains (for example, S. planned to abstain from alcohol use, journaling for 10 min a day, begin volunteering, and doing daily relaxation or yoga). A patient-generated review of what was learned and what worked is included in the final session. While resolution of abnormal movements may be *a* desired goal, this is not *the* sole objective, acknowledging that symptoms may still occur in chronic conditions. Relapse prevention should be discussed, and the patient's work in a therapy manual, worksheets and their notebook can be highlighted as their own "parting gift" *to themselves* that they can refer to as needed. Adequate time in the final session is important for closure, with attention devoted to the treatment termination process. Plans for next steps in treatment, such as ongoing mental health treatment, can be discussed. The overarching goal of NBT is to train a patient to become their own therapist, and the last session is a graduation onto next steps knowing they have gained tools to take control of their thoughts, feelings, movements, and life.

Summary
- Psychological treatment of FMD begins with a documented diagnosis that validates the patient's experiences, explains the symptoms in understandable terms, and offers hope for treatment.
- A complete biopsychosocialspiritual history provides the framework for exploring predisposing, precipitating, and perpetuating factors of FMD in psychotherapy.

- CBT-informed psychotherapy (Neuro-Behavioral Therapy) offers a practical, integrative approach to treating FND, calling upon multiple modalities to tailor treatment and equip the patient with tools to connect the past and present, address symptoms and schema, examine self, and develop healthy interactions in their social environment.
- Evidence supports psychotherapy treatment of FMD, but further research is needed to delineate the most effective elements of psychological treatments, highlight valid outcome measures and biomarkers, and incorporate psychotherapy into transdisciplinary treatment models.
- Ultimately, the goal of psychotherapy is to guide a patient to become more self-aware, increasing self-management, so that they may regain a sense of agency over abnormal movements, foster healthy relationships, and improve their quality of life and psychological well-being.

References

1. Baizabal-Carvallo JF, Hallett M, Jankovic J. Pathogenesis and pathophysiology of functional (psychogenic) movement disorders. Neurobiol Dis. 2019;127:32–44.
2. Beck AT, Freeman E, & Associates. Cognitive Therapy of Personality Disorders. London: The Guilford Press 1990.
3. Edwards MJ, Stone J, Lang AE. From psychogenic movement disorder to functional movement disorder: it's time to change the name. Mov Disord. 2014;29(7):849–52.
4. Gelauff JM, Dreissen YE, Tijssen MA, Stone J. Treatment of functional motor disorders. Curr Treat Options Neurol. 2014;16(4):286–014.
5. Espay AJ, Lang AE. Phenotype-specific diagnosis of functional (psychogenic) movement disorders. Curr Neurol Neurosci Rep. 2015;15(6):32.
6. American Psychiatric Association. Diagnostic and statistical manual of mental disorders. 5th ed. Arlington: American Psychiatric Association; 2013.
7. Adams C, Anderson J, Madva EN, LaFrance WC, Perez DL. You've made the diagnosis of functional neurological disorder: now what? Pract Neurol. 2018;18(4):323–30.
8. Gabbard GO. A neurobiologically informed perspective on psychotherapy. Br J Psychiatry. 2000;177:117–22.
9. Espay AJ, Ries S, Maloney T, Vannest J, Neefus E, Dwivedi AK, et al. Clinical and neural responses to cognitive behavioral therapy for functional tremor. Neurology. 2019;93(19):e1787–98.
10. Wampold BE. Theories of Psychotherapy Series. The basics of psychotherapy: an introduction to theory and practice. 2nd ed. American Psychological Association; 2019.
11. Cretton A, Brown RJ, LaFrance WC Jr, Aybek S. What does neuroscience tell us about the conversion model of functional neurological disorders? J Neuropsychiatry Clin Neurosci. 2020;32(1):24–32.
12. Hofmann SG, Asnaani A, Vonk IJ, Sawyer AT, Fang A. The efficacy of cognitive behavioral therapy: a review of meta-analyses. Cognit Ther Res. 2012;36(5):427–40.
13. Bullock KD, Mirza N, Forte C, Trockel M. Group dialectical-behavior therapy skills training for conversion disorder with seizures. J Neuropsychiatry Clin Neurosci. 2015;27(3):240–3.
14. Myers L, Vaidya-Mathur U, Lancman M. Prolonged exposure therapy for the treatment of patients diagnosed with psychogenic non-epileptic seizures (PNES) and post-traumatic stress disorder (PTSD). Epilepsy Behav. 2017;66:86–92.
15. Kabat-Zinn J. Mindfulness-based interventions in context: past, present, and future. Clin Psychol Sci Pract. 2003;10(2):144–56.
16. Holzel BK, Lazar SW, Gard T, Schuman-Olivier Z, Vago DR, Ott U. How does mindfulness meditation work? Proposing mechanisms of action from a conceptual and neural perspective. Perspect Psychol Sci. 2011;6(6):537–59.
17. LaFrance WC Jr, Wincze J. Treating nonepileptic seizures: therapist guide. New York: Oxford University Press; 2015.
18. Brown RJ. Chapter 8: Dissociation and functional neurological disorders. Handb Clin Neurol. 2016;139:85–94.
19. Goldstein LH, Robinson EJ, Mellers JDC, Stone J, Carson A, Reuber M, et al. Cognitive behavioural therapy for adults with dissociative seizures (CODES): a pragmatic, multicentre, randomised controlled trial. Lancet Psychiatry. 2020;7(6):491–505.
20. LaFrance WC Jr, Baird GL, Barry JJ, Blum AS, Frank Webb A, Keitner GI, et al. Multicenter pilot treatment trial for psychogenic nonepileptic seizures: a randomized clinical trial. JAMA Psychiat. 2014;71(9):997–1005.
21. Sharpe M, Walker J, Williams C, Stone J, Cavanagh J, Murray G, et al. Guided self-help for functional (psychogenic) symptoms: a randomized controlled efficacy trial. Neurology. 2011;77(6):564–72.

22. Pick S, Goldstein LH, Perez DL, Nicholson TR. Emotional processing in functional neurological disorder: a review, biopsychosocial model and research agenda. J Neurol Neurosurg Psychiatry. 2019;90(6):704–11.

23. Groves P. Mindfulness in psychiatry - where are we now? BJPsych Bull. 2016;40(6):289–92.

24. Espay AJ, Aybek S, Carson A, Edwards MJ, Goldstein LH, Hallett M, et al. Current concepts in diagnosis and treatment of functional neurological disorders. JAMA Neurol. 2018;75(9):1132–41.

25. Goldstein LH, Chalder T, Chigwedere C, Khondoker MR, Moriarty J, Toone BK, et al. Cognitive-behavioral therapy for psychogenic nonepileptic seizures: a pilot RCT. Neurology. 2010;74(24):1986–94.

26. Reiter JM, Andrews DJ. A neurobehavioral approach for treatment of complex partial epilepsy: efficacy. Seizure. 2000;9(3):198–203.

27. Perez DL, Dworetzky BA, Dickerson BC, Leung L, Cohn R, Baslet G, et al. An integrative neurocircuit perspective on psychogenic nonepileptic seizures and functional movement disorders: neural functional unawareness. Clin EEG Neurosci. 2015;46(1):4–15.

28. LaFrance WC Jr, Friedman JH. Cognitive behavioral therapy for psychogenic movement disorder. Mov Disord. 2009;24(12):1856–7.

29. Lidstone SC, MacGillivray L, Lang AE. Integrated therapy for functional movement disorders: time for a change. Mov Disord Clin Pract. 2020;7(2):169–74.

30. Kroenke K. Efficacy of treatment for somatoform disorders: a review of randomized controlled trials. Psychosom Med. 2007;69(9):881–8.

31. LaFrance WC Jr, Reuber M, Goldstein LH. Management of psychogenic nonepileptic seizures. Epilepsia. 2013;54(Suppl 1):53–67.

32. LaFrance WC Jr, Miller IW, Ryan CE, Blum AS, Solomon DA, Kelley JE, et al. Cognitive behavioral therapy for psychogenic nonepileptic seizures. Epilepsy Behav. 2009;14(4):591–6.

33. Reiter J, Andrews D, Reiter C, LaFrance WC Jr. Taking control of your seizures. Workbook. New York: Oxford University Press; 2015.

34. Dallocchio C, Tinazzi M, Bombieri F, Arno N, Erro R. Cognitive behavioural therapy and adjunctive physical activity for functional movement disorders (conversion disorder): a pilot, single-blinded, randomized study. Psychother Psychosom. 2016;85(6):381–3.

35. O'Connell N, Watson G, Grey C, Pastena R, McKeown K, David AS. Outpatient CBT for motor functional neurological disorder and other neuropsychiatric conditions: a retrospective case comparison. J Neuropsychiatry Clin Neurosci. 2020;32(1):58–66.

36. Sharma VD, Jones R, Factor SA. Psychodynamic psychotherapy for functional (Psychogenic) movement disorders. J Mov Disord. 2017;10(1):40–4.

37. Hinson VK, Weinstein S, Bernard B, Leurgans SE, Goetz CG. Single-blind clinical trial of psychotherapy for treatment of psychogenic movement disorders. Parkinsonism Relat Disord. 2006;12(3):177–80.

38. Kompoliti K, Wilson B, Stebbins G, Bernard B, Hinson V. Immediate vs. delayed treatment of psychogenic movement disorders with short term psychodynamic psychotherapy: randomized clinical trial. Parkinsonism Relat Disord. 2014;20(1):60–3.

39. Moene FC, Spinhoven P, Hoogduin KA, van Dyck R. A randomized controlled clinical trial of a hypnosis-based treatment for patients with conversion disorder, motor type. Int J Clin Exp Hypn. 2003;51(1):29–50.

40. Graham CD, Stuart SR, O'Hara DJ, Kemp S. Using acceptance and commitment therapy to improve outcomes in functional movement disorders: a case study. Clin Case Stud. 2017;16(5):401–16.

41. Graham CD, O'Hara DJ, Kemp S. A case series of Acceptance and Commitment Therapy (ACT) for reducing symptom interference in functional neurological disorders. Clin Psychol Psychother. 2018;25(3):489–96.

42. Nielsen G, Stone J, Matthews A, Brown M, Sparkes C, Farmer R, et al. Physiotherapy for functional motor disorders: a consensus recommendation. J Neurol Neurosurg Psychiatry. 2015;86(10):1113–9.

43. Jordbru AA, Smedstad LM, Klungsoyr O, Martinsen EW. Psychogenic gait disorder: a randomized controlled trial of physical rehabilitation with one-year follow-up. J Rehabil Med. 2014;46(2):181–7.

44. Stone J, Carson A, Hallett M. Chapter 44 – Explanation as treatment for functional neurologic disorders. In: Handbook of clinical neurology, vol. 139. Elsevier; 2016. p. 543–53.

45. Thomas M, Vuong KD, Jankovic J. Long-term prognosis of patients with psychogenic movement disorders. Parkinsonism Relat Disord. 2006;12(6):382–7.

46. Stone J, LaFrance WC Jr, Brown R, Spiegel D, Levenson JL, Sharpe M. Conversion disorder: current problems and potential solutions for DSM-5. J Psychosom Res. 2011;71(6):369–76.

47. Jung Y, Chen D, Bullock K, Ries S, Hamid H, LaFrance WC Jr. Chapter 33. Training in treatment of psychogenic nonepileptic seizures. In: LaFrance Jr WC, Schachter SC, editors. Gates and Rowan's nonepileptic seizures. 4th ed. Cambridge: Cambridge University Press; 2018. p. 344–57.

48. Williams C, Carson A, Cavanagh J, Smith S, Kent C, Sharpe M. Overcoming functional neurological symptoms: a five areas approach. 1st ed. UK: Routledge; 2011.

49. Conwill M, Oakley L, Evans K, Cavanna AE. CBT-based group therapy intervention for nonepileptic attacks and other functional neurological symptoms: a pilot study. Epilepsy Behav. 2014;34:68–72.

50. Jacob AE, Kaelin DL, Roach AR, Ziegler CH, LaFaver K. Motor retraining (MoRe) for functional movement disorders: outcomes from a 1-week multidisciplinary rehabilitation program. PM R. 2018;10(11):1164–72.

51. McHugh PR, Slavney PR. The perspectives of psychiatry. 2nd ed. Johns Hopkins University Press; 1998.

52. LaFrance WC Jr, Devinsky O. Treatment of nonepileptic seizures. Epilepsy Behav. 2002;3(5 Suppl):19–23.

53. Stone J, Carson A. Functional neurologic symptoms: assessment and management. Neurol Clin. 2011;29(1):1–18, vii.
54. Kranick S, Ekanayake V, Martinez V, Ameli R, Hallett M, Voon V. Psychopathology and psychogenic movement disorders. Mov Disord. 2011;26(10):1844–50.
55. Ludwig L, Pasman JA, Nicholson T, Aybek S, David AS, Tuck S, et al. Stressful life events and maltreatment in conversion (functional neurological) disorder: systematic review and meta-analysis of case-control studies. Lancet Psychiatry. 2018;5(4):307–20.
56. Kletenik I, Sillau SH, Isfahani SA, LaFaver K, Hallett M, Berman BD. Gender as a risk factor for functional movement disorders: the role of sexual abuse. Mov Disord Clin Pract. 2019;7(2):177–81.
57. Mack J, Quinn JF, Lobb BM, O'Connor S. Functional movement disorders in U.S. veterans: psychiatric comorbidity and health care utilization. Mov Disord. 2019;34(5):755–6.
58. Salinsky M, Evrard C, Storzbach D, Pugh MJ. Psychiatric comorbidity in veterans with psychogenic seizures. Epilepsy Behav. 2012;25(3):345–9.
59. Chen DK, Maheshwari A, Franks R, Trolley GC, Robinson JS, Hrachovy RA. Brief group psychoeducation for psychogenic nonepileptic seizures: a neurologist-initiated program in an epilepsy center. Epilepsia. 2014;55(1):156–66.
60. Mayor R, Brown RJ, Cock H, House A, Howlett S, Smith P, et al. A feasibility study of a brief psychoeducational intervention for psychogenic nonepileptic seizures. Seizure. 2013;22(9):760–5.
61. Demartini B, Petrochilos P, Ricciardi L, Price G, Edwards MJ, Joyce E. The role of alexithymia in the development of functional motor symptoms (conversion disorder). J Neurol Neurosurg Psychiatry. 2014;85(10):1132–7.
62. Hallett M, Stone J, Carson A, editors. Chapter 10: Psychologic theories in functional neurologic disorders. In: Handbook of clinical neurology, vol. 139 (3rd series) Functional neurologic disorders. Elsevier; 2016. p. 118.
63. Nahab FB, Kundu P, Maurer C, Shen Q, Hallett M. Impaired sense of agency in functional movement disorders: an fMRI study. PLoS One. 2017;12(4):e0172502.
64. Vizcarra JA, Hacker S, Lopez-Castellanos R, Ryes L, Laub HN, Marsili L, et al. Internal versus external frame of reference in functional movement disorders. J Neuropsychiatry Clin Neurosci. 2020;32(1):67–72.

Psychiatric Comorbidities and the Role of Psychiatry in Functional Movement Disorder

22

Kim Bullock and Juliana Lockman

Clinical Vignette

A 38-year-old married woman, employed as a nurse with history of fibromyalgia with no formal psychiatric diagnoses but a reported sexual assault at age 16, presents with shaking movements involving her legs and walking difficulties. She presents for psychiatric consultation in a wheelchair, accompanied by her teenage daughter who gives additional history. Her symptoms first started around the time of her daughter's birthday 6 months ago. They have slowly worsened to the point of severe impairment, resulting in resignation from her position as charge nurse.

A prior evaluation by a neurologist specializing in movement disorders concluded symptoms were due to a functional movement disorder (FMD) based on features of distractibility, entrainment and non-economical compensatory movements on gait examination. The neurologist provided 20 minutes of education regarding this diagnosis, including explaining positive signs.

She was subsequently referred for a psychiatric consultation in conjunction with physical therapy. Despite the extensive initial education provided, the patient left the session confused that her neurologist would not be involved in her

ongoing treatment. She felt her medical team seemed to be saying she had a psychological problem and it was "all in her head." She felt abandoned and wondered whether her neurologist would still be interested in her recovery.

On psychiatric interview, she reveals that she suffers from severe "anxiety," which she describes as being easily startled, having intrusive thoughts of feeling unsafe in her home and frequent periods of experiencing a pounding heart and loss of breath. Her sleep is chronically impaired, with nightmares and fears of falling asleep. An intense fear of leaving the house has also developed recently.

She notes being an "anxious kid" and feels her anxiety has become worse as an adult, especially in the past year. From an early age, the patient describes being the primary caregiver for her mother, who was wheelchair-bound from complications of diabetes. Her father had alcohol use disorder and was physically and verbally abusive towards the patient, her mother and two younger siblings. He ultimately left the home when her brothers entered adolescence.

Most of the patient's days are now spent at home watching television. Her daughter and husband have assumed all of the household chores and grocery shopping. She relies on them to help shower and get dressed in the mornings. The family is struggling financially and she has applied for disability. She feels extremely guilty for "being a burden."

K. Bullock · J. Lockman (✉)
Department of Psychiatry and Behavioral Sciences,
Stanford University School of Medicine,
Stanford, CA, USA
e-mail: kbullock@stanford.edu;
jlockman@stanford.edu

© Springer Nature Switzerland AG 2022
K. LaFaver et al. (eds.), *Functional Movement Disorder*, Current Clinical Neurology,
https://doi.org/10.1007/978-3-030-86495-8_22

She is having trouble finding a psychothera-pist and physical therapist that are familiar with FMD. She is feeling lost and abandoned regard-ing her treatment. There have been several trips to the emergency department for exacerbation of symptoms. There she encounters providers who have never heard of her diagnosis and make comments that seem as if they believe she is try-ing to get attention or take advantage of a dis-ability system. Her family does not understand her diagnosis and are becoming frustrated and angry at her doctors as well.

Introduction

At the beginning of care, patients with FMD pri-marily interface with neurological and medical specialties as the above vignette illustrates. Most patients are surprised by the seemingly sudden shift that can occur when the treatment phase of care begins. Patients are sometimes asked to move away from trusted physicians whom may have been pivotal in making the diagnosis. Following diagnostic confirmation, patients with FMD are often directed to follow up with a psy-chiatrist who they may perceive as outside of the general medical system. It can be perceived by patients as highly incongruent that in order to receive treatment, they must leave the doctors and specialty that made the diagnosis and shift to an entirely new specialty. As noted elsewhere in this book (See Chaps. 4 and 20), it is often help-ful for the neurologist to remain actively engaged in longitudinal collaborative care with psychia-trists and psychotherapists [1]. Additionally, developing shared (partially overlapping) exper-tise across the clinical neurosciences (See Chap. 4) can also aid interactions between neurological and psychiatric aspects of care [2].

Psychiatrists and other mental healthcare pro-fessionals can more broadly deliver a range of services that may include inpatient and residen-tial acute care treatment, outpatient behavioral and mental health services, education on lifestyle modification, psychotherapy, hypnotherapy, and psychopharmacology among others. In addition, interventional procedures such as Electroconvulsive Therapy (ECT) or Transcranial Magnetic Stimulation (TMS) may be offered when indicated. Psychiatric services may be imbedded in interdisciplinary programs for FMD, integrative medicine, pain programs and other mind-body programs.

Although well positioned to chaperone patients with FMD from the medicalized diag-nostic procedures to evidenced-based behavioral and psychological treatments, moving (at least partially) to a psychiatric system can be challeng-ing particularly if psychiatric services are not closely intertwined with the neurological care team. Establishing psychiatric care to help coor-dinate psychotherapy interventions is often one of the first recommendations a neurologist or medical professional makes for individuals with FMD. Making this transition to allow patients to accept and engage with psychiatric services can be challenging and confusing for both clinicians and patients. This chapter aims to help clinicians and treatment teams understand and guide FMD patients to make these additions and transitions collaboratively.

In addition, this chapter will provide an over-view of the psychiatric comorbidities that most often co-exist with and contribute to FMD. Most comorbidities are connected with elevated rates of depression, anxiety and childhood trauma, although significant heterogeneity exists across patients [3, 4]. This chapter hopes to aid neurolo-gists and other medical professionals by review-ing the most commonly encountered comorbid psychiatric illnesses and describing how they can be treated in the setting of FMD. The aim is to facilitate enhanced understanding (shared exper-tise) and multidisciplinary care for FMD. It should deepen medical specialists' understand-ing of the multifactorial nature of FMD and how psychiatric comorbidities contribute to the com-ponents of the biopsychosocial model.

Psychiatric professionals can be helpful in mitigating many predisposing, precipitating and perpetuating variables implicated in FMD-related biopsychosocial formulations. Understanding these factors can clarify treat-ment goals and plans. Collaborating with psy-chiatrists and other mental health services to address comorbidities is an important aspect of FMD care. Effectively referring to psychiatric services may be the crucial role a neurologist or primary care provider offers an FMD patient for successful treatment. A caveat, however, is that some FMD specialists (while rare) have developed expertise across neurology and psychiatry, – in which case referral to psychiatry for the psychiatrically well-informed neurologist may be somewhat less critical.

Although formal psychiatric diagnoses are reviewed in this chapter, it should be noted that many patients may not report symptoms at a frequency or severity that reach the threshold of a formal categorical psychiatric diagnosis. Nonetheless, subsyndromal symptoms are also important considerations and many of the treatment principles discussed in this chapter are also relevant in those circumstances as well. Personalized care should take precedence over standardization and inflexible categorizations.

Supporting Evidence for Early Psychiatric Engagement

Patients with FMD usually present to neurologists when movement symptoms first appear. They may spend years in various medical specialties until accurately diagnosed [5]. A long duration of untreated physical symptoms in FMD is associated with negative long-term outcomes [6]. Additionally, the longer the duration of untreated mental health symptoms, the higher the potential risk of treatment refractoriness and development of comorbid illness. This information suggests that diagnosing and treating psychiatric symptoms in FMD early is critical for optimizing outcomes. Thus, facilitation of the psychiatric diagnostic process to maximize speed in establishing psychiatric care is an important priority for medical specialists to consider. Neurologists and other medical providers with a special interest in FMD should work on developing efficient referral pathways to like-minded psychiatrists and psychotherapists within their own institution and extended network.

Risk Factors

Specific cognitive and affective processing patterns may be risk factors for developing FMD. These include abnormalities in self-directed attention, expectations, self-efficacy and agency [7–11]. Alexithymia refers to difficulties with awareness and interpretation of autonomic interoceptive sensations and as well as deficits labeling emotions using words. Alexithymia is a deficit in describing internal emotional states that may also play a role in FMD development. A case-control study evaluated 55 subjects with functional motor symptoms and compared them with a group of 33 subjects with other movement disorders and 34 healthy controls, identifying that alexithymia was significantly higher in the group with FMD (35%, 9% and 6%, respectively) [12]. Psychiatric systems are well positioned to deploy services for both emotional and cognitive dysfunction including psychotherapy, neuropsychiatry, neuropsychological assessments and pharmacological treatments targeting affective circuitry.

Psychosocial risk factors for FMD include childhood neglect, a history of sexual and physical abuse and major stressful life events [3, 13–16]. A large case-controlled study of 322 FMD patients in a UK mental health service found childhood bullying and adolescent drug use were increased in those with FMD [17]. In the same study, adults with FMD were more likely to have interpersonal problems affecting their intimate partnerships or causing academic or occupational dysfunction. These patients were also more likely to be involved in legal disputes. For motor functional neurological disorder (FND, including FMD and functional [psychogenic nonepileptic/dissociative] seizures), fearful attachment style has been associated with adverse life events, alexithymia, dissociation, depression, anxiety, impaired coping style, and functional neurological symptom severity [18].

In the weeks and months leading up to FMD symptom onset, there may be a high rate of physical injury or illness (e.g., infection, hospitalization), at times accompanied by panic attack symptoms [19]. In a study of patients with functional limb weakness, predisposing factors included the presence of medical comorbidities such as chronic back pain and irritable bowel syndrome as well as surgical procedures such as appendectomy [20]. Adverse childhood events were also common in this group but at rates lower than expected. See Chap. 3 on the biopsychosocial formulation for additional discussion of risk factors for FMD.

Psychiatric Comorbidities

Structured assessment tools for the purposes of DSM-5 classification are often utilized in research for characterizing the epidemiology of psychiatric comorbidities in FMD. In practice, however, research supports that the rich data acquired through qualitative psychiatric interviewing may be even more clinically useful [21].

Lifetime prevalences of psychiatric disorders in FMD were documented in one study of 42 FMD patients and included anxiety disorders (62%), personality disorder (45%), and unipolar depression (43%) [14]. However, another study comparing FMD patients to healthy controls did not find elevated rates of personality scales [22]. For patients with functional limb weakness specifically, one study found significant comorbidities of major depression (32%), generalized anxiety disorder (21%), panic disorder (36%) and somatization disorder (27%) [23]. This group was less likely to acknowledge a contributing role for stress and had the same self-report rate of anxiety and depression as controls. Post-traumatic stress disorder (PTSD) is estimated at 60% among all comers with FND, indiscriminate of subtype [24]. Psychotic disorders and bipolar disorder appear uncommon in FMD and related conditions [25].

Another common observation is the report of chronic pain or other somatic symptoms that may fit into the DSM-5 [26] diagnostic category of somatic symptom disorder (SSD). SSD encompasses many phenomena formerly labeled as somatoform disorders including somatization disorder, somatoform pain disorder and undifferentiated somatoform disorder in prior DSM versions. In one older study of 131 FMD patients,

Williams et al. [13] found a primary diagnosis of somatization disorder in 12.5% of subjects.

Patients that are misdiagnosed with FMD but who are actually willfully feigning are quite rare [27]. More often FMD is misdiagnosed as feigning, either factitious disorder or malingering. In contract to FMD, both involve the conscious production of symptoms and deception of caregivers. Factitious disorder is considered a psychiatric illness due to the unconscious motivation and compulsive nature of the behavior. Psychiatric treatment for this disorder is rare given most patients refuse care [28]. Malingering, in which an individual feigns illness for secondary gain (e.g., financial reward, avoidance of work or home responsibilities), is not considered a mental illness.

Management of Psychiatric Comorbidities

Psychiatric comorbidities are prevalent and elevated in FMD. The etiologies of these psychiatric comorbidities, as well as FMD more specifically, are generally accepted to be multifactorial. However, commonalities are appreciated among many of the predisposing, precipitating, perpetuating and protective factors. For example, psychological stress is commonly reported as a precipitating factor for the onset of FMD symptoms and psychiatric conditions such as PTSD. Yet, adverse life events do not automatically result in FMD or PTSD, owing to individual differences in one's biological, psychological and social makeup. Recognizing and treating underlying psychiatric comorbidities and symptoms if they exist concurrently with FMD is an important component to treatment that often involves overlapping strategies.

Below is an overview of the management of the most commonly encountered psychiatric comorbidities in FMD. Although diagnoses provide an important guiding framework, it is important to note that this psychiatric taxonomy does not always fit a patient's unique problems perfectly. Care needs to be taken to customize and personalize formulations and treatments according to each patient's problems and unique set of symptoms. Additionally, apart from the importance of categorical psychiatric diagnoses, dimensional psychopathological characteristics are also relevant (e.g., active hypervigilance and avoidance symptoms in a patient that is sub-threshold for the diagnosis of PTSD). A focus on multifactorial contributing factors rather than diagnoses is the usual approach in psychiatry. As the entire scope of psychiatric FMD care and possible comorbid diagnoses is beyond the scope of this text, we highlight some of the more relevant themes to the care of FMD to illustrate principals (See also Table 22.1 for additional details).

Post-Traumatic Stress Disorder (PTSD)

Definition/Diagnosis

First described as "shell shock" in veterans of World War I (1914–1918), post-traumatic stress disorder (PTSD) is defined in the DSM-5 as a syndrome arising from the "exposure to actual or threatened death, serious injury, or sexual violence" [26]. PTSD results from either direct or indirect exposure to a traumatic event. When PTSD results from direct exposure to a traumatic event, the event may be isolated or repeated.

Table 22.1 FMD psychiatric comorbidities

Psychiatric comorbidity	Screening	First-Line Medications	Evidenced-based psychotherapies	FMD literature
Post-traumatic stress disorder (PTSD)	PTSD Checklist for DSM-5 (PCL-5) [84]	SSRI SNRI	CBT Prolonged Exposure (PE) Eye Movement Desensitization and reprocessing (EMDR)	[24, 39, 40]
Panic disorder		SSRI SNRI	CBT	[14, 17]
Generalized anxiety disorder	Generalized Anxiety Disorder-7 (GAD-7) [51] Beck Anxiety Inventory (BAI) [53]	SSRI SNRI	CBT	[14]
Somatic symptom disorder	Patient Health Questionnaire-15 (PHQ-15) [55] Somatic Symptom Scale-8 (SSS-8) [56]	SSRI SNRI Tricyclic Antidepressant (TCA) at bedtime	CBT Regular visits with a primary care provider (contingency management)	[13, 57]
Unipolar depression	Patient Health Questionnaire-9 (PHQ-9) [54] Patient Health Questionnaire-2 (PHQ-2) [61] Beck Depression Inventory for Primary Care (BDI-PC) [62]	SSRI SNRI	CBT Interpersonal Psychotherapy (IPT) Electroconvulsive therapy (ECT) – for severe suicidality, malnutrition secondary to food refusal, and/or treatment refractory depression	[3, 14, 19, 25, 27, 65, 66]
Personality disorders	Structured Clinical Interview SCID-II for personality disorders [69] Personality Diagnostic Questionnaire [70]		Dialectical behavior therapy (DBT) Mentalization-based therapy Transference-focused therapy Cognitive-behavioral therapy (CBT) Systems Training for Emotional Predictability and Problem Solving (STEPPS) Schema-focused therapy	[14, 22, 65, 78–81]

SNRI Selective serotonin norepinephrine reuptake inhibitors, *SSRI* Selective serotonin reuptake inhibitors, *CBT* Cognitive Behavior Therapy

Indirect exposure may occur in the form of witnessing harm towards another or learning that a close friend or family member has been harmed.

The DSM-5 requires the presence of symptoms in the categories of intrusive phenomena (e.g., nightmares), avoidance (e.g., people or places associated with the event), effects on mood and cognition and higher levels of arousal and reactivity. The syndrome must be present for at least 1 month, cause significant distress and not be better explained by another mental health or medical condition. There is also a subtype of PTSD that has prominent dissociative symptoms advocated by some in the field [29].

Treatment

Treatment of comorbid PTSD has been linked to improvement in FND symptoms in the functional seizures subtype but less studied in FMD [30]. Standard of care consists of pharmacologic and/ or trauma-focused psychotherapy modalities. Patient preference and availability of specialized resources typically guide the treatment approach. Selective serotonin and serotonin norepinephrine reuptake inhibitors (SSRIs and SNRIs) are often first-line medications [31, 32]. Evidence-based trauma focused psychotherapies include cognitive therapy, prolonged exposure and eye movement desensitization and reprocessing (EMDR) [33–36].

Considerations with FMD

The global lifetime prevalence of PTSD in the general population is estimated at 0.3–6.8% from surveys of the World Health Organization [37] and a national survey [38]. The prevalence of PTSD in patients with FND was estimated at 60% in one study, indiscriminate of FND subtype [24]. Other studies suggest variability of trauma-related manifestations among subtypes, including those with motor symptoms and functional/ dissociative seizures [39, 40]. Comorbid PTSD correlates with poor quality of life, diminished social support, unemployment (with reliance on disability), anxiety and depression [24, 40]. As such, prompt recognition and management of PTSD is a key component for recovery in the management of FMD and related conditions.

Panic Disorder

Definition/Diagnosis

The DSM-5 diagnosis of panic disorder is characterized by recurrent, discrete attacks of panic or fear, with accompanying physiologic symptoms such as heart palpitations, shortness of breath, diaphoresis, nausea, shaking and paresthesias [26]. Events are of short duration, lasting minutes, and arise unexpectedly (often initially experienced as untriggered). The impact of panic attacks on quality of life can be significant, resulting from fear of having further symptoms and/or their implications. Panic disorder may or may not be accompanied by agoraphobia, avoidance of situations that may precipitate attacks (e.g., crowds) leading to restricted activities of daily life.

Treatment

Treatment with cognitive behavioral therapy (CBT) and serotonergic medications are evidence-based treatments for panic disorder. Trials suggest that the durability of CBT is superior to medications. That is patients are less likely to relapse in the year following treatment with CBT compared with patients who were treated with medication [41, 42].

CBT techniques include restructuring maladaptive (unhelpful) thoughts and behaviors and changing affective responses prompted by internal bodily sensations. Interoceptive exposure therapy has been shown to be particularly effective [43]. It involves having patients desensitize to the internal sensations that cause catastrophic thinking and fear via paradoxical exercises such as hyperventilation and intense exercise to increase heart rate and promote shortness of breath. Associated avoidance behaviors and agoraphobia are managed with exposure therapy as well, in which patients are gradually reintroduced to situations that have elicited fear of having a panic attack in order to desensitize.

Pharmacological treatments include SSRIs and SNRIs [44, 45]. In patients with chronic FMD and comorbid anxiety disorders, a small preliminary study was encouraging for the use of antidepressants [46]. However, a systematic review of broadly defined somatoform disorders that includes FMD highlighted the lack of controlled studies to support using antidepressants in the absence of psychiatric comorbidities [47].

Considerations with FMD

Many patients will describe panic attack symptoms prior to paroxysmal functional motor symptoms [17]. Unlike other anxiety disorders, the lifetime prevalence of panic disorder was found to be highest at initial FMD diagnosis, followed by a significant reduction at follow-up in one prospective study [14]. Like panic disorder, the often unpredictable nature of functional motor symptoms can lead to avoidance and reduction in independence. Treatment strategies focused on decoupling the biologic threat response from feared activities have been described to aid in the recovery of both conditions.

The ability to potentially treat both FMD and panic disorder concurrently makes CBT a potentially optimal option for those with FMD. A randomized controlled trial evaluating the use of a self-guided CBT manual found improvement for all FND subtypes, including motor type [48]. One pilot single randomized controlled trial demonstrated improvement in Psychogenic Movement Rating Scale (PMRS) for patients in CBT and CBT plus adjunctive physical activity groups [49]. The emerging role of CBT in the management of FMD (and its established role for treating panic disorder) is notable given initial data identifying biomarkers of CBT response in patients with functional tremor [50].

Generalized Anxiety Disorder

Definition/Diagnosis

The DSM-5 defines generalized anxiety disorder (GAD) as pervasive worry or anxiety lasting more than six months, which is difficult to control [26]. To meet criteria, patients must report difficulty in three of six areas including concentration, sleep, fatigue, muscle aches, restlessness or irritability. Medical causes of symptoms must been ruled out and the condition is not better explained by another entity. Screening tools such

as the Generalized Anxiety Disorder-7 (GAD-7) may be helpful in detecting this disorder [51]. Patients may not meet criteria for the full diagnosis but still have similar subclinical symptoms such as multiple worries, intolerance to uncertainty, difficulties making decisions and experiential avoidance.

Treatment

Like panic disorder, GAD is typically treated with pharmacotherapy and/or CBT. A meta-analysis of 79 randomized clinical trials with 11,002 participants with GAD compared pharmacotherapy and psychotherapy efficacy and found similar effects [52]. However, a secondary analysis showed superior outcomes for younger patients in CBT compared with pharmacotherapy. For patients who prefer medication, an SSRI or SNRI is considered first-line treatment. No individual medications in these classes have been shown to be superior for GAD.

Considerations with FMD

In one prospective study in patients with FMD, generalized anxiety disorder was estimated at 7.1% lifetime prevalence and demonstrated stability over time [14]. The presence of an anxiety disorder was found to be a predictive variable in outcomes with FMD [11]. Most studies identify anxiety in patients with FMD through questionnaires such as the Beck Anxiety Inventory (BAI) [53, 54]. While helpful for screening, this approach is limited by its inability to delineate specific anxiety disorders as classified in the DSM-5.

Somatic Symptom Disorder (SSD)

Definition/Diagnosis

Somatic symptom disorder (SSD) was introduced to the DSM-5 [26] in 2013 and eliminated, replaced and bundled the diagnoses of **somatization disorder undifferentiated somatoform disorder**, and **somatoform pain disorder**. Many patients that would have met DSM-IV criteria for a somatoform pain disorder will qualify for the SSD diagnosis. A hallmark for recognizing DSM-5 SSD is that bodily symptoms become central to an individual's life and identity, along with excessive healthcare seeking or avoiding behaviors. It can be associated with a lack of acceptance of the diagnosis and mental health treatment. SSD predominantly occurs in women and can begin in childhood. Screening tools include the Patient Health Questionnaire-15 (PHQ-15) [55] and Somatic Symtom Scale-8 (SSS-8) [56]. The pathophysiology is unknown but is associated with a heightened awareness of normal bodily sensations paired with cognitive biases (e.g., catastrophizing) that lead to misinterpretations of physical sensations as indicative of medical pathology [57].

SSD diagnostic criteria requires one or more bodily symptoms be present and accompanied by excessive thoughts, feelings, and/or behaviors related and in response to somatic symptoms [26]. The symptoms must cause significant distress and/or dysfunction. The somatic symptoms may or may not be explained by a recognized general medical condition. It is manifested by at least one of the following:

1. Thoughts and worries about the seriousness of one's symptoms
2. High levels of anxiety and fear about health or symptoms
3. Excessive time and energy devoted to these symptoms

Of note, the DSM-5 does not make a distinction between SSD occurring in the context of a general medical condition that is known to result in prominent physical symptoms versus. situations where the physical symptoms are otherwise "medically unexplained" However, we find in our experience that the SSD diagnosis using "rule in" psychological criteria based on a cognitive-affective-behavioral psychological model is most useful when applied to individuals who otherwise do not have another clear medical reason for their physical concerns. Lastly, the DSM-5 allows for the qualifier of "pain predominant" if the most notable physical concern is body pain.

Treatment

SSD patients may lack acceptance and engagement in psychiatric services and this can make this population challenging to treat. That being said, remission or improvement does occur in as many as 50% of patients [57]. Protecting this population from the risk of repetitive unnecessary diagnostic testing, invasive medical and surgical workups, and iatrogenic illness is an important element of effective interventions.

If psychiatric services are accepted by patients, mainstay treatment is largely based upon CBT strategies. For example, a study using the DSM-5 diagnosis of SSD documented the benefit of CBT in a 12-week randomized trial compared CBT with a waiting list control condition in 65 patients (86% had SSD) [58]. Post-treatment improvements in SSD were greater with CBT than the control condition and the clinical effect was large. Psychosocial functioning also improved more with CBT. In addition, the benefit of CBT was maintained at the 6-month follow-up assessment.

Patients may object to a psychiatric referral, feeling misunderstood and believe that their primary care clinician has dismissed their somatic symptoms as "all in their heads." Patients may also fear that the clinician is abandoning them, similar to feelings FMD patients report. If patients are not amenable to ongoing psychiatric services, then a one-time psychiatric referral can be an initial effective intervention and compromise. The referral can clarify the diagnosis and make specific recommendations for management, such as limiting tests.

Psychiatrists or other mental health specialists may help primary care clinicians manage patients with SSD who do not respond to initial therapy [59] and this does not necessarily require a patient meeting with a psychiatrist. A case discussion or collaborative care model that integrates psychiatric treatment into primary care practices is often an effective strategy. The consultant psychiatrist can also assist primary care clinicians in speaking with patients about the quality of the doctor-patient relationship, which is often problematic but important to maintain.

Principles for managing SSD as a primary care provider include scheduling regular visits, acknowledging symptoms, communicating with other clinicians, assessing and treating diagnosable medical and psychiatric disorders, limiting tests and referrals, reassuring the patient that major medical diseases have been ruled out, focusing on coping and acceptance and making functional improvement the goal of treatment. It is suggested that primary care clinicians schedule regular outpatient visits that are not contingent upon active symptoms.

For treatment resistant SSD patients with prominent symptoms of anxiety or depression, treatment with a SSRI in the morning or tricyclic antidepressant (TCA) at bedtime can be initiated, titrating the dose every four weeks as needed and tolerated. For treatment of pain-predominant SSD, antidepressants with both a noradrenergic and serotonergic (SNRI) profile can be helpful. Avoiding opioids is advisable.

Considerations with FMD

Prevalence rates of SSD, based on DSM-IV somatoform disorder criteria, are higher in patients with FMDs with reports ranging from 25% to 60% [57]. It is important to parse out which disorder is primary and causing the most dysfunction and target that diagnosis first. This is because the treatments for SSD and FMD are somewhat different. The degree of acceptance of the FMD diagnosis can often be a clue to which diagnosis is primary. Patients with high levels of SSD may not accept an FMD diagnosis, as demonstration of the "rule in" motor signs can be less relevant to their overall clinical picture and predominant chief complaint.

Providers that manage FMD comorbid with SSD need to keep in mind the waxing and waning levels of acceptance they will encounter regarding the FMD diagnoses. They also need to be mindful of the therapeutic alliance difficulties and ruptures that the SSD illness can cause during care due to

the lack of acceptance and intolerance of medical uncertainty. For example, some SSD patients may want to spend considerable time obtaining reassurance regarding the diagnosis of FMD. This may cause frustration and challenges in systems pressed for time. It may be important for providers to get support with psychiatric consultants or colleagues to manage their own emotions towards these patients. Additionally, for patients where SSD with pain is a major concern within the context of an FMD, consideration can be given to guiding patients towards interdisciplinary pain programs prior to revisiting the appropriateness of other FMD treatments [60]. See Chap. 14 for additional discussion regarding the intersection of FMD and other distressing physical symptoms including pain and fatigue, as well as information on Illness Anxiety Disorder.

Finally, it is important to recognize that although the misdiagnosis rate for FMD is low, SSD is a psychiatric diagnosis commonly missed and/or mislabeled as a functional neurological disorder. Education and training to differentiate these two disorders is important because the treatments are different. It is important that training curriculums focusing on FMD include education about SSD to insure quality care and skills to identify SSD when present.

Depressive Disorders

Definition/Diagnosis

A depressed mood may be a normal and adaptive response to loss. In addition, depressed mood and/or decreased enjoyment in activities (anhedonia) may be a symptom of a psychopathological syndrome or disorder or another medical disorder. Depressive disorders include unipolar major depression, persistent low grade depressed mood (dysthymia), disruptive mood dysregulation disorder, premenstrual dysphoric disorder, substance/medication-induced depressive disorder, and depressive disorder due to another medical condition. Short screening self-report instruments for these disorders include the Patient Health Questionnaire-9 (PHQ-9) [46], the Patient Health Questionnaire-2 (PHQ-2) [61] and the Beck Depression Inventory for Primary Care (BDI-PC) [62] among other questionnaires.

The assessment of patients who are being evaluated for a depressive disorder includes the history of present illness, medical, family and social histories, mental status examination, physical examination and focused laboratory tests. The history must address suicidal ideation and behavior. A screening physical examination should be performed and routine laboratory testing, typically includes complete blood count, serum chemistry panels, urinalysis, thyroid stimulating hormone, rapid plasma regain, human chorionic gonadotropin (pregnancy) and urine toxicology screen to rule out medical conditions. The differential diagnosis of unipolar depressive disorders includes neurological disorders with prominent apathy, sadness, burnout, adjustment disorder with depressed mood, attention hyperactivity disorder, bipolar disorder, borderline personality disorder, complicated grief, delirium and the negative symptoms of psychotic spectrum disorders among other conditions.

Symptoms of depression include:

- Depressed (dysphoric/negative) mood most of the day, nearly every day
- Markedly diminished interest or pleasure in all, or almost all, activities most of the day, nearly every day
- Significant weight loss when not dieting or weight gain or decrease or increase in appetite nearly every day.
- Insomnia or hypersomnia nearly every day
- Psychomotor agitation or retardation nearly every day
- Fatigue or loss of energy nearly every day
- Feelings of worthlessness or excessive or inappropriate guilt nearly every day
- Diminished ability to think or concentrate, or indecisiveness, nearly every day
- Recurrent thoughts of death (not just fear of dying), recurrent suicidal ideation without a specific plan, or a suicide attempt or a specific plan for committing suicide

Episodes of major unipolar depression require the presence of at least five depressive symptoms above, including depressed mood or loss of interest, for a minimum of two consecutive weeks. Persistent depressive disorder (dysthymia) is diagnosed in patients with three or more depressive symptoms from above for at least two consecutive years; at least one symptom must be depressed mood. Subtypes of depressive episodes include anxious, atypical, catatonia, melancholia, mixed features, peripartum, psychotic, and seasonal.

Treatment

For the initial treatment of unipolar major depression, pharmacotherapy or psychotherapy alone are reasonable options. The clinician should keep in mind that CBT psychotherapy may be superior given the durability of its results over time after therapy is discontinuation [63].

Psychotherapy: Several psychotherapies are available to treat unipolar major depression. For patients with major depression who are initially treated with psychotherapy, CBT or interpersonal psychotherapy (IPT) rather than other psychotherapies is usually the standard based on supporting evidence levels. However, reasonable alternatives include behavioral activation, family and couples therapy, problem solving therapy, psychodynamic psychotherapy and supportive psychotherapy.

Pharmacotherapy: All classes of antidepressants are used to treat unipolar major depression and the efficacy of different antidepressants is generally comparable. Choosing one is based upon safety, side effects, comorbid illness, potential drug-drug interactions, convenience, patient preference, and cost. Improvement with medication is often apparent within 2–6 weeks.

High severity and persistent symptoms:: For patients with severe unipolar major depression, pharmacotherapy plus psychotherapy is usually recommended. For patients with severe suicidality, malnutrition secondary to food refusal and/or treatment refractory depression electroconvulsive therapy (ECT)) is usually the initial treatment. Transcranial magnetic stimulation (TMS) is another FDA-approved biologic treatment for medication-resistant depression [64].

Considerations with FMD

Depression is a common comorbidity in FMD [14, 25, 65] and links between depression and prognosis have been reported [66]. Also, of note, is the recognized associations between fearful attachment style and depression in FMD [19]. In one study of FMD in Turkey, major depressive disorder was the most frequently diagnosed psychiatric comorbidity in 16 (33%) out of 49 subjects [27]. Another case-controlled study showed 64 adults with FMD had significantly higher scores on measures of depression than healthy controls and patients with focal hand dystonia [3].

Clinically, patients with FMD may have difficulty reporting mood states due to alexithymia, and their awareness may be more focused on neurovegetative or physical symptoms. Psychoeducation can be helpful in aiding patients with FMD to understand that depression can be predominantly experienced as somatic. Since depression is linked to circadian rhythm disturbance, we find these patients often respond to modifying sleep hygiene and implementing stimulus control strategies when needed.

An important consideration for FMD is that depressed mood can often be the consequence or secondary to another psychiatric disorder. Anxiety and pain disorders are common in FMD and difficult to tolerate if chronic, contributing to depression. Treating pain and anxiety disorders aggressively can often alleviate depressive symptoms altogether.

Patients may experience multiple losses and justified sadness due to the stressors and consequences of FMD itself. Loss of autonomy, driving privileges, loss of employment, financial strains, and interpersonal role changes all may take a toll and cause stress. An important differential to keep in mind that relates to normal emotional reactions is **Adjustment Disorder**. Adjustment disorder refers to the normal adaptive reactions that occur with environmental stressors. The way to differentiate it from major depressive disorder is to notice cognitions and beliefs. Depressive disorders more often involve cognitive distortions that lead to excessive guilt and rumination about the past and mistakes one has made and feelings of worthlessness.

Adjustment disorder is treated supportively. After the stressor and its consequences have ended, affective symptoms generally resolves on their own. The nuance between depressive disorders and adjustment disorder and FMD can be complex and obtaining psychiatric consultation can be helpful in this regard.

Personality Disorders

Definition/Diagnosis

The estimated international prevalence of personality disorders in the U.S. community is 11% [67] and in clinical populations 64% [68]. In general, personality disorders are more common in males and low socioeconomic status younger age groups. These disorders are highly comorbid with other psychiatric disorders. Personality disorders are characterized by personality traits that are inflexible and maladaptive across a wide range of situations, causing significant distress and impairment of social, occupational and role functioning [26]. It is important to note there is controversy and ongoing development regarding this categorical approach to personality within psychiatry. During the development of the recent DSM-5 by the American Psychiatric Association, several revisions were proposed but ultimately postponed. A new hybrid model of personality disorders is evolving which will include the first 6 of the 9 existing categories below:

- **Schizotypal** – Social and interpersonal deficits marked by acute discomfort with and reduced capacity for close relationships, as well as by cognitive or perceptual distortions and eccentric behavior
- **Antisocial** – Disregard for and violating the rights of others, including lying, stealing, defaulting on debts and/or neglect of children or other dependents
- **Borderline** – Instability of interpersonal relationships, self-image, affect and control over impulses
- **Narcissistic** – Grandiosity (in fantasy or behavior), need for admiration and lack of empathy

- **Avoidant** – Social inhibition, feelings of inadequacy and hypersensitivity to negative evaluation
- **Obsessive-compulsive** – Preoccupation with perfectionism, mental and interpersonal control and orderliness at the expense of flexibility, openness, and efficiency
- **Dependent** – Feelings of inadequacy, inability to make own decisions, submissiveness and/or avoidance of confrontation for fear of losing source of support
- **Schizoid** – Detachment from social relationships and a restricted range of expression of emotions in interpersonal settings
- **Histrionic** – Excessive emotionality and attention-seeking

While more work is needed to quantify categorically and dimensionally the presence of maladaptive personality traits in patients FMD and related FND subtypes, we have encountered based on clinical experience that avoidant, obsessive-compulsive and borderline traits are important considerations to keep in mind when evaluating psychopathology in this population. Diagnosis of a personality disorder is usually best performed by a clinical interview focusing on social history and attention to interpersonal functioning and patterns over time. Personality disorder researchers use the Structured Clinical Interview (SCID-5-PD) for personality disorders [69]. This is a structured clinical interview linked to the DSM-5 diagnostic system. It has been shown to provide reliable diagnoses when used by trained clinicians. Self-report scales such as the Personality Diagnostic Questionnaire [70] have the advantage of saving interviewer time but can yield false positive diagnoses.

Treatment

Psychotherapy is generally regarded as first-line for patients with personality disorders [71, 72]. Medication may be used as an adjunctive treatment. Several psychotherapies have been developed or adapted to treat patients with personality including [73]:

- Dialectical behavior therapy (DBT)
- Mentalization-based therapy
- Transference-focused therapy
- Cognitive-behavioral therapy (CBT)
- Systems training for emotional predictability and problem solving (STEPPS)
- Schema-focused therapy

Psychotherapies have common elements and differences in their approaches. Some emphasize skills training [74, 75] while others focus more on relationships and meanings of interactions with others (e.g., transference-focused or mentalization-based therapy) [76, 77]. The right type of therapy depends on a complex interplay of variables. Psychiatrists can help deliver or determine which psychotherapy may be best based on existing evidence and clinical presentation.

Considerations with FMD

Personality disorders are reported to occur in 45% to 74% of FND cases [14, 65, 78] and borderline personality disorder (BPD) in 34% [78, 79]. In research on FND, including patients with FMD, studies show elevated rates of personality disorders compared to those with defined neurological disease [22, 80, 81]. These most often include borderline, dependent, avoidant, and histrionic personality disorder. A prospective study by Binzer et al. in 1997 found 30 inpatients with motor disability due to FND had more comorbid personality disorder present than the same number of patients with recognizable neurologic conditions (50% versus 17%) [65]. In a 1998 study by Crimlisk et al. looking at 59 subjects with motor type FND, 31 (53%) fulfilled criteria for a personality disorder, which included "dependent", "emotionally unstable", "anxious" and "histrionic" subtypes [80]. Stone et al. 2004 found that patients with motor FND (N = 30) were older and less likely to have a borderline personality disorder compared to patients with functional seizures (N = 20) [22]. This raises the question of whether personality disorders may be associated with certain FND subtypes.

Skills training groups emphasizing CBT and DBT can be important in the first phases of treatment when unrelenting crises and prominent emotional dysregulation may be present. Since FMD can begin acutely and suddenly, it often creates a crisis for the patient and the family. Phase I of CBT consists of stabilization and skills acquisition for affective and behavioral regulation in order to create new, more adaptive patterns of coping. Deeper trauma or interpersonal focused work that requires tolerating exposure to uncomfortable emotions (i.e. distress tolerance) and affect may need to be delivered in phase II of treatment after stabilization and access to skills has been achieved. Patients with FMD are often experiencing psychosocial difficulties and only once stabilized (e.g., a lawsuit ends, social security is gained, caregiving duties are shifted or emotion regulation skills are mastered) are they able to tolerate highly negative emotions that a deeper reflective or trauma focused treatment may have to offer.

Psychiatric coordination of all pieces of care may be a vital component in FMD treatment to avoid fragmentation and enhance integration of services. Important for providers caring for FMD patients with comorbid personality disorders is managing therapeutic alliance challenges, boundary setting and therapy-interfering behaviors. Comprehensive programs which allow a team approach with group and individual therapy, case management and therapy consultation for providers can be useful to avoid burnout, compassion fatigue, and empathy failures.

Psychiatrist's Role

Models of Psychiatric Care

Indirect

From the above discussion of psychiatric comorbidities in FMD, one can see the many hats a psychiatrist may wear in the care of patients and their comorbidities. Psychiatrists can improve FMD prognosis indirectly by treating comorbid psychiatric illness. Psychiatrist involvement can also exist on a continuum of levels of engagement. They can provide consultation to medical providers with or without patients present. Psychiatrists can act as one-time consultants or ongoing consultants that may be especially important when prominent decompensated psychiatric comorbidities are present.

Psychiatrists usually treat comorbidities as psychopharmacologists. However, depending on their training, they may be able to deliver or connect patients with other evidenced-based interventions. These include psychotherapy, behavioral and lifestyle modification, exposure and trauma-focused therapy, group therapy, mindfulness and relaxation training, skills training, interpersonal communication training, occupational therapy, case management and social work. These services may be liaisoned in either intensive or outpatient ambulatory settings. If psychiatrists are not trained in an intervention, they often have networks in the community of trained professionals that can deliver the most evidenced-based options available. Psychiatrists may also have specialty training to deliver more novel experimental technology driven treatments for comorbidities including: Electroconvulsive therapy (ECT), deep brain stimulation (DBS), transcranial magnetic stimulation (TMS), virtual and immersive (also called extended reality [XR]) therapies and telepsychiatry.

Direct

Alternatively, psychiatrists can manage FMD directly if they are educated, willing and understand FMD, particularly those with advanced training in neuropsychiatry. Firstly, trained psychiatrists may play a critical role in the multidisciplinary assessment of patients with FMD. Despite medical professionals delivering psychoeducation regarding the diagnoses, a psychiatrist may have the advantage of longer sessions and time to discuss complex psychoeducation and treatment planning with the patient. This might afford the opportunity to digest and accept the diagnosis with repetition of information that was hard to process with their neurologist or other medical providers. There is evidence that proper psychoeducation can improve outcomes [86, 87].

Psychiatrists may act as chaperones and bridges from medical to more psychological/psychosocial modalities of treatment. Skilled psychiatrists may deliver evidence-based CBT psychotherapies that are modified for FMD or they may be able to find skilled therapists to deliver CBT for FMD. Psychiatrists may deliver interventions focused on executive functioning skills or changing beliefs around expectations, self-efficacy and agency. Developing emotional and interoceptive awareness and affective regulation to combat alexithymia may be a focus of psychiatric care directly related to FMD.

The delivery of trauma-focused interventions such as Prolonged Exposure, EMDR, Dialectical Behavior Therapy and mindfulness training to address the effects of childhood trauma or other adverse life events may be delivered by psychiatrists even in the absence of PTSD. Skills training for interpersonal problems impacting role functioning and helping those patients with FMD involved in legal disputes find the resources and skills to resolve litigation may be a direct intervention for FMD.

Additionally, regardless of the role of the psychiatrist in the longitudinal management of patients with FMD, medical and mental health professionals should work towards developing an element of shared (partially overlapping) expertise, such that neurologists are more psychotherapeutically informed in their interactions with patients and psychiatrists and allied mental health professions have greater understanding of the neurological diagnostic approach that is so critical to aiding diagnostic acceptance.

Developing Relationships with FMD Aware Psychiatrists

The origins of psychiatry are keenly related to FMD cases, catalyzing the development of psychotherapy by notable figures such as Sigmund Freud and Carl Jung. Sadly, many conventional psychiatry and psychotherapists have lost their connection and awareness of FMD and FND more broadly. Despite the high prevalence of FMD, very little medical, psychiatric, or clinical psychology training curriculums include FMD in their educational programs. Most mental health practitioners including psychiatrists have had little preparation for treating FMD and are often quite wary and uninformed. Some are not trained in even the difference between malingering, factitious, SSD or FND. Untrained mental health professionals often worry about imagined high rates of misdiagnosis and insist that patients pursue unnecessary second opinions [88]. They can also have trouble believing that movements that are so visually striking can be functional. Mental health providers may also worry about the liability of patients injuring themselves while symptomatic in their offices and may unfortunately deny care.

Although the minority, there are some mental health professionals including psychiatrists who have taken a special interest in this population most often due to close ties and collaboration with neurologists. Some have pursued extra training to be qualified. Often consult-liaison psychiatrists have received such education thru psychosomatic medicine subspecialty certification. Other psychiatrists who have special relationships with neurology may become certified in Neuropsychiatry and Behavioral Neurology through United Council of Neurological Subspecialties (UCNS). Professional neurology groups or societies may have FMD competent psychiatrist members. The American Neuropsychiatric Association (ANPA) and the international Functional Neurological Disorder Society (FNDS) have psychiatrist members who are knowledgeable and skilled in FMD. Patient advocacy organizations such as FND Hope also have updated lists of expert providers, including psychiatrists who are experienced in managing patients with FMD.

When looking for a skilled mental health professional, an important factor is the frequency and number of cases a provider has seen. This is the similar to a search for a skilled surgeon. In general, when you are looking for psychiatric experts you want to find a provider seeing the highest number of cases in a particular population you are interested in. The higher the amount of clinical exposure psychiatrists have to FMD, the more likely they are skilled. Some local neurologists have developed a referral base they can leverage. Communities and networks are vital to the treatment of FMD. These types of relationships create skill building feedback loops, as physicians collectively become even more experienced over time with FMD management.

Getting creative when mental health providers are unable to be found is important. Setting up local groups to improve access and training to mental health professionals may be a strategy. Creating, supporting and facilitating education and training in FMD treatment may be important. Our group at Stanford had particular success by setting up a local consortium dedicated to FND and holding monthly meetings. Engaging multidisciplinary experts to share experiences and advice can be invaluable. Inviting grand round speakers on the topic of FMD at your local hospital can spark interest and access to knowledge and experience. Finally, with the emergence of telehealth, many barriers to finding qualified mental health professionals are being lowered. Given the high level of problems with transportation for patients, telehealth may offer unique advantages for this population as health systems pivot towards more frequently providing virtual care.

Considerations for the Non-Psychiatrist

The neurologist and primary care physicians are often the first healthcare professionals to care for patients with FMD. A comprehensive assessment includes screening for commonly associated psychiatric conditions. The clinician may gently, non-judgmentally introduce the discussion of mental health, by "normalizing" the presence of these symptoms as commonly coexisting with FMD. Ideally, this is accomplished without implying causation. In discussion with patients, mental health conditions can be conceptualized as factors that independently impact FMD, along

with entities such as sleep disturbances, cognitive complaints, migraine and chronic pain. Beginning with open-ended questions and effectively validating emotional experiences are essential skills for navigating these sensitive topics.

Where time is limited, a focused mental health evaluation to identify acute issues such as suicidality and severe affective symptoms is prudent. Risk can be further characterized by obtaining past psychiatric history, including mental health hospitalizations, suicide attempts, self-injurious behaviors, relationship with a psychiatrist or therapist and the use of psychiatric medications. Suicide attempts occur in some with FND. A prospective study of 38 patients found a history of suicide attempts in 34% [82]. The National Institute of Mental Health recommends that all patients who are screened for suicidality be provided with phone numbers for the 24/7 National Suicide Prevention Lifeline and crisis text lines.

In busy neurology practices where FMD is confirmed, screening questionnaires can be helpful. Where time is limited, the PHQ-9 and National Institute of Health PROMIS scales survey general mental health [54, 83]. Otherwise, focused psychiatric screenings should include assessment for mood and anxiety disorders, as well as PTSD. Well validated measures include the GAD-7 [51] and the PTSD Checklist-5 (PCL-5) [84]. Positive findings may help guide the clinician towards areas for further exploration. Where mental health symptoms are closely intertwined with FMD symptoms or clearly impairing quality of life, referral to psychiatry is generally indicated for detailed assessment.

Questions to detect and quantify alcohol and substance use disorders (SUD) are standard in most initial interviews. Where use appears to be interfering with functioning or relevant to FMD symptoms, the clinician can assess the patient's readiness for change and offer resources as appropriate. SUD interferes with both the evaluation and treatment of all other psychiatric illnesses. Treatment of SUDs must be prioritized over many other comorbidities, as more targeted symptom management will be limited in the setting of intoxication and mood lability secondary to withdrawal states. Where chronic pain and alcohol or substance abuse are comorbid, medications such as gabapentin and naltrexone can be useful to diminish cravings, as part of a comprehensive substance rehabilitation program.

A diffusely positive review of symptoms, with the patient expressing distress and excessive attention towards symptoms should prompt the clinician to consider comorbid SSD. An excessive focus on the meaning of symptoms or time intensive healthcare seeking is another marker for SSD that might prompt using screening tools such as the PHQ-15 [55] and SSS-8 [56]. For more details on the neuropsychiatric assessment of FMD (emphasizing rule-in diagnosis based on neurological examination and psychiatric/social screenings aiding the development of a patient-centered treatment plan), see Perez et al. in collaboration with the American Neuropsychiatric Association [85].

Where medication is appropriate for sleep disturbances, migraine and chronic pain, choosing a multi-purpose medication that targets the psychiatric comorbidity is advised. One example is the use of SNRI or TCA medication for co-treatment of both chronic pain and depression or anxiety. If insomnia is present, a sedating TCA such as amitriptyline can be tried. Another example is the use of mirtazapine in patients reporting insomnia in conjunction with depression or anxiety.

Conclusions and Calls to Action

In this chapter, we reviewed the psychiatric services and roles a psychiatrist can play in treating FMD and its comorbidities. Psychiatrists and psychiatric services are uniquely positioned to mitigate the multifactorial variables affecting FMD symptoms and individualize care. Medical professionals, if knowledgeable, can determine how to personalize the level and kind of psychiatric engagement for each patient. Allowing that

flexibility of choice for FMD involves insuring policy and reform in our healthcare system to allow access to psychiatric services.

Despite the value of psychiatric input, a major obstacle is the lack of formal training provided in FMD and other somatic symptom related disorders. This is a major barrier for good clinical care of FMD populations. Due to FMD's inherent complexity, confusion and implicit biases in the medical system and culture towards FMD exist and are historically pervasive [89]. We hypothesize that stigma and implicit biases may explain the deficits in FMD medical training [90]. The result of stigma is social exclusion and in the case of FMD it appears to be exclusion of FMD content from the medical and psychiatric training curriculums. This exclusion leads to vicious cycles of increasing stigma and ignorance. A call to action recommended is to increase FMD awareness by advocating for increased medical education on the subject, especially across psychiatry, neurology and allied disciplines.

Stigma not only affects psychiatry training but it disrupts the therapeutic alliance of providers and patients with FMD. When patients with FMD relay their experiences with the healthcare system, they often report invalidating and minimizing interactions. Stigmatized patients may have prior negative interactions that can set up mistrust or sometimes anger towards clinicians, which may in turn create defensiveness in response. Psychiatrists are well positioned to deal with these ruptures as they do with the stigma of most mental illnesses. Coordinated effort between medical providers and psychiatrists avoids fragmented care, confusion and insecurity in patients. A unified team approach involving both neurology and psychiatry often alleviates patient concerns and enhances clinician-patient alliance, which is a powerful predictor of outcome for medical and psychiatric outcomes. Combatting stigma around mental illness more broadly will go far to improve outcomes for patients with FMD.

Summary

- Shortening the duration of time from diagnosis to treatment engagement, including psychiatric care improves outcomes. Engaging psychiatric services is a priority for FMD, while ensuring that neurology and primary care, colleagues also remain actively involved.
- The prevalence of comorbid psychiatric illness is high in FMD and its treatment may improve outcomes as it addresses predisposing, precipitating and/or perpetuating factors.
- Table 22.1 presents the basic psychiatric tools and treatments provided to the most common FMD comorbidities.
- Levels of psychiatric engagement are on a continuum and can be adjusted as needed over time and based on patient's needs and available resources.
- Some psychiatrists who are trained and experienced with FMD and related mind-body disorders may be capable of treating FMD directly through psychotherapeutic modalities.
- Training deficits currently exist in psychiatric and other medical curriculums on the topic of FMD. This gap needs correcting by effective leadership, including better engagement of training and program directors, with an emphasis on a neuropsychiatric perspective.
- Combatting psychiatric stigma by increasing awareness of FMD and mental illness in crucial for long-term improvement in patient outcomes.

References

1. Perez DL, Haller AL, Espay AJ. Should neurologists diagnose and manage functional neurologic disorders? It is complicated. Neurol Clin Pract. 2019;9(2):165–7.
2. Perez DL, Keshavan MS, Scharf JM, Boes AD, Price BH. Bridging the great divide: what can neurology learn from psychiatry? J Neuropsychiatry Clin Neurosci. 2018;30(4):271–8.
3. Kranick S, Ekanayake V, Martinez V, Ameli R, Hallett M, Voon V. Psychopathology and psychogenic movement disorders. Mov Disord. 2011;26(10):1844–50.
4. Miyasaki JM. Functional movement disorders [Internet]. Uptodate.com. 2020 [cited 2020 Apr 25]. Available from: https://www.uptodate.com/.
5. Morgante F, Edwards MJ, Espay AJ. Psychogenic movement disorders. Continuum (Minneap Minn). 2013;19(5 Movement Disorders):1383–96.
6. Herzog A, Shedden-Mora MC, Jordan P, Löwe B. Duration of untreated illness in patients with somatoform disorders. J Psychosom Res. 2018;107:1–6.
7. Edwards MJ, Fotopoulou A, Pareés I. Neurobiology of functional (psychogenic) movement disorders. Curr Opin Neurol. 2013;26(4):442–7.
8. Edwards MJ, Adams RA, Brown H, Pareés I, Friston KJ. A Bayesian account of "hysteria". Brain. 2012;135(Pt 11):3495–512.
9. Pareés I, Brown H, Nuruki A, Adams RA, Davare M, Bhatia KP, et al. Loss of sensory attenuation in patients with functional (psychogenic) movement disorders. Brain. 2014a;137(Pt 11):2916–21.
10. Maurer CW, LaFaver K, Ameli R, Epstein SA, Hallett M, Horovitz SG. Impaired self-agency in functional movement disorders: a resting-state fMRI study. Neurology. 2016;87(6):564–70.
11. Newby R, Alty J, Kempster P. Functional dystonia and the borderland between neurology and psychiatry: new concepts. Mov Disord. 2016;31(12):1777–84.
12. Demartini B, Petrochilos P, Ricciardi L, Price G, Edward MJ, Joyce E. The role of alexithymia in the development of functional motor symptoms (conversion disorder). J Neurol Neurosurg Psychiatry. 2014;85(8):e3.
13. Williams DT, Ford B, Fahn S. Phenomenology and psychopathology related to psychogenic movement disorders. Adv Neurol. 1995;65:231–57.
14. Feinstein A, Stergiopoulos V, Fine J, Lang AE. Psychiatric outcome in patients with a psychogenic movement disorder: a prospective study. Neuropsychiatry Neuropsychol Behav Neurol. 2001;14(3):169–76.
15. Hinson VK, Haren WB. Psychogenic movement disorders. Lancet Neurol. 2006;5(8):695–700.
16. Thomas M, Vuong KD, Jankovic J. Long-term prognosis of patients with psychogenic movement disorders. Parkinsonism Relat Disord. 2006;12(6):382–7.
17. O'Connell N, Nicholson TR, Wessely S, David AS. Characteristics of patients with motor functional neurological disorder in a large UK mental health service: a case-control study. Psychol Med. 2020;50(3):446–55.
18. Williams B, Ospina JP, Jalilianhasanpour R, Fricchione GL, Perez DL. Fearful attachment linked to childhood abuse, alexithymia, and depression in motor functional neurological disorders. J Neuropsychiatry Clin Neurosci. 2019;31(1):65–9.

19. Pareés I, Kojovic M, Pires C, Rubio-Agusti I, Saifee TA, Sadnicka A, et al. Physical precipitating factors in functional movement disorders. J Neurol Sci. 2014b;338(1–2):174–7.

20. Stone J, Warlow C, Deary I, Sharpe M. Predisposing risk factors for functional limb weakness: a case-control study. J Neuropsychiatry Clin Neurosci. 2020;32(1):50–7.

21. Epstein SA, Maurer CW, LaFaver K, Ameli R, Sinclair S, Hallett M. Insights into chronic functional movement disorders: the value of qualitative psychiatric interviews. Psychosomatics. 2016;57(6):566–75.

22. Stone J, Sharpe M, Binzer M. Motor conversion symptoms and pseudoseizures: a comparison of clinical characteristics. Psychosomatics. 2004;45(6):492–9.

23. Stone J, Warlow C, Sharpe M. The symptom of functional weakness: a controlled study of 107 patients. Brain. 2010;133(Pt 5):1537–51.

24. Gray C, Calderbank A, Adewusi J, Hughes R, Reuber M. Symptoms of posttraumatic stress disorder in patients with functional neurological symptom disorder. J Psychosom Res. 2020;129(109907):109907.

25. Schrag A, Trimble M, Quinn N, Bhatia K. The syndrome of fixed dystonia: an evaluation of 103 patients. Brain. 2004;127(Pt 10):2360–72.

26. American Psychiatric Association. Diagnostic and statistical manual of mental disorders (DSM-5 (R)). 5th ed. Arlington: American Psychiatric Association Publishing; 2013.

27. Ertan S, Uluduz D, Ozekmekçi S, Kiziltan G, Ertan T, Yalçinkaya C, et al. Clinical characteristics of 49 patients with psychogenic movement disorders in a tertiary clinic in Turkey. Mov Disord. 2009;24(5):759–62.

28. Irwin MR BB. Factitious disorder imposed on self (Munchausen syndrome) [Internet]. UpToDate. 2020 [cited 2020 Apr 25]. Available from: www.uptodate. com.

29. Lanius RA, Vermetten E, Loewenstein RJ, Brand B, Schmahl C, Bremner JD, et al. Emotion modulation in PTSD: clinical and neurobiological evidence for a dissociative subtype. Am J Psychiatry. 2010;167(6):640–7.

30. Myers L, Vaidya-Mathur U, Lancman M. Prolonged exposure therapy for the treatment of patients diagnosed with psychogenic non-epileptic seizures (PNES) and post-traumatic stress disorder (PTSD). Epilepsy Behav. 2017;66:86–92.

31. Stein DJ, Ipser JC, Seedat S. Pharmacotherapy for post traumatic stress disorder (PTSD). Cochrane Database Syst Rev. 2006;(1):CD002795.

32. Davidson J, Baldwin D, Stein DJ, Kuper E, Benattia I, Ahmed S, et al. Treatment of posttraumatic stress disorder with venlafaxine extended release: a 6-month randomized controlled trial: a 6-month randomized controlled trial. Arch Gen Psychiatry. 2006;63(10):1158–65.

33. Committee on Treatment of Posttraumatic Stress Disorder, Institute Of. Treatment of posttraumatic stress disorder: an assessment of the evidence.

34. Committee on treatment of posttraumatic stress disorder: board on population health and public health practice. Washington, D.C.: National Academies Press; 2008.

35. Cohen PJA, Friedman MDMJ, Keane PTM, Foa PEB. Effective treatments for ptsd: practice guidelines from the international society for traumatic stress studies. New York: Guilford Publications; 2009.

36. Foa EB, Hembree E, Rothbaum B. Prolonged exposure therapy for PTSD: emotional processing of traumatic experiences, therapist guide. New York: Oxford University Press; 2007.

37. Bisson J, Andrew M. Psychological treatment of posttraumatic stress disorder (PTSD). Cochrane Database Syst Rev. 2007;(3):CD003388.

38. Kessler RC, Ustun TB, editors. The WHO world mental health surveys: global perspectives on the epidemiology of mental disorders. Cambridge, TAS: Cambridge University Press; 2011.

39. Kessler RC, Berglund P, Demler O, Jin R, Merikangas KR, Walters EE. Lifetime prevalence and age-of-onset distributions of DSM-IV disorders in the National Comorbidity Survey Replication. Arch Gen Psychiatry. 2005;62(6):593–602.

40. Ekanayake V, Kranick S, LaFaver K, Naz A, Frank Webb A, LaFrance WC Jr, et al. Personality traits in psychogenic nonepileptic seizures (PNES) and psychogenic movement disorder (PMD): neuroticism and perfectionism. J Psychosom Res. 2017;97:23–9.

41. Matin N, Young SS, Williams B, LaFrance WC Jr, King JN, Caplan D, et al. Neuropsychiatric associations with gender, illness duration, work disability, and motor subtype in a U.S. functional neurological disorders clinic population. J Neuropsychiatry Clin Neurosci. 2017;29(4):375–82.

42. Barlow DH, Gorman JM, Shear MK, Woods SW. Cognitive-behavioral therapy, imipramine, or their combination for panic disorder: a randomized controlled trial. JAMA. 2000;283(19):2529–36.

43. Butler AC, Chapman JE, Forman EM, Beck AT. The empirical status of cognitive-behavioral therapy: a review of meta-analyses. Clin Psychol Rev. 2006;26(1):17–31.

44. Lee K, Noda Y, Nakano Y, Ogawa S, Kinoshita Y, Funayama T, et al. Interoceptive hypersensitivity and interoceptive exposure in patients with panic disorder: specificity and effectiveness. BMC Psychiatry. 2006;6:32.

45. Mitte K. A meta-analysis of the efficacy of psycho- and pharmacotherapy in panic disorder with and without agoraphobia. J Affect Disord. 2005;88(1): 27–45.

46. Wilkinson G, Balestrieri M, Ruggeri M, Bellantuono C. Meta-analysis of double-blind placebo-controlled trials of antidepressants and benzodiazepines for patients with panic disorders. Psychol Med. 1991;21(4):991–8.

47. Voon V, Lang AE. Antidepressant treatment outcomes of psychogenic movement disorder. J Clin Psychiatry. 2005;66(12):1529–34.

47. Kleinstäuber M, Witthöft M, Steffanowski A, van Marwijk H, Hiller W, Lambert MJ. Pharmacological interventions for somatoform disorders in adults. Cochrane Database Syst Rev. 2014;(11):CD010628.
48. Sharpe M, Walker J, Williams C, Stone J, Cavanagh J, Murray G, et al. Guided self-help for functional (psychogenic) symptoms: a randomized controlled efficacy trial. Neurology. 2011;77(6):564–72.
49. Dallocchio C, Tinazzi M, Bombieri F, Arnó N, Erro R. Cognitive behavioural therapy and adjunctive physical activity for functional movement disorders (conversion disorder): a pilot, single-blinded, randomized study. Psychother Psychosom. 2016;85(6):381–3.
50. Espay AJ, Ries S, Maloney T, Vannest J, Neefus E, Dwivedi AK, et al. Clinical and neural responses to cognitive behavioral therapy for functional tremor. Neurology. 2019;93(19):e1787–98.
51. Spitzer RL, Kroenke K, Williams JBW, Löwe B. A brief measure for assessing generalized anxiety disorder: the GAD-7. Arch Intern Med. 2006;166(10):1092–7.
52. Carl E, Witcraft SM, Kauffman BY, Gillespie EM, Becker ES, Cuijpers P, et al. Psychological and pharmacological treatments for generalized anxiety disorder (GAD): a meta-analysis of randomized controlled trials. Cogn Behav Ther. 2020;49(1):1–21.
53. Beck AT, Epstein N, Brown G, Steer RA. An inventory for measuring clinical anxiety: psychometric properties. J Consult Clin Psychol. 1988;56(6):893–7.
54. Kroenke K, Spitzer RL, Williams JB. The PHQ-9: validity of a brief depression severity measure. J Gen Intern Med. 2001;16(9):606–13.
55. Zijlema WL, Stolk RP, Löwe B, Rief W, White PD, et al. How to assess common somatic symptoms in large-scale studies: a systematic review of questionnaires. J Psychosom Res. 2013;74(6):459–68.
56. Gierk B, Kohlmann S, Kroenke K, Spangenberg L, Zenger M, Brähler E, et al. The somatic symptom scale-8 (SSS-8): a brief measure of somatic symptom burden. JAMA Intern Med. 2014;174(3):399–407.
57. Levenson JL. Somatic symptom disorder: epidemiology and clinical presentation [Internet]. UpToDate. 2020 [cited 2020 Apr 25]. Available from: www.uptodate.com.
58. Hedman E, Axelsson E, Andersson E, Lekander M, Ljótsson B. Exposure-based cognitive-behavioural therapy via the internet and as bibliotherapy for somatic symptom disorder and illness anxiety disorder: randomised controlled trial. Br J Psychiatry. 2016;209(5):407–13.
59. Morriss R. Role of mental health professionals in the management of functional somatic symptoms in primary care. Br J Psychiatry. 2012;200(6):444–5.
60. Jimenez XF, Aboussouan A, Johnson J. Functional neurological disorder responds favorably to interdisciplinary rehabilitation models. Psychosomatics. 2019;60(6):556–62.
61. Manea L, Gilbody S, Hewitt C, North A, Plummer F, Richardson R, et al. Identifying depression with the

PHQ-2: A diagnostic meta-analysis. J Affect Disord. 2016;203:382–95.
62. Steer RA, Cavalieri TA, Leonard DM, Beck AT. Use of the beck depression inventory for primary care to screen for major depression disorders. Gen Hosp Psychiatry. 1999;21(2):106–11.
63. Hollon SD, Stewart MO, Strunk D. Enduring effects for cognitive behavior therapy in the treatment of depression and anxiety. Annu Rev Psychol. 2006;57(1):285–315.
64. Janicak PG, O'Reardon JP, Sampson SM, Husain MM, Lisanby SH, Rado JT, et al. Transcranial magnetic stimulation in the treatment of major depressive disorder: a comprehensive summary of safety experience from acute exposure, extended exposure, and during reintroduction treatment. J Clin Psychiatry. 2008;69(2):222–32.
65. Binzer M, Andersen PM, Kullgren G. Clinical characteristics of patients with motor disability due to conversion disorder: a prospective control group study. J Neurol Neurosurg Psychiatry. 1997;63(1):83–8.
66. Gelauff J, Stone J, Edwards M, Carson A. The prognosis of functional (psychogenic) motor symptoms: a systematic review. J Neurol Neurosurg Psychiatry. 2014;85(2):220–6.
67. Torgersen S. Prevalence, sociodemographics, and functional impairment. In: Oldham JM, Skodol AE, Bender DS, editors. The American psychiatric publishing textbook of personality disorders. American Psychiatric Publishing; 2014. p. 109–29.
68. Torgersen S. Epidemiology. In: Widiger TA, editor. Oxford library of psychology. The Oxford handbook of personality disorders. Oxford University Press; 2012. p. 186–205.
69. First MB, Williams JBW, Benjamin LS, Spitzer RL. SCID-5-PD: Structured clinical interview for DSM-5® personality disorders. Arlington: American Psychiatric Association; 2016.
70. Hyler SE, Skodol AE, Kellman HD, Oldham JM, Rosnick L. Validity of the personality diagnostic questionnaire--revised: comparison with two structured interviews. Am J Psychiatry. 1990;147(8):1043–8.
71. Leichsenring F, Rabung S. Effectiveness of long-term psychodynamic psychotherapy: a meta-analysis: a meta-analysis. JAMA. 2008;300(13):1551–65.
72. Matusiewicz AK, Hopwood CJ, Banducci AN, Lejuez CW. The effectiveness of cognitive behavioral therapy for personality disorders. Psychiatr Clin North Am. 2010;33(3):657–85.
73. Stoffers JM, Völlm BA, Rücker G, Timmer A, Huband N, Lieb K. Psychological therapies for people with borderline personality disorder. Cochrane Database Syst Rev. 2012;8:CD005652.
74. Linehan MM, Comtois KA, Murray AM, Brown MZ, Gallop RJ, Heard HL, et al. Two-year randomized controlled trial and follow-up of dialectical behavior therapy vs therapy by experts for suicidal behaviors and borderline personality disorder. Arch Gen Psychiatry. 2006;63(7):757–66.

75. Davidson K, Norrie J, Tyrer P, Gumley A, Tata P, Murray H, et al. The effectiveness of cognitive behavior therapy for borderline personality disorder: results from the borderline personality disorder study of cognitive therapy (BOSCOT) trial. J Personal Disord. 2006;20(5):450–65.

76. Giesen-Bloo J, van Dyck R, Spinhoven P, van Tilburg W, Dirksen C, van Asselt T, et al. Outpatient psychotherapy for borderline personality disorder: randomized trial of schema-focused therapy vs transference-focused psychotherapy. Arch Gen Psychiatry. 2006;63(6):649–58.

77. Bateman A, Fonagy P. Randomized controlled trial of outpatient mentalization-based treatment versus structured clinical management for borderline personality disorder. Am J Psychiatry. 2009;166(12): 1355–64.

78. Søgaard U, Mathiesen BB, Simonsen E. Personality and psychopathology in patients with mixed sensory-motor functional neurological disorder (conversion disorder): a pilot study. J Nerv Ment Dis. 2019;207(7):546–54.

79. Sar V, Islam S, Ozturk E. Childhood emotional abuse and dissociation in patients with conversion symptoms: child abuse, dissociation, and conversion. Psychiatry Clin Neurosci. 2009;63(5):670–7.

80. Crimlisk HL, Bhatia K, Cope H, David A, Marsden CD, Ron MA. Slater revisited: 6 year follow up study of patients with medically unexplained motor symptoms. BMJ. 1998;316(7131):582–6.

81. Fiszman A, Kanner AM. Comorbidities in psychogenic nonepileptic seizures: depressive, anxiety, and personality disorders. In: Schacter S, LaFrance Jr WC, editors. Gates and Rowan's nonepileptic seizures. 3rd ed. Cambridge: Cambridge University Press; 2010. p. 225.

82. Sar V, Akyüz G, Kundakçi T, Kiziltan E, Dogan O. Childhood trauma, dissociation, and psychiatric comorbidity in patients with conversion disorder. Am J Psychiatry. 2004;161(12):2271–6.

83. Cella D, Riley W, Stone A, Rothrock N, Reeve B, Yount S, et al. The Patient-Reported Outcomes Measurement Information System (PROMIS) developed and tested its first wave of adult self-reported health outcome item banks: 2005-2008. J Clin Epidemiol. 2010;63(11):1179–94.

84. Blevins CA, Weathers FW, Davis MT, Witte TK, Domino JL. The Posttraumatic Stress Disorder Checklist for DSM-5 (PCL-5): development and initial psychometric evaluation: posttraumatic stress disorder checklist for DSM-5. J Trauma Stress. 2015;28(6):489–98.

85. Perez DL, Aybek S, Popkirov S, Kozlowska K, Stephen CD, Anderson J, et al. A review and expert opinion on the neuropsychiatric assessment of motor functional neurological disorders. J Neuropsychiatry Clin Neurosci. 2021;33(1):14–26.

86. Stone J, Carson AJ, Sharpe M. Psychogenic movement disorders: explaining the diagnosis. In: Hallett M, Lang AE, Jankovic J, Fahn S, Halligan PW, Voon V, Cloninger CR, editors. Psychogenic movement disorders and other conversion disorders. Cambridge: Cambridge University Press; 2011. p. 254.

87. Duncan R, Razvi S, Mulhern S. Newly presenting psychogenic nonepileptic seizures: incidence, population characteristics, and early outcome from a prospective audit of a first seizure clinic. Epilepsy Behav. 2011;20(2):308–11.

88. Stone J, Smyth R, Carson A, Lewis S, Prescott R, Warlow C, et al. Systematic review of misdiagnosis of conversion symptoms and "hysteria". BMJ. 2005;331(7523):989.

89. Looper KJ, Kirmayer LJ. Perceived stigma in functional somatic syndromes and comparable medical conditions. J Psychosom Res. 2004;57(4):373–8.

90. Kurzban R, Leary MR. Evolutionary origins of stigmatization: the functions of social exclusion. Psychol Bull. 2001;127(2):187–208.

Physical Therapy: Retraining Movement

23

Paula Gardiner, Julie Maggio, and Glenn Nielsen

Vignette

JP, a 48-year-old male, developed sudden onset spinning vertigo and nausea, which was diagnosed as acute vestibular neuritis. Over several weeks, the vertigo changed in nature from spinning to a feeling of unsteadiness when standing or walking. His ability to walk suddenly deteriorated and he presented to the emergency department with a suspected stroke. Investigations were normal and he was discharged with an outpatient neurology referral. After a long wait and further deterioration of symptoms, JP saw the neurologist and was given a diagnosis of functional movement disorder with associated features of persistent postural perceptual dizziness (3PD). He was referred to outpatient physical therapy.

P. Gardiner
Royal Infirmary Edinburgh, Edinburgh, Scotland, UK
e-mail: paula.gardiner@nhslothian.scot.nhs.uk

J. Maggio
Department of Physical Therapy, Massachusetts General Hospital, Boston, MA, USA
e-mail: JMaggio@mgh.harvard.edu

G. Nielsen (✉)
Neuroscience Research Centre, Institute of Molecular and Clinical Sciences, St Georges University of London, London, UK
e-mail: gnielsen@sgul.ac.uk

Introduction

Physical therapy is an important component of treatment for patients with functional movement disorder (FMD). There is growing evidence that physical interventions informed by a biopsychosocial understanding of FMD can lead to clinically meaningful and lasting improvement to disability and quality of life [1]. In this chapter, we discuss the rationale for physical interventions, describe a psychologically informed approach to assessment and treatment, and consider the evidence supporting our suggestions.

The primary aim of physical therapy for FMD is to retrain normal movement patterns. Treatment can be based on the principles of applied motor learning theory in rehabilitation [2]. This approach to treatment aims to induce beneficial neuroplastic changes that reinforce normal movement patterns. Motor retraining in FMD should also be informed by an understanding of underlying mechanisms that drive FMD [3], specifically the role of *attention* and *expectation*. In brief, self-directed attention exacerbates abnormal movement and posture. Conversely, redirecting attention away from the body reduces or normalizes abnormal movement. Expectations refer to beliefs about movement and/or sensation (which may not necessarily be consciously reportable thoughts) that influence motor output and sensory perception at a subconscious level (See Chap. 2 for a more detailed discussion of the

© Springer Nature Switzerland AG 2022
K. LaFaver et al. (eds.), *Functional Movement Disorder*, Current Clinical Neurology,
https://doi.org/10.1007/978-3-030-86495-8_23

pathophysiology of FMD). Physical therapy can specifically target unhelpful attention and beliefs by: (i) education; (ii) demonstration to the patient that normal movement is possible; and (iii) motor retraining coupled with an external focus of attention. Other potential mechanisms by which physical therapy may help people with FMD include the psychological and physiological benefits of exercise and activity. Physical therapy can also help with the secondary consequences of FMD, such as joint pain and deconditioning associated with altered movement patterns. For many patients, FMD is a chronic condition, therefore treatment should also aim to help patients with the long-term management of their health and wellbeing.

What Is the Evidence Base for Physical Therapy for FMD?

A systematic review from 2013 revealed a lack of controlled evidence for physical therapy for FMD [4]. In the time since publication, 2 controlled trials [5, 6] and a number of moderately sized cohort studies [7, 8] have been published, each supporting a multidisciplinary treatment approach inclusive of physical therapy.

An early influential study of rehabilitation for FMD was a retrospective review of a specialist multidisciplinary treatment program for FMD [9]. The treatment was described as motor reprogramming and was conducted intensively over five consecutive days. The study found that 73% of 60 consecutive patients were markedly improved at the end of treatment. When followed up after 2 years, 60% continued to have markedly improved symptoms or were in remission.

Jordbru and colleagues [5] conducted a trial comparing a 3-week inpatient multidisciplinary rehabilitation program to a 4 week waiting list control for 60 patients with functional gait disorder. The trial intervention was described as "adapted physical activity with an educational and cognitive behavioral frame of reference". Treatment was carried out by a physician, physi-cal therapist, occupational therapist, nurse and exercise instructor. At the end of treatment, the intervention group showed a statistically significant improvement compared to the control in a range of physical and mental health outcome measures. The treatment effect was for the most part sustained at 12 months, however, there was some loss of treatment effect for a measure of mental health.

Nielsen and colleagues [6] conducted a controlled feasibility trial in 60 patients with FMD. Specialist physiotherapy for FMD was compared to standard neuro-physiotherapy. Participants were followed up at 6 months post randomization, with a range of outcome measures. At 6 months, 72% of the intervention group rated their symptoms as improved, compared to 18% in the control group. The trial found moderate to large treatment effects for several additional measures of physical health, but no statistical change in measures of mental health. A preliminary health economic analysis found some evidence of cost benefit with a favorable incremental cost effectiveness ratio. The larger (well-powered), multisite version of this trial is currently underway [10], due for completion in 2023. Several other trials of physical therapy for FMD are listed in trial registries and should be reported in the coming years.

The outcomes from this relatively small body of research are promising. It appears that the majority of patients (60–70%) obtain at least some benefit from physical therapy that is informed by an understanding of FMD. The effect size of treatments are moderate, and are sustained when patients are followed up at 12 months. However, treatment effects may reduce with time and are likely to reduce as patient complexity and comorbidity increase. There are some limitations in the generalizability of this literature. Patients are selected for their suitability for physical rehabilitation and those with more substantial comorbidities (such as severe chronic pain, fatigue or unstable psychiatric illness) are often excluded. Importantly, patients who disagree with the diagnosis are also typically not part of treatment studies.

Assessment and Treatment Planning

We believe that it is essential to emphasize the importance of the initial assessment in this patient population. The main aims are to (i) build trust and rapport; (ii) obtain an in-depth understanding of the patient's movement problems and other pertinent symptoms; and (iii) recognize relevant biological, psychological and social problems associated with the patient's FMD. In multidisciplinary treatment teams, joint assessments with occupational therapy and psychology colleagues can lead to additional insights, prevent conflicting information or advice, and facilitate cooperative working.

Subjective Assessment

We recommend starting by asking about the onset of symptoms. Next create a list of each of the symptoms experienced by the patient, enquiring about triggering and easing factors. When taking a social history, the process does not necessarily differ from other conditions, however, we tend to spend more time asking about a typical day, which provides additional information about the impact of symptoms and often highlights maladaptive changes such as avoidance behaviors or boom-bust patterns of activity (the tendency to take on a great deal of tasks when feeling relatively well and subsequently "crash" and increased symptoms for several days). During the assessment, explore the patient's beliefs and understanding of their symptoms.

All patients with mobility problems should be asked about falls. The conventional wisdom is that patient's with FMD rarely experience "true falls" and falls-injuries. Instead, near falls, falling towards support, or a "slow descent to the ground" are thought to be more common. This pattern of mobility impairment probably overlies anxiety related to falling. However, it is also reported that some patients fall regularly and suddenly (as can be seen in cryptogenic drop attacks), which can be associated with significant injuries [11]. Such patient's will usually tell you that they fall heavily and, in such cases, additional safety precautions should be put in place.

Persistent pain and fatigue are common in people with FMD, often acting as predisposing, precipitating and/or perpetuating factors. Physical therapists should specifically ask about these symptoms. If present, they should be considered as part of the treatment plan and their presence may influence treatment decisions. When pain and fatigue are severe, treatment intensity needs to be adjusted to avoid exacerbating these symptoms and they may need to be considered before initiation of treatment targeted towards functional movement symptoms.

Complete the subjective assessment by asking the patient about their rehabilitation goals. Long-term goals may need to be broken down into achievable short and intermediate-term goals. This helps to create an experience of success and progress. Creating goals collaboratively sets the stage for promoting self-management and encouraging the patient to take an active role in their rehabilitation.

Vignette (Continued): Subjective Assessment

When asked about the onset of his symptoms, JP reported his diagnosis of acute vestibular neuritis 14 months prior, an inflammation of the vestibular nerve that occurred shortly after a viral infection. He describes how the acute symptoms changed from "room spinning" vertigo to a constant feeling of dizziness and unsteadiness without the "spinning" quality to it, a symptom characteristic of 3PD. His dizziness led to significant impairment of his gait, which was his biggest concern.

When asked about the impact of his walking problem, JP described a fear of being in public and leaving the house alone, since his gait usually worsened outside of his home environment. Although he denied falls, he experienced a fear of falling that led to avoidance behaviors and the use of two crutches when he had to go outside.

In reviewing his 24-h routine, additional concerns included daytime fatigue, poor sleep hygiene and "boom and bust" activity patterns. In terms of his social history, he was married and employed as a compliance officer in a healthcare system. He had been unable to work over the past year, which put a considerable financial strain on his family. He and his wife had taken in his elderly father in their home 3 years prior, who died of pneumonia a few months before JP's onset of vertigo. He denied any history of anxiety or depression but reported on-going strain in the relationship with his siblings related to the sale of his father's estate.

Physical Assessment

A useful way to approach the physical assessment in FMD is to give the patient an opportunity to demonstrate their symptoms and their impact. For example, start by asking the patient, "show me what happens when you try to walk". When observing movement, note variability and incongruence of symptoms, for example muscles that appear to be paralyzed in one context (e.g. strength testing) but activated in another context (e.g. when rising from a chair). Such variability (and motor inconsistency) is a hallmark of FMD and can later be discussed with the patient to help them understand the diagnosis. During the assessment, it can help to reassure the patient that you have seen people with similar symptoms and that their symptoms are typical for FMD.

Formal strength, coordination and sensation testing in FMD does not usually correlate well with functional ability. Consider the impact of functional neurological symptoms by observing how they affect posture, movement and activities. If the patient presents with tremor, observe for variability in frequency and amplitude, at rest, during various movements and with distracting tasks (such as finger or foot tapping, see Chap. 6 for details). Hands-on assessment can help to identify over-active muscles. Muscle jerks or functional myoclonus may vary in frequency with changes in posture or movement and often become less frequent with distraction. Observe the patient's breathing pattern, as symptoms are often associated with breath-holding, "huffing and puffing" (related to increased effort) [12], or other changes in breathing pattern associated with a heighted state of arousal.

We recommend selecting and completing appropriate baseline measures at an early stage in order to monitor and measure changes with treatment. See Chap. 29 for more information on this topic.

Vignette (Continued): Physical Assessment
Observations: JP walked with crutches, in a stiff, slow gait pattern, with his head held very still. He had a short right step length and his left knee buckled during the mid-stance phase (give-way weakness). When walking backwards, his gait pattern normalized to some extent. He had a positive Hoover's sign on the left. When getting up from a chair, JP was dependent on upper limb support; he leaned towards the right side, putting little weight on the left leg.

Baseline measures: 10-m walking speed was 0.5 m/s (20 s); Five Times Sit to Stand time was 37 s.

Following a thorough assessment, the patient should feel satisfied that the physical therapist has a good understanding of their symptoms and the impact on their life. The physical therapist should be able to describe the patient's symptom onset, what they experience on a day-to-day basis and the key problem(s) for physical therapy to address.

Treatment Planning

Due to the heterogeneity of the patient population, a personalized treatment plan is necessary. Factors to consider include:

- Treatment setting. If different options are available, consider the relative benefit and limitations of each. For example, inpatient treatment allows for greater intensity, improved access to integrated multidisciplinary treatment and it removes the patient from environmental factors that may be precipitating and perpetuating their symptoms. Outpatient, day program and domiciliary (residential) treatments allow for a slower paced intervention and can directly address factors in the patient's environment that may be contributing to their problem.

- Intensity and duration of treatment. The optimal intensity and duration of physical therapy for FMD is unknown and likely to vary according presentation. There is some evidence that short duration and high intensity treatments (e.g. multiple sessions in 5 consecutive days) can be effective [6, 9]. However, intensity needs to be adjusted to accommodate for patients with severe pain and/or fatigue.
- Content of sessions. Depending on the presenting problems, the relative mix of education, movement retraining and interventions aimed at addressing co-existing symptoms (e.g. pain) should be tailored to the individual.
- Timing. Consider the social context of the patient's problems and potential barriers that may interfere with the ability to engage with treatment (e.g. work obligations, childcare, school holidays, etc.). Consider scheduling the start of treatment sessions at a date and time that facilitates the patient's full engagement with therapy.

Psychologically Informed Physical Therapy

It is not necessary for physical therapists to have additional psychological training to work with people with FMD. However, psychologically-informed physical therapy can help to build a therapeutic relationship and enhance physical therapy interventions in the spirit of shared (partially overlapping) expertise. Psychologically-informed practice is becoming increasingly common in a number of physical therapy sub-specialties such as chronic pain management [13]. Table 23.1 lists a number of evidence-based communication strategies which can be employed by physical therapists [14].

Many of the physical symptoms experienced by people with FMD are triggered and maintained by psychological phenomena such as anxiety, mood lability and dissociation. The process of physical therapy may help patients to develop insight into how their psychological state affects their movement. A proportion of people with

Table 23.1 Communication strategies with therapeutic benefit during physical therapy

Unconditional positive regard	No matter what the patient tells you. Do not judge them verbally or non-verbally.
Empathic understanding and validation	This is communicated to the patient through listening, acknowledging symptoms, summarizing regularly (to confirm understanding) and an even appropriate tone of voice.
Nonverbal communication	Consider eye contact, body position and show full engagement.
Congruence (genuineness)	Be honest and authentic. For example, acknowledge when you do not understand something that the patient is saying or if you do not know the answer to a question. Let your words, nonverbal signs and tone of voice all match.
The patient should not feel at fault	Some patients express feelings of guilt associated with their symptoms and need for health care. It is usually helpful to remind them – "This isn't your fault".

FMD (perhaps a minority) will have severe psychiatric comorbidities. In such cases, multidisciplinary support is important. Acute distressing symptoms and behaviors (including suicidality) should be monitored carefully. Withdrawing treatment during this time may cause further distress. Alternatively, it may be appropriate to offer to temporarily stop physical therapy and resume at a later date, when the patient is ready.

Cognitive Behavioral Therapy (CBT) is a particular model of behavior change [15] that has some evidence for efficacy in FMD [16]. An overarching tenet of CBT is helping the patient to link thoughts with behaviors and emotions to gain insight into what is going on in their body (see Chap. 21 for more information). Table 23.2 gives examples of how physical therapists can use CBT principles in their practice.

Treatment

Physical therapy treatment for FMD can be broken down into 3 main components, (i) education about the diagnosis; (ii) movement retraining; and (iii) supporting the patient with self-management.

Education & Understanding

Education and understanding is the foundation for effective physical therapy and self-management. Patient understanding helps to reduce the threat value of symptoms and provides a rationale for physical therapy strategies, both of which can improve treatment adherence [6]. The important principles of communicating information about the diagnosis described in Chap. 17 should also be applied to physical therapy. Below we highlight important points:

- Education can start by gauging the patient's understanding and confidence in the diagnosis. This may start with an open question, "What do you understand about your diagnosis?" You might follow this up with, "Can I explain my understanding?" A discussion can then follow.
- Help the patient make sense of the onset of their symptoms by discussing potential triggering events.
- Describe how self-focused attention is a mechanism that drives symptoms. Use exam-

Table 23.2 CBT informed strategies for physical therapy

Problem or coping strategy	Explanation	Example of CBT informed physical therapy
Unhelpful illness beliefs	People often jump to conclusion about the significance of signs, symptoms and sensations. This can lead to erroneous beliefs that unhelpfully influence behavior. An example is misinterpretation of back pain as evidence of on-going damage. There is a tendency for patients to ignore disconfirming evidence for such beliefs.	Ask about beliefs (e.g. What do you think will happen when you exercise? What do you picture in your mind? What does this stop you from doing?). Help the patient to link beliefs with unhelpful behaviors. Help them to gain a new understanding, supplemented with information from websites, pamphlets etc. Plan a treatment program that gently addresses avoidances.
Avoidance or safety behavior	Avoidance or safety behaviors allow the patient to temporarily gain relief from symptoms. However, this does not improve the outcome, but instead sets up a vicious cycle of events, leading to hypersensitivity to any potential physical, social or bodily sensations [17].	Help the patient to understand that avoidance perpetuates the problem rather than solving it. Together, set realistic goals to return to the avoided activity in a graded fashion (see graded exposure below).
Hypervigilance and self-checking behavior	Hypervigilance and self-checking behavior may be associated with previous experience of illness and fear of symptoms returning (e.g. previous palpitations that were associated with a heart attack). Self-checking behavior can often be brought on by anxiety and the increased self-focus of attention can exacerbate or trigger functional neurological symptoms (e.g. a functional tremor may increase in frequency and amplitude)	Gain a shared understanding of the problem, helping the patient to recognize the impact of hypervigilance. Demonstrate examples of how movement improves when attention is redirected away from the body. Acknowledge feelings of anxiety, if the patient recognizes them.
Perfectionist personality traits	Perfectionism can be a coping strategy developed from early childhood. Although often associated with achievement, some aspects of perfectionism often lead to negative consequences, such as feelings of failure. Rigid rules for living associated with perfectionism may lead to avoidance of situations for fear of falling short of personal standards [18]. Perfectionism may lead the patient to "try too hard" during movement, which may increase their attention towards movement.	Discuss that having very high standards can get in the way of rehabilitation. Explain the value of setting small achievable goals and celebrate "little wins" during treatment. Activity planning can help to limit over-doing things for those prone to boom and bust patterns. Encourage the patient to stop and take a break if they appear to start to "try too hard" and overly focus on their movement.

Table 23.2 (continued)

Problem or coping strategy	Explanation	Example of CBT informed physical therapy
Low mood and anxiety	Although physical therapists usually do not directly address low mood and anxiety, it is ok to ask patients about these problems and consider how they may affect the FMD problem. Anxiety and low mood can exacerbate or drive the symptoms of dizziness and tremor. They can also lead to avoidant behaviors.	Help the patient to make links between low mood and/or anxiety and their movement problem. Low mood and anxiety can be normalized by acknowledging that everybody experiences these problems when they are unwell or at different stages in our life. Consider if patients have unmet needs with regards to these problems and if a referral to psychological therapy may help. If low mood affects motivation and engagement in activities, daily planning and scheduling enjoyable activities can help. Explore opportunities for engaging in exercise that the patient may enjoy. There is good evidence that exercise is helpful for depression [19].
Therapeutic Strategies		
Socratic questioning/guided discovery	Rather than telling people what to do or think, the therapist promotes discovery through a series of open questions that draw attention to relevant information. The aim is to be a "curious therapist" who does not know the answer. This can be used throughout the assessment and treatment process to promote insight building and self-management [20].	Examples: How do you feel about going out? How do you try to cope with this problem? So, would it be right to say that the reason you don't want to go out is for fear of something happening? What do you notice when you feel fearful?
Graded exposure	Graded exposure aims to gradually reintroduce patients to activity, situations and places they may be avoiding due to symptoms or anxiety associated with them. The rationale is that anxiety reduces with repeated exposure. The patient is encouraged to "sit" with the distress, rather than avoid the situation. For patients with substantial distress, this should be considered in collaboration with psychology-trained therapists [21].	Agree on a graded step-by-step plan to get back to the activity. Work through the plan with the patient and use strategies such as deep breathing and progressive muscle relaxation to control symptoms of anxiety during exposure.
Behavior experiments/ challenge unhelpful cognitions	Behavior experiments aim to challenge unhelpful illness beliefs by obtaining new information on which to construct new beliefs. Physical therapists regularly use this technique (without necessarily describing it as a behavior experiment) by gently encouraging their patients to push boundaries [22].	Example: Many patients with low back pain avoid bending and/or getting on to the floor. The belief might be that bending will cause extreme pain, held with conviction rated 10/10. The experiment might encourage the patient to bend gently during activity, such as picking up objects while using deep breathing. Explore the outcome of the experiment with the patient. Did it feel ok? Was the pain as bad as expected? Could this be progressed? Rate the new belief. Repeat with small incremental progressions.

(continued)

Table 23.2 (continued)

Problem or coping strategy	Explanation	Example of CBT informed physical therapy
Grounding	Grounding is commonly used to combat symptoms of dissociation. Grounding strategies aim to anchor awareness in the here and now. The strategies can take several forms and require regular practice to be effective. If a patient starts to feel dissociative symptoms, encouraging the use of grounding strategies can be very helpful.	Example: Look around you and try to notice everything in the most precise detail and describe it to yourself. Use all five senses, for example, what do I see? What are the colors? What are the sounds? Example: Adopt a "grounding posture", let go of tension and find a stance that makes you feel strong.

ples specific to the patient, for example, patients often report that their walking is better when they don't think about it.

- Explain the rationale for physical therapy. For example, movement retraining aims to re-establish normal movement using various methods including distraction.
- Explain that physical therapy aims to teach the patient how to manage and improve their symptoms in the long term. That they will learn strategies which they will need to practice between sessions and after completing their treatment (i.e. introduce the concept of self-management).

Vignette (Continued): Education

JP's treatment started with a long discussion about FMD. Although the neurologist had spent time explaining the diagnosis to JP, he had forgotten some of this information and he was feeling less convinced that the diagnosis was correct. Part of the problem was reconciling the diagnosis of FMD with his initial diagnosis of vestibular neuritis. It was explained that the initial diagnosis had not been revised, but that vestibular neuritis had precipitated 3PD and FMD, which were now part of the problem. It was explained that this is very common, affecting up to 20% of people who visit specialist dizziness clinics [23]. The physical therapist explained how the brain has started to misinterpret sensory information, that the brain is stuck on high alert and reacting as though the body is under threat of an imminent fall. The physical therapist was mindful of using non-blaming language, for example, "the brain

is stuck on high alert" rather than "you are on high alert".

When helping JP to understand his left sided weakness, the explanation was built around the impact of attention. "Functional symptoms tend to get worse when the person's brain is overly focused on their body. Is this something you have noticed before?" JP had noticed that his walking was often worse the harder he tried to walk normally. Together, they watched a video of JP's walking. They noticed several moments when JP's attention was distracted by answering questions and this coincided with moments of better walking.

The physical therapist explained the aims of physical therapy for JP were to "recalibrate the balance control center" of the brain and retrain movement to make it more "automatic" with less self-focused attention.

Movement Retraining

Movement retraining aims to restore normal movements and posture. The approach can be informed by the principles of motor learning as they apply to rehabilitation [2], including task specific practice, repetition and feedback. The goal of treatment is to reinforce desired movement patterns and to prevent reinforcement of unwanted movements. There may be several mechanisms by which movement retraining helps FMDs. These include: (i) altering unhelpful beliefs about movement by demonstrating to the patient that normal movement is possible; (ii) reducing self-focused attention during movement; (iii) changing habitual maladaptive postures and movement strategies (such as an antalgic gait pattern); (iv) improving confidence in the ability to move safely; and (v) inducing neuroplastic changes associated with task acquisition/motor learning. More research is needed to determine the mechanism(s) by which physical therapy works in FMD.

An important concept of movement retraining for FMD is the redirection of the patient's focus of attention away from their body [5, 6, 9]. This is to prevent self-focused attention from exacerbating and reinforcing unwanted movement patterns. As a general rule, placing the focus on activities and "whole body movements" (such as sit to stand, transfers, and gait), can help to shift the focus away from individual components of movement and towards the goal of the movement. Conversely, interventions that work on isolated movements, such as specific strengthening exercises or trying to perfect the movement at a particular joint, can exacerbate abnormal movement patterns by increasing attention on the body. However, there will be situations where asking the patient to briefly attend to their movement is helpful or unavoidable (e.g. when giving feedback).

Asking the patient to observe their movements in a mirror appears to be a helpful rehabilitation strategy for many. This may initially appear to contradict the advice to redirect attention, but as well as providing feedback, the mirror may redirect the patient's attention away from their internal "sensorimotor state" and towards the surface of the mirror.

A useful approach to rehabilitation of functional gait disorders described in the literature is based on sequential motor learning [4, 24]. This involves breaking down the gait pattern into stages (e.g. static lateral weight shift → weight shift with a period of single limb support → stepping forwards and backwards with light upper limb support → stepping forwards with light upper limb support → walking with minimal or no upper limb support). Each stage in the sequence builds on the previous stage to progressively develop a normal gait pattern "from the ground up". The patient only advances to the next stage once they have mastered the previous stage. The emphasis is placed on the quality of movement while avoiding reinforcement of unwanted movement patterns. This graded approach can provide the patient with a sense of rehabilitation momentum and mastery of movement. Table 23.3 describes other treatment strategies that may be helpful for common FMD symptoms.

Patients often experience fewer symptoms while performing more complex tasks, such as obstacle negotiation or carrying water while walking along a narrow space. This can be used as a strategy to practice and reshape movement patterns.

In some cases, therapeutic equipment can be a useful adjunct to treatment. Transcutaneous muscle stimulation set up to produce a tingling sensation without muscle twitch has been described as a useful addition to treatment for motor symptoms [30]. It may also be useful as part of a hypersensitivity/pain desensitization program. There is currently no evidence to support the use of electrical muscle stimulation (functional electrical stimulation), but it may have a number of useful applications in FMD, such as providing sensory feedback, retraining movement in upper limb weakness, and repositioning an equinovarus (inverted and plantarflexed) foot posture secondary to fixed (functional) dystonia to allow weight bearing with improved alignment. Other potentially useful therapeutic adjuncts include biofeedback [31], transcranial magnetic stimulation [32], and the use of virtual reality.

Although prescribing home exercises for practice in between sessions can sometimes be useful, we typically encourage our patients to use their improved movement patterns and postures more consistently throughout their daily routine. This can be structured using goal setting or "homework" that is reviewed at the beginning of the next session. For example, we might ask a patient to ensure that every time they stand up and sit down, they use a particular strategy.

Participation and education of family members in the treatment process should be encouraged, although their presence in every treatment session may be counterproductive. Family members can help to remember and reinforce infor-

Table 23.3 Common FMD symptoms, typical features and treatment strategies

Symptom	Typical features	Treatment strategies
Weakness	Functional weakness commonly presents as hemiparesis or paraparesis, but any pattern is possible and weakness may vary over time.	Muscle-strengthening exercises have limited value, as functional weakness is a problem of incorrect activation, rather than strength. Instead, weakness can be addressed through retraining functional tasks (e.g. sit-to-stand and gait). Allow early weight bearing. Create a safe environment (e.g. practicing between raised plinths, parallel bars, in front of chair, or use a body-weight support harness). Prevent excessive upper limb support by encouraging "finger-tip support". Starting with a good sit-to-stand maneuver can help to activate the lower limbs and place the body in an optimal position to stand and step. Standing can be progressed toward walking by adding lateral and posterior weight-shift while gradually reducing upper limb support. Task practice for upper limb weakness can be challenging, as distraction is more difficult than for lower limb activities. Potentially helpful upper limb weight bearing exercises and activities include 4-point crawling, throwing/catching a ball and using upper limb support during standing balance exercises.
Tremor	Upper limbs are more commonly affected by tremor, followed by lower limbs and head/neck. Tremor is usually associated with proximal muscle over-activity and patients often attempt to suppress a tremor by contracting their muscles more tightly.	Treatment can include helping the patient to recognize and relax areas of muscle over-activity. Sit or stand the patient in front of a mirror and use visual feedback to "find a relaxed posture". Passively moving the patient's limb so they can feel the resistance due to the tremor can help them to recognize states of muscle tension and relaxation. Teaching relaxation of upper trapezius muscles can help upper limb and head tremors. Distracting and competing movements can help to control a tremor. Examples include use of opposite extremity movements as a distraction (e.g. tapping); make the tremor feel voluntary by making the tremulous movements larger in amplitude and gradually try to slow the movement to stillness; rhythmical weight shift; upper cervical flexion/extension, or protraction/retraction movements for a head tremor.
Gait	Common patterns of functional gait disorder include monoplegic-leg dragging, antalgic patterns of movement, excessive slowness, sudden knee buckling, scissoring steps and excessive weight through walking aids [25]. Functional gait disorders are commonly associated with a fear of falling and an experience of a frightening or painful fall.	Retraining gait using a sequential motor learning approach as described in the text is usually a helpful place to start. Walking between parallel bars or raised plinths can help to improve confidence and address fears associated with falling. Treadmill training can be helpful to trigger automatic movement patterns. A mirror placed in front of the treadmill is useful for many patients. Backwards/sideways walking and turning can help trigger automatic steps. Initiating walking by sliding feet along the ground can activate the dorsiflexion muscles for patients with a foot-drop presentation. Functional electrical stimulation may be a useful short-term treatment adjunct for some patients. Practicing in increasingly challenging environments should be considered when easier tasks are mastered (e.g. uneven pavements and busy public spaces).

Table 23.3   (continued)

Symptom	Typical features	Treatment strategies
Fixed Dystonia	Fixed dystonia most commonly presents as a clenched fist or an inverted and plantarflexed foot posture. It often overlaps with the diagnosis of complex regional pain syndrome (CRPS), with patients exhibiting hypersensitivity, and secondary changes associated with disuse and poor circulation (e.g. swelling, and skin color changes) [26].	Treatment can start by helping the patient to recognize and stop unhelpful postures. Typically, patients assume positions where the affected limb passively rests in the end range/dystonic position. The patient should be taught that this maintains the problem. Improving resting posture alignment often requires a graded approach. Early weight bearing is important (including for upper limb symptoms), with care to avoid placing strain through joints due to poor alignment. Passive stretching often results in high-level pain that is eased when the limb is returned to the dystonic position. It is therefore usually unhelpful. Instead we recommend encouraging resting postures with optimal alignment and activities that move the joint through available range (e.g. optimise leg and foot position when sitting and encouraging weight bearing and stepping). Features of CRPS should be addressed as described in the relevant rehabilitation literature [27]. Electrical muscle stimulation can be helpful as a distraction and/or to reposition the affected joint (e.g. tibialis anterior muscle stimulation for a plantarflexed foot).
Jerks or Functional Myoclonus	Functional jerks/myoclonus typically present as intermittent contractions of muscles of the trunk and or shoulder girdle. The jerking movements can often be distracted or entrained, for example, by rhythmical foot or upper limb tapping [28].	Some patients notice an urge or build up prior to a jerk, this is an opportunity to practice distraction techniques. Identifying triggers can be helpful to prevent and "unlearn" the movement. The patient may not initially be aware of triggers, but sometimes with help they are able to identify them (e.g. jerks may be more common when pain is worse, in particular postures, such as slumped sitting or after prolonged sitting). Functional abdominal jerks are often associated with breath-holding or abdominal muscle activation. In this case, deep-breathing (thoracic expansion) exercises can be helpful (e.g. place your hands on the patient's lower ribs and asking them to breathe in and think about moving your hands apart). A muscle affected by jerks may be less active when stretched and more active in the shortened/mid-range position. This can be explored together with the patient to identify some easing postures and movements.
Persistent postural-perceptual dizziness (3PD) (functional dizziness)	Although 3PD is somewhat different to FMD in that difficulties are driven by a sensory/perceptual experience, it has physical consequences in the way it affects balance and gait. Dizziness often starts from vestibular neuritis due to a viral infection (or other known causes of dizziness) but persists after the triggering pathology has resolved. The symptom of vertigo is usually replaced by a sensation of non-specific dizziness [23].	The symptoms of 3PD are thought to be related to stiffened postural control and a shift in processing sensory information to favor visual over vestibular input, which is a normal physiological response to vertigo and the threat of falling [23]. The aim of physical therapy is to "desensitize a balance control mechanism that is stuck on high alert" [29]. This can be achieved through gait and balance training, and addressing maladaptive coping mechanisms, such as avoidance of head movement and reducing reliance on vision for balance. Examples include incorporating moments of eye closure during exercises, shifting visual focus during gait (e.g. making eye contact with someone or scanning the room), picking objects up off the floor, practice walking in progressively busier and "visually challenging" environments (e.g. walking down a supermarket isle).

mation, facilitate rehabilitation plans, or be encouraged to reduce their support in order to build confidence and independence.

Paroxysmal symptoms are those that occur intermittently (e.g. once an hour/day/week). It is a challenging situation for physical therapy when movement is normal between episodes of symptoms. Sometimes, attempting to address paroxysmal symptoms can result in their exacerbation due to increasing self-focused attention. In this case, treatment may move towards identifying triggers for symptoms and strategies to ward off symptoms when the patient experiences warning signs. This may require collaboration with psychotherapists for interventions such as graded-exposure to triggering environments, grounding and distraction techniques. Paroxysmal symptoms are sometimes triggered by increased pain and fatigue, which can be addressed as part of physical therapy.

Vignette (Continued): Movement Retraining

The movement problems identified for physical therapy to address were functional weakness, gait impairment and dizziness. JP's goal was to be able to walk independently outdoors without crutches. With support from the physiotherapist, this was broken down into the following short-term goals: (i) to be able to stand from a chair with bodyweight equally distributed; (ii) to walk without an assistive device within the house, using light touch support as necessary; and (iii) to experience a 50% or greater reduction in dizziness during walking.

The treatment progression started with retraining the sit-to-stand-to-sit movement pattern. The treatment environment was set up to reduce the risk and fear of falling, by having a wall and treatment plinth on either side of JP and a chair behind him. A mirror was placed in front of JP to provide visual feedback. JP completed several sets of 4 repetitions of sit-to-stand-to-sit. After each set, the physical therapist would encourage JP to reflect on his own performance and give feedback. JP was encouraged to increase the forward momentum component of the sit to stand pattern, to use only light touch support

through his hands and he was prompted to use the mirror as feedback to keep his bodyweight equally distributed between the left and right sides. JP was pleased to see he had made progress after only a single session.

Gait retraining was introduced in the following session. The treatment strategy was to build up JP's gait pattern from more simple movement components. JP worked through the following progression, each step in the progression was "mastered" before moving on to the subsequent step: Step (i) rhythmical lateral weight shift between parallel bars with light-touch upper limb support; (ii) continue lateral weight shift with upper limb support while stepping his left foot forwards and backwards; (iii) lateral weight shift while stepping his right foot forwards and backwards; (iv) walking forwards, while maintaining lateral weight shift with light touch upper limb support; etc. The physical therapist provided occasional gentle guiding support to facilitate rhythmical movement and to help redirect JP's focus of attention. In subsequent sessions, gait retraining was progressed to using a treadmill, where speed was gradually increased. JP was encouraged to look around the room while walking on the treadmill with the aim of reducing visual fixation for balance. As JP progressed, physical therapy exercises included obstacle negotiation, getting on and off the floor without using furniture for support and walking in the busy hospital corridor. JP tried gaze stabilization exercises that are commonly used in vestibular rehabilitation, but found them less helpful, so this was discontinued.

The physical therapist taught JP to use his crutches in a way that minimized their impact on his walking quality and rhythm. As treatment progressed, the physical therapist encouraged JP to reduce his use of crutches indoors. He was initially reluctant to stop using his crutches when outdoors, however, as his confidence improved with regular outdoor walking practice, he progressed to walking with a single crutch and eventually without crutches. He found the simple strategy of stopping to take short rest and "reset" when he started to feel unsteady very helpful.

Self-Management

For many patients, FMD is a chronic condition with periods of relative relapse and remission. There is therefore a need to develop self-management skills to avoid dependence on clinicians and therapy for symptom control. The treatment period from initial assessment to discharge planning can support the patient to develop these skills. Steps to support self-management include:

- Education and understanding at each stage. The patient should understand why particular exercises and instructions are helpful and what they aim to achieve.
- A collaborative approach. Encourage the patient to be actively involved in decision-making. This includes graded goal setting, considering whether particular exercises or strategies have been helpful and how exercises can be adjusted to improve outcomes.
- Collaborative homework setting and reviewing each session.
- Development of a staying well and relapse management plan (see Chap. 24 for more details).

Secondary and Coexisiting Problems

There is some evidence to suggest that early access to treatment will lead to better outcomes [33]. Long symptom duration is thought to be associated with the accumulation and progression of secondary problems that can worsen prognosis. Secondary and coexisting problems act as symptom precipitating and perpetuating factors and therefore should be considered as part of the treatment plan. A detailed discussion of all possible secondary and coexisting problems is beyond the scope of this chapter, instead, a brief overview of common problems and treatment approaches is described in Table 23.4.

Adaptive Equipment and Adaptations

It is generally recognized that adaptive equipment such as mobility aids, splints and orthotics can be unhelpful for patients with FMD. Use of adaptive equipment can lead to further maladaptive ways of moving and prevent restoration of normal "automatic" movement patterns. Adaptive aids can also cause secondary problems, such as joint pain and physical deconditioning. Early wheelchair/mobility scooter use may deprive the patient of the opportunity to regain normal movement and reduces the opportunity for incidental exercise. Adaptive equipment should therefore be avoided if possible. With this in mind, it should be recognized that aids and adaptations are not necessarily contraindicated and, in some cases, adaptive aids may be needed to improve safety, independence and quality of life. Each situation should be considered individually. We would recommend that aids are avoided early on and during rehabilitation if possible. If an aid is deemed to be useful or necessary, the patient should be supported to make decisions regarding its use. When aids are issued, a thorough assessment should be completed, with plans put in place to mitigate the potential for harm, reassess and (where possible) wean its use.

Concluding Treatment

Concluding treatment can be challenging, especially when patients remain symptomatic. In order to facilitate a smooth discharge from physical therapy, preparation can start from the very beginning of treatment by: (i) agreeing on the number of sessions prior to starting treatment; (ii) fostering self-management skills through the treatment period, so that the patient feels they are able to continue to progress even if therapy stops; (iii) tapering the frequency of sessions; (iv) collaboratively completing a self-management plan towards the end of treatment; and (v) offering a distant follow-up appointment.

Table 23.4 Common secondary and coexisting problems in FMD

Persistent pain	Evidence-based physical therapy interventions for persistent pain are typically composed of education, exercise, and self-management [34–36]. Pain physiology education has a good evidence base for helping to reduce distress associated with persistent pain [37]. Physical therapy interventions for persistent pain are well described in the literature and the findings are relevant to people with FMD and pain.
Fatigue	Fatigue is common in FMD and in one study was found to be a more important determinant of quality of life than motor symptom severity [38]. For some patients, persistent fatigue predates the motor symptoms, but for others, fatigue appears to develop and worsen after the onset of FMD. Fatigue management strategies are discussed in Chap. 24
Sleep disturbance	Sleep disturbance is common in people with FMD [39], especially those who experience regular fatigue. Poor sleep has been found to affect both mental and physical health [40]. It is not necessary for the physical therapist to be an expert in this area, but some simple recommendations or provision of written information may help to improve sleep quality in patients with FMD. Where obstructive sleep apnea or other primary sleep disorders are suspected (for instance, the patient snores at night and experiences morning headaches and day time sleepiness), this should be discussed with the patient's physician. Some strategies that may help to improve sleep include using a sleep diary; sleep hygiene education; relaxation exercises; limiting alcohol, caffeine and nicotine; physical exercise; and developing a bedtime routine.
Muscle contracture	Muscle and joint contracture, although relatively rare, occurs in some people with FMD. It is most often seen with the specific symptom presentation of fixed-functional dystonia, where it is commonly associated with pain and hypersensitivity [26]. In our experience we have noticed that fixed dystonia and contracture is often related to habitual resting postures and movement patterns with joints "stuck" at the end of range (e.g. ankle plantarflexion/inversion, hand clenched into a fist, hip and knee flexion, etc.). Management involves postural education, considering the 24-h period. Passive stretches often cause high level pain and increased "protective-positioning" (i.e. the patient seeks comfort in the dystonic position). As an alternative, as much as is possible, we suggest encouraging weight bearing and movement of the joint through the available range within normal function (such as walking, and upper limb activities). Functional electrical stimulation holds promise as a useful adjunct to encourage movement out of dystonic positions, although more research is needed. Serial casting for patients with fixed functional dystonia has been found to be harmful or at least unhelpful in several cases within a cohort study, and therefore should be avoided if possible and where indicated, used with close monitoring and extra precautions [26].

The following suggestions can help to draw physical therapy to a close: Openly ask the patient how they feel about discharge and acknowledge their concerns. Collaboratively writing out a self-management and staying well plan. This might include a list of strategies (tool-box) developed during the intervention period that help to improve movement; as well as plans to address other problems such as persistent pain and fatigue. See Chap. 24 on occupational therapy for further ideas for developing a self-management plan.

The current evidence suggests that most patients have at least some improvement in symptoms with physical therapy, but also that up to 30% of patients will not benefit. This can be difficult for both the patient and therapist. In this situation, alternative treatment options can be discussed. Further neurologic and/or neuropsychiatric care is encouraged to reassess symptoms and examine potential treatment obstacles [41].

Most patients experience "bad days" and setbacks at some point following rehabilitation and the patient should be prepared for this possibility. Explain that setbacks are common and almost always transitory, often related to triggering factors such as "boom and bust" activity patterns, illness or stressful events. Writing out a plan in advance for bad days and setbacks can be helpful. This can be as simple as encouraging relative rest and retuning to strategies that previously helped to restore normal movement.

Concluding treatment with a formal discharge report can be used as an opportunity to positively reinforce changes made by the patient and educate others about FMD.

Summary and Conclusions

There is growing evidence that physical therapy is effective for FMD. Treatment should be individualized, guided by a thorough assessment and informed by an understanding of the mechanisms of FMD. Patients with FMD are heterogeneous, often presenting with multiple complex comorbidities and thus multidisciplinary care is often helpful as discussed in Chap. 26. Physical therapy for FMD can be challenging, but is often rewarding and can result in profound improvements to quality of life.

Summary
- There is growing evidence that physical therapy, informed by a biopsychosocial model, is an effective treatment for FMD.
- The initial assessment should be thorough, seeking to understand symptom onset, the range of symptoms, how symptoms affect activities of daily living and the patient's understanding and beliefs related to symptoms.
- Education is the foundation for physical therapy. The physical therapist should aim to help the patient understand the diagnosis, including how the diagnosis is made, the role of self-focused attention in driving symptoms, and how physical therapy can help.
- Movement retraining aims to restore normal movement patterns and postures. Sequential motor learning and task-specific practice is used alongside strategies that help to redirect the patient's focus of attention away from their body.
- Psychologically-informed physical therapy practice may help to improve patient engagement and treatment outcomes; efforts should also be made to develop elements of shared (partially overlapping) expertise across treatment team members.
- Development of self-management skills is an important part of the treatment process.
- Physical therapy may be most effective as part of a multidisciplinary treatment intervention.

References

1. Nielsen G. Physical treatment of functional neurologic disorders. In: Hallett M, Stone J, Carson A, editors. Functional neurologic disorders, Handbook of clinical neurology series, vol. 139. Amsterdam: Elsevier; 2016. p. 555–69.
2. Shumway-Cook A, Woollacott MH. Motor control: translating research into clinical practice, Fifth. Philadelphia: Lippincott Williams & Wilkins; 2007.
3. Edwards MJ, Adams RA, Brown H, Parees I, Friston KJ. A Bayesian account of "hysteria". Brain. 2012;135:3495–512.
4. Nielsen G, Stone J, Edwards MJ. Physiotherapy for functional (psychogenic) motor symptoms: a systematic review. J Psychosom Res. 2013;75:93–102.
5. Jordbru AA, Smedstad LM, Klungsøyr O, Martinsen EW. Psychogenic gait disorder: a randomized controlled trial of physical rehabilitation with one-year follow-up. J Rehabil Med. 2014;46:181–7.
6. Nielsen G, Buszewicz M, Stevenson F, Hunter R, Holt K, Dudziec M, Ricciardi L, Marsden J, Joyce E, Edwards M. Randomised feasibility study of physiotherapy for patients with functional motor symptoms. J Neurol Neurosurg Psychiatry. 2017;88:484–90.
7. Jacob AE, Smith CA, Jablonski ME, Roach AR, Paper KM, Kaelin DL, Stretz-Thurmond D, LaFaver K. Multidisciplinary clinic for functional movement disorders (FMD): 1-year experience from a single centre. J Neurol Neurosurg Psychiatry. 2018;89(9):1011–2.
8. Maggio JB, Ospina JP, Callahan J, Hunt AL, Stephen CD, Perez DL. Outpatient physical therapy for functional neurological disorder: a preliminary feasibility and naturalistic outcome study in a U.S. cohort. J Neuropsychiatry Clin Neurosci. 2020;32:85–9.
9. Czarnecki K, Thompson JM, Seime R, Geda YE, Duffy JR, Ahlskog JE. Functional movement disorders: successful treatment with a physical therapy rehabilitation protocol. Parkinsonism Relat Disord. 2012;18:247–51.
10. Nielsen G, Stone J, Buszewicz M, et al. Physio4FMD: protocol for a multicentre randomised controlled trial of specialist physiotherapy for functional motor disorder. BMC Neurol. 2019;19:242.

11. Hoeritzauer I, Carson AJ, Stone J. "Cryptogenic Drop Attacks" revisited: evidence of overlap with functional neurological disorder. J Neurol Neurosurg Psychiatry. 2018;89:769–76.

12. Laub HN, Dwivedi AK, Revilla FJ, Duker AP, Pecina-Jacob C, Espay AJ. Diagnostic performance of the "huffing and puffing" sign in functional (psychogenic) movement disorders. Mov Disord Clin Pract. 2015;2:29–32.

13. Denneny D, Frijdal (Nee Klapper) A, Bianchi-Berthouze N, Greenwood J, McLoughlin R, Petersen K, Singh A, de C. Williams A. The application of psychologically informed practice: observations of experienced physiotherapists working with people with chronic pain. Physiotherapy. 2020;106:163–73.

14. Cahill J, Barkham M, Hardy G, Gilbody S, Richards D, Bower P, Audin K, Connell J. A review and critical appraisal of measures of therapist-patient interactions in mental health settings. Health Technol Assess. 2008;12:1–47.

15. Leahy RL. Cognitive therapy techniques: a practitioner's guide. 2nd ed. New York: Gilford; 2017.

16. Goldstein LH, Mellers JDC. Psychologic treatment of functional neurologic disorders. In: Hallett M, Stone J, Carson A, editors. Functional neurological disorder, Handbook of clinical neurology series, vol. 139. Amsterdam: Elsevier; 2016. p. 571–83.

17. Butler G, Fennell MJV, Hackmann A. Cognitive-behavioral therapy for anxiety disorders: mastering clinical challenges. New York: Guilford Press; 2008.

18. Egan S, Wade T, Shafran R, Antony MM. Cognitive-behavioral treatment of perfectionism. New York: Guilford Press; 2014.

19. Schuch FB, Vancampfort D, Richards J, Rosenbaum S, Ward PB, Stubbs B. Exercise as a treatment for depression:a meta-analysis adjusting for publication bias. J Psychiatr Res. 2016;77:42–51.

20. Kazantzis N, Beck JS, Clark DA, Dobson KS, Hofmann SG, Leahy RL, Wing Wong C. Socratic dialogue and guided discovery in cognitive behavioral therapy: a modified Delphi panel. Int J Cogn Ther. 2018;11:140–57.

21. López-De-Uralde-Villanueva I, Munõz-García D, Gil-Martínez A, Pardo-Montero J, Munõz-Plata R, Angulo-Díaz-Parrenõ S, Gómez-Martínez M, La Touche R. A systematic review and meta-analysis on the effectiveness of graded activity and graded exposure for chronic nonspecific low back pain. Pain Med. 2016;17:172–88.

22. Bennett-Levy J, Butler G, Fennell M, Hackman A, Mueller M, Westbrook D. Oxford guide to behavioural experiments in cognitive therapy. Oxford: Oxford University Press; 2004.

23. Popkirov S, Staab JP, Stone J. Persistent postural-perceptual dizziness (PPPD): a common, characteristic and treatable cause of chronic dizziness. Pract Neurol. 2018;18:5–13.

24. Trieschmann RB, Stolov WC, Montgomery ED. An approach to the treatment of abnormal ambulation resulting from conversion reaction. Arch Phys Med Rehabil. 1970;51:198–206.

25. Daum C, Hubschmid M, Aybek S. The value of "positive" clinical signs for weakness, sensory and gait disorders in conversion disorder: a systematic and narrative review. J Neurol Neurosurg Psychiatry. 2014;85:180–90.

26. Schrag A, Trimble M, Quinn N, Bhatia K. The syndrome of fixed dystonia: an evaluation of 103 patients. Brain. 2004;127:2360–72.

27. Goebel A, Barker C, Turner-Stokes L. Complex regional pain syndrome in adults: UK guidelines for diagnosis, referral and management in primary and secondary care. London: RCP; 2018.

28. Espay AJ, Lang AE. Phenotype-specific diagnosis of functional (psychogenic) movement disorders. Curr Neurol Neurosci Rep. 2015;15:32.

29. Popkirov S, Stone J, Holle-Lee D. Treatment of persistent postural-perceptual dizziness (PPPD) and related disorders. Curr Treat Options Neurol. 2018;20:50.

30. Ferrara J, Stamey W, Strutt AM, Adam OR, Jankovic J. Transcutaneous electrical stimulation (TENS) for psychogenic movement disorders. J Neuropsychiatry Clin Neurosci. 2011;23:141–8.

31. Espay AJ, Edwards MJ, Oggioni GD, Phielipp N, Cox B, Gonzalez-Usigli H, Pecina C, Heldman DA, Mishra J, Lang AE. Tremor retrainment as therapeutic strategy in psychogenic (functional) tremor. Parkinsonism Relat Disord. 2014;20:647–50.

32. Pollak TA, Nicholson TR, Edwards MJ, David AS. A systematic review of transcranial magnetic stimulation in the treatment of functional (conversion) neurological symptoms. J Neurol Neurosurg Psychiatry. 2014;85:191–7.

33. Gelauff J, Stone J, Edwards MJ, Carson A. The prognosis of functional (psychogenic) motor symptoms: a systematic review. J Neurol Neurosurg Psychiatry. 2014;85:220–6.

34. The British Pain Society (2013) Guidelines for pain management programmes for adults: an evidence-based review prepared on behalf of the British Pain Society.

35. Hansen Z, Daykin A, Lamb SE. A cognitive-behavioural programme for the management of low back pain in primary care: a description and justification of the intervention used in the Back Skills Training Trial (BeST; ISRCTN 54717854). Physiotherapy. 2010;96:87–94.

36. Lamb SE, Lall R, Hansen Z, Castelnuovo E, Withers EJ, Nichols V, Griffiths F, Potter R, Szczepura A, Underwood M. A multicentred randomised controlled trial of a primary care-based cognitive behavioural programme for low back pain. The Back Skills Training (BeST) trial. Health Technol Assess. 2010;14:1–128.

37. Van Oosterwijck J, Meeus M, Paul L, De Schryver M, Pascal A, Lambrecht L, Nijs J. Pain physiology education improves health status and endogenous pain inhibition in fibromyalgia: a double-blind randomized controlled trial. Clin J Pain. 2013;29:873–82.

38. Gelauff JM, Kingma EM, Kalkman JS, Bezemer R, van Engelen BGM, Stone J, Tijssen MAJ, Rosmalen JGM. Fatigue, not self-rated motor symptom severity, affects quality of life in functional motor disorders. J Neurol. 2018;265:1803–9.

39. Věchetová G, Slovák M, Kemlink D, Hanzlíková Z, Dušek P, Nikolai T, Růžička E, Edwards MJ, Serranová T. The impact of non-motor symptoms on the health-related quality of life in patients with functional movement disorders. J Psychosom Res. 2018;115:32–7.

40. Drake CL, Roehrs T, Roth T. Insomnia causes, consequences, and therapeutics: an overview. Depress Anxiety. 2003;18:163–76.

41. Adams C, Anderson J, Madva EN, LaFrance WC Jr, Perez DL. You've made the diagnosis of functional neurological disorder: now what? Pract Neurol. 2018;18:323–30.

Occupational Therapy: Focus on Function

Clare Nicholson and Kate Hayward

Case Vignette: Part I – Presentation

Mr. A is a 37-year old full-time school teacher who presented to an Emergency Room after being hit by a car while biking to work. He suffered multiple soft tissue injuries. He was discharged home on the same day with pain medications and was advised to take a few days off work. In the days following, Mr. A noticed weakness in his left leg affecting his ability to walk and the onset of a tremor in his left hand. An evaluation by a neurologist found a positive Hoover's sign and distractible tremor and he was given a diagnosis of a functional movement disorder (FMD). As part of his treatment plan, he was referred to occupational therapy as he was struggling to manage his daily activities and had been unable to return to work.

During the initial assessment, Mr. A reported that he lived with his wife and three young step-daughters. His wife worked full-time. Despite repeated attempts, Mr. A had been unable to return to work following the accident. He was independent with personal care and light domestic tasks using adaptive aids and strategies. He was also independently mobile indoors without an aid (but tended to "furniture walk"), was able to walk 5 minutes to the local shop with one

elbow crutch (on the right side), but was otherwise reliant on his family for other daily activities. He had stopped driving and his social life was limited. He previously enjoyed spending time with his family, gardening, cooking, cycling, running and going to the gym.

Introduction

Occupational therapy is defined as a 'client centered health profession concerned with promoting health and well-being through occupation' [1]. The term 'occupation' in occupational therapy does not just refer to paid employment, but to any daily activity. The overarching aim of occupational therapy is to enable people to engage in activities that they need to, want to or are expected to do, within their societal and cultural norms [1].

Occupational therapists are dually trained in physical and mental health rehabilitation and use conceptual models of practice to guide their intervention. These models advocate seeing the person as a whole, in the context of their environment, and highlight the importance of taking into consideration the interaction between physical and psychological states [2–4]. This combined with a focus on function rather than impairment, makes occupational therapists ideally suited to working with patients with functional movement disorder (FMD) [5].

C. Nicholson (✉) · K. Hayward
Therapy Services Department, The National Hospital for Neurology and Neurosurgery, London, UK
e-mail: clare.nicholson6@nhs.net

© Springer Nature Switzerland AG 2022
K. LaFaver et al. (eds.), *Functional Movement Disorder*, Current Clinical Neurology,
https://doi.org/10.1007/978-3-030-86495-8_24

Reasons for Referral to Occupational Therapy for FMD

FMD, as with any neurological condition, often disrupts a person's ability to participate fully in their daily life. Common reasons for referral to occupational therapy include:

- Difficulties with transfers and mobility
- Difficulty using upper limbs (particularly for fine motor skills in the hands, for example when eating)
- Difficulties accessing home, education, work or community environments
- Difficulties undertaking personal care, domestic, leisure, paid or unpaid working roles
- Pain, fatigue and emotional difficulties which prevent optimal activity engagement
- Assessment of and advice regarding care needs (informal and formal care)
- Aids and adaptations (assessment, provision and/or reduction)
- Assessment and management of sensory processing difficulties

Occupational therapy for FMD should not primarily focus on the implementation of compensatory techniques to increase a person's function. Although compensatory approaches assist a person to complete a task despite difficulties, they do not necessarily support rehabilitation of these difficulties. Occupational therapists should therefore encourage patients with FMD to work on completing daily tasks in a normal movement pattern, with reduced reliance on equipment and help from others. This serves to promote independence, as well as providing opportunities for rehabilitation and recovery. Participation in daily activities should be viewed as a part of rehabilitation, as participation acts to build confidence, endurance and independence.

A multidisciplinary approach is often beneficial when working with patients with FMD [6–8], however this is not always possible due to insurance regulations or lack of access to specialized care in many regions. For occupational therapists working in isolation, it is important to recognize the scope of their role and identify

when multidisciplinary intervention is required. Clear lines of communication with the referring healthcare professional should be established, along with clear referral pathways to appropriate disciplines [5].

Occupational Therapy Theoretical Models

Occupational therapy practice is guided by overarching theoretical models. Key models of practice which can be applied when working with patients with FMD are The Model of Human Occupation (MOHO) and The Canadian Model of Occupational Performance and Engagement (CMOP-E) [5, 9, 10]. Both MOHO and CMOP-E are aligned with occupational therapy assessment tools, including the Canadian Occupational Performance Measure (COPM) [11], the Occupational Circumstances Assessment Interview and Rating Scale (OCAIRS) [12], and the Occupational Self-Assessment (OSA) tool [13]. Although not validated in an FMD population, these tools can be used by occupational therapists when working with patients with FMD to help prioritize intervention areas and to measure treatment outcomes [5].

Occupational Therapy Initial Assessment

It can be useful to undertake the initial assessment (for FMD) over a number of sessions to allow symptoms to be explored thoroughly, gain a detailed sense of symptom impact on function, and assist with the establishment of therapeutic rapport [5].

The following assessment principles can help guide the occupational therapy assessment:

1. Ask the person to discuss how their symptoms started. Do any significant life events (including physical injury) correlate with the onset of symptoms? If so, does the person think this is relevant?
2. Create a symptom list. Consider physical (e.g., sensorimotor, pain), cognitive and

affective (mood/anxiety) domains. Ask about exacerbating and easing factors for each symptom, as well as variability and severity.

3. Ascertain the persons' understanding and agreement with the diagnosis, as well as thoughts and beliefs associated with their symptoms.

4. Ask about other health problems past and present that may impact on function (including psychological health).

5. Determine the person's usual roles and responsibilities, what activities are meaningful and necessary to them.

6. Determine the impact of symptoms on function.

7. Explore their 24-hour routine. Consider self-care (bathing, grooming, sleep, nutrition), occupational engagement, structure, routines, occupational balance (i.e. are they taking on too much?).

8. Take a detailed social history and enquire about family and other social support.

9. Determine if the person has care needs. If so, are these needs being met? Who provides the care? Have their care needs changed over time?

10. Explore the use of aids and adaptations and their ability to access home and community environments.

11. Ask about their work/education history. Do symptoms impact on their vocational roles?

12. Assess the person while completing functional (activity-based) tasks (e.g. functional transfers, personal care, meal preparation). Note the impact of symptoms on activity engagement whilst also looking for 'positive signs' of FMD (variability, distractibility). Taking a baseline video (with consent) of the functional assessment can be used therapeutically as findings can be discussed to help guide treatment.

13. Ascertain the person's goals or areas of need for occupational therapy intervention. Are the goals realistic or do they need to be broken down further? Can they be achieved within the intervention period that you have to offer? Are they within the realm of occu-

pational therapy or best met by another professional?

It is important in the assessment phase to discuss the person's expectations of occupational therapy interventions. It should be highlighted that interventions will be driven by the goals or problem areas that the person identifies. The concept of self-management should be introduced early, for instance, that independent practice of goals and taught strategies will be necessary outside of sessions and implemented consistently within daily activities. If the treatment is structured within a multidisciplinary team (which can often be helpful), it may be valuable to undertake the assessment jointly with other rehabilitation specialists to avoid unnecessary repetition, share findings and build a joint management plan. An alternative, yet potentially equally helpful approach, is performing separate assessments across specialists and subsequently collaborating after the initial assessment to develop a coordinated and internally consistent treatment plan.

Graded Goal Setting

Helping patients with FMD to set realistic and achievable goals is an essential part of the occupational therapy intervention [2]. Some occupational therapists use the Goal Attainment Scale (GAS) [14] or SMART (Specific, Measurable, Achievable, Realistic, Timed) [15] tool to set goals with patients with neurological disorders (including FMD). However, these frameworks do not necessarily allow for the variability of symptoms that are common in FMD. Functional neurological symptoms can wax and wane and patients will be more prone to symptom exacerbation if they experience physical or psychological stressors. As such it can be useful to take a flexible approach to goal setting [5]:

- Goals are set by the person with FMD, in their own words and may not necessarily be time dependent.
- Functional (activity-based) rather than impairment-based goals are often helpful.

Consider "I want to be able to stand at the sink to brush my teeth twice a day" (functional goal) over "I want my legs to be stronger" (impairment-based goal).

- Setting difficult or unattainable goals can decrease confidence in abilities, resulting in disappointment and possible symptom exacerbation.
- The COPM, OCAIRS and OSA can be useful to guide goal setting as the identified occupational performance problems can be collaboratively rewritten as goals [11–13].
- Carefully graded goals and consolidation of symptom management techniques within functional tasks can help patients with FMD to build on their capacities and progress at a faster rate.

Case Vignette: Part II – Graded Goal Setting

Mr. A identified a goal of preparing the evening meal for his family. He worked with his occupational therapist to break down this goal into graded steps (after being shown how to integrate symptom management techniques into the task). Each step was repeated until Mr. A felt confident that he could increase the task complexity:

Step 1:
Mr. A sits to peel and cut up vegetables for dinner. Mrs. A then prepares and cooks the rest of the meal.

Step 2:
Mr. A alternates between sitting and standing to peel and cut up vegetables for dinner (ahead of time allowing for a rest period). Mr. A assists his wife to complete the rest of the meal (alternating between sitting and standing).

Step 3:
Mr. A alternates between sitting and standing to peel and cut up vegetables for dinner (ahead of time allowing for a rest period). Mr. A cooks the meal with his wife in the room supervising and providing assistance if required.

Step 4:
Mr. A alternates between sitting and standing to peel and cut up vegetables for dinner (ahead of time allowing for a rest period). Mr. A cooks the meal (alternating between sitting and standing) with a family member in the house but not supervising.

Step 5:
Mr. A stands to complete the meal preparation. Takes a seated rest. Mr. A cooks the meal in standing.

Step 7:
Mr. A prepares the evening meal independently, pacing the activity according to his fatigue levels.

Supported Risk Taking

Patients with FMD will often disengage from activities due to concerns that they will inadvertently harm themselves (or experience worsening of their symptoms). For example, someone with a functional tremor may avoid making a hot drink as they are concerned about the risk of spilling hot water and burning themselves. Although this may keep them safe in the short term, this avoidance can become a barrier to activity engagement and have a negative impact on mood and quality of life. Occupational therapists have a key role in supporting patients with FMD to identify and manage risk as they re-engage with their usual activities, using a graded approach [16]. The concept of supported risk taking is explored in a guidance document for occupational therapists, 'Embracing risk; enabling choice' [17] which provides a useful framework to support practice.

Symptom Management Techniques

Intervention strategies that lead the person with FMD to focus on their body or specific symptoms are likely to exacerbate symptoms and should therefore be avoided. Movement strategies that redirect attention away from the body can help to reduce motor symptoms and normalize movement [18]. Delivering therapy within the context of functional activities can help to prevent focus on symptoms. If symptoms worsen during an intervention, occupational therapists can give a prompt or cue designed to re-direct attention. If the person is looking at a cup that they are carrying, resulting in tremor and spillage, a simple cue of 'look up' or 'focus on your destination' can take the persons attention outside of their body and reduce the tremor. A brief change in activity, taking a rest or taking a moment to refocus on taught strategies ('re-set') can be helpful before continuing with the task at hand. Implementation of diaphragmatic breathing can be a useful management strategy for many symptom types to help the body relax and prevent breath holding. We would suggest implementation of this technique prior to entering into an activity/situation identified as difficult or stressful, during the activity and afterwards to bring the person back to a relaxed state. See Table 24.1 for examples of specific intervention techniques to encourage normal movement patterns.

Case Vignette: Part III – Implementation of Symptom Management Techniques

The occupational therapist explored normal movement strategies (even weight bearing, use of forward momentum, reduction of maladaptive postures) to improve efficiency of Mr. A's transfers along with diaphragmatic breathing techniques. These techniques were then integrated into personal care activities and meal preparation.

Mr. A's arm tremor was impacting on his ability to complete tasks requiring dexterity (e.g. using knives, dressing, shaving and writing). The occupational therapist assessed him completing these tasks. It was discussed that increased tension (and co-contraction) was likely a maintaining factor to his tremor and high pain levels. Mr. A was taught how to relax the muscles in combi-

nation with diaphragmatic breathing and use tremor entrainment strategies, integrated into daily activities.

Fatigue and Pain Management

Fatigue and pain are common in FMD and often have a negative impact on activity engagement [7, 23, 24]. Management of these symptoms should therefore be a priority for occupational therapy and fatigue-interventions from other chronic neurologic conditions such as energy conservation and activity pacing can be adapted for use with this client group [25–27]. Occupational therapists can assist the person with FMD to develop an understanding of the mechanisms behind pain and fatigue, exacerbating and alleviating factors and facilitate integration of management techniques into daily life [3, 5].

Case Vignette: Part IV – Implementation of Fatigue and Pain Management Strategies

Mr. A was asked to complete an activity log for three consecutive days, noting what he was doing and associated fatigue and pain levels. This was reviewed with his occupational therapist and together they identified:

- *Altered sleep/wake cycle – getting up late and difficulty getting to sleep.*
- *Tendency to miss meals.*
- *Pain and fatigue levels increasing throughout the day.*
- *Not taking rest breaks, but 'crashing' late afternoon.*
- *Over compensating for not being at work by pushing himself to do household chores at the expense of symptom exacerbation.*

The occupational therapist and Mr. A discussed how his current routine may be making it difficult to manage his FMD and worked together to explore:

Table 24.1 Specific occupational therapy interventions for FMD

Symptom	Intervention strategy
Functional tremor	Use of tremor entrainment and distraction techniques. Tremor entrainment, such as having the patient tap one hand to a set rhythm while the other arm is outstretched is helpful not only as diagnostic tool but can teach the patient to modulate and control their tremor. The task should initially be taught in isolation and subsequently be implemented into functional tasks.
	Use of a 'sensory diet'. Sensory hypersensitivity can worsen functional motor symptoms for some patients with FMD (e.g. sensitivity to bright lights or loud noises can trigger physical symptoms). For these patients use of a 'sensory diet' with identification and graded integration of stimuli into daily routines to aid sensory modulation can decrease sensory hypersensitivity and its impact on motor symptoms [19–21].
	Assist the person to relax the muscles in the limb to prevent co-contraction prior to starting a task. Discourage co-contraction or tensing of muscles as a method to suppress a tremor. Try to control a tremor with the person at rest, before moving onto activity.
	Use of gross rather than fine movements (which take more concentration) e.g. handwriting re-training; using a marker and large piece of paper or white board with big lettering or patterns / shapes rather than trying to focus on 'normal' handwriting.
	When carrying items – focus 'on the destination' rather than on items in the hand.
	Use of taught symptom management techniques whilst grading task complexity; practice pouring cold water, and progressively increase the temperature of the water until the person can manage pouring boiling water safely and confidently.
	A two-handed grip on the kettle (one on the handle, one under the base of the kettle) can initially be helpful to aid stabilization.
	When drinking from a cup; a bilateral hand grip can initially be helpful (so as to avoid learnt non-use).
Functional jerks	Addressing unhelpful pre-jerk cognitions and movement (e.g. signs of anxiety, frustration, extra effort or breath-holding). Suppression of jerks e.g. tensing the body to prevent a jerk coming on is unlikely to be helpful.
	General relaxation techniques; diaphragmatic breathing or progressive muscular relaxation can be used at rest and in function.
	If the jerks impact speech production, practice relaxation techniques and strategies to better manage breath control e.g. diaphragmatic breathing.
	Sensory grounding techniques (using the senses to bring attention back to the present moment) can be helpful if functional jerks are preceded by an urge or feeling of 'pressure'. For example, focusing on visual or auditory stimuli in the environment, cognitive distractors such as counting backwards or focusing on the texture of an item held in the hand [22].
	Encourage learning of "slow" movement activities such as yoga, tai chi, pilates as a way of regaining movement control and redirecting attention away from symptoms.
Dystonia	Encouraging optimal postural alignment at rest and within daily activities.
	Encourage even weight bearing in sitting and within function to normalize movement patterns and muscle activity.
	Gradually increase the time that the affected limb is used (using normal movement techniques) within activity.
	Discourage prolonged positioning of joints at the end of range (e.g. full hip, knee or ankle flexion while sitting; often seen when a person sits with their leg bent underneath them).
	Discourage guarding of the affected limb and promote therapeutic resting postures and limb-use. Address associated problems of pain and hypersensitivity.
Allodynia (as a consequence of fixed dystonia or CRPS)	Graded use of the affected limb whilst reducing protective postures. Promotion of arm swing when walking. Weight bearing in sitting or standing. Bilateral upper limb use in functional tasks. Graded sensory stimulation (sensory processing re-training) e.g. wearing clothing on the affected limb, showering or bathing the affected body part, applying moisturizer, washing up in warm water.
Functional limb weakness	Encourage normal movement, good alignment and even weight-bearing within activity-based tasks e.g. functional transfers, standing or perch sitting in personal care or kitchen tasks, using the affected hand to stabilize items within function so as to avoid non-use.
	Bilateral functional leg weakness; joint sessions with physical therapy colleagues to complete tasks using the upper limbs whilst standing with the aid of a standing frame.

Adapted from [5, 18]

- *The benefits of a structured routine with proactive regular rest breaks.*
- *Maintaining good self-care (regular nutrition and hydration, graded participation in exercise and enjoyable activities).*
- *Accepting that it is okay to rest and that this is an essential part of FMD self-management.*
- *What rest meant for Mr. A: switching off mind and body – e.g. listening to music and using relaxation techniques.*
- *Sleep hygiene advice.*
- *Ways to prioritize, plan and pace activities.*
- *Integration of normal movement principles into function to increase efficiency.*
- *Mr. A was advised to discuss optimization of pain medication with his doctor.*

The above principles were then integrated into Mr. A's daily routine.

Vocational Rehabilitation

Within most societies, employment is integral to daily life, providing income, social contact, routine and independence, thus supporting physical and psychological health [28, 29]. For patients with FMD, maintaining work or study roles can be challenging and occupational therapists have a key role to play in supporting them in this endeavor [2]. Vocational rehabilitation can be described as "whatever helps someone with a health problem to stay at, return to and remain in work" [30]. When treating patients with FMD, vocational rehabilitation principles used with other neurological conditions can be applied [31, 32]. These may include;

- Support with positive disclosure of their condition to employers.
- Education on employment rights.
- Education to employers on FMD and symptom impact (via letter or face to face meeting).
- Breaking down the demands of their job role and identification of reasonable adjustments (in conjunction with occupational health).

- Supporting 'work hardening' (gradually increasing tolerance to day to day activities and simulating mock work tasks) in preparation for return to work.
- Developing a return to work plan.

Although in general work is thought to be good for health [28], in some cases it may be a symptom maintaining factor, it therefore may not be possible to maintain employment despite reasonable adjustments. In these cases, occupational therapists can support patients to positively exit their current employment and plan for alternative productive roles (in some healthcare systems such as in the United States, such support can also be performed by a social worker). It is important to recognize that for some patients with FMD it may not be the demands of the work role itself that is a symptom maintaining factor, but the work environment (for example a breakdown of relationships with their manager or colleagues). Therefore, a move to a similar role at an alternative company may be beneficial. For others, exploring the possibility of a career change, to a less physically, cognitively or emotionally demanding role may be appropriate. Exploration of these various possibilities can also be explored collaboratively across occupational therapy and psychological therapies.

Case Vignette: Part V – Vocational Rehabilitation

Mr. A was employed full-time as a school teacher. He had not been able to work since the onset of his symptoms, but was keen to return to work. As he began to manage his day to day tasks with increased efficiency and independence, the focus of his occupational therapy sessions shifted to vocational rehabilitation. This built on work he had already done to establish a consistent level of daily activity (work hardening).

Mr. A and the occupational therapist discussed his job role. This included travel to/from work, the school environment, his timetable (teaching and non-teaching demands) etc. Together they identified areas that may be challenging, for example moving quickly between classrooms at busy times and began to set out reasonable adjustments to support a successful return to work. These included:

- *A graded and structured return to work plan (taking into account hours and duties with periods of consolidation and regular review).*
- *Having an allocated classroom to avoid the need to quickly change rooms between classes.*
- *Rest breaks planned into his timetable to help manage fatigue.*

They discussed ways to positively disclose his diagnosis to his employers and his occupational therapist agreed to liaise with occupational health about the impact of his symptoms on his working role and suggested reasonable adjustments (collaborations with occupational health can also involve the treating physician). Once Mr. A started his return to work plan, he met with the occupational therapist regularly for review.

Aids, Adaptations and Splinting

In general, the use of aids and adaptations are thought to be unhelpful in FMD rehabilitation as they can interrupt normal automatic movement patterns and encourage maladaptive ways of functioning. In addition, they can lead to secondary problems such as joint pain (e.g. wrist pain from weight bearing on a walking stick) and deconditioning of muscles [18]. Occupational therapists can assist patients with FMD to use a rehabilitative approach and minimize the need for aids and adaptations. However, there are times when provision of equipment is appropriate, and occupational therapists need to carefully, on an individual basis, weigh up the pros and cons of provision. The following can be useful to guide decision making [5]:

- Consider whether the person's symptoms are presenting acutely or whether they have been long lasting.
- Are aids needed on a short-term basis? For example, to enable a safe discharge from hospital? If so, it is advisable to take a minimalist

approach and make a plan of how to reduce use over time (and it can be helpful to be transparent with the patient about the planned short-term use of such an aid).
- Major adaptations should be avoided if symptoms are recent in onset.

For patients with ongoing disability despite rehabilitation and best efforts, equipment or adaptations can increase independence and have a positive impact on quality of life.

Splinting in FMD can present similar problems and it is important to be aware that serial casting for fixed functional dystonia has been associated with worsening symptoms and the onset of complex regional pain syndrome [33, 34].

Case Vignette: Part VI – Use of Adaptive Aids

Mr. A had been using a toilet-frame and bath-board to aid his transfers. He had also been given a perching stool to use in the kitchen. Whilst using taught symptom management strategies the occupational therapist worked with Mr. A to reduce reliance on these aids.

Toilet transfers:

- *Sit to stand using forward momentum (nose over toes), even weight bearing through both legs and pushing up with hands (using toilet-frame).*
- *Sit to stand using forward momentum (nose over toes), even weight bearing through both legs and pushing up with hands on knees (toilet-frame available if required).*
- *Sit to stand using forward momentum (nose over toes), even weight bearing through both legs and pushing up through legs without the use of hands (removal of toilet-frame).*

Bath transfers:

The occupational therapist practiced bath transfers (at first with assistance) with Mr. A on a number of occasions without the use of equipment. This was done until he felt he was able to manage getting in and out of the bath on his own without equipment (bath-board removed). To build confidence with this, he was initially supervised in and out of the bath by his wife, followed by having a bath whilst she was in the house and then moving to complete independence when home alone.

Perching stool:

Mr. A was initially encouraged to complete kitchen tasks alternating between standing for short periods (evenly weight-bearing, not propping) and sitting on the perching stool to complete meal preparation tasks. The time standing within function was gradually increased until he could complete meal preparation without needing to sit (perching stool then removed).

Disability Management

Care Needs

Many patients with FMD will have care needs and occupational therapists can provide advice on the type and intensity of care required. Although the use of professional and informal caregivers may be appropriate, prolonged use can reduce self-confidence in one's own abilities, reduce endurance, decrease overall independence and engagement in daily activities, and adversely affect relationships (if care is provided by significant others).

Whenever possible, care that facilitates active engagement as opposed to passive caregiving should be encouraged. Rehabilitation with an occupational therapist can help to reduce the need for care over time.

Benefits/Insurance Claims

Occupational therapists can assist patients with FMD to complete benefits and insurance claims in some clinical settings (this may be less common in the United States where case managers and social workers may be more involved in some of these activities). Providing basic education to agencies on the diagnosis and nature of FMD can be helpful, for example, highlighting the often unpredictable and variable nature of symptoms and their impact on the person's func-

tional capacities. Occupational therapists can also advocate for the need for specialized rehabilitation on behalf of the person with FMD to their insurance or healthcare provider.

Housing

Occupational therapists and social workers may have a role in advocating for relocation on behalf of patients with FMD. For example, this may be appropriate if the person has chronic symptoms that have not responded to rehabilitation and their home environment is restricting their independence; there is overcrowding in the home (leading to tension and stress which may exacerbate/maintain functional symptoms); or there is social conflict in the local environment (neighborly disputes) which is causing stress/affecting community access.

Relapse Prevention and Management Plan

It is common for patients with FMD to have periods of symptom remission and exacerbation. It is therefore essential that a relapse prevention/management plan be discussed and documented collaboratively with the patient and treating team, prior to discharge [5, 35]. This can include:

Identification of what can lead to exacerbation of symptoms.
- Symptom management strategies they have found helpful.
- What they can do if they experience a 'bad day'.
- Identification of short and long-term goals to carry their progress forward.

Patients with FMD should be encouraged to share this plan with significant others. Additionally, a video summary of key normal movement strategies can also be helpful should the person experience a relapse in the future.

Concluding Occupational Therapy Interventions

When concluding occupational therapy interventions, it is important to maintain the therapeutic relationship and foster the person's belief in their abilities to self-manage their symptoms post discharge. Weaving self-management principles throughout treatment sessions will likely support the person to feel more adequately prepared to carry goals forward independently post discharge. A discharge session with the person with FMD and significant others is a useful way to end intervention. This gives the opportunity to discuss what has gone well, what areas need further improvement and how significant others can support the person to continue to get better.

For patients with chronic FMD symptoms, open communication with their neurologist and other treatment team members (e.g., psychiatrist, psycho therapist, physical therapist) is paramount to optimize treatment outcomes. Additional referrals to relevant specialists (e.g. pain management) and giving the person additional resources such as connections to patient advocacy groups should be considered. A discharge report can be completed and copied to the person and all professionals involved (with consent) assisting with continuity of care. Scheduling follow up appointments can be beneficial to minimize anxiety about discharge, trouble-shoot problems and reset goals.

Timing of rehabilitation is important; re-engaging in therapy at a later date may be advantageous, especially if specific obstacles towards full therapy engagement can be addressed in the meantime.

Summary
- Use a philosophical model to guide occupational therapy interventions for FMD, utilizing appropriate assessment tools and outcome measures.
- Allow time for a thorough initial assessment and development of therapeutic rapport.
- Set treatment parameters at the start of intervention.
- Use mutual goals/areas of need identified by the person with FMD to guide interventions.
- Focus on functional (activity-based) rather than impairment-based goals.
- Introduce the importance of self-management during the assessment phase.
- Provide education about the diagnosis and rationale for interventions.
- Deliver therapy within the context of real-world activities to reduce symptom focus.
- Integrate symptom management techniques into tasks of interest and demonstrate how to continue with this independently outside of sessions.
- Address pain and fatigue management.
- Support patients with FMD to identify and manage risk within their daily routine.
- Consider the need for vocational rehabilitation.
- Provision of equipment, aids, adaptations and splints should be carefully considered on an individual basis weighing up the pros and cons of provision.
- Complete a relapse prevention and self-management plan as part of treatment.
- Encourage collaboration across clinicians to emphasize team-based approaches to care.

References

1. World Federation of Occupational Therapists. Statement of occupational therapy. 2012. http://www.wfot.org/about-occupational-therapy.
2. Royal College of Occupational Therapists (RCOT). Goals of occupational therapy intervention. London: Royal College of Occupational Therapists; 2016.
3. Preston JEJ. Occupational therapy and neurological conditions. Chichester: Wiley; 2016.
4. Tyerman A, Meehan M. Vocational assessment and rehabilitation after acquired brain injury:interagency guidelines. London: British Society of Rehabilitation Medicine/Royal College of Physicians; 2004.
5. Nicholson C, Edwards MJ, Carson AJ, Gardiner P, Golder D, Hayward K, et al. Occupational therapy consensus recommendations for functional neurological disorder. J Neurol Neurosurg Psychiatry. 2020:1–9. https://doi.org/10.1136/jnnp-2019-322281.
6. Jordbru AA, Smedstad LM, Klungsøyr O, Martinsen EW. Psychogen ic gait disorder: a random ized cont rolled trial of physical rehabilitation with one-year followup. J Rehabil Med. 2014;46(2):181–7.
7. Saifee TA, Kassavetis P, Pareés I, Kojovic M, Fisher L, Morton L, et al. Inpatient treatment of functional motor symptoms: a long-term follow-up study. J Neurol. 2012;259(9):1958–63.
8. McCormack R, Moriarty J, Mellers JD, Shotbolt P, Pastena R, Landes N, et al. Specialist inpatient treatment for severe motor conversion disorder: a retrospective comparative study. J Neurol Neurosurg Psychiatry. 2014;85(8):893–8.
9. Kielhofner G. A model of human occupation. Theory and application. Baltimore: Williams & Wilkins; 1985.
10. Polatajko HJ, Townsend EA. Enabling occupation II: advancing an occupational therapy vision of health, well-being, & justice through occupation. Ottawa: CAOT Publications ACE; 2007. p. 22–36.
11. Carswell A, McColl MA, Baptiste S, Law M, Polatajko HPN. The Canadian occupational performance measure: a research and Clinical Literatrure Review. Can J Occup Ther. 2004;71(4):210–22.
12. Forsyth K, Deshpande S, Kielhofner G, Henriksson C, Haglund L, Olson L, et al. OCAIRS: the occupational circumstances assessment interview and rating scale. 4.0. Chicago: MOHO Clearinghouse; 2005.
13. Baron K, Kielhofner G, Lyenger A. The occupational self assessment (version 2.2) model of human occupation. Chicago: Clearinghouse; 2006.
14. Kiresuk TJ, Sherman RE. Goal attainment scaling: a general method for evaluating comprehensive community mental health programs. Community Ment Health J. 1968;4(6):443–53.
15. Locke EA, Latham GP. A theory of goal setting & task performance. Prentice Hall, Inc; 1990.
16. Gallagher A. Risk assessment: enabler or barrier? Br J Occup Ther. 2013;76(7):337–9.
17. Royal College of Occupational Therapists. Embracing risk; enabling choice-guidance for occupational therapists. London: Royal College of Occupational Therapists; 2017.
18. Nielsen G. Chapter 45 – Physical treatment of functional neurologic disorders [Internet]. In: Handbook of clinical neurology, vol. 139. 1st ed. Elsevier B.V.; 2016. p. 555–69. Available from: https://doi.org/10.1016/B978-0-12-801772-2.00045-X.
19. Ranford J, Perez DL, MacLean J. Additional occupational therapy considerations for functional neurological disorders: a possible role for sensory processing. CNS Spectr. 2018;23(3):194–5.
20. Ranford J, MacLean J, Alluri PR, Comeau O, Godena E, LaFrance Jr WC, et al. Sensory processing difficulties in functional neurological disorder: a possible predisposing vulnerability? Psychosomatics. 2020;61(4):343–52.
21. Jean A. Occupational therapy for motor disorders resulting from impairment of the central nervous system. Rehabil Lit. 1974;21:302–10.
22. Goldstein L, Chalder T, Chigwedere C, Khondoker M, Moriarty JTB, et al. Cognitive-behavioural therapy for psychogenic non-epileptic seizures: a pilot RCT. Neurology. 2010;74(24):1986–4.
23. Stone J, Warlow C, Sharpe M. The symptom of functional weakness: a controlled study of 107 patients. Brain. 2010;133(5):1537–51.
24. Gelauff JM, Kingma E, Kalkman J, Bezemer R, Engelen B, et al. Fatigue, not self-rated motor severity, affects quality of life in functional motor disorders. J Neurol. 2018;265(8):1803–9.
25. The British Pain Society. The British Pain Society. London: Guidelines for pain management programs for adults; 2013.
26. Thomas S, Thomas PW, Kersten P, Jones R, Green C, Nock A, et al. A pragmatic parallel arm multi-centre randomised controlled trial to assess the effectiveness and cost-effectiveness of a group-based fatigue management programme (FACETS) for people with multiple sclerosis. J Neurol Neurosurg Psychiatry. 2013;84(10):1092–9.
27. Kamper SJ, Apeldoorn AT, Chiarotto A, Smeets RJEM, Ostelo RWJG, Guzman J, et al. Multidisciplinary biopsychosocial rehabilitation for chronic low back pain: Cochrane systematic review and meta-analysis. BMJ. 2015;350(February):1–11. https://doi.org/10.1136/bmj.h444.
28. Department for Work and Pensions; Department of Health. Improving lives: the work, health and disability green paper. London: Dandy Booksellers Ltd; 2016.
29. Dorstyn DS, Roberts RM, Murphy G, Haub R. Employment and multiple sclerosis: a meta-analytic review pf psychological correlates. J Health Psychol. 2019;24(1):38–51.
30. Waddell G, Burton A, Kendall N. Vocational rehabilitation, what works for whom and when. London: The Stationary Office; 2008.

31. Sweetland J, Howse E, Playford E. A systematic review of research undertaken in vocational rehabilitation for people with multiple sclerosis. Disabil Rehabil. 2012;34(24):2031–8.

32. Kirk-Brown A, van Dijk P, Simmons R, Bourne MCB. Disclosure of multiple sclerosis in the workplace positively affects employment status and job tenure. Mult Scler J. 2014;20(7):871–6.

33. Schrag A, Trimble M, Quinn NBK. The syndrom of fixed dystonia: an evaluation of 103 patients. Brain. 2004;127:2360–72.

34. Popkirov S, Hoeritzauer I, Colvin L, Carson ASJ. Complex regional pain syndrome and functional neurological disorders: time for reconciliation. J Neurol Neurosurg Psychiatry. 2019;90:608–14.

35. Nielsen G, Stone J, Matthews A, Brown M, Sparkes C, Farmer R, et al. Physiotherapy for functional motor disorders: a consensus recommendation. J Neurol Neurosurg Psychiatry. 2015;86:1113–9. https://doi.org/10.1136/jnnp-2014-309255.

Jennifer Freeburn

Case Vignette

A 37-year-old single woman with a history of chronic back pain and no formal psychiatric history suddenly developed speech changes and right arm weakness while at work. She was sent to the hospital, where brain imaging was normal. The initial examination by the attending neurologist was notable for distractibility and variability of the patient's speech and collapsing/give-way weakness on motor examination of her right arm, raising suspicion for a functional neurological etiology. The remainder of her elemental neurological examination was non-focal and her brain MRI was normal. She was discharged home and referred for multidisciplinary outpatient care including neurology follow-up and physical and speech therapy consultations. At the speech-language pathology assessment, the patient reported variations in her speech output, sometimes presenting as stuttering, halted speech at other times sounding like an unidentifiable accent. She noted worsened symptoms coinciding with stressful speaking situations. The patient also shared that she had begun avoiding conversations with anyone outside of her immediate family, including friends and acquaintances at her son's school. On examination, her speech was notable for irregular consonant substitutions, vowel distortions, and prosodic abnormalities, along with atypical grammatical errors. The severity and frequency of the speech errors increased when attention was drawn to the patient's speech (such as during reading tasks) and less prevalent during spontaneous conversation. The clinician highlighted the aspects of her speech presentation consistent with a functional speech disorder and shared that with motivated effort she would very likely regain her normal speech pattern. The patient was initially reluctant to accept this diagnosis, expressing her continued concern that she had experienced an undetected stroke leading to the speech difficulties, but agreed to a trial of treatment. Initial treatment sessions focused on diagnostic counseling, education, and working toward increased control of her speech output through trials of imitating personally relevant phrases. The patient demonstrated intermittent improvement during these trials, although had difficulty maintaining the change when any novel text was introduced. During the third treatment session, the patient was repeatedly cued to imitate typical speech using clinician models as well as video clips of her own voice recorded prior to

Supplementary Information The online version contains supplementary material available at [https://doi.org/10.1007/978-3-030-86495-8_25].

J. Freeburn (✉)
Department of Speech, Language, & Swallowing Disorders, Massachusetts General Hospital, Boston, MA, USA
e-mail: jfreeburn@partners.org

the onset of speech changes and demonstrated a significant improvement in accuracy. She then quickly progressed to reading sentences and paragraphs while maintaining the accurate speech pattern, until finally moving to spontaneous conversation with typical articulation and prosody. She arrived at her fourth session having reverted to the altered functional speech pattern; however, she was easily cued by the clinician to return to accurate speech production by producing the imitated phrases again. She was encouraged to use imitation of her recorded voice as a cue for independently modifying her speech output. When she returned to the clinic for her fifth visit, her speech pattern was normal. With encouragement, the patient identified several goals for re-engaging in communication opportunities, such as returning to community yoga classes with friends and engaging with other parents at her son's soccer games. The patient returned to clinic 1 month later for follow-up reporting "about 90%" accurate speech, with occasional brief episodes of slurred articulation in the setting of stress.

Introduction

Changes in communication as a form of a functional movement disorder (FMD) may represent alterations in speech motor function alone or include a far more complex constellation of symptoms [1, 2]. The impact of communication dysfunction is widespread, affecting an individual's vocational outcomes, social interactions, and overall quality of life [3]. This chapter provides an overview of clinical strategies for managing both functional speech and voice disorders, as well as functional cognitive symptoms as contributors to overall communication impairments. Diagnostic considerations in functional speech/voice disorders are addressed in Chap. 13.

Speech-language pathologists (SLPs) have expertise in anatomical, physiological, and neurological aspects of communication and are well-positioned to assess and treat patients with functional speech/voice disorders. As the number of patients diagnosed with FMD continues to

rise, it is essential that SLPs develop comfort and expertise in providing symptomatic treatment for patients with functional speech/voice and/or cognitive disorders.

The treatment strategies described within this chapter represent an approach informed by available literature and expertise across the rehabilitative sciences including physical therapy, occupational therapy, and cognitive behavioral therapy. While intended as guidance for SLP interventions, the principles are applicable to any healthcare professional encountering a patient with functional communication deficits. This chapter is also relevant to physicians longitudinally following patients with functional speech and voice disorders, facilitating the development of shared expertise allowing physicians to reinforce basic SLP principles with their patients.

Considerations for Initiating Treatment

Any treatment plan must aim to optimize the patient's outcome through consideration of logistical, clinical, and personal variables. Several factors should be taken into account when formulating a treatment plan for patients presenting with functional speech/voice and/or cognitive symptoms.

Timing

As with other rehabilitative efforts in FMD, intervention for functional speech/voice disorders and cognitive dysfunction is best initiated after the patient has received a clinically-established FMD diagnosis as typically performed by a neurologist or neuropsychiatrist. A thorough assessment of the communication difficulty is also foundational to treatment and can often have therapeutic value in itself (see Chap. 13 for a detailed description of assessment tasks). Additionally, within the scope of a multi-disciplinary clinic, it may be useful to consider the timing of a patient's participation in other therapies. The purposeful alignment of speech, physical, occupational, and cognitive behavioral therapy may serve to reinforce a patient's trajectory of progress. Even so, patients with significant comorbidities such as pain and fatigue may benefit from a more paced or even sequential approach to engaging in therapies.

Frequency

Similar to considerations for treatment timing, patient variables such as tolerance for the physical and cognitive demands of treatment must be considered in determining a plan for treatment frequency. Logistical factors such as the patient's proximity to the clinic and support for transportation are also inevitable considerations. However, there is great value in framing treatment as an opportunity for intensive motor retraining, which is best completed at a high level of frequency, with treatment sessions spaced out no more than weekly if possible.

Patient Readiness

While always relevant in gauging a patient's readiness to fully engage in therapy, patient-specific attitudes and beliefs are particularly relevant in the management of FMD. A patient's acceptance of the FMD diagnosis is considered to be one of the most important factors in predicting a positive prognosis, as per a recent study that surveyed movement disorder specialists [4]. Assessing patient's readiness for change and acceptance of the diagnosis may include several components including patient self-report [5], motivational interviewing, and clinical observations.

Measuring Therapy Outcomes

The collection of outcome measures is valuable to the rehabilitative treatment process for functional speech/voice and cognitive disorders. Regular collection of progress metrics serves to support treatment planning and provides a continuous opportunity to discuss progress with the patient. At the end of treatment, patients may be encouraged to reflect on their progress by reviewing pre- and post- data including audio or video recordings. Furthermore, given the limited evidence of treatment efficacy in functional speech/ voice and cognitive disorders, collecting objective outcome measures is an important step toward future research. Recommendations for collecting treatment outcomes in FMD include the use of complimentary patient-reported subjective measures alongside performance-based or clinician-rated measures [6, 7].

Patient-reported outcome measures for functional speech/voice disorders may include validated survey tools such as the Communicative Effectiveness Survey [8] and the Voice Handicap Index [9]. In cognition, tools that capture a point-in-time patient perspective on functioning such as the Neuro-QoL Cognitive items [10] or the Functional Memory Disorder Inventory [11] may be useful.

Clinical measures for motor speech may include ratings of perceptual characteristics across tasks such as connected speech, oral reading, sustained phonation, and alternating/sequential motion rates [12]. Fluency metrics, such as formal Stuttering Severity Instrument scores [13] or simple percentage of fluency from a transcription of reading/expository speech tasks are valuable measures for functional stutter. Similarly, traditional voice measures including the clinician-rated CAPE-V [14] or acoustic voice measures may be used as appropriate to individual cases. More details on selecting outcome measures in FMD can be found in Chap. 29.

Treatment of Functional Speech and Voice Disorders

As detailed in Chap. 13, functional speech/voice disorders may present across a wide spectrum of alterations of motor speech functioning and can affect any speech subsystem. The speech disorder may present as the primary symptom, or within the context of mixed FMD. Symptoms may range from nearly undetectable atypical movements of speech structures to profound dysfluency or functional mutism. In all cases, facilitating improved spoken communication is often a critical element of a patient's recovery. For patients whose communication has been significantly decreased in the setting of functional speech/voice disorders, symptomatic improvement in speech may be a prerequisite for participation in interdisciplinary therapies.

Given that mechanisms of functional speech/voice disorders are inherently rooted in altered motor functioning, treatment paradigms share many similarities with physical therapy programs for FMD [15]. These overarching treatment principles are outlined in recent consensus guidelines as relevant to the wider spectrum of FMD-associated symptoms seen in the SLP clinic [16] and are detailed below in the context of functional speech/voice presentations.

Diagnostic Counseling and Education

Perhaps the most consistent theme across the literature discussing treatment of FMD is the importance of the provider's delivery and discussion of the diagnosis. Likewise, the confident and compassionate delivery of a positive diagnosis of functional speech/voice disorder is a foundational element of therapy. This may begin with the simple acknowledgement that the symptoms are genuine and have a clear impact on the patient's quality of life [17]. The clinician may further provide support for the patient's understanding of FMD in general, and then provide the diagnosis of a functional speech/voice disorder. It is often helpful to outline positive, rule-in evidence of the functional etiology of the speech/voice disorder gathered during the assessment (see Chap. 13 for in-depth discussion of diagnostic features), which may have therapeutic effect [18]. Patients may benefit from guided listening or viewing of recordings from the assessment to support this conversation.

Following delivery of the functional speech/voice disorder diagnosis, many patients will be left with questions regarding the underlying etiology. It is important to emphasize the focus on "what" the disorder is and examination features that rule in the diagnosis [18, 19]. The clinician may also provide an explanation of the brain-body connection (see Chap. 3 for further details on this concept). Finally, an essential component of diagnostic counseling is the assurance that treatment is available and often highly effective. It may be helpful to highlight that, despite changes in functioning, no irreversible structural damage has occurred in the speech output centers of the brain. As such, clinicians may express confidence that it is possible for the patient to regain control over the motor pattern with dedicated effort and therapeutic support.

Discussing Functional Speech/Voice Disorder Features

After engaging in supportive education about the diagnosis, it is often helpful to increase the patient's understanding of typical motor speech functioning. This both highlights the automaticity and effortlessness of many speech functions and serves as context for discussion of the patient's specific deviations from normal functioning.

Understanding Typical and Altered Motor Speech Function

Providing an overview of the typical anatomy, physiology, and functioning of speech subsystems and mechanisms in simplified terms aims to support a patient's insight and provide a foundation for facilitating change. Education must be highly tailored to topics most relevant for the individual patient. For example, a patient experiencing dysfluency as a primary symptom may benefit from education focused on the typical functioning of articulatory structures. Similarly, education for a patient with primary vocal symptoms would likely include a discussion of respiration and phonation. While not an exhaustive list, education topics by speech subsystems that often support patient education are included in Box 25.1.

Box 25.1 Education Topics by Speech Subsystem

- **Respiration**
  - Effortless tidal/resting breathing versus more purposeful speech breathing
  - Diaphragmatic breathing
- **Phonation**
  - The voice mechanism and relevant musculature
  - Relationship between breathing and voicing
- **Articulation**
  - Movement and control of articulatory structures
  - Limited articulatory muscle strength required to produce accurate speech sounds
- **Resonance**
  - Nasal airflow patterns during speech production
  - Automatic versus conscious velar control
- **Prosody**
  - Components of speech prosody, including intonation, stress, and rhythm
  - Natural variations across speakers and within a single speaker across contexts

Education regarding typical anatomy and physiology should include a focus on the limited conscious effort devoted to the motor aspects of speech. Typical speakers focus their attention on what they are saying, with only rare attention to specific movements associated with speech sounds. Conversely, some level of hypervigilance to symptoms and/or body structures appears to be an underlying factor in functional speech/voice disorders [12]. When applicable, it may be help-ful to highlight the patient's descriptions of increased effort and/or experiences of fatigue with speaking. Discussion of the body's secondary reaction of muscle tension in response to hypervigilance may also be helpful, particularly in the case of visible physical tension in the patient's face, neck, and/or jaw.

Describing Atypical Speech Features

Following a discussion of typical functioning, the clinician is well-positioned to open a discussion of the patient's altered functioning in the speech and voice mechanisms. The use of objective, specific, and non-judgmental descriptions is essential. Descriptions of speech must also be accessible to the patient, although the therapist may need to employ some terminology introduced during the discussion of typical anatomy and physiology. Patients may initially describe their symptoms vaguely (e.g. "my speech is off") or with a focus on specific motor dysfunction (e.g. "my tongue is sluggish and doesn't move well"). In these cases, it may be helpful for the clinician to describe the clinical speech features noted during the examination to invite increased awareness. For example: "I notice that you often repeat the first sound of a word, and you close your eyes tightly whenever this happens". The clinician may encourage the patient to use a mirror or review audio/video recordings of speech samples during the session to supplement insight as necessary. The clinician can then help to shape the patient's language and/or provide prompts for more specific descriptions; for example: "I hear an extra syllable inserted in the middle of words sometimes, and certain consonants are substituted with others – that may be why you are hearing your speech as sounding 'accented'". The goal of this process is to empower patients to use accurate language describing function when discussing their atypical speech features in order to promote an increased sense of volitional control.

Facilitating Change

An essential goal of therapy for functional speech/voice disorders is to elicit a purposeful change in the patient's pattern of altered speech output. This often occurs as a two-part process, during which the therapist facilitates the change in speech output through symptomatic therapy and then fosters the patient's increased awareness and volitional control. Facilitation strategies often include components of physical relaxation and trials with various sound production techniques which will be discussed in additional detail.

It is recommended that strategies to change the patient's speech motor output be initiated at the evaluation, although that may be deferred to subsequent treatment sessions as needed due to time limitations or patient-specific factors. Regardless, therapeutic attempts to facilitate change should follow a thorough and frank discussion of the functional speech/voice diagnosis as detailed above. Through the process of providing education and counseling, the clinician will be positioned as an expert and an ally (or "co-pilot") in the patient's process of regaining control over speech. The importance of continuing to exude clinical confidence and consistently employing positive, non-judgmental language throughout the treatment course cannot be overstated.

The strategies that elicit a change in the speech motor pattern vary from patient to patient. Change may occur within minutes or may be gradual and require more support. Initially, clinical efforts will likely focus on eliciting change from the engrained functional motor pattern to reinforce the concept of control. Then, cuing will focus on shaping the speech output to approximate more typical speech patterns. Detailed below are a number of strategies that may support both aspects of this process.

- **Reflexive Sounds**: A patient may naturally exhibit more natural motor functioning during production of automatic sounds, such as laughter or sighing. Reflexive sounds can

also be purposefully stimulated (e.g. audible gargle or throat clear) and may be useful for provoking a more normal speech/voice pattern. Once an improved pattern is established, the therapist may then shape the sound into a related syllable, and eventually into words.

- **Automatized Speech Patterns**: Some patients may demonstrate a change in speech pattern that naturally emerges during speech production. At times this is observed during conversation, such as during production of stereotyped phrases (e.g. "ok", "I don't know"), or may be drawn out by asking the patient to repeat highly automatic patterns (e.g. days of the week) repetitively. When present, these instances of typical speech can be used as the basis for shaping toward typical speech.

- **Singing**: For some patients, producing a familiar song or speaking to a tune may evoke a more normal speech pattern. The singing can be shaped into highly prosodic speaking, and eventually into typical prosody.

- **Relaxation Strategies**: Particularly for patients presenting with significant musculoskeletal tension, strategies overtly aimed at increasing awareness and control over muscle tension may be helpful. Diaphragmatic breathing and guided progressive muscle relaxation are often useful at the start of initial treatment to increase the patient's awareness of any tension present within the speech mechanism. The use of clinician or patient self-administered massage may also be helpful if significant tension is identified.

- **Negative Practice**: Once a patient has successfully described his or her features, it may be helpful to guide him/her in exploring what it might feel like to purposefully create the atypical speech pattern. Encourage experimentation and support the imitative attempts. Allow patients to trial the purposeful negative practice, and then challenge them to try to modify it (e.g. a low pitch turns to a high pitch; a tense face turns to an overly relaxed face).

Change Facilitation Specific to Functional Speech/Voice Disorder Subtype

For patients with a speech presentation that matches a known subtype of functional speech/voice disorders (detailed in Chap. 13), specific strategies for change facilitation and shaping may be helpful.

Acquired Functional Stuttering

Functional stuttering, particularly when accompanied by secondary struggle behaviors, may be associated with musculoskeletal tension and therefore benefit significantly from procedures for reducing tension as described above [12]. Eliciting a change in the dysfluent speech pattern may also be supported by a number of additional symptomatic strategies highlighted below.

- Introduce traditional dysfluency strategies, such as easy onset and "feather-light" articulatory touch, during the speech session. Model the exaggerated use of the strategy during production of a word and encourage the patient to trial the strategy. This likely will not sound like typical speech, but nevertheless provide positive feedback for any change in the underlying pattern of dysfluency.
- Similarly, it may be useful to cue the patient to create purposeful alternative dysfluencies. For example, if the patient has a consistent pattern of first sound blocking, encourage exaggerated prolongation of the first sound.
- Once the patient's fluency improves, the exaggerated fluency strategies and/or "replacement" dysfluencies can be shaped into typical speech.

Prosodic/Articulatory Disturbance

For patients presenting with speech patterns featuring primary prosodic and articulatory disturbances (including foreign accent syndrome and infantile speech), several additional strategies may be helpful in facilitating modified speech patterns. Of note, many patients falling into this sub-category may also present with atypical language alterations in morphology, syntax, and semantics [20]. It is not recommended that ther-

apy aim to specifically "correct" these alterations, as they are not indicative of an underlying aphasia, but rather to encourage accurate production as the speech pattern is modified.

- Encourage the patient to playfully mimic other accents/prosodic patterns. The use of videos of well-known accents may be helpful for this, as well as the use of common phrases that lend themselves to varying prosody associated with different emotions/situations (e.g. "hello" and "goodbye").
- Similarly, direct imitation of the dialectical patterns of someone with a similar baseline dialect as the patient. This may be the clinician in some cases, or a gender-matched family member or friend. (Audio samples 25.1, 25.2, and 25.3 demonstrate the therapeutic use of direct imitation in a patient with prosodic and articulatory disturbances).
- Point out and praise any change from the functional speech pattern. Any modification of the underlying atypical speech pattern, even if not fully normal, may be shaped toward typical speech.

Functional Voice Disorders

Extensive literature exists on the management of functional voice disorders. Treatment efficacy studies have demonstrated improvement in patients' functional voice symptoms following a combination of patient education and direct treatment aimed at eliciting a change in the patient's voice production [21, 22]. Included here is a brief review of strategies that may serve as the first steps to facilitating vocal changes. These strategies are covered extensively elsewhere [22, 23].

- Decrease musculoskeletal tension through manual manipulation and relaxation techniques. These are often performed by the SLP during treatment sessions, while the patient is educated on self-administration of the techniques at home.
- Support decreased vocal hyperfunction through the use of strategies such as confidential voice and/or semi-occluded vocal tract.
- Elicit typical voice through the use of vegetative (cough, throat clear, grunting, gargling) or

playful (lip trills, giggling/laughing) sounds [21]. Use any typical sound production to shape toward improved voicing.

Functional Mutism

Very limited research has chronicled patients with complete loss of speech output, or functional mutism, in the context of functional speech/voice disorders. Most case studies have shown a significant emotional component prior to the onset of functional mutism [24], highlighting the importance of psychiatric and psychological care. However, patients with functional mutism have also demonstrated similarities to patients with functional voice disorders, including the potential to benefit from symptomatic treatment [12, 23]. The use of similar voicing strategies including elicitation and shaping of vegetative sounds and focusing on muscle relaxation may be helpful.

Functional Movements of the Face

Functional movements of the face often involve the unilateral lower lip and the soft palate [25, 26], both of which may affect patient's speech output. Therapeutic methods to address facial movements are congruous with functional speech/voice disorder management strategies including diagnostic counseling and education regarding typical versus atypical movements of the involved muscle groups. Patients may also benefit from specific tasks targeting increased motor control of the affected muscle group, such as production of exaggerated production of vowel sounds (e.g. "eee-ooo-ahhh") or strategically chosen words to activate the targeted facial muscles or production of nasal consonants to open vowels (e.g. "ng-ah-ng-ah") for palatal tremor.

Building Independence

Throughout trials of strategies to facilitate change, the patient should receive reinforcement for any change from the altered speech pattern. When a change is observed, it is important to support the patient in identifying the differences between their changed speech production and

their atypical functional speech pattern. As the patient demonstrates increased awareness of the change in speech output, the therapist can encourage their self-identification of both accurate and inaccurate patterns. Reinforcing that recognition is a critical step to creating long-lasting change.

As the patient's accuracy increases, the therapist can gradually increase the length and complexity of speech targets used in treatment sessions. To shape a single sound produced with the new speech pattern, the patient can be guided to increase the production of single words and short phrases with that phoneme in the initial position. To move toward lengthier speech output, oral reading of conversational phrases and sentence-level text (e.g. quotations, simple poetry, children's books) may be valuable, as well as the use of structured phrase and sentence level conversational tasks. The therapist should continue to support the patient in moving through a hierarchy of tasks up to the paragraph level, with continued encouragement for self-correction of any return to the deviant speech pattern. Once the patient's speech output has reached 90% accuracy or above in these structured tasks, therapeutic tasks will move toward less structured language (e.g. short personal narratives, multi-step task descriptions). Finally, the therapist should provide prompts for spontaneous conversation while continually encouraging the patient to self-monitor speech output.

Mutual Setting of Treatment Goals

Ultimately, the long-term treatment goal for functional speech/voice disorders is to support the patient in meeting his/her communication needs across environments. Interim short-term goals for treatment may include measures of patient understanding, metrics for accuracy along a hierarchy of speech tasks, carryover of learned strategies to their natural environment, and increased participation in communication opportunities. As patients near the end of treatment, goals may include independent application of self-cuing strategies for improved speech, particularly in the case of future symptom recurrence.

Patients should be involved in the development of appropriate goals, with the clinician working to understand the patient's daily communication demands/patterns as well as any withdrawal from communication opportunities that has occurred in the setting of speech changes. Ideally, discussions of communication demands will begin at the start of treatment and remain prevalent throughout. Support the patient in setting specific goals for gradually returning to communication activities that he or she may have been avoiding. For example, if the patient had been avoiding phone conversations due to the fear of not being understood, an initial participation goal may be to call the clinician's office and leave a message. Then, a patient may make a low-stakes phone call to request information (such as calling a store to inquire about their hours) or make a brief call to a familiar communication partner while in the clinic. Sample short-term treatment goals are listed in Box 25.2.

Box 25.2 Sample Short-Term Treatment Goals in Functional Speech/Voice Disorders
Speech Intelligibility

- The patient will describe typical vs. atypical speech/voice features using accurate terminology.
- The patient will demonstrate application of strategies for modifying speech output during tasks of repetition.
- The patient will read highly salient phrases using learned strategies independently.
- The patient will read novel text at the [phrase/sentence/paragraph] level using learned strategies with minimal cuing.
- The patient will apply learned strategies during structured clinical conversation tasks.

Carryover/Participation

- The patient will engage in a 5-min phone conversation with a familiar communication partner.
- The patient will engage in a novel in-person communication opportunity with an unfamiliar communication partner.

Prognosis for Improvement of Functional Speech and Voice Disorders

A recent scoping review of existing literature confirmed that little evidence exists about the effects of interventions in functional speech/voice disorders [27]. Still, smaller studies and case samples from SLPs treating functional speech/voice disorders have demonstrated significant potential for patients to improve through symptomatic therapy. For example, in a study of patients receiving symptomatic speech therapy for functional stuttering, over 70% were shown to improve rapidly with few treatment sessions [28]. This is aligned with outcome data examining the efficacy of physical therapy programs for FMD, which have shown symptom improvement in 60–87% of participants [29, 30, 31]. Certainly, anecdotal evidence and recommendations from experts across the field support physical rehabilitation as a first-line treatment across FMD presentations [4, 16]. However, further evidence is needed to better understand the trajectory of patient improvement through participation in therapy for functional speech/voice disorders.

Clinicians are encouraged to assess patient prognosis for functional speech/voice disorder treatment based on individual variables including readiness to change and stimulability for alterations to the disordered speech pattern at assessment. Patients who demonstrate immediate change in the underlying speech pattern are generally excellent candidates for treatment. Negative prognostic factors identified during the interview may include patient presentations that are particularly episodic and therefore cannot be addressed directly during the therapy session, as well as low patient insight or frank denial of the presence of speech abnormality [32]. Additionally, a number of other variables such as duration of symptoms, baseline psychiatric comorbidities, and pending litigation may also affect treatment prognosis [33], although more research in this area is needed.

Functional Cognitive Disorder Affecting Communication

Alongside speech output changes and FMD symptoms more broadly, patients' communication may also be affected by cognitive dysfunction. Functional cognitive disorder (FCD) is defined as subjective cognitive complaints with internal inconsistencies that cannot be directly attributed to other neurological conditions. Patients with FCD describe a constellation of cognitive symptoms that prominently include memory deficits, word retrieval problems, and decreased attention [34, 35]. The underlying mechanisms for FCD may often reflect multi-factorial contributions including mood, pain, fatigue, and excessive inward attention to cognitive processes [36]. Functional cognitive symptoms are common in neurology clinics and the cause of significant patient distress and reduced functioning [34, 37]. In the rehabilitative setting, patient complaints often include difficulty comprehending and/or remembering the educational materials provided by therapists and significant cognitive fatigue resulting from therapeutic tasks.

Under the umbrella of neurocognitive disorders, it is within the SLP scope of practice to provide support for patients experiencing functional cognitive difficulties [38]. In many cases and clinical contexts, occupational therapists and/or cognitive behavioral therapists may also play a role in addressing cognitive symptoms. Regardless of the primary clinician, close coordination with a multidisciplinary team including neurology, neuropsychology, occupational therapy, and behavioral health is important in the management of FCD. Notably, a neuropsychological evaluation can be helpful in the assessment of FCD and ideally will be conducted prior to a patient's initiation of treatment. The initial assessment is strongly recommended to include measures of effort and internal validity and may also include patient-reported scales measuring mood, stress, and/or somatic symptoms [39]. While treatment of FCD is underdeveloped and under-investigated in comparison to the role of SLP for the management of functional speech/voice disorders, several guiding therapeutic principles based on clinical experience are detailed below.

Shared Goal-Setting as Treatment

A primary goal in managing FCD is supporting the patient's return to increased independence in meeting his or her daily cognitive demands. An initial discussion of the patient's home responsibilities and independence for instrumental activities of daily living is helpful in determining the full impact of cognitive concerns on his or her overall functioning. Upon presenting for therapy, many patients may report increased reliance on family and friends and avoidance of cognitively demanding activities [35]. As such, it may be helpful to involve close friends and family members alongside the patient in developing initial goals for gradually increasing independence. Some examples of practical goals may include the patient's independent use of a notebook to record the recommendations from medical appointments or implementation of a system to manage medications with reduced support. Goals that support cognitive communication functioning, such as the application of word retrieval strategies in conversational contexts, are often also relevent. Involving the patient in goal setting should be considered an inherent part of the treatment itself, useful for reinforcing the metacognitive concept of goal-directed behavior as well as increasing patient commitment.

Therapeutic Management of FCD

Given the wide variability in presentation and underlying neuropsychiatric factors that may contribute to the overall cognitive dysfunction, there is no singular approach for the therapeutic management of functional cognitive symptoms. In general, intervention should focus on training the patient's use of external tools and metacognitive strategies to support his or her increased participation and independence.

Cognitive rehabilitation strategies are detailed in the literature on recovery from neurogenic cognitive impairments, including mild traumatic brain injury, and are potentially applicable in management of FCD. Resources for specific tools and educational materials to be used in the clinical setting go beyond the scope of this chapter but are included as references [40, 41]. In addition, offering supportive education and strategies for management of concomitant symptoms such as fatigue, sleep disturbance, and headache may be critical to a patient's holistic rehabilitation as further detailed in the mild traumatic brain injury literature [42]. Some patients may also benefit from participating in cognitive retraining tasks for attention processing (either computerized or paper-based), primarily to build confidence and support gradual re-integration of focused activities. The patient's overall tolerance for cognitive engagement must be considered during task selection, and cognitive tasks should be offered with an intentionally paced and highly individualized approach.

Summary
- Speech-language pathologists play an important role in the treatment of functional speech/voice and functional cognitive disorders, both of which may affect a patient's communication abilities.
- Clinicians are encouraged to consider the most advantageous timing and frequency of treatment sessions, as well as the patient's readiness to change prior to initiating a therapy course.
- Outcome measures for therapy should include patient self-report on validated surveys, clinician ratings, and performance-based measures as relevant to the patient's primary presenting symptoms.
- Core elements of functional speech/voice therapy include counseling around the diagnosis, patient education, change facilitation, and shaping of the change for increased self-monitoring.
- Therapeutic techniques to stimulate improvement in a patient's atypical speech pattern should be individualized where possible.
- Beyond supporting a patient's improved intelligibility, the goals of functional speech/voice therapy also include carryover across settings and a return to participation in everyday communication opportunities.
- The management of functional cognitive symptoms requires more research to better evaluate good treatment practices.

References

1. Baizabal-Carvall JF, Jankovic J. Speech and voice disorders in patients with psychogenic movement disorders. J Neurol. 2015;262(11):2420–4.
2. Chung DS, Wettroth C, Hallett M, Maurer CW. Functional speech and voice disorders: case series and literature review. Mov Disord Clin Pract. 2018;5(3):312–6.
3. Neumann S, Quinting J, Rosenkranz A, de Beer C, Jonas K, Stenneken P, et al. Quality of life in adults with neurogenic speech-language-communication difficulties: a systematic review of existing measures. J Commun Disord. 2019;79:24–5.
4. LaFaver K, Lang AE, Stone J, Morgante F, Edwards M, Lidstone S, et al. Opinions and clinical practices related to diagnosing and managing functional (psychogenic) movement disorders: changes in the last decade. Eur J Neurol. 2020;27(6):975–84.
5. Maggio JB, Ospina JP, Callahan J, Hunt AL, Stephen CD, Perez DL, et al. Outpatient physical therapy for functional neurological disorder: a preliminary feasibility and naturalistic outcomes study in a U.S. cohort. J Neuropsychiatr Clin Neurosci. 2019;32(1):85–9.
6. Nicholson TR, Carson A, Edwards M, Goldstein LH, Hallett M, Mildon B, et al. Outcome measures for functional neurological disorder: a review of the theoretical complexities. J Neuropsychiatr Clin Neurosci. 2020;32:1.
7. Pick S, Anderson DG, Asadi-Pooya AA, Aybek S, Baslet G, Bloem BR, et al. Outcome measurement in functional neurological disorder: a systematic review and recommendations. J Neurol Neurosurg Psychiatry. 2020;91(6):638–49.
8. Donovan NJ, Kendall D, Young ME, Rosenbek J. The communicative effectiveness survey: preliminary evidence of construct validity. Am J Speech Lang Pathol. 2008;17:335–47.
9. Jacobson BH, Johnson A, Grywalski C, Silbergleit A, Jacobson G, Benninger MS, et al. The voice handicap index: development and validation. Am J Speech Lang Pathol. 1999;6:66–70.
10. Hanmer J, Jensen RE, Rothrock N. A reporting checklist for HealthMeasures' patient-reported outcomes: ASCQ-Me, Neuro-QoL, NIH Toolbox, and PROMIS. J Patient Rep Outcomes. 2020;4(21):1–7.

11. Schmidtke K, Metternich B. Validation of two inventories for the diagnosis and monitoring of functional memory disorders. J Psychosom Res. 2008;67:245–51.

12. Duffy JR. Motor speech disorders: substrates, differential diagnosis, and management. 4th ed. St. Louis: Elsevier; 2019.

13. Riley GD. Stuttering severity instrument. 4th ed. Torrance: WPS; 2009.

14. Zraick RI, Kempster GB, Connor NP, Thibeault S, Klaben BK, Bursac Z, et al. Establishing validity of the Consensus Auditory-Perceptual Evaluation of Voice (CAPE-V). Am J Speech Lang Pathol. 2011;20(1):14–22.

15. Nielsen G, et al. Physiotherapy for functional motor disorders: a consensus recommendation. J Neurol Neurosurg Psychiatry. 2015;86:1113–9.

16. Baker J, Barnett C, Cavalli L, et al. Management of functional communication, swallowing, cough, and related disorders: consensus recommendations for speech and language therapy. J Neurol Neursurg Psychiatry. 2021;92(10):1112–25.

17. Stone J. Functional neurological disorders: the neurological assessment as treatment. Pract Neurol. 2015;16(1):7–17.

18. Stone J, Edwards M. Trick or treat? Showing patients with functional (psychogenic) motor symptoms their physical signs. Neurology. 2012;79:282–4.

19. Stone J, Carson A. Functional neurologic disorders. Continuum. 2015;21:818–37.

20. McWhirter L, Miller N, Campbell C, Hoeritzauer I, Lawton A, Carson A, et al. Understanding Foreign Accent Syndrome. J Neurol Neurosurg Psychiatry. 2019;90(11):1265–9.

21. Ruotsalainen J, Sellman J, Lehto L, Verbeck J. Systematic review of the treatment of functional dysphonia and prevention of voice disorders. Otolaryngol Head Neck Surg. 2008;138:557–65.

22. Baker J. Functional voice disorders: clinical presentations and differential diagnosis. In: Handbook of clinical neurology functional neurologic disorders. Amsterdam: Elsevier; 2016. p. 379–88.

23. Aronson A, Bless D. Clinical voice disorder. 4th ed. New York: Thieme; 2009.

24. Spengler FB, Becker B, Kendrick KM, Conrad R, Hurlemann R, Schade G. Emotional dysregulation in psychogenic voice loss. Psychother Psychosom. 2017;86:121–3.

25. Fasano A, Valadas A, Bhatia KP, Prashanth LK, Lang AE, Munhoz RP, et al. Psychogenic facial movement disorders: clinical features and associated conditions. Mov Disord. 2012;27:1544–51.

26. Lehn A, Gelauff J, Hoeritzauer I, Ludwig L, McWhirter L, Williams S, et al. Functional neurological disorders: mechanisms and treatment. J Neurol. 2016;263:611–20.

27. Barnett C, Armes J, Smith C. Speech, language and swallowing impairments in functional neurological disorder: a scoping review. Int J Lang Comm Dis. 2018;54(3):309–20.

28. Duffy JR, Baumgartner J. Psychogenic stuttering in adults with and without neurologic disease. J Med Speech Lang Pathol. 1997;5(2):75–95.

29. Czarnecki K, Thompson JM, Seime R, Geda YE, Duffy JR, Ahlskog JE. Functional movement disorders: successful treatment with a physical therapy rehabilitation protocol. Parkinsonsim Relat Disord. 2012;18:247–51.

30. Nielsen G, Buszewicz M, Stevenson F, Hunter R, Holt K, Dudziec M, et al. Randomised feasibility study of physiotherapy for patients with functional motor symptoms. J Neurol Neurosurg Psychiatry. 2017;88(6):484–90.

31. Jacob AE, Kaelin DL, Roach AR, Ziegler CH, LaFaver K. Motor retraining (MoRe) for functional movement disorders: outcomes from a 1-week multidisciplinary rehabilitation program. PM R. 2018;10(11):1164–72.

32. Duffy JR. Functional speech disorders: clinical manifestations, diagnosis, and management. In: Handbook of clinical neurology functional neurologic disorders. Amsterdam: Elsevier; 2016. p. 379–88.

33. Gelauff J, Stone J, Edwards M, Carson A. The prognosis of functional (psychogenic) motor symptoms: a systematic review. J Neurol Neurosurg Psychiatry. 2014;84:220–6.

34. McWhirter L, Ritchie C, Stone J, Carson A. Functional cognitive disorders: a systematic review. Lancet Psychiatry. 2020;7(2):191–207.

35. Stone J, Pal S, Blackburn D, Reuber M, Thekkumpurath P, Carson A. Functional (psychogenic) cognitive disorders: a perspective from the neurology clinic. J Alzheimers Dis. 2015;48(1):5–17.

36. Teodoro T, Edwards MJ, Isaacs JD. A unifying theory for cognitive abnormalities in functional neurological disorders, fibromyalgia and chronic fatigue syndrome: systematic review. J Neurol Neurosurg Psychiatry. 2018;89:1308–19.

37. Pennington C, Hayre A, Newson M, Coulthard E. Functional cognitive disorder: a common cause of subjective cognitive symptoms. J Alzheimers Dis. 2015;48(1):S19–24.

38. American Speech-Language-Hearing Association. Scope of practice in speech-language pathology [Scope of Practice]. 2016. Available from www.asha.org/policy/. https://doi.org/10.1044/policy.SP2016-00343.

39. Alluri PR, Solit J, Leveroni CL, Goldberg K, Vehar JV, Pollak LE, et al. Cognitive complaints in motor functional neurological (conversion) disorders: a focused review and clinical perspective. Cogn Behav Neurol. 2020;33(2):77–89.

40. Ehlhardt LA, Sohlberg MM, Kennedy M, Coelho C, Ylvisaker M, Turkstra L, et al. Evidence-based practice guidelines for instructing individuals with neurogenic memory impairments: what have we learned in the past 20 years? Neuropsychol Rehabil. 2008;18(3):300–42.

41. Sohlberg MM, Turkstra LS. Optimizing cognitive rehabilitation: effective instructional methods. New York: The Guilford Press; 2011.

42. van Gils A, Stone J, Welch K, Davidson L, Kerslake D, Caesar D, et al. Management of mild traumatic brain injury. Pract Neurol. 2020;20:213–21.

Interdisciplinary Rehabilitation Approaches in Functional Movement Disorder

Kathrin LaFaver and Lucia Ricciardi

Clinical Vignette, Part I

Michael is a 21-year-old college student on a baseball scholarship. Over the past few months, he felt increasing pressure by his coach due to poor performance in several games. He also overheard two of his teammates questioning his role in the team in the school cafeteria. During the next game, he felt intense pain in his lower back. By the end of the game, he had trouble walking off the field and was sent to the Emergency Department for an evaluation. Over the next hour, he was barely able to move either leg and lost all feeling below the hips, however noticed trembling movements in his leg when trying to activate his muscles. Urgent magnetic resonance imaging (MRI) of his thoracic and lumbar spine showed no spinal cord compression or other structural changes explaining his problems. A neurologist evaluated him and admitted him to the hospital with a suspected diagnosis of Guillain-Barre syndrome. His past medical history was unremarkable except for a mild concussion a few years ago and low back pain. He was single, lived in a dorm, was a non-smoker, with alcohol use on weekends and no illicit drug use. There was no family history of neurological disorders. Over the following days, additional tests including a lumbar puncture were performed and showed normal results. He was observed to move his legs while supine and sitting, but continued to be unable to bear weight, stand or walk, and leg tremors were frequently triggered by touch or unexpected sounds. He was suspected to have Guillain-Barre syndrome, treated with intravenous immunoglobulin (IVIG) therapy and admitted to a rehabilitation hospital for a few weeks without making any progress in his neurologic function. When a new attending came on the service, his case was reviewed and he was suspected to have a functional movement disorder (FMD). Given little explanation about the new diagnosis, his parents were told in a private conversation that malingering could not be excluded, which led to hospital discharge without further follow-up recommendations. Through his primary care physician, he obtained adaptive equipment including a wheelchair and power scooter, allowing him to continue going to college. He felt increasingly frustrated by the lack of improvement in his symptoms and researched online for additional treatment avenues.

Supplementary Information The online version contains supplementary material available at [https://doi.org/10.1007/978-3-030-86495-8_26].

K. LaFaver (✉)
Movement Disorder Specialist, Saratoga Hospital Medical Group, Saratoga Springs, NY, USA
e-mail: klafaver@saratogahospital.org

L. Ricciardi
Neurosciences Research Centre, Molecular and Clinical Sciences Research Institute, St George's University of London, London, UK

© Springer Nature Switzerland AG 2022
K. LaFaver et al. (eds.), *Functional Movement Disorder*, Current Clinical Neurology,
https://doi.org/10.1007/978-3-030-86495-8_26

Introduction

Functional neurological disorder (FND) represents up to one-third of adult outpatient visits to neurologists [1], and 9% of acute admissions to inpatient neurology services [2]. In specialized movement disorder clinics, up to 20% of patients were found to carry a diagnosis of FMD [3]. Despite these staggering numbers and high costs associated with FND care, there often is a considerable delay in diagnosis and poor access to treatment services in the US and around the world [4, 5]. While FMD was previously seen as primarily psychiatric condition, with treatment confined to the realms of psychotherapy [6], there has been growing evidence for the role of multi- and interdisciplinary care models, offering comprehensive treatments to address physical and mental health aspects [7–9]. Following detailed outlines of treatment planning, psychological, physical, occupational and speech therapies for FMD in previous chapters, we will focus here on specific treatment considerations involving specialists from multiple disciplines. In regards to terminology, "multidisciplinary" teams draw on knowledge from different disciplines, each staying largely within their boundaries. "Interdisciplinary" teams analyze, synthesize and harmonize knowledge between different disciplines into a coordinated and coherent whole – encouraging elements of shared expertise [10]. For the purpose of this chapter, we will refer to "interdisciplinary treatment" with the stated goal of combining insights and perspectives from diverse healthcare professionals to create comprehensive FMD treatment services – acknowledging also that optimal treatment initiatives in FMD should likely leverage both multidisciplinary and interdisciplinary perspectives.

Planning Interdisciplinary Treatment for FMD

Treatment of FMD begins with establishing the diagnosis and explaining it to the patient within a biopsychosocial framework, addressing risk factors and triggers for symptoms and outlining next steps [11, 12]. It is important to explore patients' beliefs and understanding of the diagnosis, which can often be negatively shaped by prior healthcare encounters. There is a high degree of stigma perceived by many patients with FMD [13], also manifested in self-reported negative attitudes towards this diagnosis by about a third of movement disorder specialists in a recent survey [4]. Many neurologists perceive their role as establishing the diagnosis and referring patients to treatment, but do not wish to remain engaged longitudinally in their clinical care, often citing lack of expertise in FND and time constraints [14]. There is currently a paucity of best practice guidelines for FMD care, with the "stepped care model for functional neurological symptoms" established in Scotland in 2012 as a notable exception (http://healthcareimprovementscotland.org). According to this model, the local neurologist makes the diagnosis and provides patient education (Step 1), followed by brief interventions provided by local therapists (Step 2). If patients require additional interventions, referral to neuropsychiatric assessment and specialized FMD treatment programs and services are provided (Step 3) [15].

In creating specialized FMD clinics, comprehensive assessment of neurological function and limitations, neuropsychiatric and psychosocial histories are at the core of developing a biopsychosocial case formulation and treatment plan (see Chap. 3) [16]. For this purpose, the patient either spends dedicated time with several specialists individually or is seen by healthcare professionals with different expertise (e.g. a neurologist and a neuropsychologist) in a joint visit [17, 18]. We suggest a "core team" of a neurologist with expertise in movement disorders, a (neuro)psychologist and a physical therapist for the initial assessment and treatment planning visit, with additional participation of occupational and speech therapists if available (an alternative approach could also be to include a (neuro)psychiatrist and/or a master's level social worker as core team members). In one version of this approach, patients spend a total of 3 h in assessments, followed by an interdisciplinary team meeting of all healthcare providers to discuss

	FMD specialists	Patient 1	Patient 2	Patient 3
9am	Neurologist (N)	N	PSY	PT
10am	Physical therapist (PT) (+/-Occupational and speech therapists)	PT	N	PSY
11am	(Neuro)psychologist (PSY)	PSY	PT	N
12pm	INTERDISCIPLINARY	TEAM	MEETING	

Fig. 26.1 Example for an interdisciplinary FMD clinic schedule template

treatment planning (Fig. 26.1) [17]. To facilitate the neuropsychological assessment, patients are asked to complete a set of standardized questionnaires ahead of the visit that include screening for depression, anxiety, stressful life events, physical functioning and disability (Table 26.1). Patients are encouraged to have a family member or care partner accompany them to their visit to provide additional history and participate in education about FMD and treatment planning.

The role of the neurologist is to (1) confirm a diagnosis of FMD, (2) provide education about the disorder and set expectations for the treatment process, and (3) assess patients' and family members' understanding of FMD, agreement with the diagnosis and potential treatment obstacles. Open questions such as "What have you been told about FMD?", "What are your treatment goals?" and "Is this a good time for you to engage in treatment?" are important to work towards a shared decision making process. Assessing agreement with the diagnosis and confidence in treatment are important, as patients should fully commit to engaging in therapy, and ongoing pursuits of additional diagnostic opinions can be distracting and detrimental to treatment progress. This can be done with a 10-point Likert scale, e.g. "On a scale from 1 to 10, how confident are you that FMD is the correct diagnosis for your symptoms?" and "On a scale from 1-10, how confident are you that you will be able to get better with treatment?". If diagnostic agreement and treatment confidence are low, the

underlying reasons should be explored further and inform next steps. Motivational interviewing has been shown to help with treatment adherence and outcomes for patients with functional seizures and is explored in detail in Chap. 18 [19]. During the allied rehabilitative team assessment (physical therapist and if available, occupational and speech therapist), history is focused on current limitations and strengths of the patient, past treatment interventions, symptom triggers and alleviating factors, history of prior musculoskeletal injuries and surgeries, and pain assessment. This is followed by a standardized functional assessments of physical function and communication skills. Lastly, the (neuro)psychologist performs a psychiatric and social history including early development and education, family relationships, current/past psychiatric diagnoses and treatment interventions and current living circumstances. As mentioned before, it is helpful to have patients complete screening tools for mood disorders, anxiety, life stressors and functional disability before the visit to avoid test fatigue. Although there is currently not a standardized "FMD Inventory", many clinicians perform a selection of measures as outlined in Table 26.1. A patient-centered, qualitative interview performing a focused psychiatric interview can complement to self-report questions, particularly since it has been shown that these approaches provide only partially overlapping information [20]. A standardized video of the patient may capture typical examination features and serve as tool to

Table 26.1 Examples of potential assessment tools for patients with FMD

Patient-reported scales

Clinical Global Impression Scale, self-reported (CGI-SR)

Beck Depression Inventory II (BDI-II)

Beck Anxiety Inventory (BAI)

Patient Health Questionnaire-15 (PHQ-15), a brief instrument for identifying and monitoring somatic symptoms

Life Event Checklist for DSM-5 (LEC-5)

PROMIS-29, a short assessment containing four items from each of seven PROMIS domains (depression, anxiety, physical function, pain interference, fatigue, sleep disturbance, and ability to participate in social roles and activities)

Sheehan Disability Scale (SDS), a brief, 5-item tool assessing functional impairment in work/school, social life, and family life

Short-Form (SF-36) Health Survey, a 36-item instrument designed to capture patients' perceptions of their own health and well-being across physical and emotional domains

Brief Illness Perceptions Questionnaire (BIPQ), assessing an individual's perceptions and cognitions regarding their illness

Clinician-obtained measures

Clinical Global Impression Scale (CGI)

Simplified Functional Movement Disorder Rating Scale (S-FMDRS)

Timed Up and Go (TUG) test, a performance-based measure of functional mobility

10-m timed walking test

The Nine-Hole Peg Test (9-HPT), a standardized, quantitative assessment used to measure finger dexterity

Montreal Cognitive Assessment (MoCA), a screening tool for cognitive function

Iowa Personality Disorders Screen (IPDS), an 11-item mini-structured interview designed to detect the presence of personality disorders

document symptom severity and change over time, although the inherent nature of FMD with distractibility and variability of symptoms is a complicating factor [21, 22]. For further details on symptom monitoring over time and outcome measurements in FMD, please refer to Chap. 29.

In cases with prominent cognitive complaints, especially if past medical history suggests learning disabilities, traumatic brain injuries or other disorders with potential impact on cognitive functions, a separate visit may be needed to per-

form comprehensive neurocognitive testing prior to treatment initiation to better gauge overall cognitive strengths and relative limitations. After assessments are completed, patients are discussed in an interdisciplinary team meeting and treatment recommendations are made based on input from all team members. Depending on local availability of FMD specific treatment, pathways may include brief courses of physical, occupational or speech therapy alone or in combination with focused psychotherapy interventions, multidisciplinary interventions in an outpatient or day rehabilitation setting, or admission to a specialized inpatient rehabilitation service [9, 23–26]. Setting of mutually agreed upon treatment goals and providing a clear timeline for therapy may be helpful for patients in providing a framework and encouraging maximal engagement, although the needs especially for intensity and duration of psychotherapy will vary.

Clinical Vignette, Part II

Through online research, Michael had found a clinic offering specialized FMD treatment and was scheduled for an assessment visit. At time of his appointment, his symptoms had been present for 13 months and he was using crutches, a wheelchair, an electronic scooter and handicap-equipped car for mobility and transportation. During his neurological assessment, his strength in both upper and lower extremities was found to be normal when he was in a sitting position, as were his reflexes and sensory function. When asked to stand up, he developed irregular tremulous movements in both legs, which stopped once he sat down again. He stated that he was unable to walk independently due to leg weakness and tremor, but was able to ambulate with an unusual gait pattern by using his crutches and propelling both legs forward at the same time (see Videos 26.1 and 26.2). A diagnosis of FMD was confirmed based on typical exam findings of variable and distractible tremor and weakness. A physical therapist assessed functional abilities and limitations including current adaptive equipment use as well as typical patterns of activity throughout the day. Both he and his parents were asked about their understanding about the diagnosis of FMD and treatment expectations. His mother expressed her frustrations about the long waiting time to get professional help and previous negative experiences with some medical professionals, including the accusation that Michael was malingering. During the psychological assessment, no prior psychiatric history was reported. He was noted to have perfectionistic tendencies and had felt under stress over his athletic performance in the months prior to onset of his neurological symptoms over fear of losing his college scholarship. He was not involved in a romantic relationship and reported no problematic drinking or illicit substance use. Self-reported screening questionnaires showed no symptoms of depression or anxiety. He indicated high confidence in the accuracy of his FMD diagnosis (9/10) as well as belief that he could get better with treatment (8/10). His most important goals for treatment were to relearn normal control over his gait and handwriting, which was intermittently also impacted by tremor. The interdisciplinary team felt that he was a good candidate for a week-long, intensive FMD-specific inpatient rehabilitation program and perceived no major treatment barriers. His reliance on extensive adaptive equipment was noted and it was explained that use of his crutches and wheelchair would be minimized throughout the treatment week. A model of FMD as a brain connectivity disorder with intermittently "faulty connections" and loss of normal control over movement patterns was used to help him and his parents understand his experience. The neurologist furthermore explained that many patients in the program were able to reach significant improvements and that the goal of treatment would be retraining of normal movement patterns. Additional educational materials and an overview of the treatment program were provided.

Contraindications for FMD Treatment

It is important to note that not every intervention is suitable for every patient at a given time. Common reasons to advise against intensive interdisciplinary FMD treatment include (1) chronic pain or chronic fatigue as the most disabling symptom; (2) presence of severe and unstable psychiatric conditions including depression with suicidality, post-traumatic stress disorder (PTSD) or alcohol/drug misuse; (3) predominance of functional seizures, purely sensory or cognitive complaints. Of note, the comorbidity of functional seizures may not necessarily be an absolute contraindication in some instances – particularly in patients who have identifiable triggers/warning signs AND have active FMD symptoms that would otherwise warrant intensive motor-specific treatments. In many of the above cases, other treatment approaches are often more suitable such as chronic pain rehabilitation programs, psychotherapy and/or intensive psychiatric care. Following a team discussion, treatment recommendations should be communicated to the patient and care partner and provided in written form, and any questions or concerns should be addressed. Other treatment obstacles may include financial or time constraints, pending litigation or other legal action and may necessitate a delay in treatment initiation. Social workers and case managers also have an important role in providing additional resources if treatments other than those directly available at a given center are recommended. To ensure adequate care, follow-up visits in the FMD clinic should be offered to all patients to monitor treatment progress. Patients initially triaged to undergo chronic pain rehabilitation or intensive psychiatric therapies should be reassessed and may benefit from FMD specific therapies at a later date.

What Is the Evidence for Interdisciplinary FMD Treatment?

Throughout this book, a strong focus on interdisciplinary (and multidisciplinary) approaches in the treatment of FMD is emphasized. As acknowledged earlier, there remains a paucity of FMD treatment studies, especially of well-designed randomized controlled treat-

ment (RCT) trials. In Table 26.2, we provide an ferences in patient selection, the treatment set-
overview of select multi- and interdisciplinary ting (e.g. outpatient versus inpatient), duration
treatment programs in the literature. Due to dif- and intensity of treatment, specifics of therapies

Table 26.2 Examples of multidisciplinary rehabilitation programs for FMD

Study	Design and sample size	Setting and duration	Multidisciplinary program	Results
Delargy et al. (1986) [31]	Not specified, $n = 6$ with functional leg weakness	Inpatient neurology and spinal injuries units; duration not stated	Physical therapy, nurse and consultant inputs	All six patients were wheelchair bound before admission and were able to walk within a mean of 41 days (range 10–70 days). They continued to be independent at follow-up at mean of 10 months.
Speed (1996) [32]	Retrospective; $n = 10$ with CD, all with gait problems	Inpatient rehabilitation unit (4–22 days)	PT, OT, recreational therapy, psychological treatment	All improved at discharge, measured with the Functional Independence Measure gait score. At follow-up, 7/9 had maintained improvement.
Heruti et al. (2002) [33]	Retrospective; $n = 34$ with functional weakness	Inpatient in a rehabilitation unit (duration not stated)	PT, OT, psychological therapy, nurse, social worker, psychiatric consultation	26% complete, 29% partial recovery, 44% unchanged.
Moene et al. (2002) [27]	Randomized controlled trial, multidisciplinary therapy with/without hypnosis. $n = 45$ with motor CD	Inpatient in general psychiatric unit (12 weeks)	PT and psychological therapy +/− hypnosis Team: nurse, group therapist, creative therapy therapist, sports therapist, PT	65% in both groups very much improved. 83% improved at 6 months, hypnosis was not influencing outcome.
McCormack et al. (2013) [34]	Retrospective; $n = 33$ with motor CD	Inpatient neuropsychiatric ward (mean stay 101 days)	PT, OT, SLT, psychological therapy, neuropsychiatrist evaluation	Significant improvement in modified Rankin Scale.
Aybeck et al. (2013) [35]	Part prospective and part chart review ($n = 23$ with CD, 12 intervention versus 11 standard care)	Outpatient neurology and psychiatry consultations (2.4 mean number of visits)	Multidisciplinary intervention (neurology and psychiatry)	83% of cases and 36% of controls had a good subjective outcome. Cases had a significantly better improvements of SF-36.
Saifee et al. (2012) [36]	Retrospective; $n = 26$ patients with FMD	Inpatient treatment in neuropsychiatric unit (4 weeks)	PT, OT, CBT, nursing care, neurologist and psychiatrist evaluations	58% reported that the program had been useful at follow-up (mean 7 years).
Demartini et al. (2014) [37]	Prospective; $n = 66$ patients with FMD	Inpatient treatment in neuropsychiatric unit (4 weeks)	PT, OT, CBT, nursing care, neurologist and psychiatrist evaluations	2/3 rated better/much better by CGI.
Jordbru et al. (2014) [28]	Randomized cross-over study (4-weeks waiting list as control), $n = 60$ patients with functional gait disorder	Inpatient rehabilitation unit (3-week)	Physician, PT, OT, nurse and an educator in adapted physical activity	Significant improvement in physical function and quality of life in cases compared to controls (FMS, FIM, SF12).

Table 26.2 (continued)

Study	Design and sample size	Setting and duration	Multidisciplinary program	Results
Hubschmid et al. (2015) [29]	RCT (interdisciplinary psychotherapeutic intervention versus standard care); n = 23 patients with motor FND and functional seizures	Inpatients neurology unit (4–6 sessions over 2 months)	Interdisciplinary psychotherapeutic intervention + psychiatry and neurology consultants assessments.	Significant improvement of physical and psychological symptoms (SDQ-20, CGI, mental health component of the SF-36, Beck Depression Inventory). Reduction in new hospital stays after intervention.
Jacob et al. (2018) [38]	Retrospective; n = 32 patients with FMD	Inpatient rehabilitation unit (1-week)	Physical, occupational, and speech therapy (if applicable) and psychotherapy	At discharge, 87% of patients reported improvement in CGI, maintained in 69% at 6-months follow-up. 59% improvement in PMDRS.
Jimenez et al. (2019) [30]	Retrospective; n = 49 patients with chronic pain and functional seizures or FMD	Interdisciplinary chronic pain rehabilitation program (3–4 weeks, day rehab setting)	Pain rehabilitation experts (pain psychiatrist, psychologist, PT/OT, nurse), interventions included individual and group psychotherapy, medication management, biofeedback and PT/OT.	Significant improvements were seen in pain-related disability, depression, anxiety and timed gait measures (TUG, 6 min walk test).
Lidstone et al. (2020) [18]	Prospective; n = 11 patients with FMD	Outpatients (6-session, bi-weekly)	Therapy was simultaneously delivered by the neurologist, neuropsychiatrist and physiotherapist in 45-min appointment	7/11 (64%) of patients had "much" or "very much" improved at CGI, which was sustained at 3 months.
Petrochilos et al. (2020) [25]	Prospective; n = 78 patients with FND	Outpatient (day-unit) treatment (2 days a week for 5-week)	Neuropsychiatry, cognitive behavioural therapy, PT, OT, psychoeducation and family meetings	Significant improvements at discharge and at 6-month follow-up in somatic symptoms (PHQ15), depression (PHQ9), anxiety (GAD7), health and social functioning (HONOS), functionality (COPM), health status (EQ-5D-5L) and CGI.

Abbreviations: *CD* conversion disorder, *CBT* Cognitive behavioral therapy, *CGI* Clinical Global Impression Scale, *COPM* Canadian Occupational Performance Measure, *EQ-5D-5L* EuroQol 5 Dimension 5 Level, *FIM* Functional independence measure, *FMD* Functional Mobility Scale, *FMS* Functional Mobility Scale, *GAD-7* General anxiety disorder-7, *HONOS* Health of the Nation Outcome, *MoRE* Motor Retraining, *OT* occupational therapy, *PHQ9* Patient Health Questionnaire, *PHQ15* patient rated somatic symptoms, *PMDRS* Psychogenic Movement Disorder Rating Scale, *PT* physical therapy, *SDQ-20* Somatoform Dissociation Questionnaire, *SF-36* Short-Form health Survey, *SLP* speech and language therapy, *TUG* timed up and go test provided as well as outcome reporting, it is difficult to draw direct comparisons between programs. Despite these differences, there are many commonalities in approaches, which we will highlight in the next section. To date, there have only been a few single-center prospective RCTs looking at multi/interdisciplinary treatment interventions for FMD. A study published by Moene et al. in 2002 compared the added effects of hypnosis to a multidisciplinary rehabilitation intervention in an inpatient psychiatry setting. Both intervention groups improved to similar degrees, without added benefits shown in the hypnosis group [27]. Jordbru et al. compared a multidisciplinary intervention administered during a 3-week inpatient rehabilitation stay against a wait-list control, demonstrating significant improvements in physical function and quality of life in the treatment group [28]. In another study looking at the effects of an interdisciplinary psychotherapy intervention with combined psychiatric and neurological visits (4–6 sessions over 2 months in an inpatient setting), improvements in physical and psychological measures were found in the treatment group compared to standard care, although limitations of the study include a small case number and mixed patient population [29]. An interesting approach was taken by Jimenez et al. at the Cleveland Clinic, reporting improvements in measures of physical and mental health in a group of patients with chronic pain and comorbid FND in a recent retrospective case series. Although FND was not the treatment focus, patients seemed to benefit from intensive interdisciplinary treatments offered in a day rehab setting that included individual and group psychotherapy, medication management (detoxification from opioids and benzodiazepines), biofeedback and other relaxation techniques, and physical/occupational therapy [30]. Given the high prevalence of chronic pain syndromes in patients with FMD, treatment programs primarily targeting pain should be further studied regarding therapeutic benefit on FMD symptoms.

Treatment Principles

Specific treatment principles for psychotherapy modalities, physical, occupational and speech therapy are covered extensively in Chaps. 21, 22, 23, 24, and 25. In this section, important overarching principles will be emphasized, with a focus on strategies important within an interdisciplinary team approach. Establishing a diagnosis of FMD and communicating the diagnosis in understandable terms needs to take place prior to initiation of other treatment to help maximize therapeutic benefit. Unfortunately, it remains a common experience for many physical and occupational therapists to receive patient referrals with neurological symptoms such as weakness and "negative workup", yet without a specific diagnosis made. In these situations, patient progress is typically slow or halting, as risk or trigger factors related to symptoms remain unexplored. Similarly, patients benefit from hearing a uniform message from all healthcare professionals involved in their care regarding diagnosis and treatment goals. This deserves special mentioning, as many neurologists have experienced psychologists doubting a diagnosis of FMD if no obvious trauma history is identified in the neuropsychological assessment [4]. Indicating belief and recognition of patients' symptoms and expressing confidence in their ability to regain control over motor function can be important first steps to overcome prior negative experiences in the healthcare system, and instill trust towards the treatment process. See Table 26.3 for additional principles important in interdisciplinary FMD care.

In case of stalled treatment progress or relapses, perpetuating factors and other potential treatment obstacles should be reviewed. If no positive response to treatment is seen, reassessment for perpetuating factors and other potential treatment obstacles should take place, as outlined in Chap. 30. New symptoms may emerge over time, which are best assessed for in follow-up visits with the treating physician [39].

Table 26.3 Important principles in interdisciplinary FMD care

A diagnosis needs to be established and communicated prior to subsequent treatment

Patient and family/caregiver education and shared goal setting is a crucial step towards successful treatment and relapse prevention

Patients should be treated respectfully and empathetically, recognizing and acknowledging prior negative experiences in the healthcare system

The diagnosis of FMD should be normalized and understood within a biopsychosocial formulation, outlining steps towards getting better

Consistent messaging on diagnosis and treatment goals from all healthcare professionals is important

Positive reinforcement is an important principle in supporting treatment gains

Regular communication between members of the treatment team is important for optimal information flow and treatment consistency

Patient independence and self-management strategies should be fostered

Relapse and emergency planning is important to reduce ER and urgent care visits

Recognizing and addressing frequent comorbidities, specifically chronic pain, fatigue, somatic symptom disorder, health anxiety and mood disorders is covered in Chaps. 14 and 22. The common co-occurrence of autonomic dysfunction including postural orthostatic tachycardia syndrome (POTS) and functional gastrointestinal disorders in FMD is thought to be related to shared imbalances in activity of the sympathetic and parasympathetic nervous systems, but has not been extensively studied in adult patients [40, 41]. Recognizing autonomic dysfunction and referring patients to specialists such as cardiologists or gastroenterologists for additional assessment and management is important [42, 43]. Patients with untreated POTS will continue to experience symptoms including dizziness, headaches, and exercise intolerance, actively impeding treatment progress or limiting their ability to participate in physical therapy. Assessment of chronic fatigue may include evaluations for sleep disorders, mood disorders, other medically contributing factors (e.g. anemnia, hypothyroidism, Vitamin B12 deficiency), or sedating medication effects. If other factors have been excluded, optimizing sleep schedules, regular exercise individualized to the patient's abilities and dietary interventions may have promise in addressing this often disabling symptom. Overall, more research is needed – including how to best therapeutically address the range of non-motor symptoms that are frequently concurrent in patients with FMD.

Clinical Vignette, Part III

Several weeks after his initial assessment, Michael was admitted for a 1-week long, specialized inpatient FMD treatment program. After being oriented to the treatment facility, his first day included detailed assessments and goal setting with his physical and occupational therapists, as well as his first session with a rehabilitation psychologist. Over the next 5 days, he re-established control over simple movements with his legs such as weight shifting and tapping his toes. Motor imagery, a commonly used intervention in stroke rehabilitation and training of athletes, was used prior to each training session. His therapists guided him to visually imagine his goal activities as if he was performing them, breaking down movement patterns in small steps. He was also introduced to deep breathing techniques and mindful meditation. By using relaxation methods in his physical therapy sessions, he was able to quickly progress from foot tapping exercises to supported walking on bars, independent walking and finally high-level gait activities including running and navigating an obstacle course (see Videos 26.3 and 26.4). His five treatment sessions with the psychologist were based on the self-guided workbook entitled "Overcoming Functional Neurological Disorders: A Five Area Approach [44]", and covered topics such as identification of symptom triggers, mind-body connections, challenging unhelpful thinking and planning behavioral changes. He recognized that he had always struggled with expressing negative emotions and took to journaling as a way of organizing his thoughts and processing daily events. Discussing his identity as an athlete and perceived threats towards this role by physical injury and other factors started a process of self-exploration and different options of addressing difficult situations. Throughout the week, a physiatrist was overseeing his treatment, working together with the rest of the team on outlining the treatment process and providing positive reinforcement of therapy gains. Furthermore, he addressed his chronic low back pain and helped in formulating a plan on his return to school and social activities without adaptive equipment. There was a separate meeting with Michael's parents towards the end of the treatment week to address their questions and provide advice on how to best support him, fostering his independence and preventing relapses.

Follow Up Planning and Relapse Prevention

Following completion of the FMD-specific treatment program, assessments performed during the initial visit should be repeated to provide objective measures of improvement. Taking standardized videos at the beginning and end of therapy and sharing them with the patient can also provide a helpful tool of reinforcing treatment success. Providing home exercises and an individualized relapse prevention plan, focusing on aspects of physical and mental health, is a crucial step in helping patients develop confidence as they return in their home environments and expand their activities. The need for regular rest periods to avoid "boom and bust" patterns needs to be emphasized, and a gradual return to previous work and social activities is important to avoid overexertion and allow for adaptation to increased stimulation.

Planning for regular follow-up care is important to monitor symptoms longitudinally, especially in cases where ongoing symptoms are present. Exploration of perpetuating factors as well as potentially new precipitating factors, facilitating therapy engagement by active listening and inquiring about obstacles to treatment can all fall within the realm of ongoing neurological care [39], while other aspects of treatment may continue to be provided by psychiatrists, psychologists, social workers or rehabilitation specialists. Taking therapy breaks and setting limits to treatment can also be an important concept to foster independence and self-management of symptoms. Once FMD-specific treatment is completed, it is often possible for the patient's local neurologist or primary care physician to take over care of ongoing needs, e.g. management of comorbid conditions such as migraines.

Treatment Modalities Under Development

Since the onset of the COVID-19 pandemic, many healthcare providers have rapidly adopted telemedicine services, which can provide effective ways for patients to stay connected with specialized FMD services that are often not available in their immediate geographical area [45]. Further research is needed to study the appropriateness and effectiveness of telemedicine visits as long-term care models, although results from the treatment of functional seizures via telemedicine have been encouraging [46]. In a pilot study testing the delivery of physical therapy through telemedicine, significant improvements were seen in ratings of functional movements, general health, vitality, social functioning and mental health [47]. Delivery of psychoeducation or therapy interventions in a group setting also holds promise and may address the lack of mental health professionals readily available to deliver FMD treatment [48, 49]. Other treatment modalities currently under development include virtual reality-delivered mirror visual feedback and exposure therapy [50] and neuromodulation approaches to specifically target sensorimotor and limbic pathways affected in FMD, as outlined in Chap. 28 [8, 51].

Insurance Coverage of FMD Treatment

In determining treatment pathways for FMD, availability of treatment services and coverage by the patient's insurance are often important considerations. In the US, many insurance carriers exclude mental health services from coverage or make them available at a high self-pay rate. Since FMD is often considered under psychiatric diagnostic coding, this can create a major barrier towards appropriate treatment services. Ongoing advocacy efforts to raise awareness for the high impact of providing adequate and timely treatment for patients with FMD is important to work towards system changes. Potential cost savings in avoiding chronic disability and high healthcare utilization in often young patients with FMD may provide a motivator for insurance companies to offer more comprehensive treatment coverage.

Summary

- There is growing evidence for the effectiveness of interdisciplinary treatment approaches for FMD.
- Treatment needs to be planned carefully and should be informed by the biopsychosocial case formulation to guide interventions.
- Treatment for FMD may be delivered in the outpatient, intensive day rehabilitation, or inpatient hospital setting.
- Specialists included in multidisciplinary treatment of FMD may include neurologists, physiatrists, psychiatrists, (neuro) psychologists, physical, occupational and speech therapists, social workers, and other rehabilitation experts.
- More research is needed to help determine the most effective treatment models in regards to treatment intensity and duration and determine long-term treatment outcomes.
- Access to treatment remains difficult for many patients in the US and around the world due to a paucity of specialized FMD treatment centers.

References

1. Stone J, Carson A, Duncan R, Roberts R, Warlow C, Hibberd C, et al. Who is referred to neurology clinics?--the diagnoses made in 3781 new patients. Clin Neurol Neurosurg. 2010;112(9):747–51.
2. Beharry J, Palmer D, Wu T, Wilson D, Le Heron C, Mason D, et al. Functional neurological disorders presenting as emergencies to secondary care. Eur J Neurol. 2021;28(5):1441–5.
3. Hallett M. Psychogenic movement disorders: a crisis for neurology. Curr Neurol Neurosci Rep. 2006;6(4):269–71.
4. LaFaver K, Lang AE, Stone J, Morgante F, Edwards M, Lidstone S, et al. Opinions and clinical practices related to diagnosing and managing functional (psychogenic) movement disorders: changes in the last decade. Eur J Neurol. 2020;27(6):975–84.
5. Stephen CD, Fung V, Lungu CI, Espay AJ. Assessment of emergency department and inpatient use and costs in adult and pediatric functional neurological disorders. JAMA Neurol. 2021;78(1):88–101.
6. Kanaan RAA. Freud's hysteria and its legacy. Handb Clin Neurol. 2016;139:37–44.
7. Espay AJ, Aybek S, Carson A, Edwards MJ, Goldstein LH, Hallett M, et al. Current concepts in diagnosis and treatment of functional neurological disorders. JAMA Neurol. 2018;75(9):1132–41.
8. LaFaver K, LaFrance WC, Price ME, Rosen PB, Rapaport M. Treatment of functional neurological disorder: current state, future directions, and a research agenda. CNS Spectr. 2020:1–7. https://doi.org/10.1017/S1092852920002138.
9. Saxena A, Godena E, Maggio J, Perez DL. Towards an outpatient model of care for motor functional neurological disorders: a neuropsychiatric perspective. Neuropsychiatr Dis Treat. 2020;16:2119–34.
10. Choi BC, Pak AW. Multidisciplinarity, interdisciplinarity and transdisciplinarity in health research, services, education and policy: 1. Definitions, objectives, and evidence of effectiveness. Clin Invest Med. 2006;29(6):351–64.
11. Carson A, Lehn A, Ludwig L, Stone J. Explaining functional disorders in the neurology clinic: a photo story. Pract Neurol. 2016;16(1):56–61.
12. Stone J, Burton C, Carson A. Recognising and explaining functional neurological disorder. BMJ. 2020;371:m3745.
13. MacDuffie KE, Grubbs L, Best T, LaRoche S, Mildon B, Myers L, et al. Stigma and functional neurological disorder: a research agenda targeting the clinical encounter. CNS Spectr. 2020:1–6. https://doi.org/10.1017/S1092852920002084.

14. Perez DL, Haller AL, Espay AJ. Should neurologists diagnose and manage functional neurologic disorders? It is complicated. Neurol Clin Pract. 2019;9(2):165–7.

15. Healthcare Improvement Scotland; National Health Service in Scotland. Stepped care for functional neurological symptoms. Healthcare Improvement Scotland; 2012.

16. Aybek S, Lidstone SC, Nielsen G, MacGillivray L, Bassetti CL, Lang AE, et al. What is the role of a specialist assessment clinic for FND? Lessons from three national referral centers. J Neuropsychiatry Clin Neurosci. 2020;32(1):79–84.

17. Jacob AE, Smith CA, Jablonski ME, Roach AR, Paper KM, Kaelin DL, et al. Multidisciplinary clinic for functional movement disorders (FMD): 1-year experience from a single centre. J Neurol Neurosurg Psychiatry. 2018;89(9):1011–2.

18. Lidstone SC, MacGillivray L, Lang AE. Integrated therapy for functional movement disorders: time for a change. Mov Disord Clin Pract. 2020;7(2):169–74.

19. Tolchin B, Baslet G, Martino S, Suzuki J, Blumenfeld H, Hirsch LJ, et al. Motivational interviewing techniques to improve psychotherapy adherence and outcomes for patients with psychogenic nonepileptic seizures. J Neuropsychiatry Clin Neurosci. 2019; https://doi.org/10.1176/appi.neuropsych.19020045.

20. Kranick S, Ekanayake V, Martinez V, Ameli R, Hallett M, Voon V. Psychopathology and psychogenic movement disorders. Mov Disord. 2011;26(10):1844–50.

21. Hinson VK, Cubo E, Comella CL, Goetz CG, Leurgans S. Rating scale for psychogenic movement disorders: scale development and clinimetric testing. Mov Disord. 2005;20(12):1592–7.

22. Nielsen G, Ricciardi L, Meppelink AM, Holt K, Teodoro T, Edwards M. A simplified version of the psychogenic movement disorders rating scale: the simplified functional movement disorders rating scale (S-FMDRS). Mov Disord Clin Pract. 2017;4(5):710–6.

23. Nielsen G, Buszewicz M, Stevenson F, Hunter R, Holt K, Dudziec M, et al. Randomised feasibility study of physiotherapy for patients with functional motor symptoms. J Neurol Neurosurg Psychiatry. 2017;88(6):484–90.

24. Duffy JR. Functional speech disorders: clinical manifestations, diagnosis, and management. Handb Clin Neurol. 2016;139:379–88.

25. Petrochilos P, Elmalem MS, Patel D, Louissaint H, Hayward K, Ranu J, et al. Outcomes of a 5-week individualised MDT outpatient (day-patient) treatment programme for functional neurological symptom disorder (FNSD). J Neurol. 2020;267(9):2655–66.

26. Gilmour GS, Jenkins JD. Inpatient treatment of functional neurological disorder: a scoping review. Can J Neurol Sci. 2021;48(2):204–17.

27. Moene FC, Spinhoven P, Hoogduin KA, van Dyck R. A randomised controlled clinical trial on the additional effect of hypnosis in a comprehensive treatment programme for in-patients with conversion disorder of the motor type. Psychother Psychosom. 2002;71(2):66–76.

28. Jordbru AA, Smedstad LM, Klungsoyr O, Martinsen EW. Psychogenic gait disorder: a randomized controlled trial of physical rehabilitation with one-year follow-up. J Rehabil Med. 2014;46(2):181–7.

29. Hubschmid M, Aybek S, Maccaferri GE, Chocron O, Gholamrezaee MM, Rossetti AO, et al. Efficacy of brief interdisciplinary psychotherapeutic intervention for motor conversion disorder and nonepileptic attacks. Gen Hosp Psychiatry. 2015;37(5):448–55.

30. Jimenez XF, Aboussouan A, Johnson J. Functional neurological disorder responds favorably to interdisciplinary rehabilitation models. Psychosomatics. 2019;60(6):556–62.

31. Delargy MA, Peatfield RC, Burt AA. Successful rehabilitation in conversion paralysis. Br Med J (Clin Res Ed). 1986;292(6537):1730–1.

32. Speed J. Behavioral management of conversion disorder: retrospective study. Arch Phys Med Rehabil. 1996;77(2):147–54.

33. Heruti RJ, Reznik J, Adunski A, Levy A, Weingarden H, Ohry A. Conversion motor paralysis disorder: analysis of 34 consecutive referrals. Spinal Cord. 2002;40(7):335–40.

34. McCormack R, Moriarty J, Mellers JD, Shotbolt P, Pastena R, Landes N, et al. Specialist inpatient treatment for severe motor conversion disorder: a retrospective comparative study. J Neurol Neurosurg Psychiatry. 2014;85(8):895–900.

35. Aybek S, Hubschmid M, Mossinger C, Berney A, Vingerhoets F. Early intervention for conversion disorder: neurologists and psychiatrists working together. Acta Neuropsychiatr. 2013;25(1):52–6.

36. Saifee TA, Kassavetis P, Parees I, Kojovic M, Fisher L, Morton L, et al. Inpatient treatment of functional motor symptoms: a long-term follow-up study. J Neurol. 2012;259(9):1958–63.

37. Demartini B, Batla A, Petrochilos P, Fisher L, Edwards MJ, Joyce E. Multidisciplinary treatment for functional neurological symptoms: a prospective study. J Neurol. 2014;261(12):2370–7.

38. Jacob AE, Kaelin DL, Roach AR, Ziegler CH, LaFaver K. Motor retraining (MoRe) for functional movement disorders: outcomes from a 1-week multidisciplinary rehabilitation program. PM R. 2018;10(11):1164–72.

39. Adams C, Anderson J, Madva EN, LaFrance WC Jr, Perez DL. You've made the diagnosis of functional neurological disorder: now what? Pract Neurol. 2018;18(4):323–30.

40. Maurer CW, Liu VD, LaFaver K, Ameli R, Wu T, Toledo R, et al. Impaired resting vagal tone in patients with functional movement disorders. Parkinsonism Relat Disord. 2016;30:18–22.

41. van der Kruijs SJ, Vonck KE, Langereis GR, Feijs LM, Bodde NM, Lazeron RH, et al. Autonomic nervous system functioning associated with psychogenic nonepileptic seizures: analysis of heart rate variability. Epilepsy Behav. 2016;54:14–9.

42. Mar PL, Raj SR. Postural orthostatic tachycardia syndrome: mechanisms and new therapies. Annu Rev Med. 2020;71:235–48.

43. Black CJ, Drossman DA, Talley NJ, Ruddy J, Ford AC. Functional gastrointestinal disorders: advances in understanding and management. Lancet. 2020;396(10263):1664–74.

44. Williams CC, Carson A, Smith S, Sharpe M, Cavanagh J, Kent C. Overcoming functional neurological symptoms: a five areas approach. 1st ed. CRC Press; 2011.

45. Perez DL, Biffi A, Camprodon JA, Caplan DN, Chemali Z, Kritzer MD, et al. Telemedicine in behavioral neurology-neuropsychiatry: opportunities and challenges catalyzed by COVID-19. Cogn Behav Neurol. 2020;33(3):226–9.

46. LaFrance WC Jr, Ho WLN, Bhatla A, Baird GL, Altalib HH, Godleski L. Treatment of psychogenic nonepileptic seizures (PNES) using video telehealth. Epilepsia. 2020;61(11):2572–82.

47. Demartini B, Bombieri F, Goeta D, Gambini O, Ricciardi L, Tinazzi M. A physical therapy programme for functional motor symptoms: a telemedicine pilot study. Parkinsonism Relat Disord. 2020;76:108–11.

48. Cope SR, Smith JG, King T, Agrawal N. Evaluation of a pilot innovative cognitive-behavioral therapy-based psychoeducation group treatment for functional non-epileptic attacks. Epilepsy Behav. 2017;70(Pt A):238–44.

49. Bullock KD, Mirza N, Forte C, Trockel M. Group dialectical-behavior therapy skills training for conversion disorder with seizures. J Neuropsychiatry Clin Neurosci. 2015;27(3):240–3.

50. Bullock K, Won AS, Bailenson J, Friedman R. Virtual reality-delivered mirror visual feedback and exposure therapy for FND: a midpoint report of a randomized controlled feasibility study. J Neuropsychiatry Clin Neurosci. 2020;32(1):90–4.

51. Pollak TA, Nicholson TR, Edwards MJ, David AS. A systematic review of transcranial magnetic stimulation in the treatment of functional (conversion) neurological symptoms. J Neurol Neurosurg Psychiatry. 2014;85(2):191–7.

Placebo Effects and Functional Neurological Disorder: Helpful or Harmful?

27

Matthew J. Burke and Sarah C. Lidstone

Case Vignette

S.V. is a 25-year-old woman who was evaluated in a Movement Disorders Clinic for painful, abnormal posturing of her legs. At age 15, she developed difficulty writing, experiencing excessive gripping of the pen and flexion of her wrist that she could not control, sometimes with a tremor. She was diagnosed with writer's cramp by a neurologist and was then lost to follow-up. Two months prior to presentation, her right ankle

M. J. Burke (✉)
Neuropsychiatry Program, Department of Psychiatry, Sunnybrook Health Sciences Centre, University of Toronto, Toronto, ON, Canada

Division of Neurology, Department of Medicine, Sunnybrook Health Sciences Centre, University of Toronto, Toronto, ON, Canada

Hurvitz Brain Sciences Research Program, Sunnybrook Research Institute, Toronto, ON, Canada

Program in Placebo Studies, Beth Israel Deaconess Medical Center, Harvard Medical School, Boston, MA, USA
e-mail: matt.burke@utoronto.ca

S. C. Lidstone (✉)
Integrated Movement Disorders Program, Toronto Rehabilitation Institute, Toronto, ON, Canada

Edmond J. Safra Program in Parkinson's Disease and the Morton and Gloria Shulman Movement Disorders Clinic, Toronto Western Hospital, University Health Network, Toronto, ON, Canada

Division of Neurology, Department of Medicine, University of Toronto, Toronto, ON, Canada
e-mail: Sarah.lidstone@uhnresearch.ca

started turning in when she tried to walk. It appeared suddenly one morning when she woke up. She developed painful spasms. When the neurologist examined her, she had variable and distractible plantarflexion and inversion of the right ankle, but it remained fixed whenever she tried to walk. Her symptoms were consistent with functional dystonia. Although there were clear positive signs, her neurologist wondered about the possibility of a primary dystonia given her prior history of writer's cramp. To clarify the diagnosis, she decided to use placebo in the guise of botulinum toxin with the added benefit that if it worked, the patient might also experience some relief from her painful spasms. She instructed the patient that she was injecting botulinum toxin into the leg to relax the overactive muscles and let the brain resume "normal" control of her ankle. There was immediate improvement of the dystonia with injection of saline into the tibialis posterior. The patient was able to regain normal walking within minutes in the clinic. She became tearful and expressed profound relief that she could once again walk normally. She was strongly encouraged to continue to focus on the leg and to walk as much as possible, to allow the brain to "rewire." She experienced fluctuating benefit over the next 3 months. At her follow-up appointment, it was revealed that she had in fact received saline and not botulinum toxin, to help with the diagnosis. She was told that the immediate improvement was indicative of functional dysto-

© Springer Nature Switzerland AG 2022
K. LaFaver et al. (eds.), *Functional Movement Disorder*, Current Clinical Neurology,
https://doi.org/10.1007/978-3-030-86495-8_27

nia. The patient became angry and felt that she had been lied to. She left the appointment in tears and did not return to clinic.

Introduction

In no other area of medicine has placebo been so seriously considered for sanctioned use in diagnosis or treatment as it has in functional neurological disorder (FND). Why is this the case? FND and placebo effects seem to be inexorably linked over medical history, their paths intertwining, each influencing the perception of the other, highlighting the fundamental medical debate about what constitutes "real" disease and "real" treatment. Placebos have been used to try to diagnose and treat FND over the last two centuries. However, as FND has evolved through its different identities – hysteria, conversion disorder, psychosomatic, and now functional neurological disorder – under the shifting terrains of neurology and psychiatry, and as placebo effects have risen in parallel to a legitimate field of study in its own right, attitudes toward placebo use in FND have remained a source of controversy. Here we provide a critical perspective and synthesis of the literature on the important considerations for the use of placebo in FND, and attempt to resolve whether placebos are helpful, or harmful.

A Primer on Placebo

Placebo effects can be defined as therapeutic benefits derived from the context surrounding administration of a treatment rather than the treatment itself. This involves a number of complex inter-relationships between environmental factors such as treatment cues and patient-physician interactions and internal factors such as the patient's expectancies, emotions and cognitive schema [1]. Much of the research investigating placebo effects to date has been in the fields of neuroscience and psychology. Neuroimaging studies have demonstrated that placebo effects are capable of meaningfully modulating brain regions/networks and neuropharmacological

studies have identified many associated neurotransmitter systems including endogenous opioids, dopamine and endocannabinoids [2]. Evolving psychological models emphasize roles for both conscious and unconscious processes in placebo effects. Conscious expectancies (expectations) may be acquired from verbal instructions/suggestion, prior experience of treatment effects, and/or social observation, while unconscious expectancies may be established through conditioning and other mechanisms [3]. We emphasize that suggestion is just one way in which placebo effects may be generated, as this will be a topic discussed extensively in the next section. The vast majority of placebo effects research to date has been based on data collected from healthy individuals studied in an experimental setting, with placebo analgesia being the most commonly used paradigm [1].

In clinical medicine, placebo effects have largely been ignored or considered a nuisance based on their role in placebo-controlled clinical trials. It is commonly ingrained into medical trainees that placebo effects are an enemy that thwart the development of treatments, rather than a potential source of therapeutic benefit for patients. A few isolated fields, including Parkinson's disease, chronic pain, mood disorders and other neuropsychiatric conditions have interrogated placebo effects in a clinical context and are shedding light on their importance in medicine [4]. Nocebo effects, briefly defined as new or worsening symptoms in response to negative expectations or beliefs, also have large impacts in clinical practice and clinical trials [3]. Much of the work on nocebo effects in medicine focuses on their potential role in the development of medication side effects (e.g., via providing patients with expectation of possible side effects during consent for a given treatment) [5]. Furthermore, conducting a review of symptoms can contribute to the generation of functional symptoms experienced by patients, demonstrating the critical role of the therapeutic interaction and expectation in the illness experience. Whether acknowledged by clinicians or not, placebo and nocebo effects are ubiquitous elements of all clinical practice and for certain patient populations may be harnessed to optimize and/or undermine treatment. In the following sections we will explore the potential role for leveraging placebo effects in the management of patients with FND. We will critically examine arguments in favor and against, weighing conceptual and neurobiological rationales with practical and ethical considerations.

Historical Context for the Use of Placebo in FND

Both FND and placebo effects date back to the oldest medical texts. Hysteria is among one of the earliest recognized neurological disorders, with case descriptions dating back to before 400 BC [6] – and persisted until the 1960s [7]. The history of medicine is the history of placebo effects, given that early medical treatments employed a wide variety of substances to treat a wide range of physical ailments with little to no specificity [8]. Both have been fixtures in the evolution of medicine, and both have struggled at various times to gain legitimacy. The use of hypnosis to treat hysteria employed by Charcot, Breuer and Freud; the employment of suggestion therapy to treat shell shock and war neuroses by Max Nonna; the rise of psychosomatic medicine in the 1920s in the German and American schools; and the shift toward holistic health in the 1970s; each of these periods in medicine illustrates the changing prevailing attitudes and beliefs encompassing the mind-body relationship, and points of convergence and overlap between FND and placebo effects.

Suggestion provides one of the most direct links between FND and placebo effects, and warrants a brief discussion. The power of suggestion has a long, complex and conflicted history, involving demonic possession, mesmerism and hypnosis, from at least the sixteenth century. Prominent Harvard medical historian Anne Harrington writes "Were these strange states of mind the product of powerful external forces – satanic, physical or psychological? Alternatively, were they the product of outright fraud? Or again, were they perhaps the result of unwitting self-

deception? No other narrative of modern mind-body medicine is as fundamentally conflicted about its own epistemological and ethical message as this one, and its history is the primary reason" [9]. Simply put, suggestion is the influence provoked by an idea suggested and accepted by the brain. Suggestibility – a natural tendency of human beings – became linked to hysteria by Hippolyte Bernheim, an internist and contemporary of Charcot in the 1880s. Bernheim strived to demonstrate that the symptoms of the "hypnotizable hysterics" of Charcot could be replicated and subsequently cured by the use of suggestion, with the implication that hysterical symptoms were therefore products of suggestion. Charcot devoted a substantial portion of his career and resources to the study of hysteria at the Salpêtrière, painstakingly using case studies and photography to document the patterns he observed in women suffering from episodic convulsions (what would be later recognized as functional seizures or paroxysmal functional movement disorders), fixed dystonia, and other symptoms [10]. Charcot saw hypnosis as a tool by which he could experimentally induce an altered state within the nervous system that enabled hysterical symptoms to manifest, which could then be rigorously studied and catalogued [11]. As a neuropathologist and fastidious clinician, suggestion did not enter into it: hysteria was as an objective physiological disorder and hypnosis was a means to study and locate the anatomical lesion [11]. Bernheim instead used verbal suggestions in patients who had entered a solemnant state akin to hypnosis, and was able to not only recreate symptoms, but remove them, telling patients that they were better. The approach worked. Hysterical symptoms were therefore produced by suggestion, and could be cured by suggestion. The link was drawn that patients suffering from hysteria were "suggestible," and this continues to persist until today, as can be seen in the diagnostic criteria for functional dystonia which is still in use [12].

On the placebo side, placebo effects were first directly linked to suggestion in Beecher's influential 1955 paper "The Powerful Placebo," a meta-analysis in which he combined the results of 15 clinical trials with a placebo arm. Placebo pills improved symptoms in about one third of the patients in the placebo group, and they were capable of producing substantial physiological changes, in some cases exceeding those of the active drug [13]. These changes were consistent with bodily phenomena produced by suggestion. His solution to this was to distribute these "suggestion effects" equally across all participants, and the randomized controlled trial (RCT) was born. It is important to note that this paper was published during the time of the pharmacological revolution in medicine. The decade following the Second World War saw a transformation in laboratory medicine, and the production of effective new drugs to treat infections (antibiotics), analgesics, and anesthetics, and it was critical to have a mechanism to neutralize any "pseudosymptoms" in order to ensure that new treatments in development worked. As previously mentioned, placebo effects were thus contextualized as a nuisance, obscuring the results of clinical trials, with the embedded understanding that any such nonspecific physiological changes were a result of the mind, or suggestion. This perspective that placebo effects equalled suggestibility would dominate the field for another 40 years.

It is therefore not surprising that placebos would be used in functional disorders, which had already been associated with suggestibility 80 years prior. Placebo use became especially employed in the diagnosis of episodic functional neurological symptoms, such as functional seizures. Provocative testing, in which a placebo is used to elicit and/or terminate symptoms, proved not only useful diagnostically, but also practically given that it substantially reduced the time required for monitoring. Triggering an attack while the patient is under video electroencephalography (EEG) proved a compelling provocative test to demonstrate functional seizures [14, 15], although more recent work indicates noninferiority of a non-placebo induction technique [16]. In the original proposed diagnostic criteria for psychogenic dystonia by Fahn and Williams, the highest degree of certainty, or "documented" psychogenic dystonia, was achieved by fullfilling the following:

...the dystonic symptoms must be persistently relieved by psychotherapy, by the clinician utilizing psychological suggestion including physiotherapy, or by administration of placebos (again with suggestion being part of this approach)...The degree of remission seen in our cases with documented psychogenic dystonia is usually the dramatic, sudden improvement occuring within a few days with supportive suggestion or placebo treatment. In a few patients with more chronic symptoms, improvement was more gradual, ocurring over weeks of "physiotherapy" which was used as the approach to have the patient relinquish the symptoms in a face-saving manner. [12]

In recent years the diagnosis of FND has shifted away from provocative measures and instead relies on the identification of postive signs [17]. It is important to note that even "organic" symptoms can improve with suggestion [18] and be placebo responsive (e.g., symptoms of Parkinson's disease) [2]. Despite this lack of specificity, placebos continue to be frequently used in aiding diagnosis [19] and we would strongly discourage such practice. The majority of this chapter will focus on potential treatment considerations for placebo in FND.

Placebo Effects in Medicine

Data from clinical trials provide strong evidence that patients randomized to placebo groups often exhibit substantial improvements in clinical outcomes. This has been most consistently observed in the clinical neurosciences, with impressive effects typically ranging from 20% to 40% [20]. It is important to be aware that overall benefits observed in patients in the placebo arm of trials are referred to as placebo responses. Placebo responses are an umbrella term that include placebo effects but also include non-specific effects such as regression to the mean, spontaneous improvement, elevation bias (higher reported symptom severity at initial/baseline assessment than actually experienced), [21] and the Hawthorne effect (changes in outcomes associated with the act of being studied/observed) [22]. In order to delineate placebo effects from overall placebo responses, one typically needs to include a third trial arm described as a "no-treatment" control [3]. These study designs are often advocated for but unfortunately are rarely conducted.

Placebo effects in medicine are not uniform. While there is a lack of head-to-head comparisons between patient populations, generally, "subjective" symptoms, including many symptoms relevant to FND such as pain, fatigue and mood may be particularly responsive [3]. A landmark placebo-focused study of asthma exemplifies this principle and demonstrates that it may stretch beyond conventionally conceived "brain" disorders. In this double-blind crossover study, patients with asthma were randomly assigned to an active albuterol inhaler, a placebo inhaler, sham acupuncture or no intervention. They found a dramatic difference in the effect profile between groups for objective versus subjective outcome measures. On objective spirometry measures, they reported that active albuterol was far superior to all three comparator groups (20% increase in FEV1 vs. approximately 7% in each other group). However, on patient's subjective reports of symptom improvement, there was no significant difference between active albuterol and the two placebo groups (50% improvement vs. 45–46%) and all were considerably better than the no treatment control (21%) [23].

Inter-individual differences in patients and healthy individuals have also been noted. The investigation of how personality factors may shape placebo effects has yielded mixed results but optimism, suggestibility, empathy, altruism and neuroticism have all been implicated [24]. More recently, genetic factors have been identified that may predict placebo responses, coined the "placebome" [25]. Genetic variation in Catechol-O-methyltransferase (COMT), an enzyme implicated in dopamine metabolism, has been the most extensively studied [25]. However, examples in other neurotransmitter systems relevant to placebo effects, such as the serotonin-related tryptophan hydroxylase-2 gene are also beginning evaluated. In patients with social anxiety disorder, the G variant of this gene's TPH2 G703T polymorphism was found to mediate placebo-induced reductions of amygdala activity and predict placebo response [26]. Interestingly, TPH2 G703T was also recently found to predict

brain connectivity changes between the right amygdala and middle frontal gyrus in functional movement disorder and interacted with childhood trauma to predict symptom severity [27].

Treatments are also not uniform in their delivery of placebo effects. Treatment intensiveness (e.g., intravenous versus oral), perceived innovation and cost are among the strongest factors associated with increasing placebo effects [28]. For example, administration of a pill at home may induce much more modest placebo effects than coming to a hospital for an elaborate treatment such as a surgical procedure or device-based treatment [28]. Much of data in support of this concept of "differential" placebo effects is based on retrospective comparative meta-analyses and few prospective studies have directly investigated this [29]. The durability of placebo effects also likely vary based on treatment characteristics such the frequency of treatments and the expectation of the length of effect, with some studies showing they can persist as long as the duration of the blinding period [30]. Durability of placebo effects remains a hotly debated topic and more studies with long-term follow-up are needed.

Data collected from clinical research trials clearly demonstrate that meaningful benefits can be derived from placebo effects and now the major unanswered question is how this can be translated in clinical settings. Generally, there are two main approaches: (i) "open-label" or honestly delivered placebo, and (ii) deceptive or misleading placebos [3]. Open-label placebo is fully transparent delivery of placebo that has full informed consent. Patients are told that they will be given inert placebos with no medication but are typically accompanied by phrases that educate them on the potential neurobiological and psychological evidence of placebo effects (specific protocols vary between studies) [31]. Open-label placebo has shown preliminary efficacy in conditions related to functional disorders including chronic pain and irritable bowel syndrome, but their potential efficacy remains controversial and future trials are underway to better delineate this [31]. Proposed mechanisms for how this may work are also controversial as they generally don't involve the traditional expectancies associated with receiving a specific medical treatment.

Deceptively delivered placebo is the main approach that most associate with placebo effects. Despite the potential well-intention of a care provider, there is no informed consent and thus it remains highly ethically contentious (as will be discussed further in later sections). Deceptive placebo use can be further divided into two categories: pure and impure. Pure placebos are completely inert substances (e.g., sugar pill) whereas impure placebos have potential specific biological activity but are probably not useful and do not have evidence for their use towards the given indication (e.g., subthreshold dosages of medications, vitamins etc) [3]. Interestingly, in a survey of 679 internists and rheumatologists in the United States, 59% said it was permissible to recommend a treatment primarily to promote patients' expectation, while an additional 31% said it was permissible only in rare circumstances [32].

Placebos in FND: Helpful or Harmful?

The use of placebos as treatment for FND remains controversial. There are many relevant factors to consider, including neurobiological rationales for efficacy, ethical implications, unique vulnerabilities of the FND population, and the lack of direct empirical evidence to date to support their use. Here we outline the current relevant arguments in favor and against this practice.

Arguments in Favor of the Therapeutic Use of Placebos in FND

A Shared Neurobiology Between Placebo Effects and FND

A growing body of neuroimaging research has demonstrated that placebo effects are associated with meaningful changes in a variety of brain regions. Most studies have been conducted using paradigms of placebo analgesia in healthy controls; however, studies also exist in fields such as Parkinson's disease and depression. Meta-analyses of placebo analgesia neuroimaging studies suggest a potential "placebo" network with most consistent activations in the dorsolateral prefrontal (PFC) cortex, nucleus accumbens, periaquaductal grey, ventrolateral PFC, ventromedial PFC and temporal-parietal junction and most consistent de-activations in the amygdala, dorsomedial PFC, anterior mid-cingulate, thalamus and supplementary sensory regions [33]. Models of placebo effects typically summarize these findings as implicating fronto-limbic circuits involved in generating expectancies, activation of reward centers and de-activation of anxiety/fear pathways [1].

As extensively discussed in other chapters of this book, FND involves changes in a similarly complex array of brain regions and networks. In fact, recent syntheses of FND neuroimaging studies [34] suggest that many of the same brain regions may be implicated. Most notably, this overlap includes the amygdala, temporal-parietal junction, anterior cingulate, dorsolateral PFC and ventromedial PFC. Focusing on the amygdala for simplicity, if patients with FND have hyperactivity (+/− abnormal connectivity) of the amygdala and placebo effects decrease activity in the amygdala, then a neurobiological mechanism emerges for how placebo effects could alter dysfunctional networks in FND and potentially improve symptoms.

Based on this reasoning, it has been argued that healthcare practitioners could potentially have ethical justification for delivering placebo to FND patients. In this context, "placebo" may have a specific effect for FND and thus not fall under the traditional, prohibited definitions used by organizations such as the American Medical Assocation (a substance that has "no specific pharmacologic effect upon the condition being treated") [35]. Furthermore, practitioners could defend themselves by considering placebo akin to other complex treatments that "work through various networks in the brain, the particulars of which no one fully understands" [36]. Such lines of argument treads on very contentious ground and we must emphasize that these models remain conceptual and there have been no prospective neuroimaging studies to date investigating whether brain changes in FND can be directly altered by placebo effects.

Anecdotes and Indirect Evidence for the Effectiveness of Placebo

As described in the *Historical Context* section, there is a longstanding history of informally reported clinical cases of high placebo responsiveness and associated expert opinions praising its potential efficacy. Information derived from such sources obviously has limited scientific rigor and needs to be interpreted very cautiously. Although likely more widely used, some published case series document using placebo and/or suggestion as formal treatment modalities in FND [11]. Another source of data comes from inferential reports of open-label FND treatment studies that attribute large and rapidly observed improvement (inconsistent with the treatment's therapeutic mechanism) to placebo effects. For example, as in the case of S.V. presented at the beginning of the chapter, dramatic and immediate response to botulinum toxin in patients with fixed dystonia has been reported [37]. The authors of this case series concluded: "The neuromuscular blocking actions of botulinum toxin take at least 72 hours to have a clinical effect. We therefore surmise that the dramatic response within minutes of injection was due to the expectation of the patient of benefit: a placebo effect." Another example comes from the use of transcranial magnetic stimulation (TMS) for patients with FND [38]. Though stimulation-based neuromodulation and cognitive-behavioral effects (e.g., demonstration of limb movement using TMS to the motor cortex in patients with functional weakness) could provide relevant therapeutic mechanisms [39], the rapid treatment response in many open-label TMS studies have led some to infer a large potential role of placebo effects [38]. As mentioned previously, the elaborate set-up and procedures for TMS may generate particularly high therapeutic expectations and yield elevated placebo effects [28]. We should also note that one sham-controlled study of TMS in patients with chronic refractory FND showed no benefit of active TMS over placebo [40]. Further discussion of TMS can be found in Chap. 28.

Considerations Relevant to Current FND Management

One of the most important aspects of the management for FND involves appropriately delivering and explaining the diagnosis to patients [41]. When one examines recommendations set forth to optimize delivery and counseling, they include many components that directly overlap with principles of placebo effects. Most notably, this includes confidently emphasizing and encouraging positive expectations for potential symptom reversibility and resolution. Providing this expectation for recovery can potentially restructure entrenched cognitive schema surrounding undiagnosed structural neurological disease (for example stroke or multiple sclerosis) that may never get better. While the label attributed to such potential therapeutic benefits may be debated, there are clear elements that share the core tenants of placebo effects.

Beyond initial diagnosis and psychoeducation of FND, much of the remaining evidence-based FND management guidelines rely on multidisciplinary care including physical therapy, psychotherapy and occupational therapy [42]. Unfortunately, there can be many barriers for patients to access these multidisciplinary services. The primary issues may vary across regions and centers but can include a lack of providers (especially in rural settings), a lack of providers educated about FND, and/or prohibitory associated costs. Arguments have been made that placebo could offer potential therapeutic benefits to patients with no or limited other treatment options [43].

Burke and colleagues have outlined critical next steps that would need to be taken in order to build on these arguments in favor of leveraging placebo effects for therapeutic use in FND [44]. They include: "(1) assess feasibility and acceptability by the relevant parties (including qualitative feedback from FND patients, families, treatment providers, etc.); (2) demonstrate target engagement (i.e., can we successfully modulate networks implicated in FND pathophysiology with placebo) and preliminary efficacy; and (3) delineate the durability of placebo effects for FND (i.e., short-term symptom relief versus long-term modification of the disease course) and at what stage(s) of management patients may benefit the most."

Arguments Against the Use of Placebo to Treat FND

Ethical Perspectives

The use of placebo – in any condition – in the guise of medication typically requires the use of deception, violating patient autonomy. Deceptive placebo use renders most practitioners uncomfortable, and it is reflected in the 2006 American Medical Association Code of Ethics. Complicating matters is evidence of the potential therapeutic benefits of *open* placebos in functional conditions such as irritable bowel syndrome, as well as other somatic symptoms [45, 46]. Conditioned placebo dose reduction has also been explored as a means of medication tapering in ADHD in children, in which placebos were openly given as "dose extenders" [47]. As discussed previously, there are a number of other considerations, for example, what if the practitioner believes a placebo to be effective? In this case, does the placebo truly qualify as a placebo? Deception necessitates violation of the patient's autonomy – or does it, if patients are supportive of their use and also believe them to have potential benefit without harm? [35] These questions remain unanswered and may never be answered. The necessary lack of consent to treatment also undermines a patient's sense of agency, which has been demonstrated as a potential impairment in FND [48]. However, in research settings, placebos are often administered with patient consent under the ethically acceptable caveat that they will undergo deception in the study, but the nature of the deception is not revealed until the end of their participation [49]. Thus, it is clear that the

issue of clinical deception is multifaceted and warrants further exploration.

Perhaps clearer are the ethical principles of beneficence and nonmaleficence. Placebo use can cause patient harm, and undermine the patient's trust in their provider, particularly with the use of deceptive placebos. One should also consider the potential harm to patients who suffer from multiple somatic symptoms as can been seen co-morbidly with FND, as placebo use in the guise of medications or procedures can serve to further medicalize their symptoms into a framework that overall is unhelpful to acheiving potential recovery for FND.

Unique Vulnerabilities of the FND Population Related to Placebo Use

Patients with FND often feel invalidated within the health care system due to the limited availability of treatments, stigmatization of disorders involving psychological factors and frequent grouping of these disorders with conditions such as malingering or secondary gain. Many have been the subjects of unintentional iatrogenic harm, either in the form of explanations for their symptoms as being attributed solely to psychological factors, not being believed, or possibly even undergoing unnecessary procedures, and can feel mistrustful of practitioners as a result [50]. Many have a history of trauma [51]. From a neurobiological perspective, an impaired sense of agency, an external locus of control can be relevant elements of the illness process, [52] which can be made worse by deceptive use of placebo. Instead the therapeutic goal should be to support self-management and a return of sense of agency. Finally, FND can be a chronic and relapsing condition, outliving potential placebo effects so long-term use may not be suitable.

Lack of Evidence Supporting Placebo Use in FND

Despite the long history of placebo and FND, direct empirical evidence for the efficacy of placebo effects in FND is very limited. As described above, most information on this topic is relatively weakly derived from indirect or anecdotal sources.

To date, there have been no prospective studies directly investigating placebo effects as a potential treatment for FND (either delivered deceptively or honestly/"open-label"). The next best source of information likely comes from retrospectively analyzing responses from the placebo arms of RCTs in FND. Unfortunately, there have been very few trials in FND in which a control group is administered a placebo. A recent RCT of botulinum toxin for chronic jerky and tremulous functional movement disorder reported very large placebo responses. They reported that 57% of patients randomized to placebo (saline injection) had improvement of motor symptoms (CGI-I score 1, 2 or 3), which was not statistically different from the botulinum toxin group (64%). Their conclusion was that their finding "underlines the substantial potential of chronic jerky and tremulous FMD patients to recover and may stimulate further exploration of placebo-therapies in these patients" [53].

These findings are contrasted with a pilot RCT of antidepressant medication for functional seizures in which a notable placebo response (inert oral pill) was not observed [54]. The data from this trial is complicated to interpret as there were large differences in the baseline mean seizure frequency between the two treatment groups (placebo group = 11.3 and active group = 19.9) and the seizure frequency at the end of the study were essentially the same (11.6 and 11.7 respectively). As previously discussed, the placebo response includes not only placebo effects but also spontaneous improvement, regression to the mean and other factors. Given the data profile described above, a placebo response may not have been observed due to capturing the patients randomized to placebo in a relative trough of their symptoms at the baseline timepoint. Finally, it should also be noted that when trying to understand the magnitude of placebo effects from RCT data, patients randomly assigned to placebo receive a 50% expectation of receiving active treatment. This is different from the clinical scenario (as reported in anecdotal cases) where the expectation of receiving active treatment would typically be 100%.

Conclusion

A longstanding history of anecdotal reports and potential overlap in neurobiological substrates may indicate a signal of opportunity for the use of placebo in the treatment of patients of FND. However, currently there is insufficient empirical evidence to suggest that placebo may offer meaningful therapeutic benefits and there are many ethical concerns surrounding placebo effects and this vulnerable patient population. More research is clearly needed and should leverage existing lines of placebo-focused research among patients with related functional syndromes, such as irritable bowel syndrome [20]. The discussion of placebo effects and FND sheds light on the central importance of practitioner-patient relationships and ultimately the search for understanding placebo effects and their potential utility is really a search for understanding the complexities of healing.

Summary
1. FND and placebo effects have a long-standing, interwoven and controversial history that date back to the origins of both entities.
2. There is a shared neurobiology between brain regions/networks implicated in FND and placebo effects that conceptually offers a potential therapeutic mechanism.
3. Anecdotal reports and expert opinion suggest that placebo could provide a beneficial treatment for patients with FND; however, there is currently a lack of evidence to support such claims.
4. Ethical principles surrounding the use of placebo in FND (and medicine more broadly) is a source of ongoing debate but deceptive use is generally discour-

aged, particularly given the unique vulnerabilities of patients with FND.

5. Future research is needed to further explore shared neurobiological substrates, prospectively investigate potential efficacy and determine if placebo could be ethically permissible to patients and care-providers in certain circumstances.

Funding and Acknowledgements MJB was supported by funding from the Liu Fu Yu Charity Foundation.

SCL is supported in part by an anonymous donation to the Movement Disorders program at the University Health Network, University of Toronto.

Declarations of Interest MJB has nothing to disclose.

SCL has nothing to disclose.

References

1. Wager TD, Atlas LY. The neuroscience of placebo effects: connecting context, learning and health. Nat Rev Neurosci. 2015;16(7):403–18.
2. Benedetti F. Placebo effects: from the neurobiological paradigm to translational implications. Neuron. 2014;84(3):623–37.
3. Colloca L, Barsky AJ. Placebo and nocebo effects. Ropper AH, editor. N Engl J Med. 2020;382(6):554–61.
4. Kaptchuk TJ, Miller FG. Placebo effects in medicine. N Engl J Med. 2015;373(1):8–9.
5. Barsky AJ. Nonspecific medication side effects and the nocebo phenomenon. JAMA. 2002;287(5):622.
6. Trimble M, Reynolds EH. Chapter 1 – A brief history of hysteria: from the ancient to the modern. In: Hallett M, Stone J, Carson A, editors. Handbook of clinical neurology [Internet], Functional neurologic disorders, vol. 139. Elsevier; 2016. p. 3–10. Available from: http://www.sciencedirect.com/science/article/pii/B9780128017722000011.
7. Kanaan RAA, Wessely SC. The origins of factitious disorder. Hist Hum Sci. 2010;23(2):68–85.
8. Shapiro AK, Shapiro E. The powerful placebo: from ancient priest to modern physician. London and Baltimore: The Johns Hopkins University Press; 1997.
9. Harrington A. The cure within: a history of mind-body medicine. W.W. Norton & Company; 2008. 354 p.
10. Goetz CG. Chapter 2 – Charcot, hysteria, and simulated disorders. In: Hallett M, Stone J, Carson A, editors. Handbook of clinical neurology [Internet], Functional neurologic disorders, vol. 139. Elsevier; 2016. p. 11–23. Available from: http://www.sciencedirect.com/science/article/pii/B9780128017722000023.
11. Harrington A. Mind fixers: psychiatry's troubled search for the biology of mental illness. W.W. Norton & Company; 2019. 384 p.
12. Fahn S, Williams DT. Psychogenic dystonia. Adv Neurol. 1988;50:431–55.
13. Beecher HK. The powerful placebo. J Am Med Assoc. 1955;159(17):1602–6.
14. Stagno SJ, Smith ML. The use of placebo in diagnosing psychogenic seizures: who is being deceived? Semin Neurol. 1997;17(03):213–8.
15. Devinsky O, Fisher R. Ethical use of placebos and provocative testing in diagnosing nonepileptic seizures. Neurology. 1996;47(4):866.
16. Chen DK, Dave H, Gadelmola K, Jeroudi M, Fadipe M. Provocative induction of psychogenic non-epileptic seizures: noninferiority of an induction technique without versus with placebo. Epilepsia. 2018;59(11):e161–5.
17. Stone J. Functional symptoms in neurology: THE BARE ESSENTIALS. Pract Neurol. 2009;9(3):179–89.
18. Baik JS. Attention in Parkinson's disease mimicking suggestion in psychogenic movement disorder. J Mov Disord. 2012;5(2):53–4.
19. Espay AJ, Goldenhar LM, Voon V, Schrag A, Burton N, Lang AE. Opinions and clinical practices related to diagnosing and managing patients with psychogenic movement disorders: an international survey of movement disorder society members. Mov Disord. 2009;24(9):1366–74.
20. Weimer K, Colloca L, Enck P. Placebo effects in psychiatry: mediators and moderators. Lancet Psychiatry. 2015;2(3):246–57.
21. Shrout PE, Stadler G, Lane SP, McClure MJ, Jackson GL, Clavél FD, et al. Initial elevation bias in subjective reports. Proc Natl Acad Sci. 2018;115(1):E15–23.
22. McCambridge J, Witton J, Elbourne DR. Systematic review of the Hawthorne effect: new concepts are needed to study research participation effects. J Clin Epidemiol. 2014;67(3):267–77.
23. Wechsler ME, Kelley JM, Boyd IOE, Dutile S, Marigowda G, Kirsch I, et al. Active albuterol or placebo, sham acupuncture, or no intervention in asthma. N Engl J Med. 2011;365(2):119–26.
24. Peciña M, Azhar H, Love TM, Lu T, Frederickson BL, Stohler CS, et al. Personality trait predictors of

placebo analgesia and neurobiological correlates. Neuropsychopharmacology. 2013;38(4):639–46.

25. Hall KT, Loscalzo J, Kaptchuk TJ. Genetics and the placebo effect: the placebome. Trends Mol Med. 2015;21(5):285–94.

26. Furmark T, Appel L, Henningsson S, Ahs F, Faria V, Linnman C, et al. A link between serotonin-related gene polymorphisms, amygdala activity, and placebo-induced relief from social anxiety. J Neurosci. 2008;28(49):13066–74.

27. Spagnolo PA, Norato G, Maurer CW, Goldman D, Hodgkinson C, Horovitz S, et al. Effects of *TPH2* gene variation and childhood trauma on the clinical and circuit-level phenotype of functional movement disorders. J Neurol Neurosurg Psychiatry. 2020;91(8):814–21.

28. Burke MJ, Kaptchuk TJ, Pascual-Leone A. Challenges of differential placebo effects in contemporary medicine: the example of brain stimulation: Neurology Grand Rounds. Ann Neurol. 2019;85(1):12–20.

29. Kaptchuk TJ, Stason WB, Davis RB, Legedza ART, Schnyer RN, Kerr CE, et al. Sham device *v* inert pill: randomised controlled trial of two placebo treatments. BMJ. 2006;332(7538):391–7.

30. McRae C, Cherin E, Yamazaki TG, Diem G, Vo AH, Russell D, et al. Effects of perceived treatment on quality of life and medical outcomes in a double-blind placebo surgery trial. Arch Gen Psychiatry. 2004;61(4):412–20.

31. Kaptchuk TJ, Miller FG. Open label placebo: can honestly prescribed placebos evoke meaningful therapeutic benefits? BMJ. 2018;363:k3889.

32. Tilburt JC, Emanuel EJ, Kaptchuk TJ, Curlin FA, Miller FG. Prescribing "placebo treatments": results of national survey of US internists and rheumatologists. BMJ. 2008;337(2):a1938.

33. Ashar YK, Chang LJ, Wager TD. Brain mechanisms of the placebo effect: an affective appraisal account. Annu Rev Clin Psychol. 2017;13(1):73–98.

34. Voon V, Cavanna AE, Coburn K, Sampson S, Reeve A, LaFrance WC, et al. Functional neuroanatomy and neurophysiology of functional neurological disorders (conversion disorder). J Neuropsychiatry Clin Neurosci. 2016;28(3):168–90.

35. Rommelfanger KS. The role of placebo in the diagnosis and treatment of functional neurologic disorders. Handb Clin Neurol. 2016;139:607–17.

36. Shamy MCF. The treatment of psychogenic movement disorders with suggestion is ethically justified: suggestion is an ethical treatment for PMDs. Mov Disord. 2010;25(3):260–4.

37. Edwards MJ, Bhatia KP, Cordivari C. Immediate response to botulinum toxin injections in patients with fixed dystonia. Mov Disord. 2011;26(5):917–8.

38. Pollak TA, Nicholson TR, Edwards MJ, David AS. A systematic review of transcranial magnetic stimulation in functional (conversion) neu-

rological symptoms. J Neurol Neurosurg Psychiatry. 2014;85(2):191–7.

39. Burke MJ, Isayama R, Jegatheeswaran G, Gunraj C, Feinstein A, Lang AE, et al. Neurostimulation for functional neurological disorder: evaluating longitudinal neurophysiology. Mov Disord Clin Pract. 2018;5(5):561–3.

40. McWhirter L, Ludwig L, Carson A, McIntosh RD, Stone J. Transcranial magnetic stimulation as a treatment for functional (psychogenic) upper limb weakness. J Psychosom Res. 2016;89:102–6.

41. Stone J. Functional neurological disorders: the neurological assessment as treatment. Pract Neurol. 2016;16(1):7–17.

42. Espay AJ, Aybek S, Carson A, Edwards MJ, Goldstein LH, Hallett M, et al. Current concepts in diagnosis and treatment of functional neurological disorders. JAMA Neurol. 2018;75(9):1132.

43. Kaas BM, Humbyrd CJ, Pantelyat A. Functional movement disorders and placebo: a brief review of the placebo effect in movement disorders and ethical considerations for placebo therapy: placebo for functional movement disorders. Mov Disord Clin Pract. 2018;5(5):471–8.

44. Burke MJ, Faria V, Cappon D, Pascual-Leone A, Kaptchuk TJ, Santarnecchi E. Leveraging the shared neurobiology of placebo effects and functional neurological disorder: a call for research. J Neuropsychiatry Clin Neurosci. 2020;32(1):101–4.

45. Kaptchuk TJ, Friedlander E, Kelley JM, Sanchez MN, Kokkotou E, Singer JP, et al. Placebos without deception: a randomized controlled trial in irritable bowel syndrome. PLoS One. 2010;5(12):e15591.

46. Park LC, Covi L. Nonblind placebo trial: an exploration of neurotic patients' responses to placebo when its inert content is disclosed. Arch Gen Psychiatry. 1965;12:36–45.

47. Sandler AD, Glesne CE, Bodfish JW. Conditioned placebo dose reduction: a new treatment in attention-deficit hyperactivity disorder? J Dev Behav Pediatr. 2010;31:369–75.

48. Edwards MJ. Chapter 12 – Neurobiologic theories of functional neurologic disorders. In: Hallett M, Stone J, Carson A, editors. Handbook of clinical neurology, Functional neurologic disorders, vol. 139. Elsevier; 2016. p. 131–7.

49. Lidstone SC, Schulzer M, Dinelle K, Mak E, Sossi V, Ruth TJ, et al. Effects of expectation on placebo-induced dopamine release in Parkinson disease. Arch Gen Psychiatry. 2010;67(8):857–65.

50. Lidstone SC, MacGillivray L, Lang AE. Integrated therapy for functional movement disorders: time for a change. Mov Disord Clin Pract. 2020;7(2):169–74.

51. Roelofs K, Pasman J. Chapter 13 – Stress, childhood trauma, and cognitive functions in functional neurologic disorders. In: Hallett M, Stone J, Carson A, editors. Handbook of clinical neurol-

ogy [Internet], Functional neurologic disorders, vol. 139. Elsevier; 2016. p. 139–55. Available from: http://www.sciencedirect.com/science/article/pii/ B9780128017722000138.

52. Edwards MJ, Adams RA, Brown H, Parees I, Friston KJ. A Bayesian account of "hysteria". Brain. 2012;135(11):3495–512.

53. Dreissen YEM, Dijk JM, Gelauff JM, Zoons E, van Poppelen D, Contarino MF, et al. Botulinum neuro-toxin treatment in jerky and tremulous functional movement disorders: a double-blind, randomised placebo-controlled trial with an open-label extension. J Neurol Neurosurg Psychiatry. 2019;90(11):1244–50.

54. LaFrance WC, Keitner GI, Papandonatos GD, Blum AS, Machan JT, Ryan CE, et al. Pilot pharmacologic randomized controlled trial for psychogenic nonepileptic seizures. Neurology. 2010;75(13):1166–73.

Transcranial Magnetic Stimulation (TMS) as Treatment for Functional Movement Disorder

28

Daruj Aniwattanapong and Timothy R. Nicholson

Illustrative Case Vignette

A 35-year-old man fell from the top of a 12-foot ladder while at work. An ambulance was called by his work colleagues, and he had severe lower back and ankle pain. He was taken to a local Emergency Department (ED) and plain x-rays showed no fractures; he was discharged with pain medications after a few hours. Over the next few days, he was unable to walk due to the pain and had to stay in bed. He found that his legs became increasingly weak and 7 days later was unable to move or feel his legs at all. His primary care doctor visited him at home and sent him to the ED again, where a computed tomography (CT) spine was performed which was normal. Magnetic resonance imaging (MRI) of his whole neuroaxis was requested and he was referred to neurosurgery who reviewed the scans which were normal. Nerve conduction studies were then requested along with an outpatient neurology opinion. The neurology exam revealed non der-matomal sensory change (at the groin crease) and complete loss of power in both legs, although hip flexion was possible when flexing his trunk. Functional Neurological Disorder (FND) with features of functional limb weakness and functional sensory loss was diagnosed.

He was admitted to a neuropsychiatry inpatient rehab unit for multidisciplinary treatment including physical, psychological, and occupational therapy but after 2 months there was no change in his function. Physical therapy was limited by the fact that he could not generate any movement of his legs to work with the therapist. At this point Transcranial Magnetic Stimulation (TMS) was considered as an off-label treatment option and he was given a treatment session stimulating both legs simultaneously using a double cone coil with 10 pulses above motor threshold to the primary motor cortices leading to significant involuntary movement of both legs. After the first few pulses, the patient was encouraged to try and move with the stimuli, resulting in more movement of the legs than when not attempting to move the legs. After the TMS pulses, he was able to make spontaneous very small movements of his big toes but not able to move other muscles in his legs, but this ability faded over the next few days.

He was brought back for a second session 2 weeks later, this time with the ward physical therapist attempting to do a session of therapy during and immediately after the TMS treatment. This led to marked improvements with ability to

D. Aniwattanapong
Neuropsychiatry Research and Education Group,
Institute of Psychiatry Psychology & Neuroscience,
King's College London, London, UK

Department of Psychiatry, Faculty of Medicine,
Chulalongkorn University, Bangkok, Thailand

T. R. Nicholson (✉)
Neuropsychiatry Research and Education Group,
Institute of Psychiatry Psychology & Neuroscience,
King's College London, London, UK
e-mail: timothy.nicholson@kcl.ac.uk

© Springer Nature Switzerland AG 2022
K. LaFaver et al. (eds.), *Functional Movement Disorder*, Current Clinical Neurology,
https://doi.org/10.1007/978-3-030-86495-8_28

spontaneously flex and extend his ankles. An intensive course of physical therapy over the next few months, combined with other components of multidisciplinary treatment, allowed recovery such that he was able to walk out of the ward using a rolling walker and with normal sensation returning to the legs. He continued physical therapy as an outpatient and was soon able to walk without aids and resume normal activities of daily living.

Introduction

Functional neurological disorder (FND), also known as conversion disorder, is a neuropsychiatric condition characterised by neurological symptoms that are not compatible with other identifiable neuropathological diseases. Clinical manifestations of FND have been classified by the Diagnostic and Statistical Manual of Mental Disorders, Fifth Edition (DSM-5) [1] and the International Classification of Diseases 11th Revision (ICD-11) [2] into various symptom types: abnormal movements, weakness, sensory abnormalities, seizures, and cognitive impairment. Functional movement disorder (FMD) includes a range of functional motor symptoms including tremor, myoclonus, tics, parkinsonism, dystonia, gait difficulties and limb weakness [3]. The pathophysiology of FMD and other FND subtypes is still not yet fully understood, but there are accumulating insights into the neurophysiological and cognitive-affective (psychological) processes.

Management of FMD begins with a personalised explanation of what is generally a difficult diagnosis to understand and therefore accept. Thereafter the therapeutic approach generally builds around multidisciplinary collaborations between neurology, neuropsychiatry, psychology, physical and occupational therapy. Evidence-based interventions for FMD include specialist physiotherapy for treatment of functional motor symptoms [4] and a large scale trial is underway [5]. There is mixed evi-

dence for specialist cognitive-behavioral therapy (CBT) for FMD and functional seizures. In the most well studied FND subtype (i.e., functional seizures), there is encouraging pilot data on improving the primary outcome of seizure frequency – however this was not replicated in well powered larger study although a number of secondary outcomes improved preferentially in the CBT treatment arm [6]. There is also some encouraging evidence for some other forms of psychological therapy, including psychodynamic therapy [7] but as yet no convincing evidence for any pharmacological therapy. As such, if first line treatments do not yield positive results clinicians can be left with few additional therapeutic options.

Transcranial magnetic stimulation (TMS) is a method of "indirect" neurostimulation and another potential treatment modality for FMD which has been used therapeutically for a wide range of neurological and psychiatric disorders including stroke, movement disorders and migraine [8]. It is also licenced for major depression, migraine, and obsessive-compulsive disorder (OCD), and listed in guidelines, such as the National Institute for Health and Care Excellence (NICE) guidelines in the UK, which recommended rTMS for depression [9].

TMS devices discharge magnetic pulses on the scalp that pass through the soft tissues and skull to stimulate the underlying cerebral cortex, and as such provide an "indirect" form of neurostimulation. There are different types of magnetic coils used to deliver these pulses. Circular coils generate maximal magnetic field under the center of the coil and therefore maximal induced electrical current near the edge of the coil but lack focal specificity. Figure-of-eight or "butterfly" coils combine two maximal electrical fields together resulting in better focal specificity at the expense of strength of stimulation. A double cone coil is required to stimulate cortical areas in the interhemispheric fissure, such as the areas of primary motor cortex controlling leg movement. TMS can be delivered in single pulses (spTMS) or trains of "repetitive" pulses (rTMS) with different parameters to either stimulate or inhibit the targeted area.

TMS was first developed in 1985, using a single pulse method as a diagnostic tool for neurological conditions [10]. In 1991, repetitive stimulation paradigm of TMS (rTMS) was described along with the ability to modify cortical function, for example inducing speech dysfunction. rTMS was later also shown to induce sustained effects after the cessation of stimulation. The development from single pulse to rTMS increased the number of interventional applications of TMS for various medical conditions. The higher number and frequency of stimuli could theoretically negative impact tolerability (localized discomfort/pain or short term headaches) and safety concerns (longer term headache or the risk of triggering epileptic seizures), but if specific stimulation parameters are utilized and patients at risk of seizures excluded these risks are very low [11, 12].

There is quite a long history of other neurostimulation methods being used therapeutically for movement disorders and paralysis, including FMD. Direct neurostimulation, applying electrical stimulation directly to peripheral nerves, has a long history and Johann Kruger was thought to be the first to propose and use electricity to treat limb weakness in Germany in 1743 [13]. Of particular note, such direct neurostimulation was widely used to treat many soldiers with shell shock syndrome, a specific war trauma induced form of FND, in the aftermath of World War I [14]. However, this was often used as a deliberately painful, and therefore aversive therapy, and this unethical treatment approach was not widely adopted, especially as psychological therapies were largely the treatment of choice at this time, in keeping with the increasing dominance of Freud's psychodynamic etiological theories in the first half of the twentieth century.

Over the last two decades there has been increasing interest and accumulating evidence in using TMS to treat FND, particularly FMD. In this chapter, we summarize and critically appraise this evidence before discussing in depth the

methodological issues that arise in assessing TMS as a treatment for FND. We then consider the potential mechanisms by which TMS could have therapeutic effects in FND, before finally considering future research directions including other forms of direct and indirect neurostimulation that are either currently available or in development.

Evidence for TMS as Treatment for FND

We will briefly review the case report literature before discussing data from randomized controlled trials (RCTs).

Case Reports

The majority of case reports have been of FMD, but there have also been some cases of other functional neurological symptoms reported and we will detail these in turn.

Functional Movement Disorder

The first case report [15] was published in 1992 and since then there have been a further 12 case series reporting therapeutic use of TMS for FMD. They have described 81 patients with limb weakness, and 55 patients with abnormal movement (27 tremor, 12 dystonia, 7 jerks, 6 myoclonus, 3 gait impairment, 2 parkinsonism, 1 stereotypy, 1 blepharospasm). See Table 28.1 for methodological details and reports of efficacy.

The stimulation parameters used in these reports have varied considerably. Most used rTMS as their intervention, except for two studies [15, 16] which used single pulse (spTMS). As discussed above, spTMS is generally used to investigate brain function by causing brief transient stimulation of a cortical area and does not generally have lasting treatment effects, whereas rTMS can induce changes brain activity lasting beyond the stimulation period itself [17]. The frequency of rTMS stimulation was low (≤ 1 Hz) in all but one

Table 28.1 Case series of transcranial magnetic stimulation (TMS) treatment for functional movement disorder (FMD)

First author (year)	Symptoms	Subjects	Target	Stimulation parameters	Outcome measures	Adverse events	Follow up
Jellinek (1992)	1 paresis	Age 25 years; male	Vertex	spTMS (F8c) "Supra" MT intensity; no other details given	Effective 1/1: full recovery at 1 week (clinical examination)	N/A	Sustained at 1 month
Schönfeldt-Lecuona (2006)	4 paresis	Age 20–59 years; M:F = 2:2	MC	rTMS (F8c) HF (15 Hz, 4000 pulses/session) 110% MT, then 90% after 2 weeks 1 session/day for 4–12 weeks	Effective 3/3 with FND 2 complete recovery and 1 major improvement at 4–12 weeks. 1 patient did not improve but diagnosed with malingering (clinical examination)	N/A	Sustained at 6–12 months
Chastan (2010)	70 paresis (40 paraparesis, 26 monoparesis, 2 tetraparesis, 2 hemiparesis)	Age 8–79, mean (SD) = 24.7 (16.6) years; M:F = 26:44	MC	rTMS (Cc) LF (0.2–0.25 Hz, 30 pulses) 100% stimulator output (2.5 tesla) 1 or 2 sessions on 1 day (second given if incomplete recovery after first)	Effective in 62/70 Total recovery in 53 Dramatic improvement in 9 (clinical impression)	N/A	8/62 who improved relapsed at mean of 156 days; 6 of these responded to further treatment
Kresojevic (2010)	1 paresis (hemiparesis) 1 MD (blepharospasm)	Age 24 and 52 years; M:F = 1:1	Vertex	spTMS (Cc) 30–80% of stimulator output 12 pulses	Effective in 2/2: Complete recovery in 2 (clinical impression)	None	Recurrence of mild symptoms at 6 months
Dafotakis (2011)	11 MD (tremor)	N/A	MC	rTMS (F8c) LF (0.2 Hz, 30 pulses) 120% MT for 15, then 140% for 15 pulses 1 session	Effective in 11/11: Mean of 97% immediate reduction in tremor (kinematic motion analysis)	N/A	7/11 relapsed & 4/11 recovery sustained at 8–12 months

Study	Patients	Age	Target	Protocol	Outcome	Side effects	Follow-up
Garcin (2013)	24 MD (11 fixed dystonia, 5 myoclonus, 3 tremor, 3 jerky dystonia, 1 parkinsonism, 1 stereotypies)	Age 22–76, mean (SD) = 44.5 (13.2) years; M:F = 8:16	MC	rTMS (Cc) LF (0.25 Hz, 20 pulses) 120% MT for 250 μs 1 session	Effective in 24/24: Improved >50% in 18 "Cured" in 3 (AIMS/BFMS, CGI)	None	17/24 still improved at median 20 months and 12/24 CGI-I score of 1 or 2.
Bonnet (2015)	1 parkinsonism	Age 31 years; female	MC	rTMS (Cc) LF (0.25 Hz, 20 pulses) 120% MT for 250 μs 1 session	Effective in 1/1: Complete and immediate recovery of all the symptoms including dream acting behaviors and gambling	N/A	Still in remission at 6 months
Shah (2015)	6 MD (4 jerks, 3 tremors, 3 gaits, 1 rhythmic movement)	Age 32–56, mean = 43 years; M:F = 1:5	MC then PMC	rTMS (F8c) LF (0.33 Hz, 50 pulses) 90% MT 5 sessions over 5 consecutive weekdays to MC then repeated to PMC NB: Protocol included suggestion of recovery	Unclear if effective: Significant improvement in physical (but decrease in psychological QOL) domain after PMC (but not MC) stimulation 2 weeks post treatment No clear change in CGI (WHOQOL-BREF, CGI)	MC: 6 headache, 1 insomnia, 1 palpitation PMC: 2 headache, 1 fatigue, 1 "fluid in ear"	None
Chen (2017)	4 paresis	Age 16–48, mean = 33 years; M:F = 3:1	MC	TMS (F8c)	Effective in 2/4: 2 patients returned to normal or near-normal at discharge and 1 had residual weakness, and 1 had resistant weakness Improving score (FIM)	None	N/A
Portaro (2017)	1 paresis (flaccid paraparesis)	Age 30 years; male	MC	rTMS 1 Hz 100% stimulator output 3 sessions/week for 3 months	Effective in 1/1: Marked improvement up to resolution Able to walk independently (MMPI-2: hysteria and hypochondria items)	N/A	N/A

(continued)

Table 28.1 (continued)

First author (year)	Symptoms	Subjects	Target	Stimulation parameters	Outcome measures	Adverse events	Follow up
Prezelj (2019)	10 MD (tremor)	N/A	MC	rTMS 5 days repeated sessions	Ineffective: 3/10 had subjective improvement 5/10 had objective improvement (EMG, accelerometry)	N/A	N/A
Blades (2020)	1 MD (dystonia)	Age 29 years; female; comorbidity: dissociative PTSD	ACC, SMC, PMC	rTMS 1 Hz 36 session in 2 months	Effective in 1/1: In remission and return to active duty Improved score from 13 to 9 (TWSTRS)	N/A	After 2 months, emotional and physical symptoms subsided sufficiently
Naro (2020)	1 MD (myoclonus)	Age 50 years; female	PMC	rTMS (F8c) 1 Hz, 1200 pulses 115% MT 1 session/day (5 consecutive days with 2 rest days in between) for 6 weeks	Effective in 1/1: Reduced magnitude and frequency of symptoms (UMRS, MRC, FIM) Brain area current densities and brain connectivity were modified (EEG)	None	Significant reduction of involuntary movement frequency and intensity and the related disability burden up to the 2-month follow-up

Key: *ACC* anterior cingulate cortex, *AIMS* abnormal involuntary movement scale, *BFMS* Burke-Fahn-Marsden scale, *Cc* circular coil, *CGI* Clinical Global Impression, *F8c* figure-of-8 coil, *FIM* Functional Independence Measure, *HF* high frequency, *LF* low frequency, *MC* (primary) motor cortex, *MD* functional movement disorder, *MT* motor threshold, *PFC* pre-frontal cortex, *PMC* pre-motor cortex, *rRMS* repetitive spinal root magnetic stimulation, *rTMS* repetitive TMS, *SMC* supplementary motor cortex, *spTMS* single pulse TMS, *TWSTRS* Toronto Western Spasmodic Torticollis Rating Scale, *WHOQOL-BREF* World Health Organisation Quality of Life Brief scale study [18] which used higher frequency (≥5 Hz) stimulation. Low frequency will transiently reduce cortical excitability, whereas high frequency will enhance excitability [19]. Stimulation intensity was measured by a percentage of either resting motor threshold (RMT) or of the TMS machine's maximal output. RMT is the minimum intensity needed to activate a motor output from resting state. Most studies used "suprathreshold" (>100% RMT) stimuli, except for two studies [16, 20] which used subthreshold (<100% RMT) intensity. A high intensity suprathreshold pulse will activate cortical neurons via excitatory interneurons, leading to motor output, i.e. muscle contraction corresponding to the region of motor cortex stimulated. In contrast, a low-intensity subthreshold pulse will potentially excite cortical interneurons but will not result in a motor output [21].

The sample sizes were generally small; five single cases, one study of two cases, two studies of four cases and one each of six, 10, 11 and 24 cases. There was one outlier with a larger sample size of 70 cases [22]. The quality of these studies was appraised in a previous systematic review [23] using a standardized system [24] assessing specified inclusion/exclusion criteria, subject characteristics, reliability and validity of outcome measures. TMS quality was also scored by checklist of TMS parameters such as coil type, frequency, intensity. Most case reports had low overall quality scores (<50%), but acceptable TMS quality scores.

The outcome measures used were mainly clinical examination or subjective clinical impression (e.g. using the Clinical Global Impression (CGI) of severity and/or improvement) but some studies reported other measures such as the Functional Independence Measure, behavioural motor analysis (measured by accelerometry), and neurophysiologic tools such as electromyography (EMG) and electroencephalography (EEG). Improvements after TMS were reported by 12/13 studies for 112 of 136 (82%) patients, and sustained improvement after follow-up, for variable time periods, in 82/106 (77%) patients. There was limited data available on adverse events, but of the five studies detailing this four reported no adverse events and one study reported headache, insomnia and fatigue.

Other FND Symptoms

There have also been five studies [25–29] reporting TMS treatment of other functional neurological symptoms; see Table 28.2 for details. Overall, there were 53 patients with seizures, 12 patients with visual impairment, 12 patients with sensory loss. There was also one patient with aphonia – which could also be seen as a case of FMD. Stimulation parameters of TMS for these patients were similarly heterogeneous but mostly used rTMS, only one study [28] used spTMS. Regarding stimulation frequency, three studies used low frequency (≤1 Hz) stimulation [25–27], whereas two studies used high frequency (≥5 Hz) stimulation [28, 29].

The motor cortex and prefrontal cortex were targeted for the aphonia case [26] but for the other studies different anatomical targets were used; fronto-central [27] and temporoparietal [25, 29] areas were targeted for seizures and occipitoparietal [27] and occipital [28] areas were targeted for visual loss. Outcome measures were again mostly clinical assessment [26–29]. Furthermore, one study [25] objectively evaluated symptoms using rating scales. In terms of the results, improvements were reported in 48/53 (91%) of patients with seizure, 9/12 (75%) of patients with visual impairment, 9/12 (75%) of patients with sensory loss, and 1/1 patient with aphonia. No adverse events were reported by one study [25], some side effects e.g. headache were reported by one study [29], but no data was reported for the others studies. Improvements were seemingly sustained after variable follow-up lengths in 44/48 (92%) seizure, 7/9 (78%) visual impairment, and 1/1 aphonia cases.

In summary there has been a slowly accumulating body of case report evidence since 1992 indicating high rates of improvement with TMS for FMD and some other FND symptoms. These reports built the case for needing RCTs to provide a higher quality evidence base that could account for placebo effects and other key factors such as the impact of concurrently present factors influencing recovery (e.g. reduction in stressors or other treatments) or potential spontaneous natural recovery.

Table 28.2 Transcranial magnetic stimulation (TMS) treatment for other functional neurological disorder (FND) presentations

First author (year)	Symptoms	Subjects	Target	Stimulation parameters	Outcome measure	Adverse events	Follow up
Case series							
Chastan (2009)	1 aphonia	Age 18 years; female	MC (& PFC)	rTMS (Cc) LF (0.33 Hz, 50 pulses) 100% stimulator output (2.5 tesla) 2 sessions 1 week apart (first session to left PFC, second session to right MC)	Effective 1/1: Dramatic improvement within few days after MC stimulation only *(clinical impression)*	N/A	Sustained at 6 months
Parain (2014)	10 visual loss (5 bilateral VA, 2 unilateral VA, 2 bilateral VF, 1 monocular diplopia)	Age mean 18 years; M:F = 4:6	Midline & occipito-parietal area	rTMS (Cc) LF (approx. 1 Hz, 60 pulses) "50% intensity" (unclear if of machine output or MT) 2 sessions (first & second days after communication of diagnosis)	Effective in 9/10: Immediate total recovery in 6 Dramatic improvement in 3 *(clinical impression)*	N/A	2/9 who improved relapsed "some months later" but responded to further treatment
	12 sensory loss (3 complete unilateral, 3 unilateral brachio-facial, 2 one arm, 4 both legs)	Age 17–48 mean 31 years; M:F = 5:7; comorbidities: 2 paresis, 1 dystonia	Centro-parietal area (midline or contralateral to symptoms)	rTMS (Cc) LF (approx. 1 Hz, 60 pulses) "Above" MT 1 session	Effective in 9/12: Immediate total recovery in 6 Dramatic improvement in 3 *(clinical impression)*	N/A	N/A
	45 seizure	Age 12–52, mean 27.9 (9.3) years; M:F = 13:32	Fronto-central area in midline	rTMS (Cc) LF (approx. 1 Hz, 60 pulses) "Above" MT Multiple sessions: all had 2 sessions (first & second days after communication of diagnosis) with extra sessions if symptoms no initial effect or relapse (max 8 sessions/month for 3 months)	Effective in 40/45: 2 months symptom free in 34 (80%) 50% reduction in seizures in 40 *(seizure frequency)*	N/A	Improvements sustained at 6 and 12 month follow-up. 4/40 improved relapsed but responded to further treatment

Peterson (2018)	7 seizure	Age 33–56, mean 43.1 (8.8) years; M:F = 1:6; comorbidities: depression, anxiety disorders	TPJ	rTMS (F8c) HF (10 Hz, 3000 pulses) 110% MT 30 sessions: twice per day over 3 weeks	Effective in 7/7 2 months symptom free in 4 A notable decrease in weekly seizure in 7 (*seizure frequency*)	5 headache or migraine 3 vivid/altered dreams 2 fatigue	Improvements sustained at 1, 2, 3 month follow-up in 7/7
Agarwal (2019)	1 seizure	Age 22 years; female; pregnant; comorbidities: depression	TPJ	rTMS (F8c) LF (0.33 Hz, 600 pulses) 80% MT 10 sessions (2 sessions/day for 1 week)	Effective 1/1: Significant improvement immediately and improving trend after 1 week (PNES scale)	None	Attack frequency reduced to "1 every 2 days" post 1 week and no attacks in the second and third week
Yeo (2019)	2 visual	Age 18 and 43 years; M:F = 1:1	Occipital	spTMS HF (10 Hz, 10 pulses/second for 10 seconds) 3 sessions (at 1, 2, and 6 weeks) for case 1 and 6 sessions for case 2	Ineffective: No significant change in vision (*clinical impression*)	N/A	1/2 transiently increased perception of light intensity from week 1 to week 2.

Key: *Cc* circular coil, *F8c* figure-of-8 coil, *HF* high frequency, *LF* low frequency, *MC* (primary) motor cortex, *PFC* pre-frontal cortex, *PMC* pre-motor cortex, *PNES* psychogenic non-epileptic seizure, *TPJ* temporoparietal junction, *MT* motor threshold, *rTMS* repetitive TMS, *spTMS* single pulse TMS, *VA* visual acuity, *VF* visual field

Randomized Controlled Trials (RCTs)

At present there have been five small RCTs with
the number of randomized patients ranging from
10 to 33. Trials with such small numbers would
generally best be described as "feasibility" studies as they will only be powered to detect excep-
tionally large treatment effect sizes and are
generally the first stage of trial design to test out
the study design works before conducting a pilot
study – which is usually the first step in assessing
efficacy and safety before progressing to a fully
powered definitive trial. The studies also varied
substantially in many aspects from trial design
(e.g. parallel armed or "cross over" design) to
TMS protocols (e.g. sham or real TMS control
intervention and brain area targeted) and the primary and key secondary outcome measures used.
We will now review these studies in turn – see
Table 28.3 for comparisons of key methodological issues and results.

The first RCT published [30] was of 11 subjects with functional paralysis of at least one
hand in a single-blind cross-over study. Subjects
were randomized to either the active rTMS or
control first and then, 2 months later, the other
intervention. The active intervention was a 15 Hz
figure-of-8 coil rTMS at 80% of resting motor
threshold (RMT) delivered over the hand area of
the primary motor cortex contralateral to the
affected side, with a train length of 2 seconds and
an intertrain interval of 4 seconds for 30 minutes
once daily for two periods of 5 consecutive days.
The control intervention was sham using a "real
electromagnetic placebo" (REMP) device placed
in front of the TMS coil to stimulate the scalp
sensation with small electric current and identical
TMS parameters. The primary outcome was
objective muscle strength measured by dyna-
mometry, and secondary outcomes included
patients' subjective report of changes in muscle
strength (0–100% premorbid functioning). A significant increase was reported in objective
strength comparing active rTMS to sham TMS
(24% vs 6%, $P < 0.04$) in patients who received
both interventions. However, no significant difference of subjective strength ratings was
detected (7% vs 1%, $P = 0.4$). The authors did not

follow up the outcomes after immediate results
and no available data for adverse events were
reported from both interventions.

The next RCT published [31] was and
unblinded study of ten participants with upper
limb weakness randomized to immediate ($n = 7$)
or delayed (3 months) ($n = 3$) TMS treatment. A
circular coil was used to deliver 46–70 spTMS
stimuli at 120–150% of motor threshold over the
hand area of primary motor cortex at ≤ 0.3 Hz in
sets of 4–5 pulses 3–4 seconds apart for both
groups. The primary outcomes were self (SF-12)
and clinician (Modified Rankin Scale) rated disability and self-reported symptom severity
(5-point Likert Scale) without one of these been
specified as the single key (primary) outcome
measure. Secondary outcomes were objectively
measured hand grip strength using a hand dyna-
mometer and tapping frequency (maximum taps
of the spacebar within 10 seconds). Comparison
between active and control groups was not done
due to the small number of subjects. However,
differences before and after TMS were analysed
for both groups; marginally significant reductions in self-reported symptom severity were
found ($P = 0.05$) but no significant differences in
grip strength ($P = 0.28$) or tapping frequency
($P = 0.89$). They followed up participants for
3 months and found no significantly sustained
improvements. Adverse effects were noted by
some patients both immediately after treatment
(mild headache, mild tingling and mild difficulty
concentrating), and at follow-up (severe headache, difficulty writing and a "severe 2-week dissociative regression").

Garcin et al. studied 33 patients with FMD
(tremor, dystonia, myoclonus, or parkinsonism)
in a single-blind cross-over design [32]. Subjects
were randomized to first receive either active
TMS or control, followed by the other treatment
after a minimal interval of 18 hours. Active treatment was 30–80 pulses of rTMS at was 0.25 Hz
and 120–150% of RMT over the lateral or medial
primary motor cortex, while control treatment
was nerve "root magnetic stimulation" (RMS)
using same stimulation parameters but applied
over the cervical or lumbar spinal roots. The primary outcome measure was an objective expert

Table 28.3 Randomized controlled trials (RCTs) of transcranial magnetic stimulation (TMS) treatment for functional movement disorder (FMD)

First author (year)	Symptoms	Subjects	Target	Stimulation parameters	Outcome measures	Adverse events	Follow up
Broersma (2015)	11 paresis	Age 34–64, mean = 50.8 years; M:F = 4:8	MC	*Study design:* Primary outcome: dynamometry at immediately before and after TMS Cross-over (2 months between condition) 11 received active, 8 received control TMS Single blind Limited communication with the patients during the treatments *Active treatment:* rTMS (F8c) HF (15 Hz, 4000 pulses/session) 80% MT 1 session/day for 2 blocks of 5 consecutive days (with 2 rest days in between) *Control treatment:* sham with above protocol	Effective Objective: significant ($P < 0.04$) higher increase in active (24%) > control (6%) (*Dynamometer*) Subjective: non-significant higher increase in active (7%) > control (1%)	N/A	None

(continued)

Table 28.3 (continued)

First author (year)	Symptoms	Subjects	Target	Stimulation parameters	Outcome measures	Adverse events	Follow up
McWhirter (2016)	10 paresis	Age 23–52, median = 35 years; M:F = 4:6; comorbidities: 2 dissociative seizures, 1 hemi-anaesthesia, 1 dysarthria, 1 visual impairment, 1 depression, 1 bipolar disorder	MC	*Study design:* Primary outcome: disability (SF-12 and MRS) and self-reported symptom severity Using a computerised random number generator Assessed by the doctor not blinded to group allocation or treatment effect. *Active treatment:* spTMS (Cc) 0.3 Hz (4–5 pulses 3–4 seconds apart) 120–150% MT Immediate treatment *Control treatment:* above protocol with delayed treatment	Ineffective Subjective: Significant reduction in severity immediately No patient reported delayed improvement Objective: No significant difference in grip strength or tapping frequency	1 severe headache, 1 "a thumping sore head" 1 increased difficulty writing, 1 dissociative regression	None
Garcin (2017)	33 MD (13 tremor, 11 dystonia, 4 jerky dystonia, 2 myoclonus, 2 stereotypies, 1 parkinsonism)	Age median (IQR) = 45 (28.6–54.9); M:F = 7:26; comorbidities: 7 motor deficits, 7 sensory deficits, 8 pain, 20 depression and/or anxiety	MC	*Study design:* Primary outcome: Clinical assessment Cross-over (18 hours between session) Prospectively randomized in Excel Raters were blinded *Active treatment:* rTMS LF (0.25 Hz) 120–150% MT *Control treatment:* rRMF	Ineffective Objective: No significant difference in the final percentage improvement between two groups (AIMS/BFMS)	N/A	At 3, 6, 12 months follow-up, no CGI statistical difference 56% of the patients were still much or very much improved 12 relapsed

First author (year)	Symptoms	Subjects	Target	Stimulation parameters	Outcome measures	Adverse events	Follow up
Taib (2019)	18 MD (tremor)	Age 24–64, mean = 48.9 years; M:F = 8:10; comorbidities: seven other functional motor symptoms, six history of depression and or anxiety	MC	*Study design:* Primary outcome: Psychogenic Movement Disorder Rating Scale (PMDRS) at month 1 compared with baseline. Double-blind Randomized by computer *Active treatment:* rTMS (F8c) 5 daily sessions 1 Hz, 1600 pulses 90% MT *Control treatment:* sham	Effective Objective: Significant change of score in active group (PMDRS: total and tremor subscores) Subjective: Active group rated 3–4 and control group rated 2–3 (CGI-Improvement)	N/A	Results sustained at 2, 6 & 12 months
Pick (2020)	21 paresis	(Active TMS) Age median (IQR) = 38 (32.5–46.5); M:F = 3:18	MC	*Study design:* Primary outcome: patient-rated symptom change (CGI-Improvement scale) Double-blind Randomized online Hours *Active treatment:* spTMS (Cc) 120 pulses/session 120% MT 2 sessions *Control treatment:* sham Below MT	Ineffective (but study explicitly not powered for efficacy) Subjective: No statistically significant differences but at TMS visit 2 (67% v 20%) & 3 month follow-up (44% v 20%), those in Active arm reported being "much improved" more frequently (CGI-I) Objective: Not significant change (Dynamometer)	Headaches (3 active, 5 control)	At 3-month follow-up, there were still more patients reporting "much improvement" in the active treatment; however, the difference was smaller that at TMS visit 2.

Key: *AIMS* abnormal involuntary movement scale, *BFMS* Burke-Fahn-Marsden scale, *Cc* circular coil, *CGI* Clinical Global Impression, *F8c* figure-of-8 coil, *FIM* Functional Independence Measure, *HF* high frequency, *LF* low frequency, *MC* (primary) motor cortex, *MD* functional movement disorder, *MT* motor threshold, *rRMS* repetitive spinal root magnetic stimulation, *rTMS* repetitive TMS, *spTMS* single pulse TMS assessment of FMD symptoms using blinded video recordings of clinical symptoms. Additional outcomes were depression and anxiety ratings and psychiatric comorbidity screenings. Overall improvement was reported at 70% post treatment, with significantly larger effects after the first session compared to the final session ($P = 0.03$), but no significant difference between rTMS and RMS after first session (37.5% vs 23.6%, $P = 0.29$) and final session ($P = 1$). Participants were followed up for 3, 6 and 12 months and found improvements in CGI scores but no statistical difference between day 3 and the follow up points.

Taib et al. studied 18 patients with functional tremor in a double-blind, two-arm, parallel, controlled study [33]. Patients were randomized to either active or inactive TMS for five consecutive daily sessions. The active group received rTMS using a figure-8 coil delivering 1600 biphasic pulses at 1 Hz at 90% of RMT applied to the lateral or medial primary motor cortex contralateral to a single affected limb (or bilaterally if the tremor was bilateral). The control (inactive) TMS was a sham coil providing an acoustic stimulus comparable to that of the active rTMS. The primary outcome was objectively measured symptoms within the Psychogenic Movement Disorder Rating Scale (PMDRS) [34] assessed by three experts using blinded video recordings. Secondary outcomes were changes in the total PMDRS and tremor subscores alongside subjective disability (SF-36) and both anxiety and depression (HADS) scales and the clinician rated CGI (severity) scale assessed at months 1, 2, 6, and 12. One month after the intervention, the mean PMDRS scores had decreased in both groups, but the differences from baseline were only significant in the active group ($P < 0.001$). This remained significant at month 2 ($P < 0.001$). The significant decrease of the total PMDRS and tremor subscores were maintained at months 6 and 12 for the active group. For the control group, the PMDRS had returned almost to its baseline value by month 2 and remained unchanged at months 6 and 12.

The most recent RCT to date [35] was of 21 participants with functional limb weakness in a double-blind (patient and outcome assessor) two parallel-arm, controlled trial. Participants were randomized to active or inactive TMS for two sessions, 4 weeks apart. The active intervention was 120 pulses of spTMS at 120% of RMT delivered to the primary motor cortex of the weakest limb. The inactive TMS was the same (real) spTMS at 80% of RMT thereby not resulting in movement of the affected limb. The primary outcome was subjectively measured symptoms using the patient rating of CGI (improvement), and secondary outcomes included objective clinician-rated symptom change, subjective psychosocial functioning and disability questionnaires. The percentage of participants who rated themselves as "much improved" immediately after the first session in the active group compared with control was 0% vs 9%, changing to 67% vs 20% comparing before and after second session, and 44% vs 20% at 3-month follow-up. Effect sizes were small to moderate (Cliff's delta = −0.1 to 0.3), reflecting a more positive outcome for the active treatment. Adverse events were lower in active group compared with control (26 vs 37) and no serious adverse events occurred immediately following TMS. Blinding was successful in that there was no statistical evidence for patients being able to guess whether they received active or inactive TMS.

In summary there have been five small RCTs with some encouraging results for both efficacy and safety, but no clear or consistent statistical evidence, as would be expected with studies of this size.

Methodological Issues

There are several key methodological issues which warrant further discussion.

Control Intervention

There is currently no consensus regarding the optimal control intervention. A key aspect of any control intervention is that the patient should not be able to tell if receiving the active or inactive intervention. One of the most commonly used controls in TMS studies are "sham" TMS stimulators which produce minimal or no actual magnetic pulses, but aim to produce a near-identical treatment experience. The most basic sham stimulation is achieved by rotating the magnetic coil away from the target site so as to not stimulate it when the pulse is discharged. However, most commonly a specific "sham coil" is used which is designed to look, sound and feel identical to a real coil but which produces no magnetic pulse. Such devices can produce sensory experience such as audible click [36] and more advanced coils can now produce a scalp sensation that is potentially similar to real TMS stimulation [37]. However, sham devices are not always perfect in that subjects can sometimes guess whether they have had real or sham treatment so it is critical that the success of blinding is assessed by asking subjects to guess if they have had real or sham interventions. Alternatively, as used by Pick et al. [35], TMS can be delivered at below RMT intensities, if it is considered that movement of the limb is the "active ingredient" of the TMS treatment.

Parallel or Cross-Over Design

Two studies used a method where subjects receive both the active and the control intervention one after the other, known as a cross-over design, while the others used a parallel group method where they receive just one of the interventions. Although cross-over trial can have advantages in that more statistical power is created for the same number of patients recruited, there are some disadvantages for TMS, especially in the context of FND, with regard to the issue of "carry-over effects", i.e. the potential for persistent effects of the first intervention given that carries over to the time period when the second intervention is given therefore contaminating the assessment of the second intervention. As such, one should be cautious about cross-over design used in this context.

Outcomes Measures

Outcome measure selection is important in trials and there needs to be single pre-specified primary outcome [38]. This needs to be clinically meaningful to patients, but also one which can realistically expected to change with the intervention. There are various types of outcome measures used which can be subjective or objective, patient-rated or clinician-rated, general or symptom specific. Objective outcomes are generally preferred in most clinical trials for most disorders as they are considered more robust markers of improvement. However, an argument can be made that subjective measures are important for patients with FND and potentially equally valid [39]; see Chap. 29 for more details. Furthermore, consensus is needed amongst researchers, clinicians, patients, carers, funders and other stakeholders on "core outcome sets" so that trials can collect the same measures, at least in part, to allow comparison and collation and this work is underway in FND [40].

Potential Mechanisms

There are several potential mechanisms that could explain how TMS might improve FMD symptoms, over and above placebo effects which can occur as at least part of the mechanism of improvement for almost all treatments for all conditions. We will briefly review the three main possibilities that are, of course, not mutually exclusive, and could occur either alone or in combination.

Neuromodulation

As mentioned in the introduction, TMS can influence cortical function in the area directly stimulated but also potentially alter the connectivity, or the function of, other brain areas indirectly. These changes can therefore potentially restore normal functioning. TMS has been shown to enhance motor learning by increasing motor cortex excitability with long-term potentiation (LTP)-like mechanisms in healthy humans [41–43] and also in patients with stroke [44]. However, there is still limited evidence of TMS for FND acting via neuromodulation and some of the very rapid responses reported in case would be less compatible with such a mechanism. Moreover, we still have very limited and preliminary understandings of the mechanisms of FND [45, 46], specifically regarding the role of different cortical structures that could be modulated by TMS for the disorder as a whole, let alone for a given individual. Consequently, we would expect a lot more research to be needed to identify critical dysfunction, modifiable by TMS, of specific cortical areas at the level of individual patients before we would expect this to be postulated as the key mechanism.

Belief and Expectation

A key contemporary neurobiological theory of brain function is that it is a hierarchical Bayesian inference machine, for example predicting sensory input based on past experience [47]. Symptoms in FND have been proposed to arise from dysfunction of the brain's integration of motor and sensory activity, mediated by dysfunctional attention to bodily symptoms and therefore driven by "attentional and belief-driven processes" [48]. Beliefs are therefore important information for sensorimotor processing at a neuronal level, and prior beliefs, or expectation, play a crucial role in modifying sensory experiences and motor function. Beliefs of patients with FND are influenced by several possible factors after TMS, particularly if applied to the motor cortex creating "artificial" movement of a weak limb or interrupting a movement disorder. This demonstrates the possibility of normalisation of function, with certainty at the time of stimulation, and the possibility of longer-term changes and return of function.

Perception of Action

Perception, in terms of somatosensory feedback, is crucial for learning (or re-learning) movements and optimizing synaptic activity and the integrity of brain connectivity. The process of action observation activates brain areas not only in visual centers in the occipital lobe but also neural systems of action execution, including motor areas in the frontal lobe and somatosensory areas in the parietal lobe [49]. To make and improve new movement, the brain needs somatosensory feedback from body motion. After TMS, a movement of body perceived to be dysfunctional is a new sensory input for the brain. Perceptual learning drives improvements in motor learning and neural changes in the motor systems. This phenomenon is seen in everyday situations such as learning to speak a new language by observing others' speaking – perceptual and motor learning occur together [50]. Moreover, there is some evidence patients with FND need less information to form a decision and were more likely to change their probability estimates in the direction suggested by the new evidence [51]. Therefore, re-experiencing normal movement triggered by TMS could help with (re)learning normal movement.

Future Directions

Research Methodology

There are still considerable challenges in optimizing the methodology for RCTs of TMS for FMD and other FND symptoms. As discussed above, we caution against the use of cross-over designs as it is possible, indeed likely, that the potential mechanism(s) of action can persist beyond any cross-over point in the trial to contaminate subsequent data. Until perfect sham devices are developed, which are physiologically inert with regard to the mechanism(s) of action of TMS on FND, but not detectably different to real TMS, another potential control treatment is subthreshold TMS (delivered at below RMT intensities), e.g. that used in the Pick et al. RCT [35]. Such control interventions are not likely to induce physiological changes in cortical excitability or long-lasting neuromodulatory effects but will potentially allow successful blinding of a control intervention. Other control arms, for example, treatment as usual or wait list controls could be used but these are considered suboptimal in terms of discerning treatment effects, particularly if a control intervention is available. There are also ethical questions about how much suggestion of recovery is appropriate to use in trials, or indeed clinical practice.

Most studies of TMS for FMD applied the magnetic coil over the primary motor cortex (M1) as an anatomical target area. However, other locations thought to be mechanistically involved in all, or particular, FND symptoms could be targeted; for example the supplementary motor area (SMA) is implicated in motor initiation/planning, temporoparietal junction (TPJ) implicated in motor intention/self-agency perceptions [29], anterior insula and bilateral middle cingulate cortex implicated in assigning emotional salience [52], and anterior cingulate cortex and insula implicated in suppression of fear response [25].

Combining TMS with other treatment modalities either individually or as part of a multidisciplinary intervention could be particularly effective, especially concomitant physical therapy which could be combined in the same session, such that small initial gains in voluntary movement could be built on and reinforced following TMS induced involuntary movement. The case vignette at the start of this chapter provided an example of such potential synergistic effects. TMS could also be combined with psychological interventions, such as CBT, or pharmacological approaches such as psychedelics which have been used in the past and which there is renewed interest in FMD and other FND symptoms [53, 54].

TMS might also have a particular role when there is complete limb paralysis, such that physical therapy, a cornerstone of contemporary management, is not possible or exceedingly limited. TMS might also be indicated when all other treatment modalities, have failed. Further work is clearly needed to see if other FND symptoms, particularly visual, might be effective. Work also needs be done alongside trials of TMS to identify which patients might benefit from TMS, particularly with regard to other variables such as lengths of symptoms, risk factors and comorbidities which could be predictors of response. The sys-

tematic review by Pollak et al. [23] reported that length of disorder duration was associated with poorer response, compatible with other studies found that longer duration of FND symptoms was a negative predictor of recovery [55]. Therefore, further research investigating predictors of TMS response is urgently needed.

Other Types of Neuromodulation

Novel TMS methods have been developed that rapidly induce synaptic plasticity, using protocols known as Theta-burst stimulation (TBS). It produces short bursts of high-frequency (50 Hz) stimulation repeated at 5 Hz. There are two types of TBS: intermittent TBS (iTBS), associated with long-term potentiation–like activity, and continuous TBS (cTBS) associated with long-term depression–like activity [56]. One recent study investigated TBS [25] as treatment for a female patient with functional seizures by applying iTBS over the TPJ with 80% RMT for ten sessions within 7 days and reported significant improvement.

In addition to TMS, there have been a variety of brain stimulation therapies that can alter neural activity via different approaches. One of the most common techniques is transcranial direct current stimulation (tDCS), producing low amplitude of direct current through the skull to the brain. While TMS depolarizes neurons and modulates cortical excitability, tDCS modifies the transmembrane neuronal potential and influences level of cortical excitability. Therefore, tDCS is a neuromodulation technique, whereas TMS is both neurostimulation and neuromodulation therapy. One study of tDCS [57] has been published in FND using a double-blinded two-period crossover trial. Nine patients with functional motor symptoms and seven age- and sex-matched healthy control were randomized to either active stimulation or sham first and then, at 2 days later, having the other intervention. An active stimulation was a single session of anodal tDCS over right posterior parietal cortex at 1.5 mA intensity for 20 minutes, whereas sham stimulation used same parameters as the active intervention except for duration at only 30 seconds to make subjects feel similar itching or tingling sensation as the active stimulation. Interoceptive sensitivity was assessed using heartbeat detection task and spatial attention assessed using the Posner paradigm. Significant differences in interoceptive sensitivity after active and sham stimulation were found and remained significant in patients with FND when separately considering the two groups. No adverse events were reported.

Another, older, electrical stimulation method is electroconvulsive therapy (ECT) which has proven efficacy for a range of severe psychiatric disorders although of course has potential risks, especially those due to the anesthesia required and potential medium and longer term memory impairments. However, the severity and chronicity of disability experienced in some FND cases could potentially make ECT a therapeutic option if all else has failed. A systematic review of non-invasive brain stimulation (NIBS) for functional weakness found two successful case reports of ECT [58]. The first study [59] reported a male elderly patient with functional hand paralysis for 11 months treated with bilateral ECT 3 times a week for 2 weeks, then 2 times a week for 6 weeks. His FND symptoms improved after the first ECT without relapse during follow-up. A second study [60] reported a male young adult with fluctuating quadriplegia for 3 years who was treated with ECT 2–3 times a week, then once a week. Again, the functional weakness symptoms improved after 9 sessions with full independent function after 25 sessions but relapsed after a while during follow-up. However, muscle activity remained better than baseline. Both studies assessed improvement using CGI-I, it was rated as 2 (much improved) after ECT and 3 (minimally improved) after follow-up.

Additionally, there have been other neurostimulation techniques that have some evidence of efficacy for neurological disease and are potential options for FND treatment. Stimulation of other targets apart from the central nervous system has been applied, for example, repeated root magnetic stimulation (RMS) applied over the cervical or lumbar spinal roots demonstrated similar FND motor symptom improvement compared to TMS [32]. Peripheral nerve stimulation (PNS), a technique delivering electrical impulse to peripheral nerve has shown its efficacy to improve paretic upper limb after stroke either with or without functional training [61]. One case report [62] noted an adult patient with right upper limb functional weakness treated with peripheral electrical stimulation (PES) and measured clinical outcome using grip strength and neurophysiological outcomes using TMS. Stimulation parameters were a 30 Hz single stimulation over the right median, ulnar, and radial nerves with a train length of 4 seconds and an intertrain interval of 6 seconds for 30 minutes. Clinical symptoms with neurophysiological outcomes did not change immediately after stimulation but did change over weeks and full recovery by 6 months. No adverse events were reported.

Another new potential modality of indirect neuromodulation utilizes ultrasound waves, using a technique known as focused ultrasound (FUS) which can be applied transcranially (tFUS). Importantly this has the potential for higher spatial resolution and can reach deeper structures than TMS and other indirect neurostimulation methods allowing more precise stimulation of more structures, including subcortical structures such as the limbic/paralimbic system for which there is mounting evidence of mechanistic relevance in FND [45]. Stimulation parameters can also be varied to cause a wide spectrum of effects from suppression or facilitation of neuronal activity through to tissue ablation. It has been approved for various medical diseases, including refractory essential tremor [63], and potentially improves symptoms and the quality of life in patients with essential tremor [64]. Further studies of other techniques for neuromodulation would be interesting to explore its efficacy and potential mechanisms for FND.

Conclusions

There is accumulating evidence that TMS is a potentially effective, well-tolerated and safe treatment for FMD and other subtypes of FND. TMS is a cheap and potentially rapidly scalable treatment modality given that TMS machines are generally available in clinical neuroscience departments – where they are most prominently used for the treatment of major depression. However, there have been no large RCTs to fully evaluate its efficacy and safety. Furthermore, optimal TMS therapeutic protocols and the methodology for trials to assess this treatment, and for which patients it might be effective for, is still not clear.

Relatedly the mechanisms by which TMS could improve functional neurological symptoms are also unclear but these are likely to be a mixture of placebo, other more complex changes in belief and expectation or perception of action. It also possible that there are neuromodulatory effects, depending on the TMS stimulation protocol and brain area targeted.

More studies of TMS for FND are needed to optimize protocols for treatment, including studies of mechanism of action, as well as studies to help achieve consensus on optimal trial design. This will pave the way for definitive trials to assess efficacy and safety. It is possible that other currently available neurostimulation methods, or new neurostimulation methods, could also be applied therapeutically to FND in the future, particularly in response to emerging mechanistic insights into the neurobiology of FND.

Summary

- TMS is a promising, off-label treatment option for patients with FMD and other functional neurological symptoms.
- TMS warrants additional research as a treatment used in isolation, as well as part of a multidisciplinary treatment package.
- When effective, potential mechanisms of action include neuromodulation, perception of action, alterations of beliefs/expectations, and placebo among other possibilities.
- While only feasibility randomized controlled trials using TMS have been conducted to date, larger-scale efforts will need to carefully consider appropriate control interventions.

References

1. American Psychiatric Association. Diagnostic and statistical manual of mental disorders. 5th ed. Arlington: American Psychiatric Association; 2013.
2. World Health Organization. International statistical classification of diseases and related health problems. 11th ed. Geneva: World Health Organization; 2020.
3. Espay AJ, Aybek S, Carson A, Edwards MJ, Goldstein LH, Hallett M, et al. Current concepts in diagnosis and treatment of functional neurological disorders. JAMA Neurol. 2018;75(9):1132–41.
4. Nielsen G, Stone J, Matthews A, Brown M, Sparkes C, Farmer R, et al. Physiotherapy for functional motor disorders: a consensus recommendation. J Neurol Neurosurg Psychiatry. 2015;86(10):1113–9.
5. Nielsen G, Stone J, Buszewicz M, Carson A, Goldstein LH, Holt K, et al. Physio4FMD: protocol for a multi-centre randomised controlled trial of specialist physiotherapy for functional motor disorder. BMC Neurol. 2019;19(1):242.
6. Goldstein LH, Robinson EJ, Mellers JDC, Stone J, Carson A, Reuber M, et al. Cognitive behavioural therapy for adults with dissociative seizures (CODES): a pragmatic, multicentre, randomised controlled trial. Lancet Psychiatry. 2020;7(6):491–505.
7. Gutkin M, McLean L, Brown R, Kanaan RA. Systematic review of psychotherapy for adults with functional neurological disorder. J Neurol Neurosurg Psychiatry. 2021;92:36–44.
8. Lefaucheur JP, Aleman A, Baeken C, Benninger DH, Brunelin J, Di Lazzaro V, et al. Evidence-based guidelines on the therapeutic use of repetitive transcranial magnetic stimulation (rTMS): an update (2014–2018). Clin Neurophysiol. Elsevier Ireland Ltd. 2020;131:474–528.
9. National Institute for Health and Care Excellence. Depression in adults: recognition and management. Clinical guideline [Internet]. 2009 [cited 2021 Apr 26]. Available from: www.nice.org.uk/guidance/cg90.
10. Barker AT, Jalinous R, Freeston IL. Non-invasive magnetic stimulation of human motor cortex. Lancet. 1985;325(8437):1106–7.
11. Rossi S, Hallett M, Rossini PM, Pascual-Leone A, Avanzini G, Bestmann S, et al. Safety, ethical considerations, and application guidelines for the use of transcranial magnetic stimulation in clinical practice and research. Clin Neurophysiol. NIH Public Access. 2009;120:2008–39.
12. Horvath JC, Perez JM, Forrow L, Fregni F, Pascual-Leone A. Transcranial magnetic stimulation: a historical evaluation and future prognosis of therapeutically relevant ethical concerns. J Med Ethics. 2011;37(3):137–43.
13. McWhirter L, Carson A, Stone J. The body electric: a long view of electrical therapy for functional neurological disorders. Brain. 2015;138(Pt 4):1113–20.
14. Tatu L, Bogousslavsky J, Moulin T, Chopard J-L. The "torpillage" neurologists of World War I: electric therapy to send hysterics back to the front. Neurology. 2010;75(3):279–83.

15. Jellinek DA, Bradford R, Bailey I, Symon L. The role of motor evoked potentials in the management of hysterical paraplegia: case report. Paraplegia. 1992;30:300–2.

16. Kresojevic N, Petrovic I, Tomic A, Svetel M, Radovanovic S, Kostic V. Transcranial magnetic stimulation in therapy of psychogenic neurological symptoms: two case reports. Mov Disord. 2010;25:S220–S.

17. Hallett M. Transcranial magnetic stimulation and the human brain. Nature. 2000;406(6792):147–50.

18. Schönfeldt-Lecuona C, Connemann BJ, Viviani R, Spitzer M, Herwig U. Transcranial magnetic stimulation in motor conversion disorder: a short case series. J Clin Neurophysiol. 2006;23(5):472–5.

19. Fitzgerald PB, Fountain S, Daskalakis ZJ. A comprehensive review of the effects of rTMS on motor cortical excitability and inhibition. Clin Neurophysiol. 2006;117(12):2584–96.

20. Shah BB, Chen R, Zurowski M, Kalia LV, Gunraj C, Lang AE. Repetitive transcranial magnetic stimulation plus standardized suggestion of benefit for functional movement disorders: an open label case series. Parkinsonism Relat Disord. 2015;21(4):407–12.

21. Daskalakis ZJ, Christensen BK, Fitzgerald PB, Chen R. Transcranial magnetic stimulation: a new investigational and treatment tool in psychiatry. J Neuropsychiatry Clin Neurosci. 2002;14(4):406–15.

22. Chastan N, Parain D. Psychogenic paralysis and recovery after motor cortex transcranial magnetic stimulation. Mov Disord. 2010;25(10):1501–4.

23. Pollak TA, Nicholson TR, Edwards MJ, David AS. A systematic review of transcranial magnetic stimulation in the treatment of functional (conversion) neurological symptoms. J Neurol Neurosurg Psychiatry. 2014;85(2):191–7.

24. Walburn J, Gray R, Gournay K, Quraishi S, David AS. Systematic review of patient and nurse attitudes to depot antipsychotic medication. Br J Psychiatry. 2001;179:300–7.

25. Agarwal R, Garg S, Tikka SK, Khatri S, Goel D. Successful use of theta burst stimulation (TBS) for treating psychogenic non epileptic seizures (PNES) in a pregnant woman. Asian J Psychiatr. 2019;43:121–2.

26. Chastan N, Parain D, Vérin E, Weber J, Faure MA, Marie JP. LETTERS psychogenic aphonia: spectacular recovery after motor cortex transcranial magnetic stimulation. J Neurol Neurosurg Psychiatry. 2009;80(1):94.

27. Parain D, Chastan N. Large-field repetitive transcranial magnetic stimulation with circular coil in the treatment of functional neurological symptoms. Neurophysiol Clin. 2014;44(4):425–31.

28. Yeo JM, Carson A, Stone J. Seeing again: treatment of functional visual loss. Pract Neurol. 2019;19(2):168–72.

29. Peterson KT, Kosior R, Meek BP, Ng M, Perez DL, Modirrousta M. Right temporoparietal junction transcranial magnetic stimulation in the treatment

30. of psychogenic nonepileptic seizures: a case series. Psychosomatics. 2018;59(6):601–6.

30. Broersma M, Koops EA, Vroomen PC, Van der Hoeven JH, Aleman A, Leenders KL, et al. Can repetitive transcranial magnetic stimulation increase muscle strength in functional neurological paresis? A proof-of-principle study. Eur J Neurol. 2015;22(5):866–73.

31. McWhirter L, Ludwig L, Carson A, McIntosh RD, Stone J. Transcranial magnetic stimulation as a treatment for functional (psychogenic) upper limb weakness. J Psychosom Res. 2016;89:102–6.

32. Garcin B, Mesrati F, Hubsch C, Mauras T, Iliescu I, Naccache L, et al. Impact of transcranial magnetic stimulation on functional movement disorders: cortical modulation or a behavioral effect? Front Neurol. 2017;8:338.

33. Taib S, Ory-Magne F, Brefel-Courbon C, Moreau Y, Thalamas C, Arbus C, et al. Repetitive transcranial magnetic stimulation for functional tremor: a randomized, double-blind, controlled study. Mov Disord. 2019;34(8):1210–9.

34. Hinson VK, Cubo E, Comella CL, Goetz CG, Leurgans S. Rating scale for psychogenic movement disorders: scale development and clinimetric testing. Mov Disord. 2005;20(12):1592–7.

35. Pick S, Hodsoll J, Stanton B, Eskander A, Stavropoulos I, Samra K, et al. Trial of Neurostimulation in Conversion Symptoms (TONICS): a feasibility randomised controlled trial of transcranial magnetic stimulation for functional limb weakness. BMJ Open. 2020;10(10):e037198.

36. Herwig U, Cardenas-Morales L, Connemann BJ, Kammer T, Schönfeldt-Lecuona C. Sham or real-post hoc estimation of stimulation condition in a randomized transcranial magnetic stimulation trial. Neurosci Lett. 2010;471(1):30–3.

37. Duecker F, Sack AT. Rethinking the role of sham TMS. Front Psychol. 2015;6:210.

38. Schulz KF, Altman DG, Moher D. CONSORT 2010 statement: updated guidelines for reporting parallel group randomised trials. BMJ. 2010 Mar 27;340(7748):698–702.

39. Nicholson TR, Carson A, Edwards MJ, Goldstein LH, Hallett M, Mildon B, et al. Outcome measures for functional neurological disorder: a review of the theoretical complexities. J Neuropsychiatry Clin Neurosci. 2020;32(1):33–42.

40. Pick S, Anderson DG, Asadi-Pooya AA, Aybek S, Baslet G, Bloem BR, et al. Outcome measurement in functional neurological disorder: a systematic review and recommendations. J Neurol Neurosurg Psychiatry. BMJ Publishing Group. 2020;91:638–49.

41. Ilić TV, Ziemann U. Exploring motor cortical plasticity using transcranial magnetic stimulation in humans. Ann N Y Acad Sci. 2005;1048:175–84.

42. Kim YH, Park JW, Ko MH, Jang SH, Lee PKW. Facilitative effect of high frequency subthreshold repetitive transcranial magnetic stimulation on complex sequential motor learning in humans. Neurosci Lett. 2004;367(2):181–5.

43. Schambra HM, Sawaki L, Cohen LG. Modulation of excitability of human motor cortex (M1) by 1 Hz transcranial magnetic stimulation of the contralateral M1. Clin Neurophysiol. 2003;114(1):130–3.

44. Hoyer EH, Celnik PA. Understanding and enhancing motor recovery after stroke using transcranial magnetic stimulation. Restor Neurol Neurosci. 2011;29(6):395–409.

45. Pick S, Goldstein LH, Perez DL, Nicholson TR. Emotional processing in functional neurological disorder: a review, biopsychosocial model and research agenda [Internet]. J Neurol Neurosurg Psychiatry. BMJ Publishing Group. 2019 [cited 2021 May 7];90:704–11. Available from: https://doi.org/10.1136/jnnp-2018-319201.

46. Drane DL, Fani N, Hallett M, Khalsa SS, Perez DL, Roberts NA. A framework for understanding the pathophysiology of functional neurological disorder. CNS Spectr. 2021;26(6):555-61.

47. Friston K. The free-energy principle: a rough guide to the brain? Trends Cogn Sci. 2009;13(7):293–301.

48. Edwards MJ, Adams RA, Brown H, Pareés I, Friston KJ. A Bayesian account of "hysteria". Brain. 2012;135(Pt 11):3495–512.

49. Lametti DR, Watkins KE. Cognitive neuroscience: the neural basis of motor learning by observing. Curr Biol. 2016;26(7):R288–90.

50. Ostry DJ, Gribble PL. Sensory plasticity in human motor learning. Trends Neurosci. 2016;39(2):114–23.

51. Pareés I, Kassavetis P, Saifee TA, Sadnicka A, Bhatia KP, Fotopoulou A, et al. "Jumping to conclusions" bias in functional movement disorders. J Neurol Neurosurg Psychiatry. 2012;83(4):460–3.

52. Voon V, Brezing C, Gallea C, Hallett M. Aberrant supplementary motor complex and limbic activity during motor preparation in motor conversion disorder. Mov Disord. 2011;26(13):2396–403.

53. Butler M, Seynaeve M, Nicholson TR, Pick S, Kanaan RA, Lees A, et al. Psychedelic treatment of functional neurological disorder: a systematic review. Ther Adv Psychopharmacol. 2020 Jan 11;10:2045125320912125.

54. Bryson A, Carter O, Norman T, Kanaan R. 5-HT2A agonists: a novel therapy for functional neurological disorders?. Int J Neuropsychopharmacol. Oxford University Press. 2017;20:422–7. Available from: https://pubmed.ncbi.nlm.nih.gov/28177082/.

55. Gelauff J, Stone J, Edwards M, Carson A. The prognosis of functional (psychogenic) motor symptoms: a systematic review. J Neurol Neurosurg Psychiatry. 2014;85(2):220–6.

56. Rounis E, Huang YZ. Theta burst stimulation in humans: a need for better understanding effects of brain stimulation in health and disease. Exp Brain Res. 2020;238:1707–14.

57. Demartini B, Volpe R, Mattavelli G, Goeta D, D'Agostino A, Gambini O. The neuromodulatory effect of tDCS in patients affected by functional motor symptoms: an exploratory study. Neurol Sci. 2019;40(9):1821–7.

58. Schönfeldt-Lecuona C, Lefaucheur J-P, Lepping P, Liepert J, Connemann BJ, Sartorius A, et al. Non-invasive brain stimulation in conversion (functional) weakness and paralysis: a systematic review and future perspectives. Front Neurosci. 2016;10:140.

59. Giovanoli EJ. ECT in a patient with conversion disorder. Convuls Ther. 1988;4(3):236–42.

60. Gaillard A, Gaillard R, Mouaffak F, Radtchenko A, Lôo H. Case report: electroconvulsive therapy in a 33-year-old man with hysterical quadriplegia. Encéphale. 2012;38(1):104–9.

61. Obiglio M, Mendelevich A, Jeffrey S, Drault E, Garcete A, Kramer M, et al. Peripheral nerve stimulation effectiveness in the upper limb function recovery of patients with a stroke sequel: systematic review and meta-analysis. Rev Neurol. 2016;62(12):530–8.

62. Burke MJ, Isayama R, Jegatheeswaran G, Gunraj C, Feinstein A, Lang AE, et al. Neurostimulation for functional neurological disorder: evaluating longitudinal neurophysiology. Mov Disord Clin Pract. 2018;5(5):561–3.

63. Elias WJ, Lipsman N, Ondo WG, Ghanouni P, Kim YG, Lee W, et al. A randomized trial of focused ultrasound thalamotomy for essential tremor. N Engl J Med. 2016;375:730–9.

64. Mohammed N, Patra D, Nanda A. A meta-analysis of outcomes and complications of magnetic resonance-guided focused ultrasound in the treatment of essential tremor. Neurosurg Focus. 2018;44(2):E4.

Measuring Symptoms and Monitoring Progress in Functional Movement Disorder

29

Glenn Nielsen, Susannah Pick, and Timothy R. Nicholson

Clinical Vignette

A neurorehabilitation unit has received additional funds to set up a specialist multidisciplinary treatment program for patients with FMD. Ongoing funding of the service is dependent on the unit being able to demonstrate that the service is effective. The neurorehabilitation team meet to plan the outcome measurement strategy for their new service. They sought to follow recently published recommendations for assessing outcome in FMD [1, 2]. Additional considerations guiding their decisions included the following:

- *Aim: The primary aim was to demonstrate effectiveness of the clinical service.*
- *Time burden: The team recognized that it was important to keep the data collection procedure as brief as possible, to reduce clinician and patient burden as well as minimize the chance of missing data.*
- *Simplicity: The chosen measures should be simple enough so that each member of the team could participate in the data collection without needing lengthy training.*
- *Generalizability: The patients were known to be heterogeneous, therefore specific symptom assessment tools (e.g. for gait, tremor, or fatigue), although useful for individuals and subgroups, were not relevant to all individuals and therefore had limited value for assessing the service as a whole.*

The team chose measures to assess core FMD symptom severity (using the Clinical Global Impression Scale of Improvement (CGI-I)), psychological symptoms (using the Hospital Anxiety and Depression Scale (HADS)), as well as activity and participation (using the Work and Social Adjustment Scale (WSAS)). In addition, the team developed a custom patient satisfaction survey and recorded adverse events associated with treatment.

The CGI-I, as rated by patients, was chosen to measure change in FND symptom severity. Alternative options were considered too time consuming (e.g. the Psychogenic Movement Disorders Rating Scale) or lacking in relevance to all patients (e.g. gait speed). In using the CGI-I, patients were asked to rate the change in their

G. Nielsen (✉)
Neuroscience Research Centre, Institute of Molecular and Clinical Sciences, St Georges University of London, London, UK
e-mail: gnielsen@sgul.ac.uk

S. Pick
Institute of Psychiatry, Psychology and Neuroscience, King's College London, London, UK
e-mail: susannah.pick@kcl.ac.uk

T. R. Nicholson
Neuropsychiatry Research and Education Group, Institute of Psychiatry Psychology & Neuroscience, King's College London, London, UK
e-mail: timothy.nicholson@kcl.ac.uk

© Springer Nature Switzerland AG 2022
K. LaFaver et al. (eds.), *Functional Movement Disorder*, Current Clinical Neurology,
https://doi.org/10.1007/978-3-030-86495-8_29

motor symptoms on a 5-point Likert scale, using the following options: Much improved, Improved, No change, Worse, or Much worse. A limitation of the CGI-I is that the data lacks meaning in terms of absolute values, an advantage of the CGI-I is that it is easily interpretable. On reviewing outcomes of the first cohort of patients, it was found that 70% of patients reported their motor symptoms had improved following treatment.

Mean anxiety and depression scores did not change after treatment. The aggregate scores were not especially useful for evaluating the service. However, exploring an individual's scores may help to understand their outcome. For example, one patient's lack of treatment response may have been related to his or her high anxiety and depression. If this had been identified at baseline, it could have become a focus of treatment. Alternatively, if there had been a post-intervention improvement in anxiety and depression scores, this might have suggested a possible mechanism for the intervention.

The team chose to assess quality of life using the Work and Social Adjustment Scale (WSAS). The WSAS has several advantages over other scales (such as the Short Form 36), including being relatively brief, easy to score and free to use. An important disadvantage is that it is less commonly used and so there is less data for comparing the service outcomes. The SF36 would be a reasonable alternative as the scale is widely used in FND research and other patient populations, although certain versions have license fees that need to be considered. The EQ-5D-5L is free for some uses, however the scoring system is less straightforward than the WSAS.

Interim recommendations from the FND-COM Outcome Measurement group suggest measuring other physical symptoms, such as fatigue, headache and dizziness. This domain of measurement has value in describing clinical presentation, however its value as a measure of treatment outcome or as a mediator of change is uncertain. It therefore arguably has greater research than clinical utility and so was not included in the measurement strategy. Also omitted from these outcomes are data related to health care utilization. This would have been valuable data to convince the hospital administrators and or insurance companies to fund the service, however it would have required follow up assessment (e.g. to determine change in health care utilization at 12 months).

Introduction

Accurately measuring outcomes is vitally important in clinical practice and research. There are unique features associated with FMD that make measurement particularly complex [3]. These include the heterogeneity of the patient population, temporal variability in symptom severity and the high prevalence of multicomorbidity. How outcome is best measured in FMD is therefore an unresolved question. Key challenges are to identify the most relevant outcome domains and measurement tools that are reliable and valid for these constructs. To date, there has been limited research activity devoted to developing specific assessment tools for FMD, or assessing the validity and reliability of currently available outcome measures.

A recent surge in research interest in FMD and functional neurological disorder (FND) more broadly has provided an impetus to improve outcome measurement. Pick et al. (2020) recently completed a systematic review of outcome measurement in clinical trials of FND interventions. An important limitation of the literature was the substantial divergence in the primary outcomes adopted and the scales used to measure relevant outcome domains (e.g., symptom severity, quality of life, disability, psychological distress, etc). Furthermore, it was noted that there were few FND-specific outcome measures available, and none that had been rigorously validated in large-scale research studies or across cultural contexts. The generic outcome measures that were frequently used also lacked validation in FND samples, therefore their psychometric properties in this population are unclear.

An international multidisciplinary group of FND specialists (FND-Core Outcome Measures, FND-COM) formed in 2017, with the aims of improving outcome measurement in clinical studies, starting the process of developing consensus on a core set of outcome measurements for FND, and pooling data between intervention studies [1, 3]. Here we summarize the findings of this work to date and discuss the clinical implications for patients with functional motor symptoms.

Principles of Outcome Measurement

The basic principles of outcome measurement are important to consider when selecting assessment tools for clinical practice. The scientific study of the attributes of an outcome measure is termed *psychometrics*. Important psychometric and other properties to consider when selecting an outcome measure are detailed in Box 29.1 [4, 5].

Box 29.1 Outcome Measure Attributes

Validity	The degree to which the assessment tool measures what it sets out to measure.
Reliability	The degree to which a measurement tool is error free. This includes the concepts of inter-rater reliability: the degree to which two or more different rater's scores will agree for the same patient; and intra-rater reliability: stability of an instrument over time when rated by the same individual (test-retest).
Responsiveness	This includes sensitivity to detect change, and the concepts of ceiling and floor effect, where a measurement tool loses sensitivity towards the top or bottom end of the scale.
Interpretability	The degree to which the scores of an assessment tool can be understood.

Validity	The degree to which the assessment tool measures what it sets out to measure.
Burden	The time and effort required to complete the assessment tool(s). This includes administrative tasks such as scoring and inputting data. The burden on both patient and clinician should be considered. In general, the higher the burden, the lower the resulting quality and completeness of the data.
Cultural relevance	This includes language and relevance of the tasks being measured to the individuals.
Mode of administration	This can include: (i) Performance based measures, such as time to complete a task or qualitative assessment of a task (e.g. timed walk). (ii) Clinician reported, based on clinical judgement (e.g. Functional Independence Measure) (iii) Observer reported, which may be completed by a parent or carer (e.g. a seizure diary). (iv) Self-report, often called Patient-Reported Outcome Measures (PROMs). PROMs measure change as experienced by the patient (e.g. Short Form 36).
Cost	The cost of an outcome measure may be an important factor to consider. While many are free, some assessment tools require the purchase of a per use license.

What to Measure?

The International Classification of Functioning, Disability and Health (ICF), is one of a number of different measurement classification systems that provide a conceptual basis for defining and measuring health and disability [2]. Mapping chosen outcome measures onto the ICF framework is advised to help ensure the broad context of the impact of FMD is considered in measurement. Dimensions of measurement listed in the ICF are [6]:

- *Body structure and function*: This pertains to anatomical parts of the body and physiological function of body systems, inclusive of psychological function. Problems with body structure and function are referred to as impairments. Examples of measurement at this level include assessment of anxiety, depression and physical symptom severity (e.g. Psychogenic Movement Disorders Rating Scale).
- *Activity*: The execution of a task by an individual. Examples of measurement at this level include assessment of balance and gait.
- *Participation*: Involvement in life situations. Examples of measurement at this level include assessment of health-related quality of life.
- *Environmental and personal factors:* Issues which affect activity and participation, either as facilitators or barriers.

In additional to the ICF, other domains of measurement that may be of interest include [7]:

- *The economic impact of illness and cost benefit of an intervervention:* This can measured using the metrics quality-adjusted life years (QALYs), health resource use, and social costs of illness (e.g. health-related unemployment).
- *Adverse medical events associated with illness and treatment:* Collecting these data is particularly important in clinical research, but the data are also valuable when auditing clinical practice.
- *Patient satisfaction with treatment:* This metric is of particular interest when evaluating a clinical service.
- *Factors that may mediate outcome:* This relates to collecting data that help to explain outcomes. Examples of this type of data in FMD include patient understanding, patient confidence that their diagnosis is correct, and measures of self-efficacy.

Purpose of Measurement

The purpose of measurement will influence the choice of appropriate assessment tools. Common reasons for measuring outcome include charting progress for patient motivation, research, clinical audit and justifying intervention costs. Assessments for patient motivation and goal achievement will prioritize outcomes that are meaningful to the patient and easy to interpret. For patients with FMD, this is most likely to relate to their movement (e.g. measures of gait speed). Assessments for research and audit purposes will prioritize measures that have proven reliability and validity, as well as measures that are in common usage to allow for comparisons. Data collected for healthcare commissioners and insurance companies will focus on costs versus benefit and the potential for cost savings.

Complexity of Measurement in FMD

FMD has a unique set of characteristics that make accurate measurement of symptoms and health outcomes complex. Complicating factors include the temporal variability of symptoms, symptom heterogeneity, discrepancy between subjective report and objective measures, and a lack of validated assessment tools.

Temporal Variability of Symptoms

Variability of symptom severity is an inherent property of functional neurological symptoms. FMD is, in part, defined by the ability of the abnormal movement to transiently resolve or improve with distracting maneuvers [8]. Conversely, movement worsens when the patient's attention is drawn towards their symptoms. Clinical assessment may also trigger additional or new abnormal movements that may not be part of the patient's usual list of symptoms. For example, a study of 101 consecutive patients with FND found that routine assessment of eye-tracking triggered abnormal movement, such as convergence spasm, in 46% [9]. Functional motor symptoms also typically vary as a consequence of fluctuating pain, fatigue and changes in other coexisting health problems. The resulting temporal variability of symptoms presents challenges for accurate and reliable measurement.

Implications of temporal symptom variability include:

- Observation and the act of clinical assessment may exacerbate symptom severity.
- Outcome measures that are based on single point observations may overestimate (or underestimate) the burden of a patient's symptoms.
- The validity and test-retest reliability of single point measurements is questionable, although data to support or detract from their use is currently lacking.
- Patient reported measures that include a recall period can mitigate the issue of temporal variability. For example, the Short Form-36 questionnaire [10] asks patients to reflect on the previous four weeks and the patient can take into account periods when symptoms are at their best and worst. However, there are potential issues with accuracy of memory recall and and bias due to current mood and symptom severity.

Disabling Symptoms Are Experienced Across Multiple Domains of Measurement

Patients typically experience a cluster of symptoms in addition to their FMD. Common coexisting symptoms in patients with FMD include persistent pain, fatigue, low or fluctuating mood, anxiety, impaired cognition, functional [psychogenic nonepileptic / dissociative] seizures and bladder/bowel impairment. Nicholson et al. (2020) conceptualised the symptoms of FND as three groups: (1) core symptoms (including abnormal movements, weakness, sensory dysfunction and seizures), (2) other physical symptoms and (3) psychological symptoms (see Fig. 29.1).

Each symptom contributes to the overall illness burden in proportions that may vary between individuals and within an individual over time. It is possible that core FND symptoms are not the most disabling or distressing and this clearly presents a challenge for selection of the most

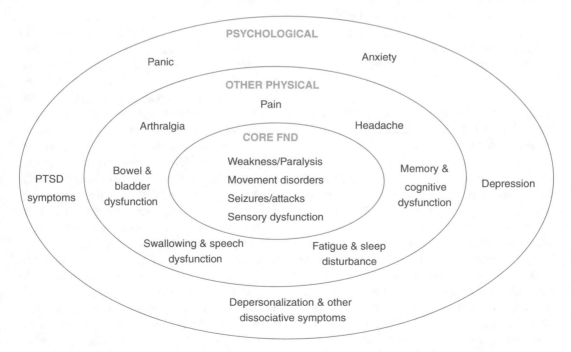

Fig. 29.1 Schematic diagram of symptom domains in functional movement disorder and related functional neurological disorder presentations

clinically meaningful measurement(s) [11, 12]. For example a patient's tremor may resolve, but there may be no overall change to measures of quality of life and health and social care costs if 'non-core' symptoms (e.g. persistent pain, fatigue or impaired cognition) continue to cause distress and disability.

Implications of multisymptom comorbidity include:

- Measurement should take into account common coexisting symptoms.
- Attempting to measure all possible symptoms is impractical, would increase the burden of measurement, and not all symptoms will be relevant to all patients.
- Measures of activity and participation can take into account the impact of multiple symptoms.
- However, measures of activity and participation are prone to lack of responsiveness (sensitivity to change) when multiple different symptoms and health conditions contribute to the illness-burden.
- Attempts to create a single all-inclusive measure with multiple domains must address the challenge of how to account for different symptoms and how to weight the scales for each symptom/domain measured.

Discrepancy Between Subjective Report and Objective Measurements of Symptoms

Some patients with FMD may have difficulty accurately reporting the severity and frequency/duration of their symptoms [13, 14]. Discrepancy between subjective and objective symptom measurement was highlighted in a study by Parees et al. [14]. In subjective ratings, patients with functional tremor (n = 8) overestimated how often their tremor was present when compared to objective measurement from an actigraph watch. However, a subsequent study attempting to replicate these findings in a larger sample (n = 14 FMD) did not find the same discrepancy [15]. If a discrep-

ancy between subjective report and objective measurement is a common feature in FMD, it could potentially, at least in part, be explained by confirmation bias, the tendency to interpret information in a way that supports pre-existing beliefs. People with FMD may be particularly susceptible to confirmation bias when it comes to reporting symptoms because abnormal movement is more likely to be present when they are aware of their body (due to the effect of attention on symptoms) and they are less likely to notice symptom-free moments because this usually coincides with distracted attention.

The implication of the potential for discrepancy between subjective and objective measures:

- Patient perception of symptom severity and frequency may differ from observer reported measurements.

Objective Versus Subjective Measurements

Objectivity is prized in outcome measurement and subjective measurement (such as patient reported measures) are often considered inferior and less informative due to the risk of bias. However, as described above, the temporal variability of FMD complicates objective measurement, with the potential for compromised validity and reliability. It has been argued that subjective or patient-reported measures may be a more valid measure of health state in FMD, particularly because FMD is, in part, defined by the presence of subjective symptoms or distress [16]. Moreover, there is growing recognition of the importance of patient-reported outcome measures (PROMs), as part of a broader move towards more inclusive, patient-centered delivery of healthcare interventions [17]. PROMs have several advantages, such as being time and labor saving. More importantly, they can measure changes that can only be perceived by the patient, such as subjective symptom severity, quality of life and symptom-related distress.

Implication:

- Objective measurement in FMD is challenging and potentially prone to problems with reliability and validity.
- PROMs have arguably greater face-validity in FMD than many objective measures because they can assess key phenomenological aspects of the disorder, such as subjective symptom severity, quality of life and distress.

Outcome Measures Used in FMD Clinical Research

Pick et al. (2020) systematically reviewed the use of outcome measures in prospective intervention studies. Those measures with clinical application for patients with FMD are presented in Table 29.1. This study highlighted two assessment tools designed specifically for the measurement of FMD, the Psychogenic Movement Disorder Rating Scale (PMDRS) [18] and the Simplified Functional Movement Disorder Rating Scale, (S-FMDRS) [19]. Both scales require further validation and reliability assessment. The PMDRS aims to provide a symptom severity score. Scoring works by identifying movement abnormality in 14 body regions; classifying the abnormal movement as one of 10 movement disorder phenomena (resting tremor, dystonia, chorea, athetosis, etc.); and then scoring the movement according to perceived severity, duration, and incapacitation. The authors of the S-FMDRS suggested there were theoretical and design flaws with the PMDRS and produced a simplified version of the scale (S-FMDRS). Changes include removal of the requirement to classify the phenomenology of the observed movement disorder and introduction of a simplified scoring scale. Both scales are scored by clinicians observing a video recording of the patient performing a standardized sequence of movements. Time requirements and the need for video may limit the clinical/research utility of both measures.

Assessment tools for physical and psychological comorbidity are also important to consider. These may include measures of additional physical symptoms (e.g., pain, fatigue, seizures), anxiety, depression, dissociative experiences, among others. However, in the studies reviewed by Pick et al. (2020), a wide range of different measures were used for each additional symptom domain and greater consistency is needed.

Some studies report symptom resolution as a primary outcome. This is commonly seen in retrospective studies, where there is no consistent use of outcome measures. A major limitation of this approach is how resolution is defined in a condition that is known to fluctuate, with periods of exacerbation and remission. In some studies, no explicit definition of symptom resolution was reported (i.e. time scale, assessment method, etc), which is problematic in terms of validating or replicating findings across studies. Additionally, given that FMD commonly coexists with other chronic conditions, it may sometimes be impossible to determine the relative impact of FMD as compared to that of comorbidities such as anxiety and persistent pain.

Outcome measures designed for other populations have been used in FMD, for example, the Functional Mobility Scale (designed for children with cerebral palsy) [20] and Modified Rankin Scale (designed for stroke) [21]. Such measures have face validity due to the shared nature of the observable symptoms and their impact on activity and participation in FMD as well as other neurological disorders. However, strictly speaking, these measures require validation for use in an FMD population, particularly because of the major differences in underlying pathophysiology and the probable subtle differences in symptom presentation.

Table 29.1 Outcome measures that have been used in FMD research. Data for this table is based on a systematic review of outcome measures used in clinical trials of FND [1], with additional suggestions from the authors. Other measures not listed here may have similar or greater value

Domain of Measurement	Assessment Tools
FMD Symptom Severity	*Clinical Global Impression - Improvement (CGI-I) scale* [22] The CGI-I scale is a patient, carer or clinician rated scale of improvement. Improvement is usually rated on a 7 point Likert scale with qualifiers: Very much improved, Much improved, Minimally improved, No change, Minimally worse, Much worse, Very much worse. When using the CGI, the question posed is important to consider. For example, the question, "How would you describe your improvement?", may be answered differently from "How would you describe change to your movement?". The CGI-I is one of the most commonly used outcome measure in FND research as well as other disorders, particularly mental health. *Psychogenic Movement Disorders Rating Scale (PMDRS)* [18] The PMDRS aims to provide a clinician-rated symptom severity score, based on video observation. Scoring works by identifying movement abnormality in 14 body regions; classifying the abnormal movement as one of 10 movement disorder phenomena (resting tremor, dystonia, chorea, athetosis, etc.); and then scoring the movement according to perceived severity, duration, and incapacitation. Gait and speech are also assessed. Sub-scores are added to produce a total severity score. *Simplified Functional Movement Disorders Rating Scale (S-FMDRS)* [19] The S-FMDRS is a simplified version of the PMDRS. Modifications include removal of requirement to classify movement phenomenon and a simplified scoring system. The authors argue that these changes improve the validity and usability of the scale. The CGI-I has the advantage of being quick to complete, sensitive to change and easy to interpret. However, it lacks meaning in terms of absolute values. The PMDRS and S-FMDRS attempts to quantify severity, however it is time consuming to complete.
Psychological Symptoms	*Anxiety Scales* The most commonly used scales of anxiety include: *Beck Anxiety Inventory* [23], *Hamilton Anxiety Rating Scale* [24] and *Generalised Anxiety Disorder-7* (GAD-7) scale [25]. *Depression Scales* The most commonly used scales of depression include: *Beck Depression Inventory* [26], *Hamilton Depression Rating Scale* [27] and *Patient Health Questionnaire-9* (PHQ-9) [28]. Each scale has its own set of strengths and weaknesses. *Anxiety and Depression* The *Hospital Anxiety and Depression Scale* (HADS) [29], is a commonly used tool that yields both a depression and anxiety score. *Psychological Distress* The *Clinical Outcomes in Routine Evaluation-10* (CORE-10), [30] is a 10-item, self reported measure of psychological distress. In a large RCT of CBT for functional seizures [31], the CORE-10 showed a statistically significant difference between the intervention and control group, where specific assessments for anxiety and depression were not different. Many of the psychological scales listed here require the purchase of a license in order to use them. At the time of publication the GAD-7, PHQ-9, CORE-10 were free to use.
Physical Symptom Count	*Patient Health Questionnaire-15* (PHQ-15) is a free to use, patient-reported screening tool for somatic symptom severity. Fifteen somatic symptoms are scored from 0 ("not bothered at all") to 2 ("bothered a lot") [32]. Alternative measures include the *Symptom Checklist-90* (SCL-90) and *Revised SCL-90* [33] somatization scales.
Other Symptoms	*Pain* Pain has been assessed in FMD research using the Bodily Pain domain of the *Short Form 36* [34], the Pain dimension of the EQ-5D-5L [35] and specific Pain visual analogue or numeric rating scales. *Fatigue* Fatigue is assessed as part of the *Short Form 36* questionnaire with the Vitality domain. The *Checklist Individual Strength Scale* [36] was used to assess the impact of fatigue in patients with FMD and found that fatigue had a greater impact on quality of life than motor symptom severity.

Table 29.1 (continued)

Domain of Measurement	Assessment Tools
Physical Disability	*Modified Rankin Scale* A commonly used outcome in stroke medicine, the Modified Rankin Scale is a simple clinician-rated, 6-point scale of physical disability [37]. *Gait, Mobility and Balance* Gait, mobility and balance scales used in FMD research include the *Functional Mobility Scale* [20], 10-meter timed walk (walking speed) [38], *Berg Balance Scale* [39], *Modified Gait Abnormality Rating Scale* (m-GARS) [40] and *Five Times Sit to Stand* [41]. The Functional Mobility Scale was shown to be a sensitive measure of change in two controlled trials of physical rehabilitation for FMD [42, 43]. It is a quick and free measure where the clinician rates on an ordinal scale the support required for the patient to mobilize over 5 meters, 50 meters and 500 meters. *Upper Limb Function* Few measures of upper limb function have been used in FMD research. The Physical Function domain of the Short Form 36 considers upper limb function with questions relating to ability to carry groceries and wash/dress. One example of a specific upper limb assessment tool is the *Disabilities of the Arm Shoulder and Hand* (DASH) [44], which showed a treatment effect in trial of 60 patients with FMD receiving specialist physiotherapy compared to treatment as usual [43].
Participation and Quality of Life	*Quality of Life* Commonly used scales include *Short Form 36* [45], *Work and Social Adjustment Scale* [46] and *EQ-5D-5L* [35]. The EQ-5D-5L has a dual function, in that it is often used in health economics to generate quality adjusted life years (QALYs). The Short Form 36 (or abbreviated versions) has been used widely in FND treatment studies and there is evidence of good responsiveness in these samples [1]. The *Canadian Occupational Performance Measure* (COPM) [47], is a assessment tool commonly used by occupational therapists. It aims to assess patient's perceived performance in areas of self-care productivity and leisure.
Health Economics	*Client Service Receipt Inventory (CSRI)* [48]. A standardized, yet adaptable assessment of health service utilization (i.e. visits to the primary care physician or hospital), informal care, and social benefits. It is commonly used in health economic analysis, but limited utility in clinical practice due to the in-depth nature of the questionnaire and specialist health economic skills required to apply appropriate costs to the reported service use and analyze the data. The CSRI was developed in the United Kingdom and may require adaptation for use in other health and social care systems. As an alternative to the CSRI, health economic benefit can be inferred by reporting change to employment status, work days lost due to sickness, receipt of disability benefits and health care contacts, etc. *Cost Utility Analysis and Quality Adjusted Life Years (QALYs)* A cost utility analysis is a standardized way of comparing the cost benefit of interventions by providing the cost per QALY gained with treatment. QALYs are a measure of quality of life over time, calculated by weighting each year of life lived using a utility score (ranging from 0 to 1, or a negative score which indicates a state worse than death). One QALY is equal to one year lived in perfect health. The EQ-5D-5L is the most commonly used outcome measure for generating QALYs [49].
Other Measures	*Other Domains of Measurement* Other potential domains of measurement include: Illness beliefs (e.g. using the *Illness Perception Questionnaire* (IPQ) or *Brief-IPQ* [50, 51]); acceptance of the diagnosis (e.g. using a visual analogue scale [52]); compliance with treatment (e.g. reporting session attendance); satisfaction with treatment (e.g. a custom made questionnaire); and reporting the occurrence of adverse medical events affecting health and safety.

Recommendations and Future Directions

There are currently insufficient data to definitively recommend one assessment tool over another. However, it is clear that there is a need to measure the impact of primary ('core') FMD symptoms and non-core symptoms (e.g., additional physical or psychological symptoms), either directly with a symptom scale or using a scale of disability. Measures administered at one point in time should be supported with the use of measures capable of accounting for temporal variability of symptoms (e.g. self-reported measures of activity and participation as well as health-related quality of life). An additional option to circumvent the issue of recall bias or error could be to use daily diary-based methods (albeit more time consuming), as have been used in functional seizure research [31]. Patient reported measures are valuable for FMD and should not necessarily be considered inferior to "objective measures", particularly those that are measured at a single point.

The interim recommendations from the FND-COM group for research outcome measurement are summarized in Table 29.2 below. In summary, it was recommended that outcome measures should consider the core symptoms of FND, other physical symptoms, psychological symptoms, life impact (quality of life), health economics and adverse medical events.

Based on our clinical experience, we add the following recommendations when selecting and using outcome measures for use in clinical practice:

- Consider the purpose of data collection and relevant stakeholders (e.g. patients, insurers, care providers, research funders).
- Measure outcomes that are in line with patient's values, perceived needs and priorities for treatment.
- Check for permissions and/or costs that may be required to use a particular assessment tool.
- Explain to the patient the purpose of each measurement and how the data will be used, and share the results with the patient where possible.

- Some patients have difficulty with forced choice/multiple choice questions when they feel that available answers do not apply to them; this can result in missing data. Therefore it is important to provide support for patients when completing outcome measures.
- Check completed forms for missing data.

Additional considerations when choosing assessments are cultural relevance and age. Both the cultural impact of FMD and FMD in children are under researched. Although there will be similarities, there are likely to be important differences with implications for outcome measurement. For example, social/developmental milestones, schooling, and parental care represent additional variables to consider when assessing FMD in children.

Summary
- There are unique features associated with FMD that make measurement particularly complex, this includes population heteroegeneity, the presence of comorbidities and temporal variations in symptoms.
- Both subjective and objective measurements are prone to error.
- Currently, there is insufficient data to recommend any specific assessment tool for FND overall.
- Multiple domains of measurement are required to capture the true burden of symptoms and potential change with treatment.
- Measurement should aim to assess the core symptom(s), (e.g. measure tremor with CGI-I); other physical symptoms (e.g. pain and dizziness with PHQ-15); psychological symptoms (e.g. anxiety and depression with PHQ-9 and GAD-7); and life impact (e.g. quality of life with SF-36).

Table 29.2 Interim recommendations from the FND-COM group for for core outcome measures [2]

Outcome domain	Recommended measures	Commentary
Core FND symptoms	CGI-I (patient +/− clinician +/− carer) Alternatives: S-FMDRS or PMDRS	CGI is cheap, free, easy and sensitive. S-FMDRS and PMDRS have generally good psychometric properties but limited clinical utility due to time required as well as cost and practicalities of using video. Temporal variability may limit validity and reliability.
Other physical symptoms	PHQ-15 Alternatives: Extended PHQ-15, SCL-90	Useful for research, less relevance to measuring outcome in clinical practice.
Psychological symptoms	HADS, BDI/BDI-II + BAI, HAM-D + HAM-A Alternatives: PHQ-9, GAD-7	It is unclear which are most useful in FMD. Cost implications: PHQ-9 and GAD-7 are free.
Life impact	Quality of Life SF-36 Alternatives: WSAS, EQ-5D-5L	QoL scales may have limited responsiveness and are often lengthy. They are important as they can measure the impact of ill-health irrespective of symptom phenotype of health domain (psychological, physical, etc). EQ-5L-5D uses a complicated process to calculate utility scores, however is commonly used to calculate QALYs.
Health economics / cost utility	Healthcare resource utilization Healthcare contacts (total, inpatient admissions, inpatient days, ED/outpatient visits) CSRI	The CSRI is a formalised measure measure of health care utilisation commonly used in clinical research. This level of data may not be necessary in clinical practice and the CSRI was developed for use within the UK and so may not be transferable to other nations or cultures.
Adverse medical events	Reporting adverse events with a brief description is mandatory in clinical trials.	Critical for trials in terms of safety (assessing risk versus benefit) but also valuable for evaluating clinical services.

References

1. Pick S, Anderson DG, Asadi-Pooya AA, et al. Outcome measurement in functional neurological disorder: a systematic review and recommendations. J Neurol Neurosurg Psychiatry. jnnp-2019-322180. 2020;91:638.

2. Nicholson TR, Carson A, Edwards MJ, et al. Outcome measures for functional neurological disorder: a review of the theoretical complexities. J Neuropsychiatry Clin Neurosci. 2020;32:33–42.

3. Nicholson T, Carson A, Edwards MJ, et al. Outcome measures for functional neurological (conversion) disorder. A review of the theoretical complexities. J Neurol Clin Neurosci online fir. 2020;32:33.

4. Lohr KN. Assessing health status and quality-of-life instruments: attributes and review criteria. Qual Life Res. 2002;11:193–205.

5. Prinsen CAC, Vohra S, Rose MR, Boers M, Tugwell P, Clarke M, Williamson PR, Terwee CB. How to select outcome measurement instruments for outcomes included in a "Core Outcome Set" - a practical guideline. Trials. 2016;17:1–10.

6. World Health Organisation. Towards a common language for functioning, disability and health: ICF. Int Classif. 2002;1149:1–22.

7. Dodd S, Clarke M, Becker L, Mavergames C, Fish R, Williamson PR. A taxonomy has been developed for outcomes in medical research to help improve knowledge discovery. J Clin Epidemiol. 2018;96:84–92.

8. Espay AJ, Aybek S, Carson A, et al. Current concepts in diagnosis and treatment of functional neurological disorders. JAMA Neurol. 2018;75:1132–41.

9. Teodoro T, Cunha JM, Abreu LF, Yogarajah M, Edwards MJ. Abnormal eye and cranial movements triggered by examination in people with functional neurological disorder. Neuro-Ophthalmology. 2019;43:240–3.

10. McHorney CA, Ware JE, Raczek AE. The MOS 36-Item Short-Form Health Survey (SF-36): II. Psychometric and clinical tests of validity in measuring physical and mental health constructs. Med Care. 1993;31:247–63.

11. Věchetová G, Slovák M, Kemlink D, Hanzlíková Z, Dušek P, Nikolai T, Růžička E, Edwards MJ, Serranová T. The impact of non-motor symptoms on the health-related quality of life in patients with functional movement disorders. J Psychosom Res. 2018;115:32–7.

12. Gelauff JM, Kingma EM, Kalkman JS, Bezemer R, van Engelen BGM, Stone J, Tijssen MAJ, Rosmalen JGM. Fatigue, not self-rated motor symptom severity, affects quality of life in functional motor disorders. J Neurol. 2018;265:1803–9.

13. Ricciardi L, Demartini B, Morgante F, Parees I, Nielsen G, Edwards MJ. Symptom severity in patients with functional motor symptoms: Patient's perception and doctor's clinical assessment. Parkinsonism Relat Disord. 2015;21:529–32.

14. Parees I, Saifee TA, Kassavetis P, Kojovic M, Rubio-Agusti I, Rothwell JC, Bhatia KP, Edwards MJ. Believing is perceiving: mismatch between self-report and actigraphy in psychogenic tremor. Brain. 2012;135:117–23.

15. Kramer G, Dominguez-Vega ZT, Laarhoven HS, Brandsma R, Smit M, van der Stouwe AM, Elting JWJ, Maurits NM, Rosmalen JG, Tijssen MA. Similar association between objective and subjective symptoms in functional and organic tremor. Park Relat Disord. 2019;64:2–7.

16. American Psychiatric Association. Diagnostic and statistical manual of mental disorders. 5th ed. Arlington: American Psychiatric Publishing; 2013.

17. Black N. Patient reported outcome measures could help transform healthcare. BMJ. 2013;346:1–5.

18. Hinson VK, Cubo E, Comella CL, Goetz CG, Leurgans S. Rating scale for psychogenic movement disorders: scale development and clinimetric testing. Mov Disord. 2005;20:1592–7.

19. Nielsen G, Ricciardi L, Meppelink A, Holt K, Teodoro T, Edwards MJ. A simplified version of the psychogenic movement disorders rating scale: the Simplified Functional Movement Disorders Rating Scale (S-FMDRS). Mov Disord Clin Pract. 2017;4:710–6.

20. Graham HK, Harvey A, Rodda J, Nattrass GR, Pirpiris M. The Functional Mobility Scale (FMS). J Pediatr Orthop. 2004;24:514–20.

21. Sulter G, Steen C, Jacques De Keyser J De. Use of the Barthel index and modified Rankin scale in acute stroke trials. Stroke. 1999;30:1538–41.

22. Guy W. ECDEU assessment manual for psychopharmacology, revised 1976. Maryland: US Department of Health, Education and Welfare; 1976.

23. Beck AT, Epstein N, Brown G, Steer RA. An inventory for measuring clinical anxiety: psychometric properties. J Consult Clin Psychol. 1988;56:893–7.

24. Hamilton M. The assessment of anxiety states by rating. Br J Med Psychol. 1959;32:50–5.

25. Spitzer RL, Kroenke K, Williams JBW, Löwe B, K K, W H. A brief measure for assessing generalized anxiety disorder. Arch Intern Med. 2006;166:1092–7.

26. Beck AT, Steer RA, Brown GK. Beck depression inventory-II. 1996. https://www.pearsonassessments.com/store/usassessments/en/Store/Professional-Assessments/Personality-%26-Biopsychosocial/Beck-Depression-Inventory-II/p/100000159.html. Accessed 4 Jun 2020.

27. Hamilton M. A RATING SCALE FOR DEPRESSION. J Neurol Neurosurg Psychiatry. 1960;23:56 LP – 62.

28. Kroenke K, Spitzer RL, Williams JBW. The PHQ-9: validity of a brief depression severity measure. J Gen Intern Med. 2001;16:606–13.

29. Zigmond AS, Snaith RP. The hospital anxiety and depression scale. Acta Psychiatr Scand. 1983;67:361–70.

30. Connell J, Barkham M. CORE-10 user manual (version 1.0). In: CORE Syst. Trust CORE Inf. Manag. Syst. Ltd; 2007. http://www.mhtu.co.uk/outcome-monitoring/outcome-core-10-manual.pdf. Accessed 4 Jun 2020.

31. Goldstein LH, Robinson EJ, Mellers JDC, et al. Cognitive behavioural therapy for adults with dissociative seizures (CODES): a pragmatic, multicentre, randomised controlled trial. Lancet Psychiatry. 2020;7:491–505.

32. Kroenke K, Spitzer RL, Williams JBW. The PHQ-15: validity of a new measure for evaluating the severity of somatic symptoms. Psychosom Med. 2002;64:258–66.

33. Derogatis LR. Symptom checklist-90-revised. 1994. https://www.pearsonassessments.com/store/usassessments/en/Store/Professional-Assessments/Personality-%26-Biopsychosocial/Symptom-Checklist-90-Revised/p/100000645.html. Accessed 4 Jun 2020.

34. Jenkinson C, Coulter A, Wright L. Short form 36 (SF36) health survey questionnaire: normative data for adults of working age. BMJ. 1993;306:1437–40.

35. Herdman M, Gudex C, Lloyd A, Janssen M, Kind P, Parkin D, Bonsel G, Badia X. Development and preliminary testing of the new five-level version of EQ-5D (EQ-5D-5L). Qual Life Res. 2011;20:1727–36.

36. Vercoulen JHMM, Swanink CMA, Fennis JFM, Galama JMD, van der Meer JWM, Bleijenberg G. Dimensional assessment of chronic fatigue syndrome. J Psychosom Res. 1994;38:383–92.

37. Banks JL, Marotta CA. Outcomes validity and reliability of the modified Rankin scale: implications for stroke clinical trials: a literature review and synthesis. Stroke. 2007;38:1091–6.

38. Peters DM, Fritz SL, Krotish DE. Assessing the reliability and validity of a shorter walk test compared with the 10-Meter Walk Test for measurements of gait speed in healthy, older adults. J Geriatr Phys Ther. 2013;36:24–30.

39. Berg KO, Wood-Dauphinee SL, Williams JI, Maki B. Measuring balance in the elderly: validation of an instrument. Can J Public Health. 1992;83(Suppl 2):S7–11.

40. Vandenberg JM, George DR, O'Leary AJ, Olson LC, Strassburg KR, Hollman JH. The modified gait abnormality rating scale in patients with a conversion disorder: a reliability and responsiveness study. Gait Posture. 2015;41:125–9.

41. Bohannon RW. Reference values for the five-repetition sit-to-stand test: a descriptive meta-analysis of data from elders. Percept Mot Skills. 2006;103:215–22.
42. Jordbru AA, Smedstad LM, Klungsøyr O, Martinsen EW. Psychogenic gait disorder: a randomized controlled trial of physical rehabilitation with one-year follow-up. J Rehabil Med. 2014;46:181–7.
43. Nielsen G, Buszewicz M, Stevenson F, Hunter R, Holt K, Dudziec M, Ricciardi L, Marsden J, Joyce E, Edwards M. Randomised feasibility study of physiotherapy for patients with functional motor symptoms. J Neurol Neurosurg Psychiatry. 2017;88:484–90.
44. Hudak PL, Amadio PC, Bombardier C. Development of an upper extremity outcome measure: the DASH (disabilities of the arm, shoulder and hand) [corrected]. The Upper Extremity Collaborative Group (UECG). Am J Ind Med. 1996;29:602–8.
45. Jenkinson C, Wright L, Coulter A. Criterion validity and reliability of the SF-36 in a population sample. Qual Life Res. 1994;3:7–12.
46. Mundt JC, Marks IM, Shear MK, Greist JH. The work and social adjustment scale: a simple measure of impairment in functioning. Br J Psychiatry. 2002;180:461–4.
47. Carswell A, McColl MA, Baptiste S, Law M, Polatajko H, Pollock N. The Canadian occupational performance measure: a research and clinical literature review. Can J Occup Ther. 2004;71:210–22.
48. Chisholm D, Knapp MR, Knudsen HC, Amaddeo F, Gaite L, van Wijngaarden B. Client socio-demographic and service receipt inventory--European version: development of an instrument for international research. EPSILON study 5. European Psychiatric Services: inputs linked to outcome domains and needs. Br J Psychiatry Suppl. 2000;s28–33.
49. Hunter RM, Baio G, Butt T, Morris S, Round J, Freemantle N. An educational review of the statistical issues in analysing utility data for cost-utility analysis. PharmacoEconomics. 2015;33:355–66.
50. Moss-Morris R, Weinman J, Petrie KJ, Horne R, Cameron LD, Buick D. The revised Illness Perception Questionnaire (IPQ-R). Psychol Health. 2002;16:1–16.
51. Broadbent E, Petrie KJ, Main J, Weinman J. The brief illness perception questionnaire. J Psychosom Res. 2006;60:631–7.
52. Goldstein LH, Mellers JDC, Landau S, et al. COgnitive behavioural therapy vs standardised medical care for adults with Dissociative non-Epileptic Seizures (CODES): a multicentre randomised controlled trial protocol. BMC Neurol. 2015;15:98.

Overcoming Treatment Obstacles in Functional Movement Disorder

Megan E. Jablonski and Adrianne E. Lange

Barriers to Effective FMD Treatment

Patients with functional movement disorder (FMD), in common with all types of Functional Neurological Disorder (FND), face a multitude of challenges in the pursuit of effective treatment, as do their clinicians and caregivers. In spite of important advances made in the diagnosis, conceptualization, and treatment of FMD [1–4] and efforts to address issues of stigma attached to this illness [5], all too often, patients are unfortunately misdiagnosed, mismanaged, and subjected to delays in appropriate care [3]. Given the complexity of FMD at the intersection of Neurology and Psychiatry, many patients struggle to understand and accept this diagnosis for a variety of reasons. Some individuals with FMD can prematurely enter specialized treatment with a host of co-occurring mental and physical health problems, which can complicate the course of treatment. Lack of resources, including social, financial, and other tangible resources, and numerous obstacles along the way influence engagement with care and treatment outcomes.

Despite its prevalence [6, 7], FMD has received surprisingly little attention in terms of medical research and is largely unknown to the general public [8]. Providers vary greatly in their aptitude, skill, and confidence treating this disorder, often lacking access to appropriate facilities and collaborative teams for treating FMD [9, 10]. Likewise, patients often struggle to navigate their way through complex medical systems and the insurance maze to find both compassionate and educated providers and adequate coverage for FMD care. Working with a team of clinicians with a consistent and coherent understanding of FMD – who can express genuine empathy, connect with patient narratives, and present information in a clear and transparent manner – is vital to treatment success. This chapter seeks to increase awareness of common barriers to successful treatment and provide suggestions regarding how to overcome these treatment obstacles. We begin with a case vignette to illustrate the diversity of challenges inherent to FMD diagnosis and treatment, review several common treatment barriers, and close with a case discussion incorporating recommendations and guidance to aid in the optimal care of patients with FMD.

Clinical Vignette

"Carol" is a married white female in her mid-30s, with four school-aged children and a prior medical history of pre-diabetes, Vitamin D deficiency, irritable bowel syndrome, anemia, and low blood pressure. She has a high school education, works in childcare, and volunteers with

M. E. Jablonski (✉)
Department of Psychology & Neuropsychology, Frazier Rehabilitation Institute, Louisville, KY, USA

A. E. Lange
Private Practice, Louisville, KY, USA

© Springer Nature Switzerland AG 2022
K. LaFaver et al. (eds.), *Functional Movement Disorder*, Current Clinical Neurology,
https://doi.org/10.1007/978-3-030-86495-8_30

an animal rescue. Carol has a history of complex relational trauma (childhood emotional abuse and neglect) as well as clinical depression and anxiety. While attending a funeral following the untimely death of her sister, Carol experienced a sudden onset of dizziness, loss of balance, and weakness in her bilateral lower extremities – unable to stand or walk. She was rushed to the emergency department by her family and treated with anxiolytics and intravenous fluids in the ER. She was observed on examination to show features of motor inconsistency (e.g., markedly impaired gait on formal testing but witnessed to be able to walk to the bathroom with minimal difficulty). Her motor symptoms resolved after a few hours and she was discharged home with diagnoses of acute stress and dehydration – only to experience additional episodes which became increasingly frequent and severe over subsequent weeks. She presented multiple times for emergency care with additional diagnoses from multiple providers of "probable" Guillain-Barre Syndrome, idiopathic neurocardiogenic (vasovagal) syncope, and panic disorder.

Approximately 1 year after her first episode, Carol presented to an outpatient neurology clinic for assessment. At that point, she described "spells" occurring almost daily with complaints of fatigue, gait instability, bilateral weakness in her lower extremities, dizziness, "cloudy vision," rapid heart rate, memory loss, and poor concentration. At times, these spells were concurrent with panic symptoms of hyperventilation, "cold sweats," and anxious, ruminative thoughts. Carol became largely housebound, unable to go to work, contribute to the household, or provide routine care for her children and aging parents. She was not eligible for disability benefits, having been employed part-time when symptoms began. Her spouse had to take on additional childcare and household duties, and though coping, he was struggling and reported feeling increasingly drained. Carol acknowledged feelings of guilt and shame associated with her inability to share parenting and financial burdens. She presented as acutely anxious, tearful, and had difficulty focusing through evaluation, *during which she stated, "I can't go on living this way."*

Treatment Barrier 1: Challenges of the FMD Diagnosis

Significant challenges present themselves around diagnosis. Often, a patient has experienced considerable adversity prior to that critical moment in the consulting room where the FMD diagnosis is delivered and, of course, our patients exist within social, psychological, and cultural systems which also play critical roles in their experience and perceptions of that diagnosis. Challenges are also present within the complex healthcare system, amongst providers and specialists, in healthcare education and medical culture. Establishing the treatment frame through a comprehensive biopsychosocial assessment is not only best practice but builds confidence and rapport in the physician-patient relationship. As discussed in Chap. 17, the delivery of the diagnosis is a crucial moment in the physician-patient relationship that sets the stage for how the patient will come to view and participate in their treatment [11]. Effective communication of the diagnosis includes education as well as compassion, understanding, and sensitivity on the part of the physician [12]. Sharing with the patient their positive signs on examination can also aid understanding that the diagnosis is being made in "rule-in" fashion, rather than simply because their previously obtained tests were negative [13]. Many patients come to FMD treatment after experiencing months or years of invalidation and dismissal from various medical professionals, often with a derogatory undertone suggesting covertly that such a mysterious "zebra" of a condition must be psychiatric in nature, "all in your head," and therefore some form of manipulation or malingering. Unfortunately, these misconceptions persist among some physicians, who perceive varying degrees of feigning or intentionality among patients with FMD [9, 14]. Even if not verbalized explicitly, patients are highly attuned to this perception [15] and may present as guarded, making it difficult to fully engage with and explore the FMD diagnosis as it is presented [1]. This may be particularly true for patients who may have sought evaluation from multiple specialists as they seek answers regarding their condition; negative experiences can carry over from one appointment to the next, across providers and treatment settings, through medical records and the patient's subjective experience.

Providers should be mindful of their own thoughts and feelings around these challenging cases – feelings can be easily perceived by patients and their loved ones who are searching for answers and understanding. Providing diagnostic information in an open and non-judgmental manner, paying careful attention to one's own and the patient's nonverbal language, can help to enhance patient satisfaction and communicate clinical empathy [16, 17]. Being able to receive and hold a patient's reactive distress with an authoritative grace can help a patient to feel heard and held, at a time when they and their bodies are feeling particularly vulnerable. Taking the time to explore the patient's reactions in the moment can shed invaluable light on misunderstandings that commonly occur in a relatively brief assessment appointment. Indeed, the demonstration by physicians of nonverbal affect and attunement has been shown to facilitate patients to express concerns more openly, mitigating the detrimental impact of patient anxiety [18] and increasing self-disclosures in the consultation room [19]. At the physician level, particularly amongst neurologists who are on the front lines of FMD care, there is a need to be more psychologically-informed in the approach to this neuropsychiatrically complex population [20].

In addition, one must also be mindful of the tendency for patients to recall just a fraction of the information provided during medical appointments [21] particularly when they may already be experiencing increased anxiety, dissociation and other psychological or cognitive symptoms [22]. It is important to avoid overwhelming the patient with too much information at once or moving into a discussion of treatment planning before it is clear whether the patient is ready to hear what you have to say. Repeating key messages several times using clear language and relatable metaphors can help to solidify and consolidate the information and serve to enhance recall down the line. Further, eliciting in the patient's own words what they understood regarding the information reviewed can be helpful in identifying and clarifying misapprehensions [23]. Providing information regarding credible sources of information regarding FMD (such as https://FNDhope.org or https://neurosymptoms.org), can also provide further opportunity to enhance understanding.

For patients expressing ambivalence about the diagnosis, assessing degree of readiness for change using the transtheoretical stages of change model [24–26] may aid in the determination of treatment recommendations. What constitutes meaningful change also matters. Change for some patients may mean change in relative health or conceptualization of their ailments, while for others it may signal movement or intention towards that next phase of treatment. Numerous researchers have noted that a patient's "stage of change" was an important moderator in psychotherapy outcomes of patients with a multitude of diagnoses; in relevant examples, with anxiety [27] and somatoform disorders [28], even in the presence of high baseline impairment. As with many medical and psychological illnesses, patients themselves play a major (if not the most important role) in the catalyzation of their own clinical improvement through engagement and acceptance. Utilizing motivational interviewing techniques [29] to focus the conversation on the patient's perceptions and goals can be useful to build trust and engagement, helping move a patient towards a state of readiness and receptivity (see Chap. 18 for a detailed discussion of motivational interviewing techniques and how they can be utilized by any member of the treatment team).

It is important to acknowledge, however, that even under the most ideal circumstances in which the diagnosis has been carefully and sensitively explained, some patients may still experience this diagnosis with a negative valence. Referring patients for treatment before obtaining some degree of "buy-in" is unlikely to result in successful outcomes. Where acceptance and commitment is lacking, nascent or the patient is otherwise seriously ambivalent may result in a self-fulfilling feedback loop, where unsuccessful treatment may provide the patient with "evidence" that your diagnosis was incorrect.

In these situations, it can be helpful to allow the patient time to consider the information provided and encourage review of reputable educational resources available online (noted above and elsewhere in this book). Patients benefit from use of both intuitive (affective) and deliberative (logical) strategies to enhance confidence in medical decision-making situations [30, 31], suggesting that reactions and emotions experienced in the consulting room are as important as processing information between appointments. Further, physicians should consider shifting the view of diagnosis delivery from a single discussion with a diagnostic decree to a process-oriented approach, including education and reinforcement over time. Encouraging the patient to bring his or her partner or a close family member or friend can allow key individuals the opportunity to better understand the patient's symptoms and respond in the most helpful way. This approach will allow patients to develop their understanding of the diagnosis, thereby increasing confidence and investment and eventually influencing outcomes for the better. Relatedly, efforts to retain focus on the "what" of the diagnosis, emphasizing "rule-in" signs and strategies to target symptoms, rather than the "why" regarding the origin of the diagnosis can be helpful in the context of rehabilitative and psychological treatment [32].

Numerous implicit and explicit biases operate as patients and physicians engage in shared decision-making in health care settings [33]. It is not necessary for a patient to be 100% in agreement prior to initiating treatment for FMD (in fact, this is rarely the case); however, often "the proof is in the pudding," and experiencing a positive response to treatment can serve as a powerful determinant. As patients engage with appropriate and comprehensive FMD-specific treatments with trained providers, and, moreover, begin to see tangible results, they tend to increase their degree of identification with the diagnosis, a cog-

nitive bias known as the "sunk cost effect" [34] where increased effort and investment results in increased perceived value. Relatedly, "confirmation bias" is the tendency to seek and screen for information to support existing beliefs [34]. Harnessing these natural heuristic tendencies can enhance a patient's connection with their diagnosis and investment in their treatment program.

Treatment Barrier 2: Psychosocial and Motivational Factors

Psychosocial and contextual factors greatly influence a patient's thoughts, feelings, and behaviors. One important variable pertains to the social support network. Some patients have support networks that can be inadequate and sometimes even invalidating. Problematic family dynamics can present a considerable barrier to treatment and progress. It is well-established that there is an increased prevalence of childhood adversity (such as abuse and neglect) among patients with FMD [35, 36]; unfortunately, these early life experiences can contribute to maladaptive relational (attachment) patterns that persist into adulthood [37]. Thus, in addition to coping with FMD, some patients also experience added distress related to the critical and invalidating response of their social network regarding their symptoms and disabilities or the FMD diagnosis itself. Simple strategies like inviting the problematic individual(s) to consultations, with or without the patient present, to explain the diagnosis can often be helpful. Patients may also benefit from support and coaching focused on managing difficult interactions with individuals who respond critically to the diagnosis – or who continually pressure the patient to pursue additional medical explanations. This may also be an appropriate domain for exploration with psychotherapy providers who are schooled in family-systems theories, interpersonal communication, and relationship dynamics.

On the opposing end of the spectrum, some (loving and well-meaning) family members can engage in over-accommodation of the patient's needs – for example, assisting with tasks that the patient could perform independently or taking over stressful tasks or responsibilities of daily life altogether to reduce the patient's distress and limit pain. This phenomenon may also occur within the extended social network, with friends, co-workers, or church or community members. For some, this may develop into a form of unintended reinforcement for the illness operating on an unconscious level, a process which can and does happen with many other forms of serious illness or injury in families and social systems. In addition to becoming progressively more physically inactive and deconditioned, patients can also experience significant shame, self-blame, and grief associated with the loss of prior social roles that brought them meaning and a sense of purpose [38]. Addressing these potential issues transparently with the treatment team is important; for example, including the discussion of values, family dynamics, and various roles of responsibility in individual and family sessions across therapies, not just limited to psychotherapy sessions. For patients, the perception of "being a burden" is associated with greater risk of clinical depression [39] and suicidal ideation [40], particularly in combination with feelings of hopelessness [41]. It can be difficult to break this pattern, once established, as caregivers may find their own feelings of validation and meaning through the caregiving role [42].

Another potential barrier to recovery with psychological roots and social implications is that of secondary gain. Not unique to those with FMD, secondary gain can theoretically be any advantage or benefit that accompanies a psychological or physical symptom. Secondary gain is often psychologically rooted and a complex and controversial concept that may exist in or outside of a patient's awareness; either way, it is critical that it is not to be conflated with factitious disorder or malingering. We discuss it here as it often relates to psychosocial issues, sometimes within family systems, as above, and with financial considerations. Secondary gain need not be pathologized or maladaptive in nature, in fact, at times secondary gain effects may be viewed as a silver lining in an otherwise dark and difficult situation. However, with respect to the goal of moving

towards greater health and symptom amelioration, for some the presence of secondary gain may complicate the acceptance of the FMD diagnosis and impact engagement with and commitment to treatment. Providers and patients can be vigilant and work collaboratively to mitigate these issues as they are uncovered with the use of a compassionate and non-judgmental stance. Psychotherapy may be helpful in some cases, though oftentimes simply bringing these issues into awareness and working with them transparently and objectively with providers can be effective to address barriers to recovery associated with secondary gain.

Not to be ignored, the financial burdens of FMD often present some of the most difficult barriers to treatment and recovery. Given the severely disabling nature of these symptoms [43] many patients are not able to continue working enough to meet their financial needs [44, 45]. This results in significant barriers in obtaining care, both due to the financial hardship of unemployment or underemployment, and because having access to affordable health insurance is often predicated on full-time employment. As a result, patients may be forced to pursue disability benefits or engage in legal processes, such as worker's compensation claims.

Patients with chronic illness are often faced with extraordinary financial costs, among other resource pressures, and may pursue whatever entitlements or legal avenues necessary to meet their needs. For providers, discerning motives amidst often confusing symptom profiles and complex psychosocial history can be a real challenge. Though caution is indicated in scenarios with legal and financial gains at stake, when a patient is otherwise receptive to the diagnosis and motivated to initiate treatment, having sought (or obtained) financial supports should not be considered an exclusionary criterion for proceeding with treatment. However, recovery may not be possible until such issues – and related stress appropriate to these situations – are resolved or adequately managed.

It is, of course, entirely appropriate for patients with disabling symptoms to apply for disability benefits, just as it would be appropriate for patients with other disabling physical, neurological, or psychiatric conditions. These benefits and other entitlements offer a lifeline for financial survival and allow patients the time and the practical and emotional bandwidth to focus on their health. It is the definition of adaptive coping to utilize what resources are available to survive and work through a new and difficult reality. However, as above, we do encourage providers and patients alike to be alert to the presence of secondary gain or layered motivations which may impact engagement. After all, these issues can detract from treatment initiatives that have the potential to ameliorate disabling symptoms and move patients toward wellness and independence.

These are challenging issues to decode and work through, even for experienced and knowledgeable providers, and these situations can offer teachable moments for team members who are perhaps more skeptical regarding the validity of FMD-related disability claims. It is important to model an attitude of non-judgmental and compassionate support and educate others where possible. We believe that negative views held by some within the medical community around illness-related dependence, so-called "ulterior motivations," and issues of responsibility and agency regarding "psychogenic" or "non-organic" conditions like FMD, are tied to continued stigmatization of mental health difficulties more broadly – something we must all work to challenge.

Treatment Barrier 3: Physical, Psychological, and Cognitive Issues

Research has shown promising results for patients with FMD engaged in interdisciplinary treatment designed to reprogram physiological and psychological pathways [46, 47]. While effective for many, intensive therapy programs can be time-consuming, physically demanding, and costly. Prior to initiating treatment, it is imperative to thoroughly assess for physical, psychological, or cognitive barriers that might impact treatment.

Regarding physical readiness for treatment, chronic pain and fatigue are common barriers

which can limit a patient's ability to participate in therapy exercises [3]. This is particularly true for patients who have been living with FMD for a long time, given the decreased activity level and deconditioning commonly experienced [48]. Providing treatments tailored to the patient's unique needs can help enhance treatment response; for example, use of non-specific, graded exercise therapy can be a helpful first step, addressing both deconditioning and chronic pain [49].

Patients prescribed high doses of pain medication may find it more difficult to engage in physical or psychological therapies due to sedation or cognitive clouding. Patients dealing with severe pain issues may be well-suited for a pain-focused rehabilitation program or pain management referral to help them prepare for the physical demands of an intensive multidisciplinary treatment program [50]. In addition, research has supported the use of psychotherapy (cognitive-behavioral therapy and mindfulness/acceptance-based interventions) to enhance pain management and reduce associated emotional distress and avoidance behaviors [51]. It may be helpful to triage with the patient what are the most bothersome symptoms; for example, a patient may have a functional tremor but report that body pain is the prominent chief complaint. This may help configure collaborative treatment priorities in a stepwise fashion, serving to engage, organize and guide patients through issues of pain and fatigue and to mitigate avoidance behaviors and emotional overwhelm.

Regarding psychological barriers, depression or anxiety are common and understandable reactions to the symptoms and impacts of FMD, as are frustration, anger, and grief. Many present with emotional distress unrelated to their condition. Research suggests that people with chronic illness are more at risk for mental health disorders, and that this risk is amplified by social problems and low levels of perceived health [52]. It is also possible that for some patients such disorders could be a risk factor for FMD or an integral part of their disorder. Psychiatric comorbidities and normative stress reactions need not preclude patients from being referred for treatment; however, some patients may experience levels of psychological distress or hold maladaptive personality pathology that can present a challenge to treatment. For example, the emotional instability characteristic of some personality disorders, especially Borderline Personality Disorder (BPD), also known as Emotionally Unstable Personality Disorder, can prove particularly challenging, with the patient's heightened emotional reactivity and interpersonal difficulties having the potential to adversely impact team dynamics as well as other patients engaging in concurrent treatment. Given that both BPD and FMD (particularly in the case of functional seizures) have trauma and abuse as shared risk factors [53], there will be some overlap among these patient groups; again, this does not suggest that these personality factors play a causative role in the presence of FMD.

In another example, for patients with debilitating anxiety, it may be a struggle to tolerate a busy therapy gym environment – leading to avoidance behaviors, difficulty with engagement, or early termination of treatment. Patients with anxiety sensitivity may be overly attuned to their somatic experience and react strongly to normal sensations of physical exertion [54]. The increased cognitive load that results from anxiety can make it difficult to focus during therapy and retain information. Likewise, patients with depression may struggle with diminished motivation, poor concentration, and lack of energy, causing them to feel overwhelmed by therapy demands or pessimistic regarding the likelihood of treatment success. At times, patients may even begin to question whether life is worth living or experience thoughts about suicide. Importantly, suicidal ideation need not preclude a patient's participation or suggest that they are unable to engage with rehabilitative care, though the discovery of these thoughts should be immediately and fully addressed.

Proper screening and referrals to mental health providers can help to identify and care for patients at risk for poor outcomes due to psychiatric comorbidities. Table 30.1 contains several brief screening measures which may be helpful in identifying patients who could benefit from a

Table 30.1 Screening instruments

Domain	Measure	Length/type
Depression & anxiety	Patient Health Questionnaire (PHQ-9) [56]	9-item SR
	Beck Depression Inventory (BDI-II) [57]	21-item SR
	Generalized Anxiety Disorder (GAD-7) [58]	7-item SR
	Hospital Anxiety and Depression Scale (HADS) [59]	14-item SR; 2 subscales
Suicidal ideation	Columbia Suicide Severity Rating Scale (C-SSRS) screening version [60]	6-item CA
	Patient Safety Screener (PSS-3) [61]	3-item CA
Emotional regulation	Cognitive Emotional Regulation Questionnaire (CERQ-short) [62]	18-item SR; 9 subscales
Personality pathology	Iowa Personality Disorder Screen (IPDS) [63]	11-item CA
Trauma/PTSD	Primary Care PTSD Screen for DSM-5 (PC-PTSD-5) [64]	5-item CA
	Stressful Life Events Screening Questionnaire (SLESQ) [65]	13-item SR
	Adverse Childhood Experiences-Questionnaire (ACE-Q) [66]	10-item SR
Social support	Multidimensional Scale of Perceived Social Support [67]	12-item SR; 3 subscales
Somatization	Patient Health Questionnaire (PHQ-15) [68]	15-item SR
	Schedule for Evaluating Persistent Symptoms (SEPS) [69]	9-item SR
Substance abuse	Alcohol Use Disorders Identification Test-Concise (AUDIT-C) [70]	3-item SR
	Drug Abuse Screening Test (DAST-10) [71]	10-item SR

SR self-report measures, *CA* clinician-administered measures/brief structured interviews

referral for mental health services; however, we offer the caveat here that though these measures are widely used among medical populations, they are not specifically validated or normed with patients with FMD and therefore may require contextual interpretation. Interested readers can also review the systematic review by Pick et al. [55] with recommendations regarding assessment instruments pertaining to all FND subtypes. We must emphasize here that mental health screening tools and brief assessments, while helpful, are blunt instruments and are not a replacement for comprehensive psychological or psychiatric evaluation by a mental health professional. We present these tools as useful scaffolding toward the preliminary assessment of mental health issues and relevant within the biopsychosocial model.

Collaborative consultation among physicians, physical and occupational therapy providers, and mental health clinicians can be quite helpful to problem-solve and work through psychological treatment barriers, enabling other team members to reinforce the techniques being discussed in psychotherapy, and vice versa. Additionally, it is worth pointing out that in the context of the biopsychosocial formulation (see Chap. 3 for additional discussion), even the most optimal initial intake will be relatively incomplete in terms of depth and appreciation of relevant psychological or social difficulties. As such, providers should view exploration of precipitating and perpetuating factors as a longitudinal process, with some details emerging with time and development of therapeutic rapport [72]. Reliance on the biopsychosocial model to frame barriers to progress and recovery can be useful in our experience.

As mentioned above, patients may also exhibit more severe psychiatric symptoms, including suicidal thoughts. Physicians should routinely screen for suicidal thoughts, and when identified, conduct a thorough safety assessment. Utilizing an empirically-supported suicide risk assessment instrument, such as the Columbia Suicide Severity Rating Scale (C-SSRS) [60], can help guide this conversation and determine how to best address the patient's immediate safety needs. In settings where mental health professionals are embedded within the treatment team, an immediate consultation can greatly assist with safety planning and rapidly facilitating the appropriate

level of follow-up care. In settings where this is not possible, patients should be provided with referrals for crisis services, counseling, and psychiatric services for optimal management of these concerns. This may include arranging for emergency psychiatric evaluation, when warranted. Following a sustained period of psychiatric stability, these patients can be safely referred for interdisciplinary FMD treatment.

These details reinforce the critical importance of attending to the intersections between FMD symptoms and psychological factors, particularly when mental illness is prominent, multi-factorial, or not well-managed. For example, patients with severe major depression, acute or post-traumatic stress disorder, ongoing alcohol or substance use disorders, suicidality and/or self-injurious behaviors, among other possibilities, may first warrant robust psychiatric treatment engagement (e.g., acute inpatient hospitalization or intensive outpatient treatment program).

In addition to the physical and psychological factors detailed above, cognitive symptoms can present a significant challenge to treatment and recovery. Cognitive complaints are common to FMD, and FND more broadly, and can have profound impact on our patients' lives. At times, these symptoms can negatively affect treatment engagement and outcomes, particularly in the presence of increased anxiety and stress [73]. Beginning with Breuer and Freud (1895/1955), patients with "conversion symptoms," then known as "hysteria," have complained of cognitive impairment such as functional forms of amnesia, confusion, mutism and loss of language [74]. Janet (1901) noted deficits in attention ("a retraction of the field of consciousness") and increased distractibility exacerbated by stress in his patients with functional neurological symptoms [75]. Present-day patients with FMD may have impairments in working memory, short-term memory, long-term memory loss, memory lapses, concentration, focus, and fatigue, as well as reduced stamina and attention, verbal tics, or even loss of language or speech [76–80]. When anxiety and stress exacerbate cognitive impairment such that cognition presents a barrier, initial work with a neuropsychologist or psychotherapist designed to decrease anxiety, improve emotion regulation, and develop more adaptive coping skills may pave the way for eventual work with a speech-language pathologist, among other therapies. Alternative treatments include referral to speech and language therapists or occupational therapists (preferably those familiar with FMD) that have training in cognitive remediation or retraining, which can be an important component of treatment in such patients (see Chap. 25 for additional details).

It is important to have a transparent conversation regarding concerns about readiness for treatment and provide clear and specific recommendations designed to enhance treatment readiness. If critical issues are not addressed proactively, the risks of FMD treatment may outweigh the potential benefits. At best, the patient might not respond to treatment if it is not framed with that patient's unique needs in mind; at worst, they could experience further declines and a potential psychological crisis, should treatment prove unsuccessful. Further, in the age of managed care, therapy benefits are limited, and patients may be unable to afford the financial and social burdens of multiple rounds of intensive treatment, whether inpatient or outpatient, interdisciplinary or targeted. As such, thorough consideration of treatment potential, including a multi-domain stepwise approach, will help ensure that the patient receives the right treatment at the right time to be most effective.

Treatment Barrier 4: Treatment Expectations

There is great (and often misplaced) clarity and security in the curative view of medical science, and this misapprehension can present another critical treatment barrier. Many people are accustomed to illnesses that can be easily identified with a swab, bloodwork, or imaging technology and treated with concrete interventions such as medication or surgery – a conceptualization that places the onus to "cure" the disease primarily on the medical team or the intervention itself. In this view, medicine is a service industry with tradi-

tional hierarchies of power and agency. This view has more than a few cracks in our contemporary medical landscape with its emerging lean towards a holistic and patient-centered care model. Treatment expectations on the part of both provider and patient must be carefully examined for such views and challenged with education and support where necessary.

FMD is a condition that requires the patient to play a particularly critical role in their own treatment [81], and requires ongoing collaborative effort for optimal symptom management, even following a successful treatment course. Here, the service metaphor breaks down and a "fix it and forget it" mentality falls painfully short. Motivational themes of external vs. internal locus of control and beliefs about illness and medicine are important elements of the clinical biopsychosocial formulation and should be confronted and explored in the consulting room, when relevant. For some patients with FMD, following intensive multidisciplinary treatment, additional courses of outpatient therapy may be necessary, with relapses expected and therapeutic "tune ups" required [49, 82]. Patients should also be prepared at the outset that symptoms might initially worsen as they enter the active treatment phase, given the increased physical and emotional demands, a nonlinear trajectory of change that has also been noted in the psychotherapy literature [83]. Ensuring that the patient and their loved ones are well-prepared for the variable nature of treatment response can help them have realistic expectations and remain more resilient to possible relapses in the future [82].

In shaping expectations, clinicians should carefully consider the full picture of the patient's medical problems, avoiding the presumption that all aspects of their illness are "functional" in nature without full examination and investigation. It is common for a patient to experience co-occurring functional neurological symptoms alongside other medical problems, including other neurological ailments [84]. In addition, some medical problems can result from the atypical movement patterns characteristic of FMD; for instance, after years of altered gait patterns or other unusual movements, patients can develop orthopedic or pain problems which require further assessment and treatment outside of FMD care. Clarifying in the initial diagnosis discussion that some symptoms may respond to treatment earlier, while others may take longer and/or require further intervention may also help to shape accurate expectations.

Early education should include an introduction to the concept of mind-body connection as a segue into the recommendation for psychological services, in addition to physiotherapy services. Providers must be aware of the unfortunate impact of stigma in this conversation, as some patients may perceive a recommendation for mental health treatment as evidence that their physician does not believe in the legitimacy of their symptoms [14]. Physicians must be careful to avoid the oversimplification of FMD as being "due to stress" while gently reinforcing that stress can, at least for some patients, exacerbate symptoms, just as it does with numerous other diseases. A framing of FMD and related FND presentations as conditions at the intersection of neurology and psychiatry can be helpful, including comments that the brain does not separate into "neurological" and "psychiatric" circuits and that mind-body approaches are helpful for a range of conditions. Using other chronic ailments as examples of the body-mind connection may also help; for example, there is ample evidence illustrating the impact of emotional factors on cardiovascular disease [85] and a plethora of other medical conditions [86, 87]. Patients should be reminded that psychological services are encouraged during the treatment process, both to aid in symptom management and coping with the stress associated with any pervasive chronic illness.

Treatment Barrier 5: Access to Treatment

Though further research is needed, there is growing evidence that an interdisciplinary treatment team model is particularly helpful when working with FMD patients [46, 88]. However, in some settings, this may not be feasible, due to the often-fragmented nature of the medical system. For medical providers who do not have access to a treatment team within their setting, it is important to cultivate an educated referral network of community therapists (physical, occupational, and speech) and mental health providers to ensure optimal treatment. An inexperienced clinician without sufficient training and expertise in FMD might inadvertently undo the difficult work of establishing "buy-in," thereby setting the patient back. A study of physical therapists indicates that although they are receptive to treating FMD, they often feel unsure how to help [89] – sometimes resulting in the patient being discharged prematurely due to lack of progress. This outcome can be demoralizing for patients; for those who remain ambivalent regarding their diagnosis, lack of improvement further fuels doubts and increases emotional distress. Fortunately, there are ongoing efforts at increasing awareness of best practices for FMD across disciplines. Recently, a paper detailing consensus recommendations for physical therapists has been published with guidance on optimal treatment approaches for physiotherapy [49] and resources for occupational therapists are also available [90, 91]. When referring a patient to a new therapist, sending a copy of these guidelines and basic educational information about FMD is advisable, as is opening the channel for ongoing cross-disciplinary conversations about care.

Psychological services have long been considered an important component of FMD treatment [3]; unfortunately, patients may experience difficulty finding an appropriate mental health provider who is familiar with the diagnosis or current terminology, models, and their nuances and sensitivities. There is a great deal of variability among community psychotherapists in terms of training and experience in rehabilitation psychology and medical patients, and few work, in particular, with FMD. Despite the increasingly accepted move away from the "psychogenic" and "conversion" diagnostic labels in favor of "functional movement disorder" within the medical field [92], this transition has been slow to spread among the mental health community [93]. When patients reach out to mental health providers and request assistance addressing FMD, they are often met with a puzzled response, with some providers lacking familiarity with updated diagnostic terminology and with limited understanding of the diagnosis itself. Though the DSM-5, the primary codified reference manual used by psychiatrists and psychologists, has updated its language and concepts, replacing "Conversion Disorder" with "Functional Neurological Symptom Disorder" and removing the requirement for an identifiable psychological conflict or stressor [94], the presumption of a psychological basis remains embedded within the diagnostic conceptualization of many clinicians [95].

Though some patients identify strongly with the role that emotional factors or trauma play in their illness, for others a presumption that these factors are primary or even present at all may leave them feeling misunderstood and contribute to their ambivalence toward, or even rejection of the diagnosis. One study found that 39% of patients with FMD exhibited no psychiatric comorbidities [96]. When a patient presents for mental health treatment without any discernible trauma or emotional distress, they may be advised that psychological services will not be helpful – or assured that their problems are "not psychological." This can foreclose on a nuanced understanding of psychophysiology and may limit future engagement with the recommended integrative mind-body-behavior psychotherapy approaches. Alternately, patients with minimal psychiatric history may be assumed by misinformed providers to be withholding critical details from their history or minimizing their distress – implicitly or even explicitly admonished to "tell the truth" so that they can recover. Experiences of this nature can severely damage not only the patient's relationship with that specific provider but lead to difficulty establishing relationships of trust with medical and mental health professionals, more broadly, and negatively influence their identification with the FMD diagnosis.

Like their physical therapy colleagues, mental health professionals report feeling underprepared to help patients manage functional neurological symptoms [10]. Ironically, cognitive-behavioral therapy (CBT) – a standard and quite common therapeutic approach focused on bringing greater awareness and alignment to thoughts and behaviors – is the treatment most frequently utilized for FMD [97–100]. Though work remains to be done to improve the efficacy of psychological therapies to reduce symptom frequency and severity, it does appear that CBT can reduce subjective distress associated with symptoms and other secondary outcomes (see results of the recently completed CODES trial for further details) [101]. Interested providers are encouraged to review Chap. 21 in this text for an overview of psychological treatment approaches.

Overcoming Functional Neurological Symptoms: A Five Areas Approach [102] includes practical and clearly communicated education regarding FMD as well as workbook modules focused on enhancing symptom management. These modules can be completed by patients independently or incorporated into psychotherapy to provide a helpful framework for treatment. Many mental health providers are surprised (and relieved) to review this text, recognizing that the core principles utilized are foundational to CBT. Clinicians trained in CBT techniques likely routinely treat anxiety, depression, and somatic symptoms and should therefore take comfort that their "bread and butter" interventions form a solid foundation from which to build their skills with FMD patients.

There are some special considerations for clinicians who are new to working with FMD to bear in mind. Understanding the diagnosis is requisite, though each case is unique in its presentation. Strong collaboration and records sharing between the referring physician and mental health treatment provider will facilitate consistent messaging and communication, particularly for clinicians unfamiliar with this patient group. Mental health providers are generally trained in patient-centered care models which allow the clinician to join with and understand the perspective of the patient. Balancing this position with that of treatment steward and collaborator must be done carefully, critically, and judiciously. The psychotherapist must simultaneously maintain the therapeutic alliance and collaborative frame, facilitate catharsis and processing of emotional strife, guide the patient toward important skills and personal insights, and promote the patient's sense of agency and ownership of their health and treatment. A healthy awareness of common pitfalls to this mission (such as "splitting" within the treatment team or a well-meaning therapist's undermining of a patient's confidence in the diagnosis) should be carefully tended and mitigated where appropriate, typically well done through increased collaboration and communication across the team.

In addition, presenting motor symptoms, sometimes confusing in nature, can initially be quite alarming for those who are unfamiliar with FMD or medical rehabilitation patient populations. For mental health professionals engaged in FMD care, it is important to remain poised and calm, careful to avoid a response that would provoke greater self-consciousness for the patient. With patients who experience episodic (rather than continuous) symptoms, there may need to be some proactive contingency planning with the patient, should an episode occur during a session that renders them unable to return home independently or which might require in vivo intervention or other safety planning. This kind of contingency planning with a psychotherapist can be therapeutic in and of itself, involving important treatment goals of elucidating symptoms, learning to address symptoms with CBT strategies in the moment, and helping both patients and clinicians assist caregivers to better manage episodes when they do occur.

Treatment Barrier 6: Patient Engagement and Plateaus

As with any patient population, challenges may arise with treatment adherence and follow-through with recommendations. Treatment plateaus and relapses are expected, as trajectories of change are inherently variable [103], with numerous characteristics influencing motivation in the rehab setting [104]. Considering the significant effort and investment required for FMD treatment, adherence can prove challenging, even for the motivated patient. When a patient returns to the clinic having made little progress in treatment – or having not followed-up with treatment recommendations at all – this presents a unique window of opportunity to further explore perceived barriers [72]. Lack of engagement could suggest that the patient may still be struggling with doubts or unresolved insecurities pertaining to the diagnosis. Lack of finances, social support, or even something as basic as transportation issues may be uncovered, which may suggest a referral for case management is needed. Likewise, any of the barriers addressed previously may be at play and interacting with one another, highlighting the importance of graceful, yet tenacious, inquiry by the physician.

When a treatment plateau is discovered, once again, it is critical for clinicians to model empathic, nonjudgmental, and transparent communication to facilitate the patient's engagement and inspire a sense of collaborative inquiry. Motivational interviewing may again be utilized in this spirit to reconnect with the trajectory of change [105]. When appropriate, exploring alternative or non-traditional treatment modalities can also be useful to break through this barrier. Active communication among the patient's treatment providers across disciplines can also help overcome plateaus in progress, allowing the individual providers to consistently address problems that may arise in treatment and reinforce congruent messaging regarding the patient's illness and the path toward recovery. Similarly, all members of the treatment team can help reshape unhelpful illness-related beliefs when they arise in the moment, more effectively done in concert. Emphasizing that therapy progress requires ongoing practice and effort, while conveying confidence and an expectation for recovery, can help the patient remain invested in the treatment process. Enacting patient-driven, meaningful, and variable-term goals for regaining control and function in daily living can help break through the monolithic task of recovery, thereby easing the path forward [106, 107].

Case Discussion

Consider Carol's story: a woman with a history of caretaking and generosity, blindsided by grief, and fraught with unresolved trauma and numerous medically undifferentiated symptoms, who was stricken without warning by worsening episodes of acute weakness with cognitive impairment. Several features stand out as potential barriers including acute emotional distress with possible suicidal ideation, lack of financial resources, and an overwrought spouse, issues which should be triaged and approached in order of risk and severity. Following the diagnosis, she evidenced a concerning degree of emotional reactivity and stated, "I can't live this way;" this warrants a thorough safety assessment which may be done by reviewing the Columbia Suicide Severity Rating Scale (C-SSRS; see Table 30.1) with her verbally, with gentle and direct follow-up inquiries. Her responses will help clarify whether there are indeed high acuity safety concerns, which will guide further crisis and mental health referrals on the spot. The patient's history suggests she has unresolved grief over her sister's untimely death affecting her mood and emotion regulation capacities as well as unresolved childhood trauma, both of which may be explored and stabilized in psychotherapy. Her acute psychiatric symptoms of depression may also be addressed with antidepressant medication handled by a provider with appropriate expertise and capacity to follow-up regularly.

Once these issues are clarified and appropriate mental health referrals have been provided, it is then time to focus on the next challenge. Financial concerns may warrant a referral to case management services, who can assist with entitlements and financial aid programs to help the family to meet basic needs while the patient is out of work, thereby lessening practical strains on the household. It may also benefit the family to bring Carol's spouse into a follow-up session and inquire about their social support network, helping them to brainstorm how they might utilize the supports they have to better cope with daily living. For example, perhaps one of their friends or community members from Church or animal-rescue may be able to help with childcare, groceries, or a meal train. Taking the time to collaborate with the patient demonstrates compassion and validation of impactful stressors, which helps the patient to feel understood, increasing rapport and alignment with your recommendations. As has been suggested previously, multiple follow-up sessions may be needed to uncover and resolve these concerns following the initial presentation of the diagnosis, allowing additional opportunity to reinforce the patient-doctor relationship and build trust in the diagnosis and recommendations [72].

Conclusion

To conclude, despite progress in recent years toward improving the diagnosis and treatment of FMD, there are still numerous obstacles to successful treatment. Anticipating and preparing for these challenges can help enhance the competence and confidence of all members of the treatment team – and thereby influence patient engagement and treatment success. Beginning with a comprehensive biopsychosocial assessment, and through collaborative and empathic care and an individualized treatment approach, effective providers are astutely aware of each patient's distinct presentation and life circumstances. When patients receive appropriate treatments at the right time, provided by compassionate and skilled clinicians who are ready and able to manage the complexities of FMD, the outcomes in our patients can be optimized.

Summary

- Management of FMD is complex and requires sensitivity and transparency on the part of the physician and other members of the treatment team.
- Understanding and acceptance of the diagnosis – and medical/psychological stability – are key factors that must be assessed (and addressed) prior to initiating other FMD-specific treatments.

- Education and support of key individuals in the patient's social network is also critical.
- Moving forward too quickly into the treatment phase may result in poor outcomes, but well-timed and appropriate intervention can be highly effective.
- Patients respond best to a collaborative, multidisciplinary approach in which each provider reinforces clear and consistent messages regarding the diagnosis and optimal treatment plan.
- Communication between treating clinicians across disciplines can greatly enhance treatment success.

References

1. Stone J. The bare essentials: functional symptoms in neurology. Pract Neurol. 2009;9(3):179–89.
2. Stone J, Reuber M, Carson A. Functional symptoms in neurology: mimics and chameleons. Pract Neurol. 2013;13(2):104–13.
3. Espay A, Aybek S, Carson A, Edwards M, Goldstein L, Hallett M, et al. Current concepts in diagnosis and treatment of functional neurological disorders. JAMA Neurol. 2018;75(9):1132–41.
4. Hallett M. The most promising advances in our understanding and treatment of functional (psychogenic) movement disorders. Parkinsonism Relat Disord. 2018;46(Suppl 1):S80–S2.
5. Rommelfanger K, Factor S, LaRoche S, Rosen P, Young R, Rapaport M. Disentangling stigma from functional neurological disorders: conference report and roadmap for the future. Front Neurol. 2017;8(106):1–7.
6. Carson A, Ringbauer B, Stone J, McKenzie L, Warlow C, Sharpe M. Do medically unexplained symptoms matter? A prospective cohort study of 300 new referrals to neurology outpatient clinics. J Neurol Neurosurg Psychiatry. 2000;68:207–10.
7. Stone J, Carson A, Duncan R, Roberts R, Warlow C, Hibberd C, et al. Who is referred to neurology clinics? The diagnosis made in 3781 new patients. Clin Neurol Neurosurg. 2010;112(9):747–51.
8. Popkirov S, Nicholson T, Bloem B, Cock H, Derry C, Duncan R, et al. Hiding in plain sight: functional neurological disorders in the news. J Neuropsychiatry Clin Neurosci. 2019;31(4):361–7.
9. Kanaan R, Armstrong D, Wessely S. Neurologists' understanding and management of conversion disorder. J Neurol Neurosurg Psychiatry. 2011;82(9):961–6.
10. McMillan K, Pugh M, Hamid H, Salinsky M, Pugh J, Noël P, et al. Providers' perspectives on treating psychogenic nonepileptic seizures: frustration and hope. Epilepsy Behav. 2014;37:276–81.
11. Stone J, Carson A, Hallett M. Explanation as treatment for functional neurologic disorders. Handb Clin Neurol. 2016;139:543–53.
12. Hall-Patch L, Brown R, House A, Howlett S, Kemp S, Lawton G, et al. Acceptability and effectiveness of a strategy for the communication of the diagnosis of psychogenic nonepileptic seizures. Epilepsia. 2010;51(1):70–8.
13. Stone J, Edwards M. Trick or treat? Showing patients with functional (psychogenic) motor symptoms their physical signs. Neurology. 2012;73(3):282–4.
14. Kanaan R, Ding J. Who thinks functional neurological symptoms are feigned, and what can we do about it? J Neurol Neurosurg Psychiatry. 2017;88(6):533–4.
15. Nettleton S, Watt I, O'Malley L, Duffey P. Understanding the narratives of people who live with medically unexplained illness. Patient Educ Couns. 2005;56(2):205–10.
16. Brugel S, Postma-Nilsenová M, Tates K. The link between perception of clinical empathy and nonverbal behavior: the effect of a doctor's gaze and body orientation. Patient Educ Couns. 2015;98(10):1260–5.
17. Mast M. On the importance of nonverbal communication in the physician-patient interaction. Patient Educ Couns. 2007;67(3):315–8.
18. Bensing J, Verheul W, van Dulmen A. Patient anxiety in the medical encounter: a study of verbal and nonverbal communication in general practice. Health Educ. 2008;108(5):373–83.
19. Duggan A, Parrott R. Research note: physicians' nonverbal rapport building and patients' talk about the subjective component of illness. Hum Commun Res. 2000;27(2):299–311.
20. Perez D, Keshavan M, Scharf J, Boes A, Price B. Bridging the great divide: what can neurology learn from psychiatry? J Neuropsychiatry Clin Neurosci. 2018;4:271–8.
21. Godwin Y. Do they listen? A review of information retained by patients following consent for reduction mammoplasty. Br J Plast Surg. 2000;53(2):121–5.
22. Nguyen M, Smets E, Bol N, Bronner M, Tytgat K, Loos E, et al. Fear and forget: how anxiety impacts information recall in newly diagnosed cancer patients visiting a fast-track clinic. Acta Oncol. 2019;58(2):182–8.
23. Watson P, McKinstry B. A systematic review of interventions to improve recall of medical advice in healthcare consultations. J R Soc Med. 2009;102(6):235–43.
24. Prochaska J, DiClemente C. Transtheoretical therapy: toward a more integrative model of change. Psychol Psychother. 1982;19(3):276–88.
25. Norcross J, Krebs P, Prochaska J. Stages of change. J Clin Psychol. 2011;67:143–54.

26. Krebs P, Norcross J, Nicholson J, Prochaska J. Stages of change and psychotherapy outcomes: a review and meta-analysis. J Clin Psychol. 2018;74(11):1964–79.

27. Boswell J, Sauer-Zavala S, Gallagher M, Delgado N, Barlow D. Readiness to change as a moderator of outcome in transdiagnostic treatment. Psychother Res. 2012;22(5):570–8.

28. Heider J, Köck K, Sehlbrede M, Schröder A. Readiness to change as a moderator of therapy outcome in patients with somatoform disorders. Psychother Res. 2018;28(5):722–33.

29. Miller W, Rollnick S. Motivational interviewing: helping people change. New York: Guilford Press; 2013.

30. de Vries M, Fagerlin A, Witteman H, Scherer L. Combining deliberation and intuition in patient decision support. Patient Educ Couns. 2013;91(2):154–60.

31. Davis E, McCaffery K, Mullan B, Juraskova I. An exploration of decision aid effectiveness: the impact of promoting affective vs. deliberative processing on a health-related decision. Health Expect. 2014;18(6):2742–52.

32. Stone S, Vuilleumier P, Friedman J. Conversion disorder: separating "how" from "why". Neurology. 2010;74(3):190–1.

33. Chapman G, Sonnenberg F, editors. Decision making in health care: theory, psychology and applications. Cambridge: Cambridge University Press; 2003.

34. Hardman D. Judgment and decision making: psychological perspectives. Chichester: Wiley; 2002.

35. Kranick S, Ekanayake V, Martinez V, Ameli R, Hallett M, Voon V. Psychopathology and psychogenic movement disorders. Mov Disord. 2011;26(10):1844–50.

36. Ludwig L, Pasman J, Nicholson T, Aybek S, David A, Tuck S, et al. Stressful life events and maltreatment in conversion (functional neurological) disorder: systematic review and metaanalysis of case-control studies. Lancet Psychiatry. 2018;5(4):307–20.

37. Williams B, Ospina J, Jalilianhasanpour R, Fricchione G, Perez D. Fearful attachment linked to childhood abuse, alexithymia, and depression in motor functional neurological disorders. J Neuropsychiatry Clin Neurosci. 2019;31(1):65–9.

38. Dosanjh M, Alty J, Carol M, Latchford G, Graham CD. What is it like to live with a functional movement disorder? An interpretative phenomenological analysis of illness experiences from symptom onset to post-diagnosis. Br J Health Psychol. 2021;26(2):325–42.

39. Dempsey L, Karver M, Labouliere C, Zesiewicz T, De Nadai A. Self-perceived burden as a mediator of depression symptoms amongst individuals living with a movement disorder. J Clin Psychol. 2012;68(10):1149–60.

40. Hill R, Pettit J. Perceived burdensomeness and suicide-related behaviors in clinical samples: cur-

41. Nalipay M, Ku L. Indirect effect of hopelessness on depression symptoms through perceived burdensomeness. Psychol Rep. 2019;122(5):1618–31.

42. Cohen C, Colantonio A, Vernich L. Positive aspects of caregiving: rounding out the caregiver experience. Int J Geriatr Psychiatry. 2002;17(2):184–8.

43. Anderson K, Gruber-Baldini A, Vaughan C, Reich S, Fishman P, Weiner W, et al. Impact of psychogenic movement disorders versus Parkinson's on disability, quality of life, and psychopathology. Mov Disord. 2007;22(15):2204–9.

44. Carson A, Stone J, Hibberd C, Murray G, Duncan R, Coleman R, et al. Disability, distress and unemployment in neurology outpatients with symptoms "unexplained by organic disease". J Neurol Neurosurg Psychiatry. 2011;82(7):810–3.

45. Gelauff J, Stone J, Edwards M, Carson A. The prognosis of functional (psychogenic) motor symptoms: a systematic review. J Neurol Neurosurg Psychiatry. 2014;85(2):220–6.

46. Jacob A, Kaelin D, Roach A, Ziegler C, LaFaver K. Motor retraining (MoRe) for functional movement disorders: outcomes from a 1-week multidisciplinary rehabilitation program. PM R. 2018;10(11):1164–72.

47. Czarnecki K, Thompson J, Seime R, Geda Y, Duffy J, Ahlskog J. Functional movement disorders: successful treatment with a physical therapy rehabilitation protocol. Parkinsonism Relat Disord. 2012;18(3):247–51.

48. Nielsen G. Physical treatment of functional neurologic disorders. In: Stone J, Carson A, Hallett M, editors. Handbook of clinical neurology, vol. 129. Boston: Elsevier; 2016. p. 543–53.

49. Nielsen G, Stone J, Matthews A, Brown M, Sparkes C, Farmer R. Physiotherapy for functional motor disorders: a consensus recommendation. J Neurol Neurosurg Psychiatry. 2015;86(10):1113–9.

50. Jimenez X, Aboussouan A, Johnson J. Functional neurological disorder responds favorably to interdisciplinary rehabilitation models. Psychosomatics. 2019;60(6):556–62.

51. Khoo E, Small R, Cheng W, Hatchard T, Glynn B, Rice D, et al. Comparative evaluation of group-based mindfulness-based stress reduction and cognitive behavioural therapy for the treatment and management of chronic pain: a systematic review and network meta-analysis. Evid Based Ment Health. 2019;22(1):26–35.

52. Verhaak P, Heijman M, Peters L, Rijken M. Chronic disease and mental disorder. Soc Sci Med. 2005;60(4):789–97.

53. Schmaling K, Fales J. The association between borderline personality disorder and somatoform disorders: a systematic review and meta-analysis. Clin Psychol Sci Pract. 2018;25(2):1–17.

54. Farris S, Uebelacker L, Brown R, Price L, Desaulniers J, Abrantes A. Anxiety sensitivity pre-

dicts increased perceived exertion during a 1-mile walk test among treatment-seeking smokers. J Behav Med. 2017;40(6):886–93.

55. Pick S, Anderson D, Asadi-Pooya A, Aybek S, Baslet G, Bloem B, et al. Outcome measurement in functional neurological disorder: a systematic review and recommendations. J Neurol Neurosurg Psychiatry. 2020;91(6):638–49.

56. Kroenke K, Spitzer R, Williams J. The PHQ-9: validity of a brief depression severity measure. J Gen Intern Med. 2001;16(9):606–13.

57. Beck A, Steer R, Brown G. Manual for the Beck depression inventory-II. San Antonio: Psychological Corporation; 1996.

58. Spitzer R, Kroenke K, Williams J, Löwe B. A brief measure for assessing generalized anxiety disorder: the GAD-7. Arch Intern Med. 2006;166(10):1092–7.

59. Zigmond A, Snaith R. The hospital anxiety and depression scale. Acta Psychiatr Scand. 1983;67(6):361–70.

60. Posner K, Brown G, Stanley B, Brent D, Yershova K, Oquendo M. The Columbia-suicide severity rating scale: initial validity and internal consistency findings from three multisite studies with adolescents and adults. Am J Psychiatry. 2011;168(12):1266–77.

61. Boudreaux E, Jaques M, Brady K, Matson A, Allen M. The patient safety screener: validation of a brief suicide risk screener for emergency department settings. Arch Suicide Res. 2017;21(1):52–61.

62. Garnefski N, Kraaij V. Cognitive emotion regulation questionnaire – development of a short 18-item version (CERQ-short). Pers Individ Differ. 2006;41(6):1045–53.

63. Langbehn D, Pfohl B, Reynolds S, Clark L, Battaglia M, Bellodi L, et al. The Iowa personality disorder screen: development and preliminary validation of a brief screening interview. J Personal Disord. 1999;13(1):75–89.

64. Prins A, Ouimette P, Kimerling R, Cameron R, Hugelshofer D, Shaw-Hegwer J. The primary care PTSD (PC-PTSD): development and operating characteristics. Prim Care Psychiatr. 2003;9(1):9–14.

65. Goodman H, Corcoran C, Turner K, Yuan N, Green B. Assessing traumatic event exposure: general issues and preliminary findings for the stressful life events screening questionnaire. J Trauma Stress. 1998;11(3):521–42.

66. Felitti V, Anda R, Nordenberg D, Williamson D, Spitz A, Edwards V, et al. Relationship of childhood abuse and household dysfunction to many of the leading causes of death in adults: the adverse childhood experiences (ACE) study. Am J Prev Med. 1988;14(4):245–58.

67. Zimet G, Dahlem N, Zimet S, Farley G. The multidimensional scale of perceived social support. J Pers Assess. 1988;52(1):30–41.

68. Kroenke K, Spitzer R, Williams J. The PHQ-15: validity of a new measure for evaluating the severity of somatic symptoms. Psychosom Med. 2002;64(2):258–66.

69. Tyrer H, Ali L, Cooper F, Seivewright P, Bassett P, Tyrer P. The schedule for evaluating persistent symptoms (SEPS): a new method of recording medically unexplained symptoms. Int J Soc Psychiatry. 2013;59(3):281–7.

70. Bush K, Kivlahan D, McDonell M, Fihn S, Bradley K. The AUDIT alcohol consumption questions (AUDIT-C): an effective brief screening test for problem drinking. Arch Intern Med. 1998;158:1789–95.

71. Skinner H. The drug abuse screening test. Addict Behav. 1982;7(4):363–71.

72. Adams C, Anderson J, Madva E, LaFrance W, Perez D. You've made the diagnosis of functional neurological disorder: now what? Pract Neurol. 2018;18(4):323–30.

73. Chutko L, Surushkina S, Yakovenko E, Anisimova T, Karpovskaya E, Vasilenko V. Impairments of cognitive control in patients with somatoform disorders and their treatment. Zh Nevrol Psikhiatr Im S S Korsakova. 2019;119(4):32–7.

74. Breuer J, Freud S. Studies on hysteria. Oxford: Basic Books; 1957.

75. Mace C. Reversible cognitive impairment related to conversion disorder. J Nerv Ment Dis. 1994;182(3):186–7.

76. Liberini P, Faglia L, Salvi F, Grant R. Cognitive impairment related to conversion disorder: a two-year follow-up study. J Nerv Ment Dis. 1993;181(5):325–7.

77. Al-Adawi S, Al-Zakwani I, Obeid Y, Zaidan Z. Neurocognitive functioning in women presenting with undifferentiated somatoform disorders in Oman. Psychiatry Clin Neurosci. 2010;64(5):555–64.

78. Brown L, Nicholson T, Aybek S, Kanaan R, David A. Neuropsychological function and memory suppression in conversion disorder. J Neuropsychol. 2014;8(2):171–85.

79. Ball H, McWhirter L, Ballard C, Bhome R, Blackburn D, Edwards M, et al. Functional cognitive disorder: dementia's blind spot. Brain. 2020;143(10):2895–903.

80. McWhirter L, Ritchie C, Stone J, Carson A. Functional cognitive disorders: a systematic review. Lancet Psychiatry. 2020;7(2):191–207.

81. Edwards M, Bhatia K. Functional (psychogenic) movement disorders: merging mind and brain. Lancet Neurol. 2012;11(3):250–60.

82. Gilmour G, Nielsen G, Teodoro T, Yogarajah M, Coebergh J, Dilley M, et al. Management of functional neurological disorder. J Neurol. 2020;267(7):2164–72.

83. Swift J, Callahan J, Heath C, Herbert G, Levine J. Applications of the psychotherapy phase model to clinically significant deterioration. Psychotherapy (Chic). 2010;47(2):235–48.

84. Kutlubaev M, Xu Y, Hackett M, Stone J. Dual diagnosis of epilepsy and psychogenic nonepileptic seizures: systematic review and meta-analysis of frequency, correlates, and outcomes. Epilepsy Behav. 2018;89:70–8.

85. Cohen B, Edmondson D, Kronish I. State of the art review: depression, stress, anxiety, and cardiovascular disease. Am J Hypertens. 2015;28(11):1295–302.

86. Bica T, Castelló R, Toussaint L, Montesó-Curto P. Depression as a risk factor of organic diseases: an international integrative review. J Nurs Scholarsh. 2017;49(4):389–99.

87. Kanaan R, Pariante C, Reuber M, Nicholson T. Stress and functional neurological disorders: mechanistic insights. J Neurol Neurosurg Psychiatry. 2019;90(7):813–21.

88. Hubschmid M, Aybek S, Maccaferri G, Chocron O, Gholamrezaee M, Rossetti A. Efficacy of brief interdisciplinary psychotherapeutic intervention for motor conversion disorder and nonepileptic attacks. Gen Hosp Psychiatry. 2015;37(5):448–55.

89. Edwards M, Stone J, Nielsen G. Physiotherapists and patients with functional (psychogenic) motor symptoms: a survey of attitudes and interest. J Neurol Neurosurg Psychiatry. 2012;83(6):655–8.

90. Gardiner P, MacGregor L, Carson A, Stone J. Occupational therapy for functional neurological disorders: a scoping review and agenda for research. CNS Spectr. 2018;23(3):205–12.

91. Nicholson C, Edwards M, Carson A, Gardiner P, Golder D, Hayward K, et al. Occupational therapy consensus recommendations for functional neurological disorder. J Neurol Neurosurg Psychiatry. 2020;91(10):1037–45.

92. Edwards M, Stone J, Lang A. From psychogenic movement disorder to functional movement disorder: it's time to change the name. Mov Disord. 2014;29(7):849–52.

93. Dent B, Stanton BR, Kanaan RA. Psychiatrists' understanding and management of conversion disorder: a bi-national survey and comparison with neurologists. Neuropsychiatr Dis Treat. 2020;16:1965–74.

94. American Psychiatric Association. Diagnostic and statistical manual of mental disorders. 5th ed. Arlington: American Psychiatric Press; 2013.

95. Kanaan R, Armstrong D, Wessely S. The role of psychiatrists in diagnosing conversion disorder: a mixed-methods analysis. Neuropsychiatr Dis Treat. 2016;12:1181–4.

96. van der Hoeven R, Broersma M, Pijnenborg G, Koops E, van Laar T, Stone J, et al. Functional (psychogenic) movement disorders associated with normal scores in psychological questionnaires: a case control study. J Psychosom Res. 2015;79(3):190–4.

97. Goldstein L, Chalder T, Chigwedere C, Khondoker M, Moriarty J, Toone B, et al. Cognitive-behavioral therapy for psychogenic nonepileptic seizures: a pilot RCT. Neurology. 2010;74(24):1986–94.

98. Sharpe M, Walker J, Williams C, Stone J, Cavanagh J, Murray G, et al. Guided self-help for functional (psychogenic) symptoms: a randomized controlled efficacy trial. Neurology. 2011;77(6):564–72.

99. LaFrance W, Baird G, Barry J, Blum A, Webb A, Keitner G, et al. Multicenter pilot treatment trial for psychogenic nonepileptic seizures: a randomized clinical trial. JAMA Psychiat. 2014;71(9):997–1005.

100. Liu J, Gill N, Teodorczuk A, Li Z, Sun J. The efficacy of cognitive behavioural therapy in somatoform disorders and medically unexplained physical symptoms: a meta-analysis of randomized controlled trials. J Affect Disord. 2019;245:98–112.

101. Goldstein L, Robinson E, Mellers J, Stone J, Carson A, Reuber M, et al. Cognitive behavioural therapy for adults with dissociative. Lancet Psychiatry. 2020;7(6):491–505.

102. Williams C, Kent C, Smith S, Carson A, Sharpe M, Cavanagh J. Overcoming functional neurological symptoms: a five areas approach. New York: Routledge; 2011.

103. Owen J, Adelson J, Budge S, Wampold B, Kopta M, Minami T, et al. Trajectories of change in psychotherapy. J Clin Psychol. 2015;71(9):817–27.

104. Guthrie S, Harvey A. Motivation and its influence on outcome in rehabilitation. Rev Clin Gerontol. 1994;4(3):235–43.

105. Yang W, Strodl E. Motivational interviewing changes the treatment trajectory of group cognitive-behavioural therapy for anxiety. In: Boag S, Tiliopoulos N, editors. Personality and individual differences: theory, assessment, and application. Hauppauge: Nova Science Publishers; 2011. p. 237–48.

106. Hurn J, Kneebone I, Cropley M. Goal setting as an outcome measure: a systematic review. Clin Rehabil. 2006;20(9):756–72.

107. Dekker J, de Groot V, Ter Steeg A, Vloothuis J, Holla J, Collette E, et al. Setting meaningful goals in rehabilitation: rationale and practical tool. Clin Rehabil. 2020;34(1):3–12.

Management Considerations for Pediatric Functional Movement Disorder

31

Kasia Kozlowska

This chapter focuses on management considerations for children and adolescents with functional movement disorder (FMD). As treatment is closely interwoven with the presenting symptoms, diagnosis, and biopsychosocial formulation, important concepts introduced in Chap. 15 on pediatric patients with FMD are illustrated in a case vignette before discussing specific treatment strategies. The term "child" is used to refer to both children and adolescents.

Part I: Presentation, Assessment, and Diagnosis

Grace, a 12-year-old girl, lived with her mother, father, 22-year-old brother and 15-year-old sister. She became ill at the beginning of sixth grade, experiencing intermittent nausea, abdominal pain and constipation, recurring bouts of chest pain, and daily headaches. Repeated visits to the family doctor—which included 24-h Holter monitoring via a cardiologist—failed to find any

identifiable medical condition. Grace and the family were told that all the tests were normal.

Two months later, Grace told her parents that she could not feel her toes properly and that she felt a strange tingling numbness in her feet. These symptoms were attributed to ill-fitting shoes. Some weeks later, she experienced a fall, fractured her right foot, and was prescribed a supportive boot for 6 weeks. Following the injury, the tingling and numbness in her right foot progressed to the right ankle. After removal of the boot 6 weeks later, Grace experienced a constant burning sensation in both feet. The burning increased in intensity, moved up her legs to the knees, and was accompanied by weakness in both legs and a wobbly gait.

Grace's father had worked as a builder but was on long-term disability due to diabetes-related complications. On his side of the family, there was a history of anxiety and depression. Grace's mother had worked as a librarian but was now a full-time caregiver to her husband and the family. Grace's brother had a full-time job, and her sister was in ninth grade of high school.

Grace's developmental history was unremarkable. Grace reported that as a little girl she had spent many hours with her father planting seedlings and attending to the vegetable garden. When Grace was 8 years old, her father began to suffer from medical complications of diabetes, neuropathy, and cardiomyopathy. The infections in the feet led to repeated hospitalizations and

K. Kozlowska (✉)
The Children's Hospital at Westmead, Westmead, NSW, Australia

Discipline of Psychiatry and Discipline of Child & Adolescent Health, University of Sydney, Medical School, Sydney, NSW, Australia

Westmead Institute for Medical Research, Westmead, NSW, Australia
e-mail: kkoz6421@uni.sydney.edu.au

© Springer Nature Switzerland AG 2022
K. LaFaver et al. (eds.), *Functional Movement Disorder*, Current Clinical Neurology,
https://doi.org/10.1007/978-3-030-86495-8_31

procedures, and alongside the progressing cardiomyopathy, led to dependence on a wheelchair. When Grace was 9 years old, her older brother found it increasingly difficult to cope with his father's deteriorating health. He became anxious and depressed, and attended weekly psychotherapy for more than a year. When Grace turned 11, her sister Cathy was diagnosed with leukemia, requiring chemotherapy and home tutoring. At this time, Grace's mother left her job to look after the ill members of the family, and the family became dependent on welfare payments.

Neurology assessment at the local hospital included a physical examination, a spine MRI scan, nerve conduction studies, and skin biopsy (for small-fiber neuropathy) all of which were normal. The report from the local hospital stated "no stress described." No diagnosis was given, but Grace was referred for physiotherapy to the local hospital therapist, who scheduled weekly sessions.

In the ensuing month the hospital physiotherapist reported that Grace's gait was getting worse, not better. Because Grace's school was worried that Grace might hurt herself if she fell, the physiotherapist recommended that Grace use a wheelchair. Grace became more and more wheelchair dependent. Her burning sensation in the legs worsened, and she now described it as crawling up from her feet to her thighs. During this period of time her father's health remained poor with frequent outpatient visits and medical procedures.

Nine months after symptom onset—Grace presented to a tertiary care hospital with the new symptom of intermittent jerking in the upper limbs. Typically, the jerking began when Grace tried to stand up. Occasionally the jerking took over Grace's whole upper body and terminated only when Grace became unresponsive and slumped in her wheel chair. In addition, Grace was now finding it difficult to sleep, and she would lie awake for hours. She was still confined to the wheelchair.

On neurological exam Grace showed normal tone and reflexes, was able to stand on heels and toes with assistance, and demonstrated loss of touch sensation and vibration in a stocking distribution from the hips down. Strength was more difficult to assess because it fluctuated with attention and effort (specifically, features of motor inconsistency). Grace's jerking episodes, captured on video EEG, had no electrographic correlate. PCO2 monitoring during the EEG showed a mild hypocapnia (pCO2 of 32 mmHg before the formal hyperventilation challenge), consistent with the elevated respiratory rate of 28 breaths/min. During the hyperventilation challenge Grace's PCO2 dropped to 22 mmHg, and she complained of chest pain—the same that she had been experiencing intermittently at home. A standing test for the assessment of orthostatic intolerance was normal. The neurology team made a diagnosis of functional neurological disorder (FND) with mixed features.

Grace's presenting history and her pathway through the health system highlight a number of key themes that characterize pediatric presentations with FMD and, more generally, FND presentations in children, including adolescents. Henceforth we use the terms "functional neurological disorder" (FND) or the even broader term "functional somatic symptoms" because as the reader can see, Grace's functional symptoms went beyond core neurological symptoms of an FMD. Each theme is discussed under a subheading.

The Child's Body Signals Stress and Distress: The Somatic Narrative

A common pattern of presentation is one where the child's presentation begins with commonplace functional somatic symptoms—frequent headaches, intermittent abdominal pain, disturbed sleep, and so on—which can mark the body's neurophysiological response to stress or to adverse life events in the child's life. Typically, the symptoms are investigated, the child and family are told that there is no clear medical condition, and nothing more is done. The significance of the body's neurophysiological response—the somatic narrative—is lost, as is the opportunity to provide early intervention, so as to help the child both regulate her body and to help her manage (together with the family) the stress that triggered the symptoms in the first place.

In a parallel process, families of children who present with FND—and functional somatic symptoms more generally—are typically unable to make a connection between the somatic narrative (the child's symptoms) and the stressful events in the child's life. Typically, families see the symptoms as an independent entity, disconnected from the child's emotional life and from the child's psychosocial context. What is striking in the case of Grace is that the medical professionals were unable to help make this connection more explicit for the family. In the medical report, the statement "no stress described" was written adjacent to a statement detailing the medical events—stress events—that had taken place in the family.

Whilst many children's functional symptoms may reflect a transient response to stress, others will go on to develop layer upon layer of functional somatic symptoms with increasing functional impairment and school absenteeism. Grace followed the second pathway. In this case, if the family doctor and pediatric cardiologist (who saw Grace in the early phase of her illness) had listened carefully to the somatic narrative, had connected Grace's somatic symptoms with the stress in the family (and an appropriate initial first-pass negative workup), and had made a referral for implementation of regulation strategies and psychological support—for Grace and for her family—her symptoms may have settled, and her health and well-being could have been supported. As such, the medical profession contributed to the process by which Grace's functional somatic symptoms became severe and chronic, and went on to impair the Grace's physical function and her health and well-being.

Unfortunately, Grace's story is not unique. Many pediatricians are unfamiliar with and fail to recognize the somatic narrative [1]—also known as body language [2], talking with the body [3], body narrative [4], or, in intolerable predicaments, "the body speak[ing] what the tongue cannot utter" (p. 38) [5]. In the science literature the somatic narrative is seen as involving interocep-

tion [6, 7], homeostatic emotions [8], or physiological feelings [9]. Because they do not identify or attend to the somatic narrative, many pediatricians fail to take appropriate action and to refer the child for appropriate treatment with a therapist (mental health clinician) who can help the child regulate and who can work with the child, family, and school to help the child manage her stress [10, 11]. Across specialties—in both pediatrics and adult practice—there is now a concerted effort to raise awareness of functional disorders; to ensure that pediatricians include functional disorders as part of their differential diagnosis; and to promote the provision of a positive functional diagnosis based on the pattern of neurological symptoms (in FND) [12] or consensus diagnostic criteria (for other functional disorders) [13–18].

The Importance of the Psychosocial History

Children are very sensitive to their family context [19], to the stress that takes place in the context of the family; the acquisition of a good psychosocial history is therefore at the core of good pediatric practice [20] (see Table 31.1). In the case of Grace, when a comprehensive psychosocial history was taken (as described in the opening paragraphs of the case), the cumulative adverse life events that formed the backdrop to Grace's functional symptoms, as well as the high levels of stress and distress experienced by all members of the family, were clearly evident to everyone—the family and the treating team.

The psychosocial history is particularly important when assessing children with functional neurological symptoms—and functional somatic symptoms more generally—because the association between adverse childhood experiences (ACEs) and functional presentations has been reported across functional disorders [24]. In Grace's case the adverse childhood experiences included: a parent with a life-threatening illness, a sibling with a life-threatening illness, a family member with a mental health disorder, and

Table 31.1 Psychosocial history [21–23]

Taking a developmental history		
Developmental stage	Relevant themes to explore[a]	Other events affecting family health and well-being
Prenatal	Pregnancy, delivery	↑
Infancy	Feeding, sleeping, settling, milestones How child and child's body responded to any family stress	Track any other events, including family events, that affected the well-being of the family at all developmental stages, and bring them into the history-taking process. ↓
Preschool years	Separating from parents (separation anxiety) Starting preschool/childcare Feeding & sleeping, and other milestones How child and child's body responded to any family stress	
Primary school	Starting school Making friends Issues of teasing/bullying Academic difficulties or high expectations Difficulties with teachers Any change of school Out-of-school activities (including sports) Response to newborn siblings Eating & sleeping, and other milestones How child and child's body responded to any family stress Was the child able to communicate distress to mother/father, or did she keep the distress to herself?	
High school	Transition to high school Making new friends Issues of teasing/bullying Boyfriend/girlfriend How the adolescent/family are handling independence and individuation Academic difficulties or high expectations Difficulties with teachers Any change of school Out-of-school activities (including sports) Eating, sleeping, emotional regulation, and other milestones Social media and technology use How adolescent and adolescent's body responded to any family stress Is the adolescent able to communicate distress to mother/father, or does she keep the distress to herself?	

© Kozlowska 2020

[a]This table provides the reader with question themes that help the child and family tell the child's developmental story and the story of the symptoms. The child and siblings are involved in telling the story from the point in it where they have access to episodic memories. This collaborative process strongly enhances engagement [21–23]. An informal way to think about this table is that the questions enable the therapist, family, and child to understand the family's stress level at any point in time or, if depicted on a visual representation of a thermometer, to concretely depict the family's temperature level

household poverty. When the adverse childhood events are made explicit and added up, it is not surprising that Grace became ill with a stress-related FND.

Stress Can Be Physical or Emotional: Physical Stress Events Often Trigger FND Symptoms

Grace's story also highlights the role of both physical and psychological stressors as an antecedent to pediatric FND. In our research in mixed FND cohorts, we have consistently found that approximately 50% of children and families report a physical trigger event—a viral illness, a minor injury, a medical event, or a series of medical events—as one of the stressors that preceded the child's illness [25, 26]. Common psychological stressors include family conflict, bullying, separation from a family member, death of a friend or family member, family illness, and sporting/school/learning stressors [27]. In pediatric practice, if a good history is taken, the connection between the child symptoms is usually obvious to the clinician, and it is very rare for the child or family to report no antecedent stress events—physical or psychological. Helping the child and family make this connection is a goal of the assessment and engagement process [21, 22].

Grace's story also highlights the common pattern of cumulative, commonplace adverse life events, versus the presence of a single event (see also section below). Grace initially coped with her father's illness and operations; she then also coped with her brother's depression; but then, when her father continued to deteriorate and her sister was diagnosed with cancer, and the family became dependent of welfare payments, the stress was more than she or her body could manage. She became symptomatic.

Maltreatment Occurs in a Subset of Cases Only

While the association between adverse childhood experiences and functional somatic symptoms is very robust, pediatric studies suggest that commonplace, cumulative stress events—family conflict, bullying, academic stress—are much more common than maltreatment (sexual abuse, physical abuse, and emotional abuse). That said, maltreatment—and questions as to whether the child is safe or not safe, or whether past trauma needs to be processed—is an issue for some children and families.

Illness Models in the Family

The idea of an illness model—for example, from a family member, whether "current or historical, real or contrived, chronic or ephemeral"—is an idea postulated by David Taylor in the 1980s (p. 40) [5]. With the exception of pain modelling by parents [28], there have been no published studies examining this hypothesis. Nonetheless, illness modelling is an important theme in some presentations. In the case of Grace, both her father and her sister suffered from symptoms involving the legs—neuropathic pain (father) and a tumor in behind the knee that led to the diagnosis of leukemia (sister). It is interesting to consider this perspective in the case of Grace. It is possible that the tingling sensations in Grace's legs progressed because she paid the symptoms significant attention, potentially due to anxiety that she, like her father and sister, could be developing a medical problem in her legs. It is well known that attention to bodily symptoms amplifies them [12].

Multiple FND Symptoms, Migrating Symptoms, and Comorbidity with Complex Pain and Other Functional Somatic Symptoms Is Common

Grace's case also highlights that in pediatric practice, FND symptoms typically present alongside pain and other functional somatic symptoms [27]. Very often, the child's symptoms shift and change during a single presentation or between presentations. In Grace's story, the reader can see how the symptoms continued to layer one over the other.

The Need to Provide a Positive Diagnosis of a Functional Disorder

The failure to provide a timely diagnosis of a functional disorder leads to a delay in treatment and can cause the child and the family significant harm. For Grace, had the initial symptoms been given an appropriate diagnostic label—functional nausea, abdominal pain and constipation, hyperventilation-related chest pain, and tension headaches—and if these had been connected to Grace's family situation, then the appropriate treatment could have been provided at the onset. The diagnosis of a functional illness took 3 months to make, and it was made only at a tertiary care hospital following the development of new motor symptoms.

Part II: Co-constructing a Formulation

After the diagnosis of FND was made, a family assessment interview with the mind-body team—a child psychiatrist, a child psychiatry fellow, and a pediatric resident—took place with Grace, her mother, and her brother and sister. Grace's father was unable to get to the appointment due to his poor health. The family told the story of Grace's development, symptoms, and the context in which they had emerged. The interactions between family members—and between the family and the team members—during the telling of the family's story were warm and open.

Following the information-gathering component of the interview, the clinical team and family co-constructed a formulation—a synthesis of Grace's story and the neurobiology of functional somatic symptoms. The child psychiatrist provided the family with information about FND and the greater spectrum of functional somatic symptoms, along with a simple explanation of their neurobiology. She explained the symptoms in the same order as they had occurred in Grace's story, so that the family knew that she had heard the story and that she was weaving what she knew into the story that the family had told.

As the psychiatrist spoke she used a number of visual metaphors, which she drew as she talked. She explained the autonomic nervous system, how stress—in Grace's case the illness of Grace's father and then the illness of her sister—may have activated Grace's autonomic nervous system and generated symptoms of nausea, abdominal pain, and constipation (see Fig. 31.1). She explained how hyperventilation—another common body response to stress—could affect arteries in the heart and was a common cause of stress-related chest pain. Here John, Grace's brother, spoke up and said that he had also suffered from chest pain as part of his depression. The psychiatrist explained that the body's pain system functioned like an alarm system that signals the presence of threat. Sometimes the threat was physical (for example, when Grace had fractured her foot), but sometimes it was emotional (for example, the distress Grace had experienced with the illness of her father and sister). Hence the onset of daily headaches. She also told the family that abdominal pain and headaches were the most common symptoms of stress experienced by children. She said that in contemporary medicine this type of pain—the body's response to threat in general—was called complex/chronic pain.

The child psychiatrist then went on to discuss the FND symptoms and the burning pain in Grace's legs. She drew a red ball to represent the stress systems in the brain—the brain systems that underpin salience detection, arousal, pain, and emotional state, and that activate in the context of stress (see Fig. 31.2). She explained that activation of the brain stress systems could interfere with motor, sensory, and pain processing, resulting in motor weakness, loss of sensation, and pain. Grace's mother looked relieved and stated that it was a relief to understand what was happening. She said that Grace had been worried that the team would tell her that she was mentally ill. Grace laughed with relief, and everyone laughed with her. Grace asked if she could keep the pictures that the psychiatrist had drawn so that she could explain what was happening to her father, when she next saw him.

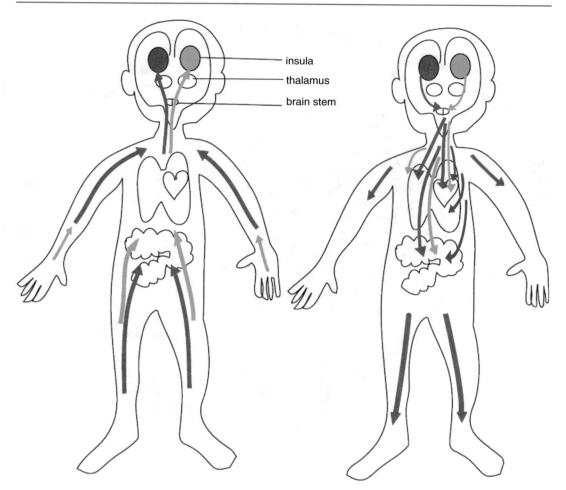

insula

thalamus

brain stem

Fig. 31.1 Functional visual representation of autonomic nervous system. Afferent signals from the body to the brain provide the brain with interoceptive information about the state of the body (figure on the left). Efferent signals from the brain to the body—involving both the *sympathetic* (depicted in red) and *restorative parasympathetic systems* (depicted in blue)—provide second-by-second fine-tuning of body state (figure on the right). In addition, when needed (as in response to threat), the *sympathetic nerves* (depicted in red) *up* body arousal by increasing heart rate, activating the secretion of adrenalin (from the adrenal glands), adjusting vascular tone, and so on. Activation of the sympathetic system by stress can switch off the gut's digestive programs and, as experi-enced by Grace, cause constipation). Likewise, *restorative parasympathetic nerves* (depicted in blue) *down* body arousal (for example, by decreasing heart rate). The *defensive parasympathetic* nerves (depicted in purple) work alongside the sympathetic system in response to threat by activating defensive programs in the gut (nausea, vomiting, and diarrhea) and in the heart (threat-induced fainting) [23]. Abdominal pain commonly accompanies the activation of defensive programs to the gut, as experienced by Grace. (This figure was first published in "Stress, distress, and bodytalk: co-constructing formulations with patients who present with somatic symptoms" [23]. © Kozlowska 2013)

The conversation then turned to treatment. Grace accepted that she would stay in hospital for 2 weeks to complete a multidisciplinary rehabilitation program. The family accepted the conditions of the program: daily school, daily physiotherapy, daily psychology sessions, weekly family sessions, and daily family visits in the afternoon after Grace had finished the program for each day. Grace would also have a one-night leave during the intervening weekend to spend the weekend at home.

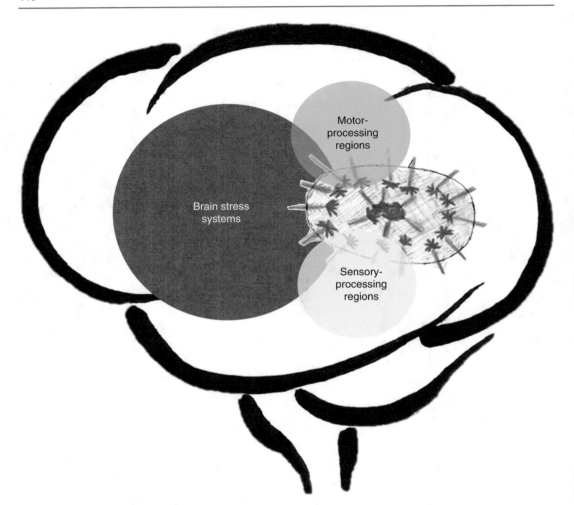

Fig. 31.2 The red ball represents the *brain stress systems*. The pink ball on the top right represents *motor-processing regions*; the yellow ball represents *sensory-processing regions*; and the spiky ball represents *pain maps*. When the *brain stress systems* are activated by infection, illness, injury, or emotional stress, they become overactive and over-dominant, and they disrupt motor- and sensory-processing regions, and amplify pain-processing regions, causing functional sensorimotor symptoms and amplifying feelings of pain. (This figure was first published in *Functional Somatic Symptoms in Children and Adolescents: The Stress-System Approach to Assessment and Treatment* [22]. © Kozlowska 2019)

Grace's mother was given an opportunity to talk to the team on her own. In this conversation without the children, Grace's mother informed the team that her husband's health was deteriorating and that the stress at home was likely to get worse. Her own sadness and distress was expressed openly in tears that rolled down her face. She described in detail how the stress of her husband's illness and that of her daughter had affected all family members. She informed the team that she had noticed that when Grace became overwhelmed that she had a tendency to "shut down." During this conversation it also became evident that the family's financial situation was tight, to the point that it was not possible for Grace to pursue normal activities, such as going to the movies with her friends. The team, in turn, acknowledged that the problems facing Grace were more than she could manage on her own and that this sort of unresolvable predicament was something that was quite often seen in children with FND. The team also validated the high stress faced by Grace's mother.

Providing an Explanation and Co-constructing a Formulation

When working with children and families, the FND diagnosis needs to be accompanied by an explanation pertaining to the neurobiology of the child's functional symptoms, as well as a clear formulation that connects together the symptoms with the child's psychosocial context [29]. When the diagnosis, explanation, and the process of co-constructing the formulation are done in a way that the child and family can understand—and that connects with the child's experience—most children and families will understand the diagnosis and accept appropriate treatment.

In the case of Grace, once the diagnosis had been made and the symptoms were clearly explained, Grace was immensely relieved, and her functional (dissociative) seizures ceased without any further intervention. Because functional seizures are associated with high levels of arousal (increased cortisol levels, lower heart rate variability, and increased heart rate) and activation of the motor respiratory system [30–32], our working hypothesis in the mind-body team is that paroxysmal exacerbations of cortical arousal lead to time-limited changes in the prefrontal cortex and to the release of reflex motor programs in the basal ganglia and brain stem, which manifest as functional seizures [33]. In the case of Grace, the formulation process was therapeutic in and of itself, decreasing Grace's level of arousal and her

propensity for further functional seizures. For other patients, discussion of the formulation may prove insufficient for a robust treatment response, and other therapeutic approaches may be indicated (see below) [34, 35].

Mental Health Comorbidities

Although Grace was often sad—as when she thought about her father's illness—and was potentially at risk of developing a depression, she did not meet clinical criteria for major depression, generalized anxiety disorder, or panic disorder at the time of presentation. In our research cohorts, however, up to four-fifths of children meet criteria for a mental health disorder, with mood and anxiety disorders being the most common [25]. Very often anxiety—either the child's or the parents'—comes to the forefront when entry into the program requires that the child to separate from the parent and to take responsibility for managing herself in the different treatment elements that make up the program.

Part III: Treatment

Patient-centered, multidisciplinary, multimodal treatment using a stepped care model—where the level of specialist treatment required by each patient varies depending on the level of functional impairment—is the treatment of choice for children presenting with FND and other functional somatic symptoms [35, 36]. What this means in practice is that specific areas of difficulty/dysfunction on multiple system levels—the body, mind, family, and school system levels—are identified during the assessment process and that the treatment program is made up of multiple treatment components, delivered concurrently or sequentially, that target the identified areas of difficulty/dysfunction [37]. When the child's symptoms are severe and when functional impairment is significant, inpatient treatment may be required. Alternatively, when the child's symptoms are less severe, then the same treatment program can be set up in the community using a combination of local resources.

In the author's tertiary care hospital setting, this multidisciplinary approach—known as the Mind-Body Program[1]—provides a state-wide clinical service for children who present with significant functional impairment and who do not have access to appropriate care in their own local communities. The program—as well as outcome data—has been described in detail in previous publications [37, 40], as have been data pertaining to other programs [35, 41–43].

Grace was admitted for inpatient rehabilitation into the Mind-Body Program for the standard 2-week period, during which time she and her family participated in the treatment interventions discussed below.

Psychoeducation

Grace's individual therapist (the child psychiatry fellow) took time to go back through the explanation and visual metaphors—pertaining to the neurobiology of Grace's functional symptoms—to make sure that Grace had the opportunity to clarify any points of uncertainty. For more information about visual metaphors that can be used in psychoeducation with children with FND and other somatic symptoms, see Kozlowska et al. [22].

Stabilizing the Circadian Clock

Grace's sleep was stabilized with melatonin. This medication was continued throughout the admission and for 3 months after discharge.

---

[1]The Mind-Body Program was set up in 1994 in Sydney, Australia, by child and adolescent psychiatrist Prof. Kenneth Nunn in response to children presenting with functional impairment secondary to FND and pervasive refusal syndrome [38, 39].

The circadian clock is often dysregulated in children with FND [22] and in adults [44]. In this context, stabilization of sleep is often the first intervention implemented in the Mind-Body Program.

Daily Psychotherapy Sessions

Grace attended daily psychotherapy sessions with her therapist (see also Text Box 31.1). The sessions initially focused on helping Grace read her body—her somatic narrative—and notice warning signs marking increased levels of stress-system activation. To facilitate this process, the therapist used "body maps", on which Grace was able to denote her body state using marks made with colored felt pens, and a "stress thermometer", where different levels on the thermometer represented different levels of activation. Grace became skilled at representing her body's level of activation or her felt sense of stress on both tools (see Figs. 31.3 and 31.4). She and the therapist then experimented with a range of de-arousal strategies to see which strategies were most effectively decreasing Grace's level of activation and which Grace enjoyed most (for more information on such strategies, see Kozlowska et al. [22]). The therapist tracked Grace's levels of activation via her breathing rate, via a heart rate variability biofeedback device designed to identify Grace's resonant breathing rate [45], and by noticing at what points in the session Grace became overwhelmed and used her shut-down strategy (withdrawing into herself).

Over the course of 2 weeks, Grace and the therapist worked to put together a "strategy toolbox" that Grace would take home and continue to use—and practice on a daily basis—to manage her arousal [47]. The key regulation strategy in Grace's toolbox proved to be using the biofeedback device to reach her resonant breathing rate of 10 breaths/min (see Fig. 31.5). This device was an effective motivator because it allowed Grace to visualize how her effort to attain her resonant, slow breathing rate (like other de-

Text Box 31.1 Core psychological treatment components across inpatient and outpatient settings [46]

Helping the child read her or his body
Body map (to help build awareness of body) (see Fig. 31.3)
Feelings jar that depicts feelings/homeostatic feelings (to help build awareness of thoughts, feelings, and body sensations)
Helping the child regulate her body and manage pain (bottom-up regulation strategies[a])
Body scan
Slow breathing/HRV biofeedback to achieve resonant breathing (see Fig. 31.5)
Progressive muscle relaxation
Sensory and motor (movement-related) regulation strategies
Mindfulness (bottom-up mindfulness strategies)
Trauma-specific interventions (when loss or trauma is a contributing factor)
Eye movement desensitization and reprocessing (EMDR)
Radical exposure tapping (RET)
Trauma-focused cognitive-behavioral therapy (CBT)
Somatic experiencing (SE)
Helping the child make connections between situations, body-states, emotions, and thoughts
Sociogram (diagram depicting the closeness of different relationships in the child's life)
Safety plan (if indicated for mood or for functional seizures)
Thermometer metaphor (allows child to quantify subjective stress levels or stress levels in the family) (see Fig. 31.4)
Drawings that are used to help the child depict situations visually and make connections with body states
Helping the child manage difficult emotions, thoughts, and pain (top-down regulation strategies[a])
Attentional refocussing (including distraction, shifting attention to music, and so on)
Visualization exercises
Mindfulness (top-down mindfulness strategies)
Hypnosis
CBT interventions, including activity scheduling (for depression, fatigue, pain)
Maintaining daily activities of function (via a daily timetable)
Interventions that help the family support the child in her individual work (e.g., attentional refocusing away from symptoms and away from pain)
Interventions that address family issues—identified problem areas—that distress the child or that activate the child's body stress system
Supporting family members to address physical, mental health, or psychosocial issues that affect the well-being of the child
Working with the school to address issues in the child's school or peer context that distress the child or that activate the child's body stress system
Safety plan for the school for functional seizures or cormorbid low mood, or suicidal ideation
Subsequent referral to other established programs or therapists for specific anxiety, pain, or trauma-focused interventions
CBT or Acceptance and Commitment Therapy (ACT) for anxiety, depression
Trauma-focused-CBT, EMDR, radical exposure tapping, somatic experiencing for trauma symptoms

© Kozlowska 2020

[a]In the psychotherapy world, *top-down regualtion strategies* are those that involve use of the mind and that engage the prefrontal cortex, which in turn, regulates—top-down—phylogenetically older regions. By contrast, *bottom-up regulation* strategies, which include sensory strategies, movement, mindfulness to body sensations, biofeedback, and therapeutic touch, are interventions inducing change via inputs, from the body, via homeostatic afferents and the thalamo-insula-cortical system. For bottom-up strategies, cortical areas do not need to be engaged [46]. For more information about top-down and bottom-up regualtion strategies, and for more detail about the material presented in this text box, see Kozlowska et al. [22]

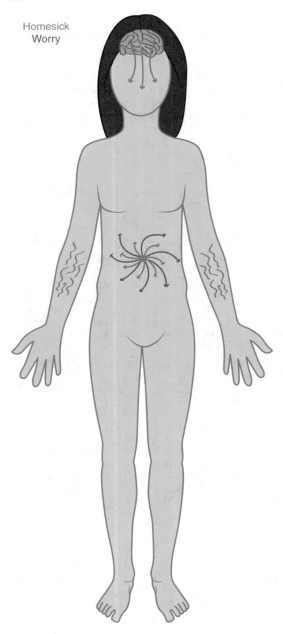

Homesick
Worry

Fig. 31.3 Body map depicting the felt sense of the body—a churning stomach—associated with worry and feelings of home sickness. (© Kozlowska 2019)

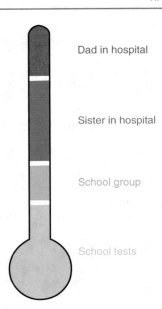

Dad in hospital

Sister in hospital

School group

School tests

Fig. 31.4 A visual depiction of the stress thermometer which Grace used to mark her level of activation (and the trigger for the activation). (© Kozlowska 2019)

arousal strategies) led to concrete changes in her body, in this case the autonomic nervous system. Other useful, more active strategies—ones that used movement to regulate—included boxing,

kicking a ball against a wall, progressive muscle relaxation, and calf and fist squeezes (tensing the large muscles in the legs in a rhythmical manner at 10-s intervals induces an increase in heart rate variability [48]).

Grace also did some work pertaining to difficult feelings. During the admission, she worked on identifying feelings of anger, annoyance, homesick, and worry in relation to events that happened during her hospital admission. She was able to visually represent her feelings on body maps; she and the therapist used the "stress thermometer" to identify feelings that could activate the stress system; and they were able to determine which strategies Grace could use to settle her body and feelings at these times (see Figs. 31.3 and 31.4). During these therapy sessions, it became apparent that Grace was not able to access her feelings regarding her father's declining health and the family's precarious financial circumstances, both of which were fraught with uncertainty. When the therapist probed these issues, Grace would go into her shut-down mode, or she would sidestep the issue by smiling at the therapist and saying, "I am a

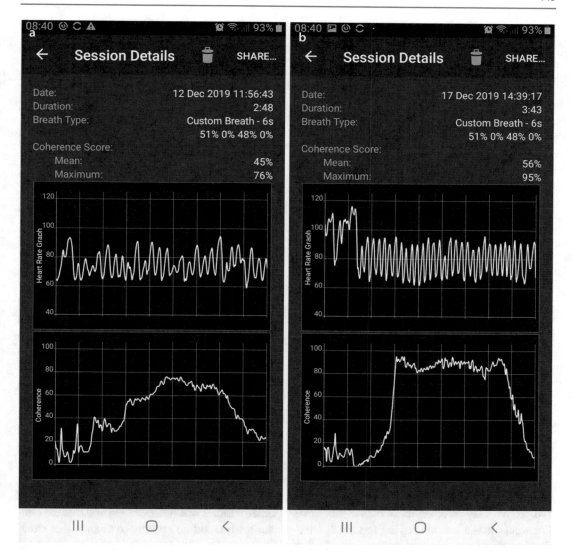

Fig. 31.5 The two screen shots from the biofeedback device document Grace's efforts to slow her breathing rate to her resonant frequency rate of 10 breaths/min. The first day of treatment is compared to the fifth day of treatment (after 5 days of practice, four times a day, 5 min/session). The top graph, a heart rate tachogram, shows Grace's heart rate during the breath training. The tachogram waveform takes on the characteristic sine pattern seen when the patient achieves a state of coherence—that is, a state of coupling between the autonomic and respiratory system that is associated with maximal restorative parasympathetic function (highest heart rate variability). The bottom graph depicts the increase in restorative parasympathetic function—or heart rate variability—also termed coher-ence. The second screen shot also demonstrates that the increase in restorative parasympathetic activity is associated with a decrease in sympathetic activation as reflected via heart rate. Autonomous heart rate—of approximately 100 beats/min—is generated, independent of autonomic control, by the sinoatrial node—a neuron bundle in the heart's right atrium [25]. Tonic vagal activity lowers this rate to normal values of approximately 60–80 beats/min, whereas withdrawal of tonic restorative parasympathetic (vagal) activity or increases in sympathetic activity raise the heart rate. With training Grace's heart rate shifting down from 70–115 to 65–95 beats/min and heart rate variability increased

chill person. I don't worry about these things." As had been discussed with Grace's mother, these situations were more than Grace could manage or hold in mind, and it remained to be seen how she would fare when her father's health deteriorated further. Ongoing psychotherapy with an outside therapist—a clinical psychologist—from a welfare organization was organized so that Grace would continue to be supported in the work that she had begun in the hospital setting.

Grace did not need specific interventions for her pain because her pain settled. Many children, however, do require pain-management strategies as part of their interventions. Common strategies used include: changing the focus of attention away from the pain (distraction, mindfulness interventions, visualization, listening to music, sensory strategies, and so on); hypnosis; heart rate variability biofeedback; cognitive-behavioral interventions; and implementation of regular exercise [45, 49, 50] (see also Text Box 31.1).

Physiotherapy

Akin to adults, children with FND symptoms show better outcomes with FND-specific physiotherapy [51–53]. Grace's case highlights that when treatment is provided by therapists with no experience with, or working knowledge of, FND, symptoms may worsen rather than improve. Potential pitfalls include paying too much attention to FND symptoms, unnecessary use of adaptive equipment, and difficulties in managing FND-seiz and the risk of falls.

Grace's daily physiotherapy sessions were goal oriented—transferring from wheelchair to bed, standing, taking steps—or they were delivered, instead, in the form of games. During physiotherapy, all tasks were done with the therapist focusing Grace's attention *away* from the weakness in her legs or away from the intermittent jerking in her upper limbs, and *toward* something else: a topic of conversation, a piece of music, or the goal of the particular game. Within 2 weeks, Grace could mobilize independently—although the tempo of her gait was still abnormally slow—

and she was discharged home with no aids. Her jerking episodes were no longer occurring. She had also stopped complaining of pain in her legs. The physiotherapist provided Grace with a home program that included mobilizing with no aids and normal activities such as swimming. The physiotherapist also emphasized that Grace's gait would continue to improve and would soon return to normal.

Six weeks later, when Grace returned to school following the holidays, the school counselor reported that she did not walk, but skipped, into her new high school.

Family Intervention

A family intervention pertaining to the role of attention was implemented. The clinical team began by explaining the role of attention in functional somatic symptoms and, in particular, in relation to pain. The family members were asked not to enquire about Graces' pain and, instead, to notice, but not attend to, her other symptoms. The therapist also told Grace that, because attention fed the symptoms and made them stronger and more intense, she would herself also be learning strategies that focused attention away from the symptoms.

As noted already, it was clear that the health of Grace's father was deteriorating and that the clinical team could do nothing to change that situation. As for the family's financial situation, however, a social work consult was organized to make sure that Grace's mother had accessed all potentially available resources for maintaining the family's financial stability.

A relapse-prevention plan was also implemented. The psychiatrist suggested that Grace would have good days and less good days; that this could vary with the stress at home and the worry about the father's health; and that this variation was normal. The psychiatrist also said that all children who did the program took it home with them, and continued on with it, for another 12 months, to make sure that they were doing everything to maintain health and well-being.

Grace was encouraged about her ongoing success with the home program: "You have done such a wonderful job in hospital, so we know that you and your family can keep the program up at home."

School Intervention

Resumption of normal age-appropriate activities is a key part of the treatment. The Mind-Body Program always involves attendance at hospital school either to maintain the child's normal function or, if the child had not been attending school, to facilitate reintegration back to school. During the 2-week inpatient treatment, Grace attended the hospital school every day. The teachers reported that she was a capable and cooperative student. For the approaching school year, the clinical team made contact with the school counselor at Grace's new high school to apprise her of Grace's situation and to ask the counselor to schedule regular meetings with Grace to make sure that she had sufficient support.

For children in high school or those enrolled in sports programs, excessively high expectations from parents, coaches, or from the child her- or himself may need to be managed. Likewise, stress related to peer relationships—including romantic relationships, loss of important relationships, bullying, and cyberbullying—is common and require a targeted intervention with the child, family, and school.

Conclusion

Through the example of Grace, this chapter has highlighted many key themes and issues that arise in the assessment and treatment of children and adolescents with FND. Stress and distress is part of the human condition, and children with functional somatic symptoms—including FND—will continue to present for help to medical settings. In pediatrics, the integration of functional somatic symptoms into clinical practice builds on the "the role of the pediatrician in providing increased attention to the prevention, early detection, and management of the various behavioral, developmental, and social functioning problems encountered in pediatric practice" (p. 731) [20, 54]. The multidisciplinary management of children and adolescents with functional symptoms by clinicians working with children in the pediatric setting—pediatricians, child psychiatrists, physiotherapists, and occupational therapists—dovetails with this important goal [55].

Acknowledgements The case history has been de-identified and is an amalgam of two very similar cases. We thank one of the family's for permission to use Grace's artwork for teaching and for publication in scientific books and journals.

Summary
- Children and adolescents presenting with functional movement disorders often manifest a broad range of other functional somatic symptoms—other FND symptoms, pain, symptoms reflecting autonomic dysregulation, and fatigue—as well as comorbid anxiety or depression.
- The functional symptoms of children and adolescents may shift and change across time and across presentations, and without respecting the boundaries of medical specialties. Their management requires a holistic multidisciplinary approach.
- Stress activates the brain-body stress system. The child/adolescent's "somatic narrative"—the symptoms, signs, and subjective experience that mark an activated or dysregulated stress system—provides the clinician with information about the physiological condition of the body. The somatic narrative—the physiological condition of the body—is also referred to as interoception, homeostatic emotions, or physiological feelings.
- Functional disorders are often triggered by identifiable stressors. In pediatric

practice approximately 50% of children/ adolescents and families report an emotional trigger event, and a similar percentage report a physical trigger event—a viral illness, a minor injury, a medical event or a series of medical events—as one of the stressors that preceded the presenting illness.

- A comprehensive assessment with the child/adolescent and the family enables the clinician to elicit a detailed developmental history and to understand the emergence of functional somatic symptoms in the context of the patient's life story and the adverse childhood experiences (ACEs) that have activated their stress system.

- With prompt (positive) diagnosis and appropriate multidisciplinary, multimodal treatment, children and adolescents presenting with FMD and other functional symptoms generally have good clinical outcomes.

References

1. Sharpe Lohrasbe R, Ogden P. Somatic resources: sensorimotor psychotherapy approach to stabilising arousal in child and family treatment. Aust N Z J Fam Ther. 2017;38:573–81.
2. Maisami M, Freeman JM. Conversion reactions in children as body language: a combined child psychiatry/neurology team approach to the management of functional neurologic disorders in children. Pediatrics. 1987;80(1):46–52. Epub 1987/07/01.
3. Lask B, Fosson A. Childhood illness: the psychosomatic approach: children talking with their bodies. Chichester: Wiley; 1989.
4. Levine PA, Blakeslee A, Sylvae J. Reintegrating fragmentation of the primitive self: discussion of "somatic experiencing". Psychoanal Dialogues. 2018;28(5):620–8.
5. Taylor DC. Hysteria, play-acting and courage. Br J Psychiatry. 1986;149:37–41.
6. Craig AD. How do you feel? Interoception: the sense of the physiological condition of the body. Nat Rev Neurosci. 2002;3(8):655–66.
7. Craig AD. Interoception: the sense of the physiological condition of the body. Curr Opin Neurobiol. 2003;13(4):500–5.
8. Craig AD. A new view of pain as a homeostatic emotion. Trends Neurosci. 2003;26(6):303–7.
9. Pace-Schott EF, Amole MC, Aue T, Balconi M, Bylsma LM, Critchley H, et al. Physiological feelings. Neurosci Biobehav Rev. 2019;103:267–304.
10. Tot-Strate S, Dehlholm-Lambertsen G, Lassen K, Rask CU. Clinical features of functional somatic symptoms in children and referral patterns to child and adolescent mental health services. Acta Paediatr. 2016;105(5):514–21.
11. Garralda ME. Hospital management of paediatric functional somatic symptoms. Acta Paediatr. 2016;105(5):452–3.
12. Stone J. Functional neurological disorders: the neurological assessment as treatment. Neurophysiol Clin. 2014;44(4):363–73.
13. Roenneberg C, Sattel H, Schaefert R, Henningsen P, Hausteiner-Wiehle C. Functional somatic symptoms. Dtsch Arztebl Int. 2019;116(33–34):553–60.
14. Drossman DA, Hasler WL. Rome IV-functional GI disorders: disorders of gut-brain interaction. Gastroenterology. 2016;150(6):1257–61.
15. Hyams JS, Di Lorenzo C, Miguel Saps M, Shulman RJ, Staiano A, van Tilburg M. Childhood functional gastrointestinal disorders: child/adolescent. Gastroenterology. 2016;150(6):1456–1468.e2.
16. Wells R, Spurrier AJ, Linz D, Gallagher C, Mahajan R, Sanders P, et al. Postural tachycardia syndrome: current perspectives. Vasc Health Risk Manag. 2018;14:1–11.
17. Knight S, Elders S, Rodda J, Harvey A, Lubitz L, Rowe K, et al. Epidemiology of paediatric chronic fatigue syndrome in Australia. Arch Dis Child. 2019;104(8):733–8.
18. American Pain Society Task Force on Pediatric Chronic Pain Managment. Assessment and management of children with chronic pain. A position statement from the American Pain Society. Available online: http://americanpainsociety.org/uploads/get-involved/pediatric-chronic-pain-statement.pdf. Accessed 7 Dec 2016.
19. Flaherty EG, Thompson R, Litrownik AJ, Zolotor AJ, Dubowitz H, Runyan DK, et al. Adverse childhood exposures and reported child health at age 12. Acad Pediatr. 2009;9(3):150–6.
20. American Academy of Pediatrics Committee on Psychosocial Aspects of Child Family Health. Pediatrics and the psychosocial aspects of child and family health. Pediatrics. 1982;70:126–7.
21. Kozlowska K, English M, Savage B. Connecting body and mind: The first interview with somatizing patients and their families. Clin Child Psychol Psychiatry. 2013;18(2):223–45.
22. Kozlowska K, Scher S, Helgeland H. Functional somatic symptoms in children and adolescents: the stress-system approach to assessment and treatment. Dallos R, Vetere A, editors. London: Palgrave Macmillan; 2020.
23. Kozlowska K. Stress, distress, and bodytalk: co-constructing formulations with patients who pres-

ent with somatic symptoms. Harv Rev Psychiatry. 2013;21(6):314–33. Epub 2013/11/10.

24. Fischer S, Lemmer G, Gollwitzer M, Nater UM. Stress and resilience in functional somatic syndromes--a structural equation modeling approach. PLoS One. 2014;9(11):e111214.

25. Kozlowska K, Scher S, Williams LM. Patterns of emotional-cognitive functioning in pediatric conversion patients: implications for the conceptualization of conversion disorders. Psychosom Med. 2011;73(9):775–88. Epub 2011/11/04.

26. Kozlowska K, Griffiths KR, Foster SL, Linton J, Williams LM, Korgaonkar MS. Grey matter abnormalities in children and adolescents with functional neurological symptom disorder. Neuroimage Clin. 2017;15:306–14.

27. Perez DL, Aybek S, Popkirov S, Kozlowska K, Stephen CD, Anderson J, et al. A review and expert opinion on the neuropsychiatric assessment of motor functional neurological disorders. J Neuropsychiatry Clin Neurosci. 2021;33(1):14–26.

28. Stone AL, Walker LS, Guest Editors: Cynthia A. Gerhardt CABDJW, Grayson NH. Adolescents' observations of parent pain behaviors: preliminary measure validation and test of social learning theory in pediatric chronic pain. J Pediatr Psychol. 2017;42(1):65–74.

29. Ross DE. A method for developing a biopsychosocial formulation. J Child Fam Stud. 2000;1(9):106.

30. Bakvis P, Spinhoven P, Giltay EJ, Kuyk J, Edelbroek PM, Zitman FG, et al. Basal hypercortisolism and trauma in patients with psychogenic nonepileptic seizures. Epilepsia. 2009;51:752–95. Epub 2009/11/06.

31. Bakvis P, Roelofs K, Kuyk J, Edelbroek PM, Swinkels WA, Spinhoven P. Trauma, stress, and preconscious threat processing in patients with psychogenic nonepileptic seizures. Epilepsia. 2009;50(5):1001–11. Epub 2009/01/28.

32. Kozlowska K, Rampersad R, Cruz C, Shah U, Chudleigh C, Soe S, et al. The respiratory control of carbon dioxide in children and adolescents referred for treatment of psychogenic non-epileptic seizures. Eur Child Adolesc Psychiatry. 2017;26(10):1207–17.

33. Kozlowska K, Chudleigh C, Cruz C, Lim M, McClure G, Savage B, et al. Psychogenic non-epileptic seizures in children and adolescents: Part I – Diagnostic formulations. Clin Child Psychol Psychiatry. 2018;23(1):140–59.

34. Kozlowska K, Chudleigh C, Cruz C, Lim M, McClure G, Savage B, et al. Psychogenic non-epileptic seizures in children and adolescents: Part II – Explanations to families, treatment, and group outcomes. Clin Child Psychol Psychiatry. 2018;23(1):160–76.

35. Sawchuk T, Buchhalter J, Senft B. Psychogenic non-epileptic seizures in children-prospective validation of a clinical care pathway & risk factors for treatment outcome. Epilepsy Behav. 2020;105:106971.

36. Garralda ME, Rask CU. Somatoform and related disorders. In: Thapar A, Pine DS, Leckman JF, Scott S, Snowling MJ, Taylor E, editors. Rutter's

child and adolescent psychiatry. 6th ed. Chichester/ Ames: Wiley; 2015. p. 1035–54. https://onlinelibrary-wiley-com.ezp-prod1.hul.harvard.edu/doi/pdf/10.02/9781118381953.ch72.

37. Kozlowska K, English M, Savage B, Chudleigh C. Multimodal rehabilitation: a mind-body, family-based intervention for children and adolescents impaired by medically unexplained symptoms. Part 1: The program. Am J Fam Ther. 2012;40(5): 399–419.

38. Nunn K. Neuropsychiatry in childhood: residential treatment. In: Green J, Jacobs B, editors. In-patient child psychiatry; modern practice, research and the future. London: Jessica Kingsley; 1998. p. 259–83.

39. Nunn K, Thompson S, Moore SG, English M, Burke EA, Byrne N. Managing pervasive refusal syndrome: strategies of hope. Clin Child Psychol Psychiatry. 1998;3(2):229–49.

40. Kozlowska K, English M, Savage B, Chudleigh C, Davies F, Paull M, et al. Multimodal rehabilitation: a mind-body, family-based intervention for children and adolescents impaired by medically unexplained symptoms. Part 2: Case studies and outcomes. Am J Fam Ther. 2013;41(3):212–31.

41. Bolger A, Collins A, Michels M, Pruitt D. Characteristics and outcomes of children with conversion disorder admitted to a single inpatient rehabilitation unit, a retrospective study. PM R. 2018;10(9):910–6.

42. Butz C, Iske C, Truba N, Trott K. Treatment of functional gait abnormality in a rehabilitation setting: emphasizing the physical interventions for treating the whole child. Innov Clin Neurosci. 2019;16(7–8):18–21.

43. Fobian AD, et al. Retraining and control therapy for pediatric psychogenic non-epileptic seizures. Ann Clin Transl Neurol. 2020.

44. Graham CD, Kyle SD. A preliminary investigation of sleep quality in functional neurological disorders: poor sleep appears common, and is associated with functional impairment. J Neurol Sci. 2017;378:163–6.

45. Lehrer PM, Gevirtz R. Heart rate variability biofeedback: how and why does it work? Front Psychol. 2014;5:756.

46. Guendelman S, Medeiros S, Rampes H. Mindfulness and emotion regulation: insights from neurobiological, psychological, and clinical studies. Front Psychol. 2017;8:220.

47. Kozlowska K, Khan R. A developmental, body-oriented intervention for children and adolescents with medically unexplained chronic pain. Clin Child Psychol Psychiatry. 2011;16(4):575–98. Epub 2011/05/14.

48. Lehrer P, Vaschillo E, Trost Z, France CR. Effects of rhythmical muscle tension at 0.1Hz on cardiovascular resonance and the baroreflex. Biol Psychol. 2009;81(1):24–30.

49. Harrison LE, Pate JW, Richardson PA, Ickmans K, Wicksell RK, Simons LE. Best-evidence for the rehabilitation of chronic pain part 1: pediatric pain. J Clin Med. 2019;8(9):1267.

50. Khachane Y, Kozlowska K, Savage B, McClure G, Butler G, Gray N, et al. Twisted in pain: the multidisciplinary treatment approach to functional dystonia. Harv Rev Psychiatry. 2019;27(6):359–81.

51. Nielsen G, Stone J, Matthews A, Brown M, Sparkes C, Farmer R, et al. Physiotherapy for functional motor disorders: a consensus recommendation. J Neurol Neurosurg Psychiatry. 2015;86(10):1113–9.

52. Gray N, Savage B, Scher S, Kozlowska K. Psychologically informed physical therapy for children and adolescents with functional neurological symptoms: the wellness approach. J Neuropsychiatry Clin Neurosci. 2020;32(4):389–95.

53. Kim Y, et al. The role of physiotherapy in the management of functional neurological disorder in children and adolescents. Seminars in Pediatric Neurology. (in press).

54. American Academy of Pediatrics Committee on Psychosocial Aspects of Child and Family Health: the pediatrician and the "new morbidity". Pediatrics. 1993;92(5):731–3.

55. Kozlowska K, et al. Changing the Culture of Care for Children and Adolescents with Functional Neurological Disorder. Epilepsy and Behavior Reports. 2021;16:1004486.

Choosing a Career in Functional Movement Disorder

Kathrin LaFaver, Carine W. Maurer,
Timothy R. Nicholson, and David L. Perez

Introduction

Leaders in the origins of modern-day neurology and psychiatry were immensely interested in functional movement disorder (FMD) and related functional neurological disorder (FND) subtypes [1]. In the late nineteenth century, distinguished neurologists, psychiatrists and other like-minded clinicians trained alongside one another – an observation memorialized by Pierre Aristide Andre Brouillet's classic painting "*A Clinical Lesson at the Salpêtrière*". During these formative years of the clinical neurosciences, an integrated perspective that cut across the spectrum of traditionally conceptualized neurological and psychiatric conditions was proposed, most famously when Jean-Martin Charcot stated: "the

K. LaFaver
Movement Disorder Specialist, Saratoga Hospital Medical Group, Saratoga Springs, NY, USA

C. W. Maurer
Department of Neurology, Renaissance School of Medicine at Stony Brook University, Stony Brook, NY, USA

T. R. Nicholson
Neuropsychiatry Research and Education Group, Institute of Psychiatry Psychology & Neuroscience, King's College London, London, UK

D. L. Perez (✉)
Departments of Neurology and Psychiatry, Massachusetts General Hospital, Harvard Medical School, Boston, MA, USA
e-mail: dlperez@nmr.mgh.harvard.edu

neurological tree has its branches, neuroasthenia, hysteria, epilepsy, all the types of mental conditions, progressive paralysis, (and) gait ataxia" [2]. Over the next 100 years, a variety of conceptual, training, healthcare policy, and sociocultural factors pushed FMD and related conditions to the neglected borderland between neurology and psychiatry [3].

Excitingly, the last two decades have seen a renaissance in clinical and research interest in FND, particularly in patients with FMD and functional seizures [4, 5] – and increasingly for other presentations, such as functional cognitive disorder [6, 7]. FND is one of the more common outpatient neurology referrals [8], and FMD comprises approximately 20% of consultations seen by movement disorder neurologists [9]. In parallel, there has been a boom in pathophysiology and treatment research [10]. In select medical centers internationally, interdisciplinary and multidisciplinary treatment programs for FMD and related conditions have also been developed [11–13]. The formation of a new professional society (www.fndsociety.org) has also added to the momentum built over the past several decades. Despite these advancements, practical challenges remain – albeit not necessarily unique to our field. These include the intricacies of building and supporting clinical programs, which can be expensive and not well incentivized by many healthcare systems. Additionally, the gaps in our understanding of FMD and related conditions remain considerable, and funding opportunities to sustain and grow research remain limited.

As the four co-editors of this Springer case-based textbook in FMD (Drs. Kathrin LaFaver, Carine W. Maurer, Timothy R. Nicholson, David L. Perez), we have all recognized the opportunities present in working in the FMD field. The effect sizes for clinical improvement can be profound, and opportunities to transform the clinical and research landscape across diagnosis, pathophysiology and treatment initiatives remain great. In the following sections, we share our personal journeys in choosing to dedicate our careers to FMD and related conditions. Our hope is that by sharing these reflections, we will energize the next generation of clinicians and scientists to join this revitalized field.

Kathrin LaFaver MD

The patient I was about to see was a young woman, using a wheelchair following a car accident 5 months prior. Unable to move her legs and relying on help from her family, the neurological exam showed normal muscle tone and reflexes, and imaging and electrophysiological studies had not revealed injury to her brain, spinal cord, or peripheral nervous system. As a resident in my first year of neurology training, I observed my attending complete a comprehensive assessment and explain that she was affected by a functional neurological disorder, a term I had never heard before. How could this be? How could a person, perfectly capable of moving their own limbs one day, not be able to do so the next, in the absence of structural injury to the nervous system? My attending took considerable time to explain his thoughts on the diagnosis, and most importantly, referred the patient for a brief course of FMD specific physical therapy. When we saw her back in clinic 2 weeks later, she was again walking normally, and had regained full control over her leg movements. My experience that day has shaped my career since, and I have been fortunate to see many patients with FMD regain control over their bodies and their lives. Understanding brain network changes and the complex connec-

tions of emotional and motor circuits lays the theoretical groundwork for psychologically-informed physical therapy, and to date my predominant interest has been to provide pragmatic, multidisciplinary treatment approaches to patients with FMD. Having started two rehabilitation oriented treatment programs now in the US focused on motor retraining with help of physical, occupational and speech therapy as well as psychotherapy, I have learned many lessons from my colleagues and patients over the past 10 years and seen wonderful transformations take place in the lives of many under my care. I have also come to realize that recovery is not always fast, and sometimes not possible. Finding better ways to provide tailored treatments in a timely manner to a larger number of patients, identifying treatment obstacles and ways to overcome them are some of important challenges in optimizing care for individuals with FMD. My sincere hope is that our book will inspire many centers around the US and worldwide to offer dedicated FMD services and treatment programs. Having fallen "between the specialty lines" for far too long, we need to do better and work together, not only for the sake of the individuals and their families affected by FMD, but also for society as a whole.

Carine W. Maurer MD, PhD

After completing my undergraduate degree in Molecular and Cellular Biology at Cornell University, I continued my studies on the basic cellular mechanisms underlying human disease by pursuing an MD/PhD. I attended Weill Cornell's Tri-Institutional MD-PhD Program, completing my PhD at the Rockefeller University in the laboratory of Dr. Shai Shaham. In Dr. Shaham's laboratory, my research focused on the basic machinery underlying programmed cell death (apoptosis) in the nematode *C. elegans*. *C. elegans* had previously been demonstrated to be an excellent model organism for studying programmed cell death – work that had previously culminated in the Nobel Prize in Medicine. My work expanded upon these prior studies, and elucidated some of the upstream regulators of the conserved cell death machinery [14–16].

Upon completion of my graduate studies and my return to medical school, I initially thought that internal medicine would be a natural path forward given my research background. However, during my clinical clerkships I found that I was most intrigued by disorders of the brain and mind. I found the complex pathophysiology of brain disorders (psychiatric as well as neurologic) to be quite fascinating, and was very much attracted to the overall approach and thought processes of the neurologists with whom I interacted during my clinical rotations. While I toyed with the possibility of pursuing a dual neurology-psychiatry residency training program, in the end I decided residency training in neurology would be best suited to my particular interests.

During my neurology residency at University of California, Los Angeles (UCLA), I realized early on that the field of movement disorders was particularly appealing. I was attracted by the field's focus on the neurological examination, as well as by the intersection with psychiatry, behavioral neurology, and sleep neurology, given the frequency with which patients with movement disorders experience non-motor symptoms.

Following residency, I pursued clinical and research fellowship training in movement disorders at the National Institute of Neurological Disorders and Stroke (NINDS) under the mentorship of Dr. Mark Hallett. Continuing studies that had been initiated under prior fellows including Drs. Kathrin LaFaver and Valerie Voon, I began my work into the biological mechanisms underlying FMD. While I had previously encountered many individuals with FMD in the emergency room setting during my neurology residency training, it was a quite different experience to hear about patients' struggles with this oftentimes chronic disorder during encounters in the outpatient and research setting. Our work sought to better understand changes in the structural and functional neural circuitry in patients with FMD [17, 18], as well as the potential alterations of stress biomarkers in these patients [19, 20]. I found it particularly satisfying to take the knowledge gained from this research back to patients, and thereby provide them with a better understanding of their disease and the implications for their recovery.

Since beginning my faculty position in the Department of Neurology at the Renaissance School of Medicine at Stony Brook University, I have sought to establish relationships with local healthcare professionals in order to be able to provide the multidisciplinary care needed for management of patients with FMD. Despite the frequency with which we see these patients in the clinical setting, FMD remains an underserved and frequently misunderstood area of clinical medicine. I am grateful to my co-editors and all the contributors to this textbook for their collaboration in creating an accessible resource for learning more about the diagnosis and management of FMD. I am grateful to those leaders in the field of FMD whose work has paved the path, and those with whom I hope to continue to improve our understanding of and our ability to care for patients with FMD.

Timothy R. Nicholson MD, PhD

Reading Freud as a teenager inspired me to apply to medical school and after qualifying I soon realized that the interface of neurology and psychiatry was without doubt the most fascinating area of medicine and where I wanted to work both clinically and academically. I was fortunate enough to get a job as a trainee in neurology at the world renown National Hospital for Neurology and Neurosurgery at Queen Square alongside University College London's Institute of Neurology. I specifically requested a post in the neuropsychiatry team, based on Hughlings Jackson ward, named after "The Father of British Neurology" who appreciated the importance of neurology's overlap with psychiatry [21].

During this time I saw many fascinating cases, but none more than the patients diagnosed with what was then largely known as conversion disorder – reflecting the still dominant Freudian notion of trauma or other stressors being "converted" into physical symptoms. As I learnt more about this condition, and how common it was, I was baffled why I'd not been taught anything about it at medical school and became increasingly committed to studying this disorder which fell between the gaps of physical and mental health for which etiological theories touched on key neuroscientific and philosophical constructs such as consciousness, free will and agency. I had some inspirational clinical and academic mentorship from Maria Ron, Michael Trimble and Richard Frackowiak at the Institute of Neurology as I designed my first studies attempting to work out the mechanisms of the disorder and how to improve symptoms. My clinical experiences confirmed that I wanted to also train in psychiatry and I was able to benefit from the exceptional training program at the Maudsley Hospital in London.

The next stroke of good fortune was the opportunity to research this intriguing and important disorder in depth during my PhD studies under the supervision of Richard Kanaan and Tony David at the Institute of Psychiatry Psychology and Neuroscience, King's College London. The projects tested the Freudian model of this disorder at the time that the field was being revolutionized by a rebirth of interest by neurologists and the application of contemporary neuroscience to this disorder, led by Jon Stone and Mark Edwards in the UK. Another critical development was the formation of patient organizations, in no small way enabled by new terminology, models and understanding of this disorder that could accommodate physical, cognitive and psychological processes – potentially interacting in differing combinations in any given individual – to create symptoms. This has been exemplified in several key publications with colleagues investigating the complex roles of stress and trauma in this condition which remain key etiological factors for many but, critically, not the whole story for what is likely a disorder with multiple mechanisms [22, 23].

It is an honor and a privilege to work clinically with this often misunderstood and neglected patient group and to be able to work with, and learn so much from, an increasingly international and diverse research community where the exam-

ple of friendly collaboration has been so clearly set by senior colleagues, many of whom have so generously contributed to this book.

David L. Perez MD, MMSc

My academic journey began as a Columbia University undergraduate where I majored in Neuroscience & Behavior. I remember my second year taking a course entitled "Mind, Brain and Behavior," during which I first became enamored with neuroscience – the science of human behavior that bridges brain and mind. That summer I joined Eric Kandel's laboratory as a research student. Professor Kandel, a psychiatrist, received the Nobel Prize in Medicine for fundamental insights into the biology of learning and memory in the year prior to my arrival in his laboratory [24]. In the Kandel Lab, I spent 2 years working with Dr. Michael Rogan – a neuroscientist who had conducted his doctoral research with Professor Joseph LeDoux at New York University – a leading authority on the neural circuitry of emotions [25]. Following Dr. Rogan's work in classical fear conditioning, he developed a curiosity regarding how deficits recognizing instances of safety may also contribute to affective disorders. I learned to perform rodent brain surgeries, implanting depth electrodes in the lateral amygdala and dorsal striatum of mice [26]. Thereafter, we trained mice in either danger or safety associative learning paradigms, followed by a characterization of their behavioral and electrophysiological responses. This foundational research opportunity taught me the rigors of the scientific method, while also growing my interest in the clinical neurosciences.

I subsequently attended New York University School of Medicine, with an interest in learning more about both neurology and psychiatry. My momentum continued relatively undisturbed throughout my first 2 years. During my clinical clerkships, I enjoyed the scientific rigor found in neurology localizing the lesion and learning brain-symptom relationships one patient at a time. The focus on neuroanatomy and brain imaging in neurology was keenly interesting.

However, when I rotated through psychiatry the complexity of psychopathology found in brain disorders such as post-traumatic stress disorder proved equally fascinating – fueling my curiosity regarding the pathophysiology of psychiatric conditions. New York University has a dual neurology-psychiatry residency training program and it was there (working alongside their attendings and residents) that I first developed the idea to train in both specialties, allowing me to acquire the neuroanatomical and physical examination expertise found in neurology – while also gaining nuanced psychiatric skills assessing and managing patients with prominent affective disturbances. The decision to pursue dual training was also complemented by an interest in systems-level neuroscience and brain imaging research. During my fourth year of medical school, I reunited with Dr. Rogan to work alongside him as he was translating his basic science safety learning paradigm into a human task functional MRI study [27]. This all culminated in me going into residency verbalizing an interest in the intersection of "emotion and movement", yet unsure about the specific populations that I would be most interested in working with.

Training in both neurology (Massachusetts General Hospital/Brigham and Women's Hospital) and psychiatry (Brigham and Women's Hospital/Beth Israel Deaconess Medical Center/Massachusetts Mental Health Center) in the Harvard Medical School hospital system, I was struck early on in my neurology training how frequent patients with FND were in our emergency department, inpatient and outpatient services. I observed at the time that emphasis was given to "ruling-out" traditionally conceptualized neurological conditions – while a parallel process of excluding the presence of acute psychiatric diagnoses and safety concerns was being performed by psychiatry. This left a major gap – what about the entity of FND itself? What was our conceptualization of this neuropsychiatric condition that sat directly at the intersection of neurology and psychiatry (and of brain, body and mind)? Throughout residency, I also continued my neuroimaging research training in the

Functional Neuroimaging Laboratory co-directed by Drs. David Silbersweig and Emily Stern. It was there that I delved into the neurocircuitry of a range of psychiatric disorders, while also developing an initial formulation for the pathophysiology of FND [28]. I was also positively influenced by other experts at Harvard Medical School, as well as by the "heavy lifting" done by international leaders such as Professors Jon Stone, Mark Hallett, Alan Carson and W. Curt LaFrance Jr. in putting FND back on the "map" with renewed interest and scientific rigor.

Following training, I joined the Massachusetts General Hospital Departments of Neurology and Psychiatry to establish and grow clinical and research programs in FND, including across the spectrum of FMD and functional seizures. We embrace transdiagnostic and interdisciplinary approaches that span the clinical neurosciences and rehabilitation specialties, recognizing that many patients have mixed symptoms and that some can develop distinct functional neurological symptoms over the course of their illness; we also emphasize a neuropsychiatric perspective in our patient conceptualization using biopsychosocial formulations [29]. In our research, we have sought to advance both the structural and functional neurocircuitry underlying motor FND [30, 31]; we have also aimed to bridge etiological risk factors and neural mechanisms – as well as highlighting the importance of individual differences and clinical outcome biomarkers [31–33]. I am grateful to my esteemed co-editors for our work together on this textbook, as well as a recent collaboration with colleagues on a Special Issue on FND [34]. As I reflect on my present and future work in FMD and related conditions, I appeal to academics and funding bodies to increasingly make clinical work and research in this underserved yet high impact area a priority. I remain deeply passionate about the work – including inherent opportunities in FND to break down the artificial walls between physical and mental health that is pervasive in medicine and society. I know that the future is bright for our field and the patients that we diligently care for.

References

1. Bogousslavsky J. Hysteria: the rise of an enigma. Karger; 2014. x, 210 p.
2. Charcot JM. Leðcons du mardi áa la Salpãetriáere: policliniques, 1887–1888. Paris: Bureaux du Prográes Mâedical; 1887. 638 p.
3. Fend M, Williams L, Carson AJ, Stone J. The Arc de Siecle: functional neurological disorder during the "forgotten" years of the 20th century. Brain. 2020;143(4):1278–84.
4. Dworetzky BA, Baslet G. Psychogenic nonepileptic seizures: toward the integration of care. Oxford University Press; 2017.
5. Hallett M, Stone J, Carson AJ. Functional neurologic disorders. Aminoff MJ, Boller F, Swaab DF, editors. Elsevier; 2016.
6. McWhirter L, Ritchie C, Stone J, Carson A. Functional cognitive disorders: a systematic review. Lancet Psychiatry. 2020;7(2):191–207.
7. Ball HA, McWhirter L, Ballard C, Bhome R, Blackburn DJ, Edwards MJ, et al. Functional cognitive disorder: dementia's blind spot. Brain. 2020;143(10):2895–903.
8. Stone J, Carson A, Duncan R, Roberts R, Warlow C, Hibberd C, et al. Who is referred to neurology clinics?--the diagnoses made in 3781 new patients. Clin Neurol Neurosurg. 2010;112(9):747–51.
9. Carson A, Lehn A. Epidemiology. Handb Clin Neurol. 2016;139:47–60.
10. Perez DL, Edwards MJ, Nielsen G, Kozlowska K, Hallett M, LaFrance WC Jr. Decade of progress in motor functional neurological disorder: continuing the momentum. J Neurol Neurosurg Psychiatry. 2021;92(6):668–77.
11. Aybek S, Lidstone SC, Nielsen G, MacGillivray L, Bassetti CL, Lang A, et al. What is the role of a specialist assessment clinic for FND? Lessons from three national referral centres. J Neuropsychiatry Clin Neurosci. 2020;32(1):79–84.
12. Jacob AE, Smith CA, Jablonski ME, Roach AR, Paper KM, Kaelin DL, et al. Multidisciplinary clinic for functional movement disorders (FMD): 1-year experience from a single centre. J Neurol Neurosurg Psychiatry. 2018;89(9):1011–2.
13. Glass SP, Matin N, Williams B, Mello J, Stephen CD, Young SS, et al. Neuropsychiatric factors linked to adherence and short-term outcome in a U.S. functional neurological disorders clinic: a retrospective cohort study. J Neuropsychiatry Clin Neurosci. 2018;30(2):152–9.
14. Maurer CW, Chiorazzi M, Shaham S. Timing of the onset of a developmental cell death is controlled by transcriptional induction of the C. elegans ced-3 caspase-encoding gene. Development. 2007;134(7):1357–68.
15. Deng X, Yin X, Allan R, Lu DD, Maurer CW, Haimovitz-Friedman A, et al. Ceramide biogenesis is required for radiation-induced apoptosis in the germ line of C. elegans. Science. 2008;322(5898):110–5.
16. Chiorazzi M, Rui L, Yang Y, Ceribelli M, Tishbi N, Maurer CW, et al. Related F-box proteins control cell death in Caenorhabditis elegans and human lymphoma. Proc Natl Acad Sci U S A. 2013;110(10):3943–8.
17. Maurer CW, LaFaver K, Ameli R, Epstein SA, Hallett M, Horovitz SG. Impaired self-agency in functional movement disorders: a resting-state fMRI study. Neurology. 2016;87(6):564–70.
18. Maurer CW, LaFaver K, Limachia GS, Capitan G, Ameli R, Sinclair S, et al. Gray matter differences in patients with functional movement disorders. Neurology. 2018;91(20):e1870–e9.
19. Maurer CW, Liu VD, LaFaver K, Ameli R, Wu T, Toledo R, et al. Impaired resting vagal tone in patients with functional movement disorders. Parkinsonism Relat Disord. 2016;30:18–22.
20. Maurer CW, LaFaver K, Ameli R, Toledo R, Hallett M. A biological measure of stress levels in patients with functional movement disorders. Parkinsonism Relat Disord. 2015;21(9):1072–5.
21. Reynolds EH. John Hughlings Jackson and Thomas Laycock: brain and mind. Brain. 2020;143(2):711–4.
22. Ludwig L, Pasman JA, Nicholson T, Aybek S, David AS, Tuck S, et al. Stressful life events and maltreatment in conversion (functional neurological) disorder: systematic review and meta-analysis of case-control studies. Lancet Psychiatry. 2018;5(4):307–20.
23. Keynejad RC, Frodl T, Kanaan R, Pariante C, Reuber M, Nicholson TR. Stress and functional neurological disorders: mechanistic insights. J Neurol Neurosurg Psychiatry. 2019;90(7):813–21.
24. Kandel ER, Dudai Y, Mayford MR. The molecular and systems biology of memory. Cell. 2014;157(1):163–86.
25. Rogan MT, Staubli UV, LeDoux JE. Fear conditioning induces associative long-term potentiation in the amygdala. Nature. 1997;390(6660):604–7.
26. Rogan MT, Leon KS, Perez DL, Kandel ER. Distinct neural signatures for safety and danger in the amygdala and striatum of the mouse. Neuron. 2005;46(2):309–20.
27. Pollak DD, Rogan MT, Egner T, Perez DL, Yanagihara TK, Hirsch J. A translational bridge between mouse and human models of learned safety. Ann Med. 2010;42(2):115–22.
28. Perez DL, Barsky AJ, Daffner K, Silbersweig DA. Motor and somatosensory conversion disorder: a functional unawareness syndrome? J Neuropsychiatry Clin Neurosci. 2012;24(2):141–51.
29. Perez DL, Keshavan MS, Scharf JM, Boes AD, Price BH. Bridging the great divide: what can neurology learn from psychiatry? J Neuropsychiatry Clin Neurosci. 2018;30(4):271–8.
30. Perez DL, Williams B, Matin N, LaFrance WC Jr, Costumero-Ramos V, Fricchione GL, et al. Corticolimbic structural alterations linked to health status and trait anxiety in functional neuro-

logical disorder. J Neurol Neurosurg Psychiatry. 2017;88(12):1052–9.

31. Diez I, Ortiz-Teran L, Williams B, Jalilianhasanpour R, Ospina JP, Dickerson BC, et al. Corticolimbic fast-tracking: enhanced multimodal integration in functional neurological disorder. J Neurol Neurosurg Psychiatry. 2019;90(8):929–38.

32. Diez I, Larson AG, Nakhate V, Dunn EC, Fricchione GL, Nicholson TR, et al. Early-life trauma endophenotypes and brain circuit-gene expression relationships in functional neurological (conversion) disorder. Mol Psychiatry. 2021;26:3817–28.

33. Perez DL, Matin N, Barsky A, Costumero-Ramos V, Makaretz SJ, Young SS, et al. Cingulo-insular structural alterations associated with psychogenic symptoms, childhood abuse and PTSD in functional neurological disorders. J Neurol Neurosurg Psychiatry. 2017;88(6):491–7.

34. Perez DL, Aybek S, Nicholson TR, Kozlowska K, Arciniegas DB, LaFrance WC Jr. Functional neurological (conversion) disorder: a core neuropsychiatric disorder. J Neuropsychiatry Clin Neurosci. 2020;32(1):1–3.

Index

© Springer Nature Switzerland AG 2022
K. LaFaver et al. (eds.), *Functional Movement Disorder*, Current Clinical Neurology,
https://doi.org/10.1007/978-3-030-86495-8

Printed in the United States
by Baker & Taylor Publisher Services